THE GLAUCOMAS

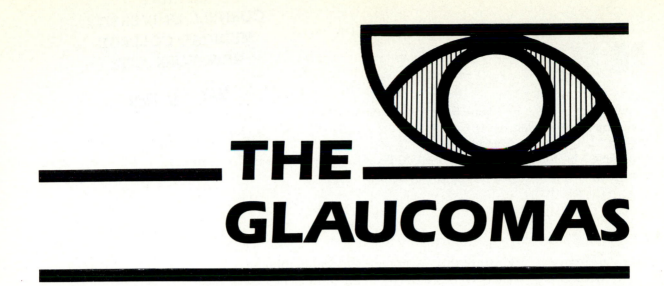

THE GLAUCOMAS

edited by

Robert Ritch, M.D.

Professor of Clinical Ophthalmology, The New York Medical College,
Valhalla, New York; Chief, Glaucoma Service, the New York Eye and Ear
Infirmary, New York, New York

M. Bruce Shields, M.D.

Professor of Ophthalmology; Director, Glaucoma Service, Duke University
Eye Center, Durham, North Carolina

Theodore Krupin, M.D.

Professor of Ophthalmology; Chief, Glaucoma Service, Scheie Eye Institute,
University of Pennsylvania School of Medicine, Philadelphia, Pennsylvania

with 1220 illustrations, including 37 illustrations in 4 color plates

THE C.V. MOSBY COMPANY

St. Louis · Baltimore · Philadelphia · Toronto   1989

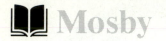

Editor: Eugenia A. Klein
Developmental Editors: Elaine Steinborn, Kathryn H. Falk
Assistant Editor: Ellen Baker Geisel
Project Manager: Teri Merchant
Production Editors: Mary Stueck, Gail A. Brower, Betty Hazelwood
Design: Rey Umali

The C.V. Mosby Company
11830 Westline Industrial Drive, St. Louis, Missouri 63146

Library of Congress Cataloging-in-Publication Data

The Glaucomas/edited by Robert Ritch, M. Bruce Shields,
  Theodore Krupin.
    p.   cm.
  Includes bibliographies and index.
  ISBN 0-8016-4116-0
  1. Glaucoma. I. Ritch, Robert. II. Shields, M. Bruce.
III. Krupin, Theodore.
  [DNLM: 1. Glaucoma—diagnosis. 2. Glaucoma—
  therapy. WN 290 5509]
RE871.G577 1989
617.7'41—dc19
DNLM/DLC

GW/MV/MV 9 8 7 6 5 4 3 2 1

CONTRIBUTORS

P. Juhani Airaksinen, M.D.
Professor and Chairman, Department of
Ophthalmology, University of Oulu, Oulu,
Finland

Stephen P. Bartels, Ph.D.
Assistant Professor of Ophthalmology, Harvard
Medical School; Boston, Massachusetts; Associate
Scientist, Department of Ophthalmology,
Ophthalmic Pharmacology Unit, Eye Research
Institute of Retina Foundation

A. Robert Bellows, M.D.
Assistant Clinical Professor of Ophthalmology,
Harvard Medical School, Boston, Massachusetts

John E. Bourgeois, M.D.
Assistant Clinical Professor, Duke University Eye
Center, Durham; Charlotte Eye, Ear, Nose, and
Throat Associates, Charlotte, North Carolina

Michael E. Breton, Ph.D.
Assistant Research Professor of Ophthalmology,
Scheie Eye Institute, University of Pennsylvania
School of Medicine, Philadelphia, Pennsylvania

Richard F. Brubaker, M.D.
Professor and Chairman, Department of
Ophthalmology, Mayo Clinic, Rochester,
Minnesota

David G. Campbell, M.D.
Professor of Ophthalmology, Dartmouth Medical
School, Hanover, New Hampshire

Louis B. Cantor, M.D.
Assistant Professor of Ophthalmology, Indiana
University; Director, Glaucoma Service,
Regenstrief Eye Clinic, Indianapolis, Indiana

Joseph Caprioli, M.D.
Associate Professor of Ophthalmology; Director
of Glaucoma Service, Yale University School of
Medicine, New Haven, Connecticut

Michael Cobo, M.D.
Associate Professor of Ophthalmology, Duke
University, Durham, North Carolina

Marshall N. Cyrlin, M.D.
Assistant Clinical Professor of Ophthalmology,
Michigan State University, East Lansing,
Michigan

Christopher J. Dickens, M.D.
Associate Professor of Ophthalmology,
University of California, San Francisco; Glaucoma
Research Consultant, The Foundation for
Glaucoma Research, San Francisco, California

Stephen M. Drance, M.D.
Professor and Chairman, Department of
Ophthalmology, The University of British
Columbia, Vancouver, British Columbia

Bruce A. Drum, Ph.D.
Assistant Professor of Ophthalmology, The Johns
Hopkins University School of Medicine,
Baltimore, Maryland

David L. Epstein, M.D.
Associate Professor of Ophthalmology, Howe
Laboratory of Ophthalmology, Harvard Medical
School; Massachusetts Eye and Ear Infirmary,
Boston, Massachusetts

Marianne E. Feitl, M.D.
Instructor of Ophthalmology, Scheie Eye
Institute, University of Pennsylvania School of
Medicine, Philadelphia, Pennsylvania

Ronald L. Fellman, M.D.
Assistant Clinical Professor of Ophthalmology,
University of Texas Southwestern Medical
School, Dallas, Texas

Kathy Felts, B.A.
Research Associate, Department of
Ophthalmology, University of Louisville School
of Medicine, Louisville, Kentucky

Robert Folberg, M.D.
Director, Eye Pathology Laboratory; Associate
Professor, Department of Ophthalmology,
University of Iowa Hospitals and Clinics, Iowa
City, Iowa

Thomas F. Freddo, M.D.
Fellow, Department of Ophthalmology,
University of Portland, Portland, Oregon

Beth R. Friedland
Clinical Assistant Professor of Ophthalmology,
University of North Carolina, Chapel Hill;
Survey of the Eye, Research Triangle Park, North
Carolina

Bruce J. Goldstick, M.D.
Fellow in Glaucoma, Department of
Ophthalmology, University of California, San
Diego, La Jolla, California

William R. Green, M.D.
Professor of Ophthalmology, Associate Professor
of Pathology, The Johns Hopkins University
School of Medicine, Baltimore, Maryland

Raymond Harrison, M.D.
Director, Glaucoma Service, Manhattan Eye, Ear,
and Throat Hospital, New York, New York

William M. Hart, Jr., M.D., Ph.D.
Associate Professor of Ophthalmology,
Washington University School of Medicine, St.
Louis, Missouri

Sohan Singh Hayreh, M.D., Ph.D.
Professor of Ophthalmology, University of Iowa,
Iowa City, Iowa

M. Rosario Hernandez, D.D.S.
Assistant Scientist, Department of
Ophthalmology, Ophthalmic Pharmacology Unit,
Eye Research Institute of Retina Foundation;
Instructor of Ophthalmology, Harvard Medical
School, Boston, Massachusetts

Jonathan Herschler, M.D.
Director, Glaucoma Service, Oregon Lions Sight
and Hearing Institute, Portland, Oregon

Helen Mintz Hittner, M.D.
Clinical Professor of Ophthalmology and
Pediatrics, Baylor College of Medicine, Houston,
Texas

H. Dunbar Hoskins, Jr., M.D.
Clinical Professor of Ophthalmology, University
of California, San Francisco, California

Shyun Jeng, M.D.
Research Fellow in Glaucoma, Department of
Ophthalmology, University of California, San
Diego, La Jolla, California

Tim Johnson, M.D.
Fellow, Department of Ophthalmology,
Washington University School of Medicine, St.
Louis, Missouri

Murray A. Johnstone, M.D.
Consultant in Glaucoma, Department of
Ophthalmology, University of Washington,
Seattle, Washington

Michael A. Kass, M.D.
Professor of Ophthalmology, Washington
University School of Medicine, St. Louis,
Missouri

L. Jay Katz, M.D.
Assistant Professor of Ophthalmology, Thomas
Jefferson University; Associate Surgeon, Wills
Eye Hospital, Philadelphia, Pennsylvania

Paul L. Kaufman, M.D.
Professor of Ophthalmology; Director, Glaucoma
Services, University of Wisconsin, Madison,
Wisconsin

Deen G. King, M.D.
Assistant Professor of Ophthalmology, University
of South Florida, Tampa, Florida

Joseph H. Krug, Jr., M.D.
Instructor of Ophthalmology, Harvard Medical
School; Ophthalmic Consultants of Boston, The
Glaucoma Consultation Service of the
Massachusetts Eye and Ear Infirmary, Boston,
Massachusetts

Theodore Krupin, M.D.
Professor of Ophthalmology; Chief, Glaucoma
Service, Scheie Eye Institute, University of
Pennsylvania School of Medicine, Philadelphia,
Pennsylvania

Yasuaki Kuwayama, M.D.
Assistant Professor of Ophthalmology, Osaka
University Medical School, Osaka, Japan

William E. Layden, M.D.
Professor and Chairman, Department of
Ophthalmology, University of South Florida,
Tampa, Florida

Julie S. Lee, M.D.
Lecturer, Department of Ophthalmology,
University of Louisville School of Medicine,
Louisville, Kentucky

Jeffrey M. Liebmann, M.D.
Clinical Instructor of Ophthalmology, the
New York Eye and Ear Infirmary, New York,
New York

Ronald F. Lowe, M.D.
Emeritus Ophthalmic Surgeon, The Royal
Victorian Eye and Ear Hospital, Melbourne,
Australia

Maurice H. Luntz, M.D.
Clinical Professor, Department of
Ophthalmology, Mount Sinai School of Medicine,
New York, New York

Elke Lütjen-Drecoll, M.D.
Professor and Chairperson, Department of
Anatomy, University of Erlangen/Nürnberg,
Erlangen, West Germany

John R. Lynn, M.D.
Professor of Ophthalmology, Univeristy of Texas
Southwestern Medical School, Dallas, Texas

Martin A. Mainster, M.D., Ph.D.
Professor of Ophthalmology, University of
Kansas Medical Center, Kansas City, Kansas

Robert M. Mandelkorn, M.D.
Clinical Assistant Instructor of Ophthalmology,
University of Pittsburgh, Pittsburgh,
Pennsylvania

Thomas H. Maren, M.D.
Graduate Research Professor of Pharmacology
and Therapeutics, University of Florida College
of Medicine, The J. Hillis Miller Health Center,
Gainesville, Florida

A. Edward Maumenee, M.D.
Emeritus Professor, Department of
Ophthalmology, The Johns Hopkins University
School of Medicine, Baltimore, Maryland

John A. McDermott, M.D.
Attending Physician, Glaucoma Service,
Department of Ophthalmology, the New York
Eye and Ear Infirmary, New York, New York

Thomas W. Mittag, Ph.D.
Professor of Ophthalmology and Pharmacology,
Mount Sinai School of Medicine, New York,
New York

Jose Morales, M.D.
Assistant Professor of Ophthalmology; Director,
Glaucoma Service, Departments of
Ophthalmology and Visual Science, Texas Tech
University Health Sciences Center School of
Medicine, Lubbock, Texas

John C. Morrison, M.D.
Assistant Professor of Ophthalmology, Oregon
Health Services, University of Portland, Portland,
Oregon

George F. Nardin, M.D.
Instructor of Ophthalmology, Kentucky Lions
Eye Research Institute, University of Louisville
School of Medicine, Louisville, Kentucky

Arthur H. Neufeld, Ph.D.
Senior Scientist and Head, Department of
Ophthalmology, Ophthalmic Pharmacology Unit,
Eye Institute of Retina Foundation; Professor of
Ophthalmology, Harvard Medical School,
Boston, Massachusetts

Randall J. Olson, M.D.
Professor and Chairman, Department of
Ophthalmology, University of Utah School of
Medicine, Salt Lake City, Utah

Paul Palmberg, M.D., Ph.D.
Associate Professor of Ophthalmology,
University of Miami School of Medicine;
Associate Professor, Bascom Palmer Eye
Institute, Miami, Florida

Richard Kenneth Parrish II, M.D.
Assistant Professor of Ophthalmology, Bascom
Palmer Eye Institute, University of Miami School
of Medicine, Miami, Florida

Jonathan E. Pederson, M.D.
Frank E. Burd Professor of Ophthalmology,
University of Minnesota, Minneapolis, Minnesota

Morris M. Podolsky, M.D.
Assistant Clinical Professor of Ophthalmology, Mount Sinai School of Medicine, New York, New York

Andrew M. Prince, M.D.
Clinical Instructor of Ophthalmology, New York University Medical Center; Director, Glaucoma Service, Catholic Medical Center of Brooklyn and Queens, New York, New York

Ronald L. Radius, M.D.
Professor of Ophthalmology, Medical College of Wisconsin, Milwaukee, Wisconsin

Alexander Reyes, M.D.
Glaucoma Fellow, the New York Eye and Ear Infirmary, New York, New York

Thomas M. Richardson, M.D.
Assistant Clinical Professor of Ophthalmology, Harvard Medical School; Assistant Surgeon, Howe Laboratory of Ophthalmology, Massachusetts Eye and Ear Infirmary, Boston, Massachusetts

Claudia U. Richter, M.D.
Clinical Assistant in Ophthalmology, Harvard University, Massachusetts Eye and Ear Infirmary, Boston, Massachusetts

Robert Ritch, M.D.
Professor of Clinical Ophthalmology, The New York Medical College, Valhalla, New York; Chief, Glaucoma Service, the New York Eye and Ear Infirmary, New York, New York

Johannes W. Rohen, M.D.
Professor and Chairman, Anatomisches Institut, Universitat Erlangen/Nürnberg, Erlangen, West Germany

Edwin M. Schottenstein, M.D.
Clinical Instructor of Ophthalmology, the New York University Medical Center; Adjunct Surgeon, the New York Eye and Ear Infirmary, New York, New York

Jeffrey Schultz, M.D.
Assistant Professor of Ophthalmology; Director, Glaucoma Service, Albert Einstein College of Medicine/Montefiore Medical Center, Bronx, New York

Carol L. Shields, M.D.
Clinical Fellow, Ocular Oncology Service, Wills Eye Hospital, Jefferson Medical College, Thomas Jefferson University, Philadelphia, Pennsylvania

Jerry A. Shields, M.D.
Director of Oncology Service, Department of Ophthalmology, Wills Eye Hospital; Professor of Ophthalmology, Thomas Jefferson University, Philadelphia, Pennsylvania

M. Bruce Shields, M.D.
Professor of Ophthalmology; Director, Glaucoma Service, Duke University Eye Center, Durham, North Carolina

Richard J. Simmons, M.D.
Associate Clinical Professor of Ophthalmology, Harvard Medical School, Boston, Massachusetts

Patricia Smith, M.D.
Assistant Professor of Ophthalmology and Pathology, University of Virginia, Charlottesville, Virginia

Ira S. Solomon, M.D.
Attending Ophthalmologist, Glaucoma Service, the New York Eye and Ear Infirmary, New York, New York

George L. Spaeth, M.D.
Professor of Ophthalmology, Thomas Jefferson University; Director, William and Anne Goldberg Glaucoma Service and Research Laboratories, and Attending Surgeon, Wills Eye Hospital, Philadelphia, Pennsylvania

Scott M. Spector, M.D.
Attending Ophthalmologist, Glaucoma Service, the New York Eye and Ear Infirmary, New York, New York

Richard J. Starita, M.D.
Assistant Clinical Professor of Ophthalmology, University of Texas Southwestern Medical School, Dallas, Texas

Walter J. Stark, M.D.
Professor of Ophthalmology, The Wilmer Ophthalmological Institute, The Johns Hopkins University School of Medicine, Baltimore, Maryland

Richard A. Stone, M.D.
Associate Professor of Ophthalmology,
University of Pennsylvania School of Medicine,
Scheie Eye Institute, Philadelphia, Pennsylvania

John V. Thomas, M.D.
Clinical Assistant in Ophthalmology,
Massachusetts Eye and Ear Infirmary, Boston,
Massachusetts

Brenda J. Tripathi, Ph.D.
Research Associate Professor of Ophthalmology
and Visual Science, The University of Chicago,
Chicago, Illinois

Ramesh C. Tripathi, M.D., Ph.D.
Professor of Ophthalmology, The University of
Chicago, Chicago, Illinois

Anja Tuulonen, M.D.
Assistant Professor of Ophthalmology, University
of Oulu, Oulu, Finland

E. Michael Van Buskirk, M.D.
Professor and Vice Chairman, Department of
Ophthalmology, Oregon Health Sciences,
University of Portland, Portland, Oregon

Martin Wand, M.D.
Assistant Clinical Professor of Ophthalmology,
University of Connecticut Medical School,
Farmington, Connecticut

Peter G. Watson, M.D.
Head, Department of Ophthalmology,
Addenbrookes Hospital, University of
Cambridge, Cambridge, England

Martin Wax, M.D.
Assistant Professor of Ophthalmology and
Pharmacology, University of Pennsylvania School
of Medicine, Philadelphia, Pennsylvania

Robert N. Weinreb, M.D.
Professor and Vice Chairman, Department of
Ophthalmology, University of California, San
Diego, La Jolla, California

Jayne S. Weiss, M.D.
Corneal and External Disease of Ophthalmology,
University of Massachusetts Medical Center,
North Worcester, Massachusetts

Elliot B. Werner, M.D.
Associate Professor of Ophthalmology,
Hahnemann University, Philadelphia,
Pennsylvania

Moustafa K. Yaqub, M.D.
Glaucoma Fellow, New England Glaucoma
Research Foundation, Inc., Boston,
Massachusetts

Alan H. Zalta, M.D.
Assistant Professor of Ophthalmology; Chief,
Glaucoma Service, University of Cincinnati
College of Medicine, Cincinnati, Ohio

Ran C. Zeimer, Ph.D.
Research Associate Professor of Ophthalmology,
University of Illinois, Chicago, Illinois

Thom J. Zimmerman, M.D., Ph.D.
Professor and Chairman, Department of
Ophthalmology, University of Louisville School
of Medicine; Kentucky Lions Eye Research
Institute, Louisville, Kentucky

PREFACE

Glaucoma has come of age. Not long ago, the glaucomas were considered to consist of essentially primary open-angle, angle-closure, and congenital types. Now we recognize the addition of a multitude of secondary glaucomas. Improvements in diagnostic techniques, advances in scientific technology, and the intellectual thrust of biochemistry, cell biology, and molecular genetics have brought us to the beginning of a new era in the elucidation of these groups of mystifying disorders.

In 1951 a textbook devoted exclusively to glaucoma, entitled *The Glaucomas*, was published by H. Saul Sugar. A second edition appeared in 1957. This excellent text comprehensively covered the knowledge and understanding of the diagnosis and management of the glaucomas at that time.

As we now offer a new textbook with the same title, we are mindful of the contributions made by earlier pioneers in the field, whose work formed the foundation of our current achievements. At the same time, a comparison of the size and content of these present volumes to those of the textbooks of the 1950s reminds us of the immense strides that have been made in the intervening generation.

Consider the discipline of glaucoma of the 1950s. The diagnosis was still based largely on indentation tonometry, poorly standardized campimetry and arc perimetry, and evaluation of the optic nerve head with a direct ophthalmoscope. Morton Grant was just beginning to apply modern tonography to questions that would revolutionize our understanding of the mechanisms of the glaucomas as well as the actions of antiglaucoma drugs. Hans Goldmann was just introducing modern applanation tonometry and standardized bowl perimetry. It would be another two decades before the application of computer technology, leading to automated perimetry and image analysis of the optic nerve head.

Concomitant with the advances in understanding of mechanisms of the glaucomas and the development of diagnostic techniques during the past three decades has been the improvement of our ability to treat this broad group of disorders. Medical therapy for glaucoma in the early 1950s was limited to topical miotics and epinephrine. The carbonic anhydrase inhibitors were introduced through the work of Bernard Becker and Thomas Maren. It would be another quarter century before the introduction of the beta-blockers.

Glaucoma filtering surgery of the 1950s had not changed significantly from the time of its introduction at the turn of the century. Advances in microsurgery, guarded filtration techniques, improved setons, and pharmacologic modulation of wound healing were still in the future. The laser had not yet been invented; by the 1980s it would become the most commonly used tool for glaucoma surgery.

In pace with other disciplines, we can expect ever more rapid advances in our understanding and treatment of the glaucomas. Many diseases that have been regarded as single entities, such as diabetes or Marfan's syndrome, are now being recognized as groups of phenotypically similar disorders with multiple etiologies based on genetically determined defects in enzymes or structural proteins or both. We can expect that the same will hold true for what we now consider as primary open-angle glaucoma. We can expect to see further elucidation of the biochemistry of the trabecular meshwork, the role of cell surface molecules in aqueous outflow, and the nature of neural and endocrine control mechanisms regulating aqueous turnover. As more and more subtypes of the glaucomas are differentiated, a clearer understanding of the molecular or genetic defect in each of these can be expected to lead to more specific forms of treatment at a more basic level.

When one considers the rapid advances and the increasing number of specialized areas of scientific research being brought to bear on the field of glaucoma, it is not surprising that a large number of experts were needed to document comprehensively the knowledge that exists today. It is this goal that we hope to have accomplished in *The Glaucomas*.

Such an undertaking would never have been possible without the help of the many contributors to this text. To each of them, and to all who assisted in the preparation of their manuscripts, we offer our most sincere thanks. We also gratefully acknowledge the expert assistance of Ms. Eugenia Klein, Elaine Steinborn, and the excellent staff at The C.V. Mosby Co.

A special thanks to all who have served as our mentors through the years, including our residents and fellows, who continue to challenge us with provocative questions and who force us continually to seek new and better answers. It is our hope that these volumes will be an accurate record of the contributions of the past and present, so that all physicians may profit from this knowledge to further our common goal of preventing blindness from glaucoma.

Robert Ritch
M. Bruce Shields
Theodore Krupin

CONTENTS

PART THREE Pharmacology

PART FOUR Laser Surgery

PART FIVE Glaucoma Surgery

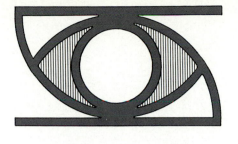

PART SIX

CLASSIFICATIONS AND MECHANISMS

40

Classifications and Mechanisms of the Glaucomas

Chapter 40

Classifications and Mechanisms of the Glaucomas

M. Bruce Shields
Robert Ritch
Theodore Krupin

The clinical forms of glaucoma have traditionally been classified as primary and secondary types. This division, although somewhat arbitrary, is based on our understanding of the pathophysiologic events that lead to obstruction of aqueous humor outflow and subsequent elevation of intraocular pressure.

The primary glaucomas (open-angle, angle-closure, and congenital) are generally defined as those in which the initiating event begins in the anterior chamber angle or conventional outflow pathway, and for which no apparent contribution from other ocular or systemic disorders has yet been discovered. These conditions usually have a genetic basis and are typically bilateral.

The secondary glaucomas can be traced a step back on the etiologic ladder and occur as distinct entities because of a recognized underlying, predisposing ocular or systemic condition. These glaucomas may be unilateral or bilateral. Some have a genetic basis, whereas others are acquired.

As our understanding of the mechanisms for both primary and secondary glaucomas has expanded, the "primary/secondary" classification has become increasingly artificial. For example, both primary angle-closure glaucoma and pigmentary glaucoma have characteristic ocular configurations that initiate a sequence of events leading to aqueous outflow obstruction. Yet the former condition is classified as a primary glaucoma, whereas

the latter is traditionally included among the secondary glaucomas. Furthermore, glaucomas caused by developmental anomalies of the anterior chamber angle do not fit neatly into either category. Nevertheless, the primary and secondary classifications are deeply ingrained in the ophthalmic literature and will be retained, and a third category of developmental glaucomas added for purposes of discussion in this text.

PRIMARY GLAUCOMAS

The primary glaucomas typically include primary open-angle glaucoma, primary angle-closure glaucoma, and primary congenital glaucoma. In primary open-angle glaucoma, the increased resistance to aqueous outflow appears to be in the trabecular meshwork or Schlemm's canal, although the precise abnormality has not been elucidated. Myopes are more susceptible to primary open-angle glaucoma, and many patients have a positive family history of the disease, although the influence of genetic factors is not fully understood. We may eventually find that this is a group of related disorders characterized by abnormalities in the trabecular meshwork or other portions of the aqueous outflow system.

Patients with primary angle-closure glaucoma have a shallow anterior chamber, which predisposes to obstruction of aqueous flow between the lens and iris (pupillary block), leading to increased pressure in the posterior chamber, forward bowing of the peripheral iris into the anterior chamber angle, and blocking of aqueous outflow. It has a genetic component in that hyperopes are more susceptible, but the probability of it becoming manifest may depend on additional genetic or other factors.

Primary congenital glaucoma results from incomplete development of the anterior chamber angle. It is typically bilateral and is believed to have a genetic basis.

DEVELOPMENTAL GLAUCOMAS

Developmental glaucomas overlap the traditional separation between primary and secondary glaucomas. They are all characterized by a developmental anomaly of the aqueous outflow system. Primary congenital glaucoma is included among the primary glaucomas because the developmental defect is limited to the anterior chamber angle with no associated ocular or systemic anomalies. Other developmental glaucomas have additional ocular or systemic abnormalities that are not directly associated with the mechanism of aqueous outflow obstruction. These have been conceptually regarded as a subset of the secondary glaucomas, and examples include aniridia, Axenfeld-Rieger syndrome, and Peters' anomaly.

SECONDARY GLAUCOMAS

For the purpose of discussion of secondary glaucomas in this book, "glaucoma" will be defined as any condition leading to a secondary rise in intraocular pressure with or without associated damage to the optic nerve head or visual field. The division that is often made between "ocular hypertension" and "glaucoma," when dealing with primary open-angle glaucoma, is not always applicable to the secondary glaucomas. Some patients with a secondary elevation of intraocular pressure are undoubtedly more resistant to glaucomatous optic atrophy than other individuals. However, it is difficult to apply general concepts to all the secondary glaucomas because of the wide variation in causes, treatments, and prognoses. In some cases, such as the pigment dispersion syndrome, the criteria for deciding whether or not to institute treatment may be quite similar to those in primary open-angle glaucoma. In other conditions, such as neovascular glaucoma, the decision to treat or not to treat rests less with the state of the optic nerve head or visual field and more with the natural history and typical progression of the underlying disorder. Therefore, all cases of secondary intraocular pressure elevation are referred to in this text as glau-

coma, and any distinctions or exceptions are discussed in the respective chapters.

The list of secondary glaucomas is long and complex, and no single classification scheme for these disorders is completely satisfactory. There is some value in considering more than one system of classification, since each offers different advantages. In this text, the secondary glaucomas have been grouped according to the underlying etiologic factors. However, it is also helpful to consider these conditions on the basis of anatomic mechanisms, a discussion of which is included in this chapter.

Etiologic Classification

The etiologic classification of secondary glaucomas is based on the underlying etiologic factor(s) that ultimately lead(s) to the elevated intraocular pressure. This classification system is limited by the fact that the primary etiologic factor is not completely understood in many forms of secondary glaucoma. However, it has the advantage of allowing discussion of a secondary glaucoma under a single heading, unlike systems based on clinical presentations or mechanisms. For example, neovascular glaucoma might be discussed with conditions that give a clinical presentation of rubeosis iridis, hemorrhage, peripheral anterior synechiae, or signs of inflammation, or with those in which the mechanism of aqueous outflow obstruction is either open-angle or angle-closure, depending on the stage of the disease.

The etiologic classification enables the clinician to think in terms of the underlying disorder and to institute treatment on that basis. Entities that are quite disparate in their manifestations may be grouped together under broader categories that allow one to think of the underlying disorders as common denominators. Such a category is the lens-related glaucomas, which include such varied entities as lens protein glaucoma and anterior dislocation of the lens. Although the mechanisms of glaucoma within this group of conditions include both open-angle and angle-closure forms, treatment may be directed at the lens rather than the secondary manifestation of the glaucoma itself.

An etiologic classification is also consistent with the ideal approach to treating secondary glaucomas, which is to eliminate the underlying disorder before the development of elevated intraocular pressure. For example, in some cases of central retinal vein occlusion, the risk of glaucoma is sufficiently high that panretinal photocoagulation can be initiated even before the development of rubeosis iridis, in the hope of avoiding this severe form of glaucoma. However, our present understanding of the sequence of events in most secondary glaucomas is insufficient to permit this therapeutic approach, and much more study is needed in this area.

Mechanistic Classification

The mechanism of intraocular pressure elevation in virtually every form of secondary glaucoma is the obstruction of aqueous outflow. Understanding the precise mechanism that leads to this obstruction in each disease provides a helpful frame-

---

MECHANISTIC CLASSIFICATION OF THE SECONDARY GLAUCOMAS*

I. The secondary open-angle glaucomas
  A. Pretrabecular (membrane overgrowth)
    1. Fibrovascular membrane (neovascular glaucoma)
    2. Endothelial layer, often with Descemet-like membrane
      a. Iridocorneal endothelial syndrome
      b. Posterior polymorphous dystrophy
      c. Penetrating and nonpenetrating trauma
    3. Epithelial downgrowth
    4. Fibrous ingrowth
    5. Inflammatory membrane
      a. Fuchs' heterochromic iridocyclitis
      b. Luetic interstitial keratitis
  B. Trabecular
    1. "Clogging" of the meshwork
      a. Red blood cells
        (1) Hemorrhagic glaucoma
        (2) Ghost cell glaucoma
      b. Macrophages
        (1) Hemolytic glaucoma
        (2) Phacolytic glaucoma
        (3) Melanomalytic glaucoma
      c. Neoplastic cells
        (1) Malignant tumors
        (2) Neurofibromatosis
        (3) Nevus of Ota
        (4) Juvenile xanthogranuloma
      d. Pigment particles
        (1) Pigmentary glaucoma
        (2) Exfoliation syndrome (glaucoma capsulare)
        (3) Uveitis
        (4) Malignant melanoma
      e. Protein
        (1) Uveitis
        (2) Lens-induced glaucoma
      f. Alpha-chymotrypsin-induced glaucoma
      g. Vitreous or exogenous hyaluronic acid in anterior chamber
    2. Alterations of the trabecular meshwork
      a. Edema
        (1) Uveitis
        (2) Scleritis and episcleritis
        (3) Alkali burns
      b. Trauma (angle recession)
      c. Intraocular foreign bodies (hemosiderosis, chalcosis)
      d. Incomplete development (Axenfeld-Rieger syndrome)
      e. Steroid-induced glaucoma

  C. Posttrabecular (elevated episcleral venous pressure)
    1. Carotid-cavernous fistula
    2. Cavernous sinus thrombosis
    3. Retrobulbar tumors
    4. Thyrotropic exophthalmos
    5. Superior vena cava obstruction
    6. Mediastinal tumors
    7. Sturge-Weber syndrome
    8. Familial episcleral venous pressure elevation
II. The secondary angle-closure glaucomas
  A. Anterior ("pulling" mechanism)
    1. Contracture of membranes
      a. Neovascular glaucoma
      b. Iridocorneal endothelial syndrome
      c. Posterior polymorphous dystrophy
      d. Penetrating and nonpenetrating trauma
    2. Contracture of inflammatory precipitates
    3. Contracture of congenital bands (aniridia)
  B. Posterior ("pushing" mechanism)
    1. With pupillary block
      a. Intumescent lens
      b. Subluxation of lens
        (1) Traumatic
        (2) Spontaneous
      c. Following lens extraction
        (1) Iris-vitreous block
        (2) Pseudophakia
      d. Iris bombé associated with intraocular inflammation
    2. Without pupillary block
      a. Ciliary block (malignant) glaucoma
      b. Following lens extraction (forward vitreous shift)
      c. Following scleral buckling
      d. Following panretinal photocoagulation
      e. Central retinal vein occlusion
      f. Intraocular tumors
        (1) Malignant melanoma
        (2) Retinoblastoma
      g. Cysts of the iris and ciliary body
      h. Retrolenticular tissue contracture
        (1) Retinopathy of prematurity (retrolental fibroplasia)
        (2) Persistent hyperplastic primary vitreous

*Clinical examples cited in this table do not represent an inclusive list of the secondary glaucomas.

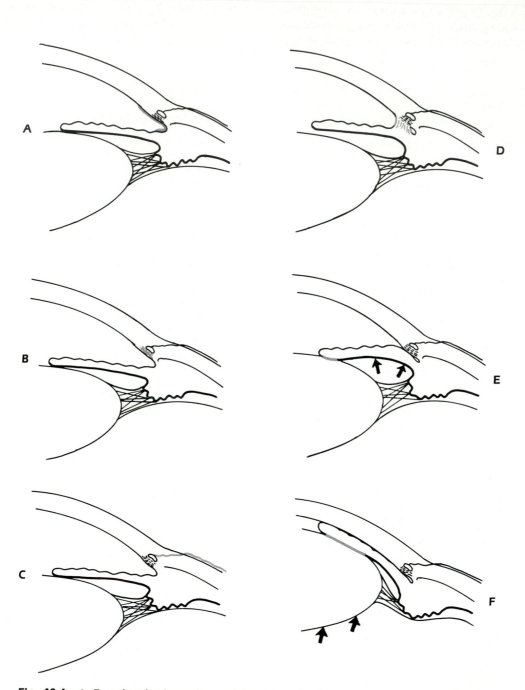

Fig. 40-1 **A,** Pretrabecular form of secondary open-angle glaucoma. **B,** Trabecular form of secondary open-angle glaucoma. **C,** Posttrabecular form of secondary open-angle glaucoma. **D,** Anterior form of secondary angle-closure glaucoma. **E,** Posterior form of secondary angle-closure glaucoma with pupillary block. **F,** Posterior form of secondary angle-closure glaucoma without pupillary block.

work on which to develop a rationale for therapy of the secondary glaucomas.

Classifying the secondary glaucomas according to the anatomic location of the aqueous outflow obstruction is helpful not only in considering the differential diagnosis, but also in determining the mechanism underlying the intraocular pressure elevation. The tabulation suggested in this chapter represents a systematic arrangement of the various mechanisms of secondary glaucoma. Particularly in the diseases that can cause glaucoma by more than one mechanism, it enables the clinician to consider systematically each possible mode of blockage to aqueous humor outflow, and thereby to select the best treatment.

The box on p. 40-3 and Fig. 40-1 present one approach to the mechanistic classification of the secondary glaucomas. In this system, all of the secondary glaucomas are arbitrarily divided into two categories on the basis of gonioscopic appearance: open-angle and angle-closure.

Secondary open-angle glaucomas

The secondary open-angle glaucomas are those in which the anterior chamber angle structures (i.e., trabecular meshwork, scleral spur, and ciliary body band) are visible by gonioscopy. However, this does not necessarily imply that the angle is free of obstructive elements.

In the "pretrabecular" form, a translucent membrane extends across the open angle, leading to the obstruction of aqueous outflow. In various cases this may be a fibrovascular membrane, an endothelial layer with a Descemet-like membrane, an epithelial membrane, a connective tissue membrane, or a membrane secondary to inflammation.

In the "trabecular form" of secondary open-angle glaucomas, the obstruction to aqueous outflow is located within the trabecular meshwork. This may be caused by a "clogging" of the meshwork with red blood cells, macrophages, neoplastic cells, pigment particles, protein, lens zonules, or vitreous. In other cases, obstruction to outflow may result from acquired alterations of the trabecular meshwork tissue, such as edema associated with inflammatory conditions, trauma with subsequent scarring, and toxic reactions associated with intraocular foreign bodies. Steroid-induced glaucoma and certain glaucomas associated with systemic disease are not well understood, but are believed

to cause obstruction to aqueous outflow in the trabecular meshwork or Schlemm's canal.

A third group of secondary open-angle glaucomas have a mechanism referred to as the "post-trabecular" form, in which obstruction to aqueous outflow results from increased resistance distal to the meshwork and Schlemm's canal. Most of these cases are caused by elevated episcleral venous pressure.

Secondary angle-closure glaucomas

The secondary angle-closure glaucomas include those conditions in which the peripheral iris is in apposition to the trabecular meshwork or peripheral cornea. The peripheral iris may either be "pulled" (anterior form) or "pushed" (posterior form) into this position.

In the "anterior" form of the secondary angle-closure glaucomas, an abnormal tissue bridges the anterior chamber angle and subsequently undergoes contraction, pulling the peripheral iris into the angle. Examples of the contracting tissue includes a fibrovascular membrane, an endothelial layer with a Descemet-like membrane, and inflammatory precipitates.

In the "posterior" form, pressure behind the iris or lens causes the peripheral iris to be pushed into the anterior chamber angle. This may occur with or without pupillary block. In the pupillary block form, there is an apposition between the pupillary portion of the iris and the lens or vitreous. The apposition may be functional, secondary to a forward shift of the lens or vitreous or following intraocular lens implantation, or it may represent synechial apposition, associated with intraocular inflammation. In either case, the apposition obstructs the flow of aqueous humor into the anterior chamber, resulting in increased pressure in the posterior chamber and causing the peripheral iris to bow forward into the anterior chamber angle.

In the posterior forms of secondary angle-closure glaucoma without pupillary block, increased pressure in the posterior portion of the eye pushes the lens-iris diaphragm or vitreous-iris diaphragm forward. Examples of initiating events include alterations in the intraocular tissues following surgery, central retinal vein occlusion, intraocular tumors, cysts of the iris and ciliary body, or contracture of retrolenticular tissue.

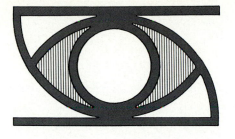

PART SEVEN

THE PRIMARY GLAUCOMAS

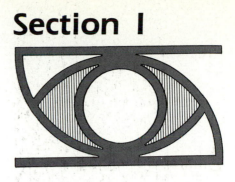

Congenital Glaucoma

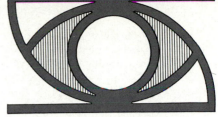

Chapter 41

Epidemiology and Pathophysiology of Congenital Glaucoma

Christopher J. Dickens
H. Dunbar Hoskins, Jr.

Primary congenital glaucoma is one of many types of developmental glaucomas, the terminology for which has been somewhat inconsistent and occasionally confusing. With increased knowledge, we have been able to define more precise terminology based on the embryology and cellular biology of congenital glaucoma. This terminology should be employed whenever possible.

HISTORY

Congenital enlargement of the eye has been recognized since the time of Hippocrates, but buphthalmos was not related to elevated intraocular pressure until the middle of the eighteenth century. At that time, congenital glaucoma was grouped together with a variety of other conditions, such as high myopia and anterior staphyloma. Von Muralt (1869) described the disease as one belonging to the glaucomas. Pathological studies in the late 1800s and early 1900s took note of congenital anomalies of the anterior chamber angle and Schlemm's canal. Descriptions were further enhanced in the early to mid 1900s by the work of Reis, Seefelder, Cross and others who demonstrated the maldevelopment of angle structures as being the primary characteristic, with inflammation playing a secondary role.

Barkan (1949) described a persisting fetal membrane overlying the trabecular meshwork. This was confirmed by Worst (1966) who termed it "Barkan's membrane." Recent pathological studies have not found evidence of Barkan's membrane but have found abnormalities within the trabecular meshwork and ciliary body.[3,24] Two classic textbooks that have been written on the subject are *Hydrophthalmia or Congenital Glaucoma*[4] and *Congenital and Pediatric Glaucomas*.[29]

DeVincentiis (1891) was the first to suggest an operation to incise the tissues of the anterior chamber angle to treat congenital glaucoma.[10,11] Good success was reported for many cases despite the limitations imposed by the technology available at that time. The incision was frequently made into Descemet's membrane or into the ciliary body rather than into the trabecular meshwork, and these incisions were unsuccessful. Scarring of the incision was also reported and could have resulted from too deep an incision of the meshwork, thus cutting into scleral tissue.

Otto Barkan perfected the procedure of goniotomy in the 1930s and, although the instrumentation has since been refined and the operating microscope now permits more precise visualization of the angle structures, the operation has remained essentially unchanged.

As late as 1939, Anderson saw little hope for

SHAFFER-WEISS CLASSIFICATION OF CONGENITAL GLAUCOMA

I. Primary congenital glaucomas (primary infantile glaucoma)
II. Glaucoma associated with congenital anomalies
   A. Late-developing primary infantile glaucoma (late developing primary congenital glaucoma)
   B. Aniridia
   C. Sturge-Weber
   D. Neurofibromatosis
   E. Marfan's syndrome
   F. Pierre Robin syndrome
   G. Homocystinuria
   H. Goniodysgenesis (iridocorneal neural crest cell dysgenesis: Axenfeld-Rieger syndrome, Peters' anomaly)
   I. Lowe's syndrome
   J. Microcornea
   K. Microspherophakia
   L. Rubella
   M. Chromosomal abnormalities
   N. Broad thumb syndrome
   O. Persistent hyperplastic primary vitreous
III. Secondary glaucomas in infants
   A. Retrolental fibroplasia
   B. Tumors
      1. Retinoblastoma
      2. Juvenile xanthogranuloma
   C. Inflammation
   D. Trauma

useful vision in these patients despite detailed evaluation of all known treatment modalities available at that time:

> The future of patients with hydrophthalmia is dark. Little hope of preserving sufficient sight to permit the earning of a livelihood can be held out to them. It progresses, as a rule, in a relentless fashion until the best setting for the patient is some institution that caters for the blind.[4]

He also stated that "one seeks in vain for a best operation in the treatment of hydrophthalmia."

A dramatic improvement in the outlook for patients with primary congenital glaucoma has occurred since Barkan introduced goniotomy. With goniotomy or trabeculotomy, there is now hope for the control of intraocular pressure and for good vision in many of these patients. Success rates, however, vary markedly among the anatomic forms of congenital glaucoma with which patients present.

A further advance in management came with the introduction of trabeculotomy by Burian and Allen and Smith, and popularized by Harms and Dannheim.[1,7,15,30] This procedure allows rupture of the malformed trabecular meshwork when corneal clouding prevents an accurate goniotomy.

TERMINOLOGY

Developmental glaucoma refers to glaucoma associated with developmental anomalies of the eye present at birth. This includes both primary congenital glaucoma and glaucomas associated with other developmental anomalies either of the eye or systemically. In all forms, it occurs in about 1 in 10,000 live births. Secondary glaucomas in infants refers to acquired ocular diseases that can cause glaucoma.

Primary congenital glaucoma refers to a specific form of glaucoma. These eyes have an isolated maldevelopment of the trabecular meshwork not associated with other developmental ocular anomalies or ocular diseases that can raise the intraocular pressure. It is the most common glaucoma of infancy, occurring in about 1 in 30,000 live births.

Infantile glaucoma is a term that has been used in a variety of contexts. Some have used it synonymously with primary congenital glaucoma, whereas others have used it to mean any glaucoma occurring during the first several years of life. Its meaning should thus be qualified or its use avoided. Primary infantile glaucoma is synonymous with primary congenital glaucoma.

Juvenile glaucoma is a nonspecific term referring to any type of glaucoma occurring in later childhood or the teenage years.

HOSKINS ANATOMIC CLASSIFICATION OF DEVELOPMENTAL GLAUCOMAS

I. Isolated trabeculodysgenesis (malformation of trabecular meshwork in the absence of iris or corneal anomalies)
  A. Flat iris insertion
    1. Anterior insertion
    2. Posterior insertion
    3. Mixed insertion
  B. Concave (wraparound) iris insertion
  C. Unclassified
II. Iridotrabeculodysgenesis (trabeculodysgenesis with iris anomalies)
  A. Anterior stromal defects
    1. Hypoplasia
    2. Hyperplasia
  B. Anomalous iris vessels
    1. Persistence of tunica vasculosa lentis
    2. Anomalous superficial vessels
  C. Structural anomalies
    1. Holes
    2. Colobomata
    3. Aniridia
III. Corneotrabeculodysgenesis (usually has associated iris anomalies)
  A. Peripheral
  B. Midperipheral
  C. Central
  D. Corneal size

Buphthalmos and hydrophthalmia are both descriptive terms that should not be used diagnostically. Buphthalmos is derived from the Greek term for "ox eye" and refers to the marked enlargement that can occur as a result of any type of glaucoma present in infancy. Hydrophthalmia refers to the high fluid content present with marked enlargement of an eye, which can occur in any type of glaucoma presenting in infancy.

CLASSIFICATION

Various classifications of the developmental glaucomas have been employed. Initial efforts at classification were directed toward eponyms and syndrome names, and many of these terms are now widely employed and recognized.

The Shaffer-Weiss disease classification divides the developmental glaucomas into primary congenital glaucoma, glaucomas associated with developmental anomalies of the eye or the body, and acquired glaucomas[20,29] (see box on p. 762).

Recently, an anatomic classification of the congenital glaucomas has been proposed[16,17] (see box at right). Clinically identifiable anatomic defects of the eye were chosen as the basis for this classification because they are readily apparent on examination of the patient and do not require supplemental information.

Identification of the anatomic defect helps in determining appropriate therapy and assessing prognostic factors, in addition to circumventing the need to differentiate between potentially confusing syndromes, which in the past have often been grouped on the bases of superficial characteristics.

Malformation of the anterior segment is the hallmark of developmental glaucoma. The goniodysgenesis that leads to glaucoma occurs in a variety of ways and may involve one or more of the three angle structures: the trabecular meshwork, the iris, and the cornea.

The extent of maldevelopment is indicated by the presence or absence and degree of trabeculodysgenesis, iridodysgenesis, and corneodysgenesis. These defects occur in a variety of combinations with attributes that have therapeutic and prognostic significance.

Isolated Trabeculodysgenesis

The classic defect found in primary congenital glaucoma, isolated trabeculodysgenesis, is the only detectable ocular anomaly in approximately 50% of infants and juvenile patients with glaucoma. This defect can present in two ways. In the most common form, the iris inserts flatly into the trabecular meshwork at or anterior to the scleral spur (Fig. 41-1). This insertion usually obscures the view of the ciliary body, although portions of the anterior ciliary body may be seen through a thickened trabecular meshwork when the angle is viewed obliquely from above. The level of iris insertion may vary along the angle circumference. In some eyes, portions of the iris may insert posterior to the scleral spur, whereas other portions may insert well anterior to it.

The surface of the trabecular meshwork may have a stippled, orange peel appearance. The peripheral anterior iris stroma may be thinned, but the central stroma and iris collarette appear normal.

In the second form of isolated trabeculodysgenesis, the iris insertion is concave. In this situation, the plane of the iris is well posterior to the normal position of the scleral spur. However, the anterior iris stroma continues upward and over the trabecular meshwork, obscuring the scleral spur and ending just short of Schwalbe's line. Thus, the iris sweeps around the angle, forming a concave or "wraparound" insertion (Fig. 41-2). This is most easily recognized in brown irides. In our experience, it is much less common than the flat iris insertion.

There is no evidence of other iris or corneal malformation in isolated trabeculodysgenesis. The elevated intraocular pressure, however, may cause stretching of these structures secondarily. The following discussion constitutes a differential diagnosis for primary congenital glaucoma.

Iridotrabeculodysgenesis

Iris anomalies may present as maldevelopment of the anterior stroma, the iris vessels, or the full iris thickness.

Hypoplasia of the iris stroma

Hypoplasia of the anterior iris stroma is the most common iris defect associated with developmental glaucoma. Because the normal infant eye has some peripheral thinning of the iris and because stretching of the iris from pressure can further thin the anterior stroma, we diagnose true hypoplasia of the anterior stroma only when there is clearly a malformation of the collarette with absence or marked reduction of the crypt layer.

This defect, when present, is easily recognized (Fig. 41-3). The sphincter muscle is quite obvious, whereas the collarette is either absent or is formed only in the far periphery. Twigs of iris stroma may be seen scattered over the surface of the iris. The iris may insert anteriorly at the level of the scleral spur, and the trabecular meshwork may appear to be thickened. Occasionally, anomalous vessels running in an irregular circumferential pattern are present in the angle. This defect, when occurring by itself, is typical of familial hypoplasia of the iris with glaucoma.[19,22,34] It should not be confused with primary congenital glaucoma since the hypoplastic iris syndrome is dominantly inherited.

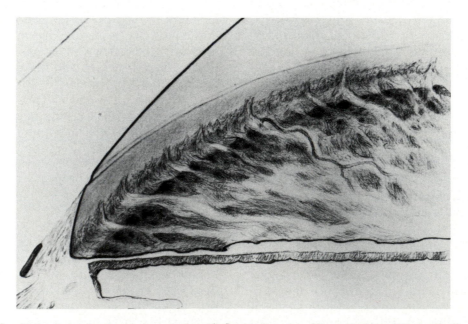

Fig. 41-1 Isolated trabeculodysgenesis with flat iris insertion. (From Hoskins, HD, Jr, Shaffer, RN, and Hetherington, J, Jr: Arch Ophthalmol 102:1333, 1984. Copyright 1984, American Medical Association)

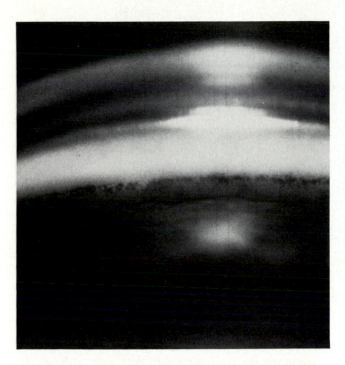

Fig. 41-2   Isolated trabeculodysgenesis with concave iris insertion. (From Hoskins, HD, Jr, Shaffer, RN, and Hetherington, J, Jr: Arch Ophthalmol 102:1334, 1984. Copyright 1984, American Medical Association)

Hyperplasia of the iris stroma

In hyperplasia of the iris stroma, the anterior stroma has a thickened, velvety, pebbled appearance. We have seen it in only two cases, both of which were associated with Sturge-Weber syndrome and developmental glaucoma.

Anomalous iris vessels

Vascular anomalies of the iris can be divided into those with some form of persistence of the tunica vasculosa lentis and those with irregularly wandering superficial anomalous iris vessels. The first condition is distinguished by the regular arrangement of the vessels looping into the pupillary axis either in front of or behind the lens. The normal radial vessels on the iris surface are also prominent because this condition is usually accompanied by hypoplasia of the anterior iris stroma. Anomalous superficial iris vessels (Fig. 41-4) wander irregularly over the iris surface, and the pupil is usually distorted. The iris surface has a whorled appearance because of the curving of the radial fibers of the iris. We have seen two patients in whom the vessels extended from the iris to attach to the peripheral cornea. The anterior iris stroma is often hypoplastic.

These vascular patterns are different from the exposure of the radial iris vessels that may be seen in normal blue-eyed infants and in patients with hypoplasia of the anterior iris stroma. In the latter

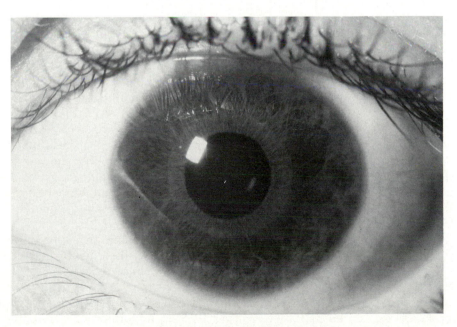

Fig. 41-3   Hypoplasia of anterior iris stroma.

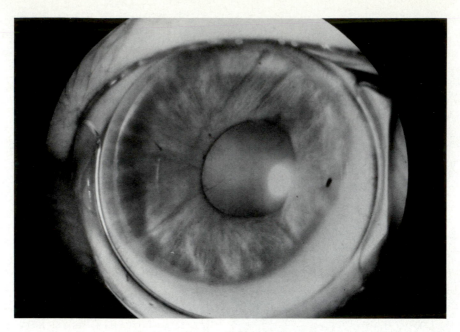

Fig. 41-4 Anomalous superficial iris vessels.

cases, although the vessels are easily seen, there is no vascular anomaly.

Anomalous vessels of the iris are seen most frequently in eyes presenting with glaucoma and cloudy corneas at birth and represent a more severe malformation of the anterior segment. Such vessels indicate a grave prognosis. These eyes behave quite differently from eyes whose only structural defect is trabeculodysgenesis. All cases we have seen have required multiple surgeries. Half of these required postoperative medical therapy to control intraocular pressure. These vessels are not associated with any particular syndrome. It is unclear whether this defect represents a more severe anomaly and, therefore, an earlier onset of primary congenital glaucoma or is an entirely different syndrome.

Structural iris defects

The last type of iridodysgenesis easily identified by clinical examination is the structural iris defect. This anatomic defect may present in the following forms: (1) a full-thickness iris hole without sphincter involvement, as seen in Rieger's anomaly; (2) a full-thickness sphincter defect or coloboma; and (3) aniridia, in which most of the iris and all of the sphincter is missing.

Corneotrabeculodysgenesis

Developmental corneal defects include peripheral, midperipheral and central defects, as well as microcornea and macrocornea. Corneal stretching

and clouding secondary to increased intraocular pressure are not considered developmental defects.

Peripheral corneal lesions occur adjacent to and concentric with the limbus and extend no more than 2 mm into clear cornea. These changes usually involve the entire corneal circumference and are most often seen as posterior embryotoxon with adherent iris tissue (Axenfeld's anomaly).

Midperipheral lesions are generally found in patients with Rieger's anomaly. These are usually sector defects, almost always opacities with iris adhesions.

Central defects are typically opacified. There may be central stromal thinning, and in two cases, we have seen a hole through the cornea, draining aqueous. Most central lesions are round, with a zone of clear cornea between the defect and the limbus. As in other corneal defects, there are frequently iris adhesions. Central defects are seen in patients with the conditions variously described as Peters' syndrome, anterior staphyloma, anterior chamber cleavage syndrome, or posterior corneal ulcer of von Hippel.

Patients with developmental glaucoma may also have microcornea or macrocornea. Microcornea is seen in patients with rubella syndrome, persistent hyperplastic primary vitreous, Rieger's anomaly, microphthalmia, and nanophthalmos.

It is important to distinguish megalocornea from the corneal stretching, which occurs as part of the glaucomatous process. It may occur primarily in patients with Axenfeld's syndrome or as X-linked recessive megalocornea in which glaucoma may occur later in life. In our experience, the prognosis for control of glaucoma in eyes with corneodysgenesis is not as good as in eyes with isolated trabeculodysgenesis.

EPIDEMIOLOGY

Incidence

Primary congenital glaucoma is not a common disease. A busy ophthalmologist may see a new case once every several years, possibly only one case every 10 years. It is estimated to affect less than 0.05% of ophthalmic patients, although patients with the disease account for a significantly higher incidence of patients in institutions for the blind (2% to 15%).[13] The disease is bilateral in approximately 75% of cases. Male patients are found to have a higher incidence of the disease, comprising approximately 65% of cases.

Heredity

The majority of cases of primary congenital glaucoma are sporadic in occurrence. In the approximately 10% of cases where a hereditary pattern is evident, it is generally believed to be autosomal recessive.[28] In this situation, both parents would usually not have the disease, but would be heterozygous carriers. Of four children, one child would be homozygous for primary congenital glaucoma and would manifest the disease. Two children would be heterozygous carriers of the disease and one child would be homozygous normal. However, investigators cite a variable penetrance between different families, with penetrance usually in the 40% to 80% range, although in certain families it has been found to be as high as 90% to 100%.* Thus in families with a low penetrance, the number of affected children would be less than 25%.

Arguments raised for autosomal recessive inheritance include a number of families in which the percentage of affected children is 25% or higher, and several cases of consanguinity of parents of affected children.[33] François states that when dealing with families whose precise background is known, the percentage of affected individuals closely approximates the theoretical figure for recessive heredity.[14]

This inheritance pattern of primary congenital glaucoma has been questioned.[25] In our experience, the percentage of affected siblings appears to be between 3% to 11%. Also, boys are affected more frequently than girls, which is more consistent with a polygenic inheritance pattern. For these reasons and others, many authors believe the inheritance pattern is polygenic.

The fact that primary congenital glaucoma occurs in families should alert the clinician to examine other children in the family for glaucoma. Parents of affected children will be most concerned about the possibility of other children being affected. Demenais et al.[9] imply a 4% to 5% likelihood of occurrence in siblings or offspring of a single affected child. Jay et al.[18] indicate a 3% risk of another sibling being affected if the affected child is male and close to 0% if the affected child is female.

HISTOPATHOLOGY

Normal Development of the Anterior Chamber Angle

Anderson[3] has described the normal development of the infant angle using the techniques of scanning electron microscopy, transmission electron microscopy, and phase contrast light microscopy. He states that the anterior surface of the iris meets the corneal endothelium at 5 months of gestation to form the peripheral aspect of the anterior chamber. Slightly posterior to this junction are cells forming the developing trabecular meshwork (Fig. 41-5). The ciliary muscle and ciliary processes overlap the trabecular meshwork, being separated by loose connective tissue.

The trabecular meshwork later becomes exposed to the anterior chamber as the angle recess deepens and moves posteriorly. Various mechanisms have been proposed to explain how this deepening process occurs, including theories proposing atrophy and absorption of tissue and another proposing that the angle is formed by a process of cleavage between two separate cell types, one of which forms the trabecular meshwork and the second of which forms the root of the iris and the ciliary body.[2,8]

Anderson[3] believes the trabecular meshwork becomes exposed to the anterior chamber by a posterior sliding of the iris, ciliary muscle, and ciliary processes (Fig. 41-6). In the normal newborn eye, the iris and ciliary body have usually recessed to at least the level of the scleral spur and usually posterior to it. Thus, on gonioscopy of a normal newborn eye, the insertion of the iris into the angle wall will be seen posterior to the scleral spur in most cases, with the anterior extension of the cil-

---

*References 12, 21, 26, 28, 35, 36.

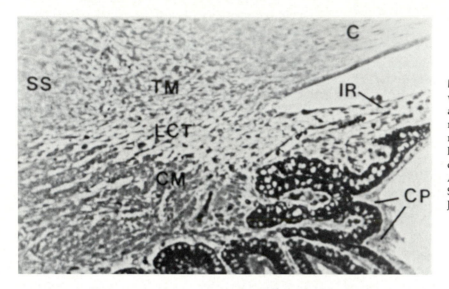

Fig. 41-5 Anterior chamber angle of 20-week-old human fetus. Ciliary muscle and ciliary processes overlap trabecular meshwork. Scleral spur *(SS)*, trabecular meshwork *(TM)*, cornea *(C)*, iris *(IR)*, loose connective tissue *(LCT)*, ciliary muscle *(CM)*, ciliary processes *(CP)*. (From Anderson, DR: Trans Am Ophthalmol Soc, 1981, vol. LXXIX, Rochester, 1982, Johnson Printing Co)

Fig. 41-6 Anterior chamber angle of 27-week-old human fetus. Uveal tract has receded to expose anterior portion of trabecular meshwork to anterior chamber. (From Anderson, DR: Trans Am Ophthalmol Soc, 1981, vol. LXXIX, Rochester, 1982, Johnson Printing Co.)

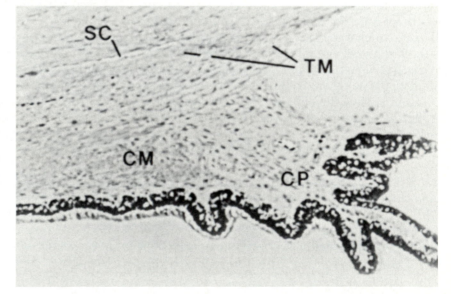

iary body seen as a band anterior to the iris insertion. The iris insertion into the angle wall is rather flat, as the angle recess has not yet formed. Continued posterior sliding of the uveal tissue occurs during the first 6 to 12 months of life, which is apparent gonioscopically as formation of the angle recess. Thus, the adult angle configuration in which the iris turns slightly posteriorly before inserting into the ciliary body is not normally present at birth but develops in the first 6 to 12 months of life.

The Anterior Chamber Angle in Primary Congenital Glaucoma

Anderson[3] states that in eyes with primary congenital glaucoma, the iris and ciliary body have the appearance of an eye in the seventh or eighth month of gestation rather than one which is at full-term development. The iris and ciliary body have failed to recede posteriorly, and thus the iris insertion and anterior ciliary body overlap the posterior portion of the trabecular meshwork (Fig. 41-7).[3]

Maumenee[24] also found an anteriorly placed insertion of the ciliary body muscle. He noted that the longitudinal and circular fibers of the ciliary muscle inserted into the trabecular meshwork rather than into the scleral spur, and that the root of the iris can insert directly into the trabecular meshwork.

Histologic abnormalities found on examination of the trabecular meshwork itself include a thickening of the trabecular beams, thickened cords of the uveal meshwork, and compression of the meshwork with a resultant decrease of trabecular spaces[3,6,16,23] (Fig. 41-8). As mentioned, the existence of Barkan's membrane has not been verified.[5,37] Anderson[3] suggested that this appearance of a membrane was due to observation of thickened, compact trabecular beams in the area of the meshwork adjacent to the anterior chamber.

Schlemm's canal is found to be open in early cases of primary congenital glaucoma.[3,23,24] It may be obliterated in advanced cases, but this is believed to be a secondary alteration from the effect of pressure elevation on the ocular tissues. A thickening of the juxtacanalicular connective tissue has been noted as has an amorphous material in the subendothelial area of the internal wall of Schlemm's canal.[3,23,32]

Causes of Elevated Intraocular Pressure

Clinical evidence supports the theory that the obstruction to aqueous flow with a resultant increase in intraocular pressure is located at the trabecular sheets. Incision into the trabecular sheets by goniotomy or trabeculotomy relieves the obstruction and normalizes the intraocular pressure in the majority of cases.

The surgical incision may relieve the compaction of the trabecular sheets and allow the trabecular spaces to open. Surgical success with goni-

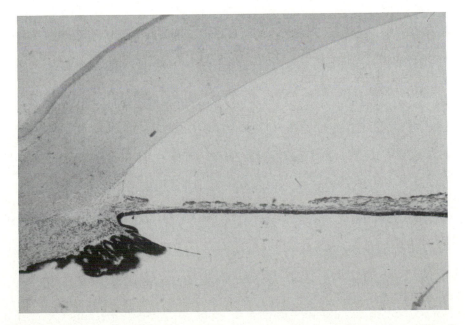

Fig. 41-7 Primary congenital glaucoma. Iris and ciliary body overlap trabecular meshwork.

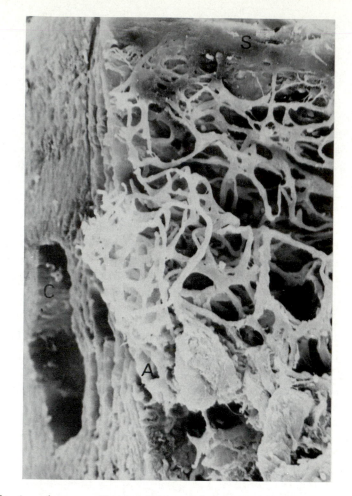

Fig. 41-8 Specimen from eye with primary congenital glaucoma and isolated trabeculodysgenesis. Onset of glaucoma at age 2 months. Note that insertion level of iris *(A)* is anterior to posterior limit of Schlemm's canal *(C)*. Thickened and abundant uveal cords appear to hold this iris forward, preventing normal separation of corneoscleral trabecular sheets. *(S)* Level of Schwalbe's line. No evidence of a membrane was found. (From Hoskins, HD, Jr, Hetherington, J, Jr, Shaffer, RN, and Welling, AM: Developmental glaucomas: diagnosis and classification. In Transactions of the New Orleans Academy of Ophthalmology: Symposium on glaucoma, St. Louis, 1981, The CV Mosby Co)

otomy is achieved by a very superficial incision into the trabecular meshwork.[29] The iris root drops backward as the blade incises the meshwork. It may be that the thickened cords of uveal meshwork hold the iris anteriorly, preventing the scleral spur from rotating posteriorly. Superficial incision of the thickened uveal meshwork will allow the iris root to drop posteriorly with accompanying posterior rotation of the scleral spur. This might allow opening of the corneoscleral trabecular sheets with improved outflow of aqueous.

Schlemm's canal has been found to be open both histologically and clinically, and does not appear to be the site of obstruction to aqueous flow.[3,24]

Tissue abnormalities adjacent to or involving the internal wall of Schlemm's canal are a less likely source for the resistance to aqueous flow as it is unlikely that goniotomy incisions consistently cut this tissue. Incisions at various heights along the meshwork have all been found to relieve the resistance to outflow.[20]

Elevated Intraocular Pressure in the Infant Eye

During the first 3 years of life, the collagen fibers of the eye are softer and more elastic than in older individuals. Thus, elevation of the intraocular pressure causes rapid enlargement of the globe, which is especially apparent as a progressive corneal and limbal enlargement. The normal neonatal horizontal corneal diameter of 10.0 to 10.5 mm may be enlarged to as much as 16.0 mm.

As the cornea and limbus enlarge, Descemet's membrane and the corneal endothelium are stretched. This can result in linear ruptures (Haab's striae), which in turn can lead to corneal stromal and epithelial edema, as well as to corneal scarring if the problem is chronic. The thinned endothelium may also decompensate in adult life, despite a normal intraocular pressure, when aging changes are superimposed upon the initial endothelial damage.[31]

As the eye enlarges, the iris is stretched and the overlying stroma may appear thinned. The scleral ring through which the optic nerve passes also enlarges with elevated intraocular pressure that could lead to an enlargement of the optic cup even in the absence of loss of optic nerve fibers.[27]

The disc is cupped far more quickly in the infant as compared to the adult eye, and reversal of the enlargement can also occur rapidly after normalization of the intraocular pressure. This is probably related to the increased elasticity of the connective tissues of the optic nerve head in the infant eye, which allows an elastic response to fluctuation in intraocular pressure.

Eyes with advanced disease are enlarged in all dimensions. The iris root and trabecular meshwork are degenerated and thinned, and Schlemm's canal may not be evident. The ciliary body is atrophic, as are the retina and choroid. The zonules may be degenerated and the lens displaced.[31] The optic nerve may show complete cupping.

SUMMARY

Goniotomy and trabeculotomy probably function by allowing separation of the trabecular sheets and flow of aqueous into Schlemm's canal. Early surgery is important in this disease to prevent prolonged apposition and scarring of these sheets. If this occurs, goniotomy or trabeculotomy cannot work, and filtering surgery has a poor prognosis because of the excellent healing capacity of the young.

Like many functions in the infant, the ciliary body probably does not reach full aqueous production until months after birth. This explains why most cases of primary congenital glaucoma have an onset 1 to 5 months after birth. Therefore, if a portion of the angle can be made to function, maturation of the rest of the angle may ultimately handle full aqueous production when it occurs.

There is still a relative scarcity of pathological specimens from patients with early trabeculodys-

genesis and further studies will be required before the exact nature of these developmental anomalies are determined. A potentially valuable aspect of this pertains to the fact that most patients who have undergone successful surgery are still in their 30s or younger. Careful clinical and pathological examination of these eyes as these individuals age will be of considerable value.

REFERENCES

1. Allen, L, and Burian, HM: Trabeculotomy ab externo, Am J Ophthalmol 53:19, 1962
2. Allen, L, Burian, HM, and Braley, AE: A new concept of the development of the anterior chamber angle, Arch Ophthalmol 53:783, 1955
3. Anderson, DR: The development of the trabecular meshwork and its abnormality in primary infantile glaucoma, Trans Am Ophthalmol Soc 79:458, 1981
4. Anderson, JR: Hydrophthalmia or congenital glaucoma, London, 1939, Cambridge University Press
5. Barkan, O: Pathogenesis of congenital glaucoma, Am J Ophthalmol 40:1, 1955
6. Broughton, WL, Fine, BS, and Zimmerman, LE: A histologic study of congenital glaucoma associated with a chromosomal defect, Ophthalmology 87:96, 1980
7. Burian, HM: A case of Marfan's syndrome with bilateral glaucoma, Am J Ophthalmol 50:1187, 1960
8. Burian, HM, Braley, AE, and Allen, L: Visability of the ring of Schwalbe and the trabecular zone, Arch Ophthalmol 53:767, 1955
9. Demenais, F, et al: Congenital glaucoma genetic models, Hum Genet 46:305, 1979
10. DeVincentiis, AU: Sulla incisione dell'angolo irideo (Taylor), Ann di Ottal, Pavia 20:92, 1891
11. DeVincentiis, AU: Incisione dell'angolo irideo nel glaucoma, Ann di ottal, Pavia 22:1893
12. Duke-Elder, S, editor: System of ophthalmology, vol 3, part 2, congenital deformities, London, 1964, Kimpton
13. Duke-Elder, S, editor: System of ophthalmology, vol 3, part 2, congenital deformities, St. Louis, 1969, The CV Mosby Co
14. François, J: Heredity in ophthalmology, St. Louis, 1961, The CV Mosby Co
15. Harms, H, and Dannheim, R: Trabeculotomy: results and problems, Advances in Ophthalmology 22:121, 1970
16. Hoskins, HD, Jr, et al: Developmental glaucoma: diagnosis and classification. In the New Orleans Academy of Ophthalmology: Symposium on glaucoma, St. Louis, 1981, The CV Mosby Co
17. Hoskins, HD, Jr, Shaffer, RN, and Hetherington, J, Jr: Anatomical classification of the developmental glaucomas, Arch Ophthalmol 102:1331, 1984
18. Jay, MR, Phil, M, and Rice, NSC: Genetic implications of congenital glaucoma, Metab Pediatr Syst Ophthalmol 2:257, 1978

19. Jerndal, T: Dominant goniodysgenesis with late congenital glaucoma, Am J Ophthalmol 74:28, 1972

20. Kolker, AE, and Hetherington, J, Jr: Becker-Shaffer's diagnosis and therapy of the glaucomas, ed 5, St. Louis, 1983, The CV Mosby Co

21. Leighton, DA, and Phillips, CI: Infantile glaucoma. Steroid testing in parents of affected children, Br J Ophthalmol 54:27, 1970

22. Martin, JP, and Zorab, EC: Familial glaucoma, Br J Ophthalmol 58:536, 1974

23. Maul, E, et al: The outflow pathway in congenital glaucoma, Am J Ophthalmol 89:667, 1980

24. Maumenee, AE: The pathogenesis of congenital glaucoma, Am J Ophthalmol 47:827, 1959

25. Merin, S, and Morin, D: Heredity of congenital glaucoma, Br J Ophthalmol 56:414, 1972

26. Phelps, CD, and Podos, SM: Glaucoma. In Goldberg, MF, editor: Genetic and metabolic eye disease, Boston, 1974, Little, Brown & Co

27. Quigley, H: Childhood glaucoma: results with trabeculotomy and study of reversible cupping, Ophthalmology 89:219, 1982

28. Shaffer, RN: Genetics in the congenital glaucomas, Trans Am Acad Ophthalmol Otolaryngol 253, 1965

29. Shaffer, RN, and Weiss, DI: Congenital and pediatric glaucomas, St. Louis, 1970, The CV Mosby Co

30. Smith, R: A new technique for opening the canal of Schlemm, Br J Ophthalmol 44:370, 1960

31. Spencer, WH: Ophthalmic pathology, an atlas and textbook, Philadelphia, 1985, WB Saunders Co

32. Tawara, A, and Inomata, H: Developmental immaturity of the trabecular meshwork in congenital glaucoma, Am J Ophthalmol 92:508, 1981

33. Waardenburg, PJ, Franceschetti, P, and Klein, D: Genetics and ophthalmology, vol. 1, Springfield, 1961, Charles C Thomas, Publisher

34. Weatherill, JR, and Hart, CT: Familial hypoplasia of the iris stroma associated with glaucoma, Br J Ophthalmol 53:433, 1969

35. Westerlund, E: On the heredity of congenital hydrophthalmus, Acta Ophthalmol (Copenh) 21:330, 1944

36. Westerlund, E: Clinical and genetic studies on the primary glaucoma disease, vol. XII, Opera ex domo biologias Heredit Hum Univ Hafniensis, Copenhagen, (Munksgaard), 1947

37. Worst, JGF: Congenital glaucoma, Invest Ophthalmol 7:127, 1968

Chapter 42

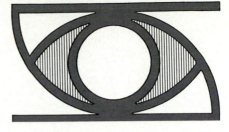

Diagnosis and Treatment of Congenital Glaucoma

Christoper J. Dickens
H. Dunbar Hoskins, Jr.

CLINICAL PRESENTATION

Epiphora, photophobia, and blepharospasm are often the first symptoms of primary congenital glaucoma. These symptoms are secondary to the corneal irritation that accompanies corneal epithelial edema caused by elevated intraocular pressure. Enlargement of the eye occurs under the influence of the elevated intraocular pressure, with the major enlargement occurring at the corneoscleral junction. A hazy appearance to the cornea can be intermittent in the early stages and precede breaks in Descemet's membrane.

As the cornea stretches, ruptures of Descemet's membrane allow influx of aqueous into the corneal stroma and epithelium, causing a sudden increase in edema and haze, and an increase of tearing and photophobia (Fig. 42-1). The child may become irritable to the point of burying his head in a pillow to avoid the pain of photophobia.

The breaks in Descemet's membrane (Haab's striae) are single or multiple and appear as elliptical, glassy, parallel ridges on the posterior cornea. They may be present in the peripheral cornea concentric with the limbus or in various orientations near or across the central visual axis (Fig. 42-2).

If the intraocular pressure is not controlled, tearing, photophobia, and blepharospasm may worsen. Continued enlargement of the cornea with more tears of Descemet's membrane may lead to corneal scarring, erosions, and ulcerations. Stretching and rupture of the zonules can cause lens subluxation. Blunt trauma in these enlarged eyes can result in hyphemas and rupture of the globe. Phthisis bulbi may be the final outcome (Fig. 42-3).

This presentation of primary congenital glaucoma is seen in children in whom the onset of pressure elevation occurs before the age of 3 years. The eye of the infant is more elastic than that of the older child; thus, signs and symptoms due to the stretching of the ocular tissues are apparent.

In children over the age of 3, the posterior sclera may still be elastic enough for elevated intraocular pressure to cause progressive myopia. Increasing myopia is commonly seen in children and is not a pathognomonic sign, but it should prompt consideration of glaucoma. Pain is unusual in the older child with glaucoma. Most commonly there are no symptoms until the patient becomes aware of visual field defects.

Routine examination of the optic nerve should be performed in all patients and tonometry performed in children who can cooperate. In children who can not cooperate for tonometry, examination of the optic nerve will reveal suspected or significant damage from intraocular pressure elevation. If such is the case, further evaluation with the aid of sedation or general anesthesia is indicated.

EXAMINATION

Depending on the age and cooperation of the patient, either an office examination or an examination under general anesthesia is required in evaluating the child with glaucoma.

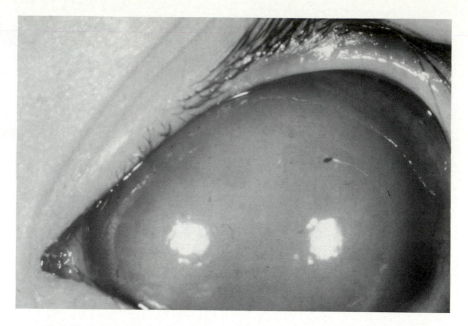

Fig. 42-1 Primary congenital glaucoma: corneal enlargement and clouding.

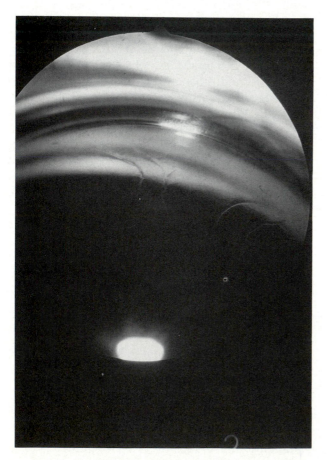

Fig. 42-2 Haab's striae.

Office Examination

Usually, a complete ocular examination, including slit-lamp examination, applanation tonometry, gonioscopy, and optic nerve evaluation, can be performed in the office in children over the age of 5 years and, with some training, in children as young as 3. If necessary, a mild sedative, such as chloral hydrate syrup (25 to 50 mg/kg body weight) can be given (chloral hydrate can mildly lower the intraocular pressure), but this is usually unnecessary if patience and gentleness are exercised.

Visual field examination can be performed at 5 to 6 years of age, but the patients' short attention span and poor fixation often prevent a detailed study. A gross confrontation examination can be performed in children by holding a toy in the peripheral fields and either moving the toy or shining a light within the toy. The older and more cooperative the child, the more detailed the examination. By the age of 8 to 10 years, most children can cooperate for a full quantitative visual field examination.

A reasonably good office examination can sometimes be performed in infants younger than 3 months using the infant diagnostic lens of Richardson and Shaffer. The lens assists in examination of the anterior segment, gonioscopy, and examination of the optic nerve. It is well tolerated when placed on the eye with topical anesthesia, and,

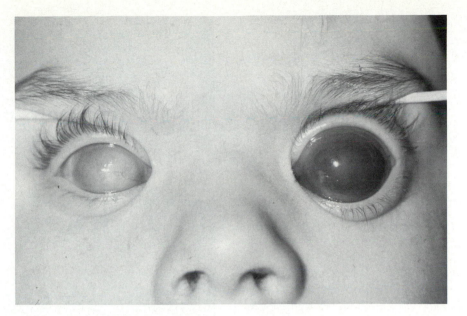

Fig. 42-3   Advanced primary congenital glaucoma.

with the use of a direct ophthalmoscope, a very good view of the posterior pole can be obtained even with small pupils and mild corneal haze.

Pacifying the child with a bottle can be helpful for obtaining pressure measurements with either a Schiøtz or hand-held electronic tonometer (TonoPen). The pneumatonometer and hand-held applanation instruments can also be useful.

General Anesthesia

General anesthesia is usually required for a thorough examination of children before 5 years of age. In a healthy child there is little risk involved when anesthesia is administered by an anesthesiologist experienced in dealing with infants. We have safely performed surgery on numerous children under 1 week of age. Usually delivery of the anesthetic by mask with an oral airway is adequate and safe for short examinations. Most general anesthetics lower the intraocular pressure variable amounts and at variable times after administration (ketamine may raise the intraocular pressure slightly). It is best to take intraocular pressure measurements as soon as the child is safely quiet. If prolonged examination or surgery is required, endotracheal intubation is performed.

Ketamine may be administered when the examination is for diagnosis only. It is not adequate for surgery, and the addition of general anesthesia to ketamine can prolong the postoperative recovery.

Special Diagnostic Techniques

Intraocular pressure measurement

Tonometry can be performed with a Schiøtz, hand-held applanation, or electronic (TonoPen) tonometer. One is usually sufficient, although in cases where uncertainty exists, checks can be performed with other instruments. In cases with microcornea, applanation pressure measurements should be used, since the smaller radius of curvature produces artifactually high intraocular pressure readings with Schiøtz tonometers.

The diagnosis of glaucoma depends on several factors, only one of which is the pressure level. Elevated intraocular pressure by itself, unless extreme, is not sufficient to confirm a diagnosis of glaucoma (Table 42-1). In our study, 9 of 74 eyes that were ultimately found to be normal had intraocular pressure levels greater than 21 mm Hg.

It is necessary to depend on signs such as increased corneal diameter, corneal haze, increased cup-to-disc ratio, or evidence of trabeculodysgenesis to confirm a diagnosis of glaucoma and justify surgery. Otherwise, it is better to reexamine the child in 4 to 6 weeks to confirm the diagnosis before performing surgery.

It is best to measure pressures early in anesthesia to reduce errors related to anesthesia. The normal intraocular pressure in an infant is slightly lower than in an adult, but 21 mm Hg remains a useful upper limit.

Table 42-1 *Intraocular pressure measurement in children*

IOP in glaucomatous eyes (N = 169)	No.	IOP in normal eyes (N = 74)	No.
Less than 21 mm Hg	14	Less than 15 mm Hg	26
21 to 24 mm Hg	0	15 to 21 mm Hg	39
Greater than 24 mm Hg	145	21 to 24 mm Hg	4
		Greater than 24 mm Hg	5

From the New Orleans Academy of Ophthalmology: Symposium on glaucoma, St. Louis, 1981, The CV Mosby Co

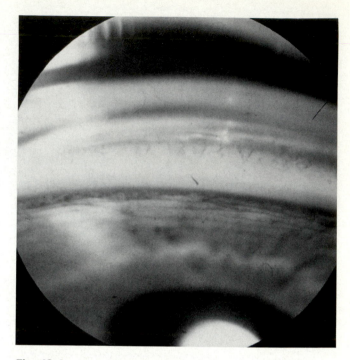

Fig. 42-4 Gonioscopy of normal infant anterior chamber angle.

Corneal diameter

The normal neonatal horizontal corneal diameter is 10.0 to 10.5 mm, increasing to 11.0 to 12.0 mm by the end of the first year of life. It is important to have a good baseline measurement for initial diagnosis and to detect subsequent change. A simple, effective method is to use calipers to measure the horizontal diameter from the first appearance of white scleral fibers on one side to the same point on the other side. This will allow a measurement accuracy of approximately 0.5 mm and, therefore, changes less than this should be considered cautiously.

Corneal clarity

An estimate of corneal clarity and corneal defects that may affect the pupillary axis should be noted. Although anisometropic amblyopia can be a cause of decreased vision because of monocular glaucoma, a tear in Descemet's can limit final acuity to the 20/40 to 20/50 range, which patching or orthoptic therapy cannot improve.

Iris and corneal anomalies

Developmental anomalies of the iris and cornea are not present in cases of primary congenital glaucoma. If they are found, a different diagnosis must be made. The anatomic classification has been discussed in Chapter 41.

Gonioscopy

The Koeppe 14 to 16 mm lens with a Barkan light and hand-held binocular microscope provides the surgeon with the view that he will have during goniotomy. The Goldmann lens can also be used for viewing the angle through the operating microscope. If corneal clouding is marked, the view may be improved by removing the epithelium with a surgical blade or applying a 70% alcohol solution with a cotton applicator.

In the normal newborn eye, the iris usually inserts posterior to the scleral spur. The anterior extension of the ciliary body is seen as a distinct band anterior to the iris insertion (Fig. 42-4). The iris insertion into the angle wall is flat, as the angle recess has not yet formed. The trabecular meshwork appears thicker and more translucent than that of the adult. The formation of the angle recess, characteristic of the adult in which the iris turns slightly posteriorly before inserting into the ciliary body, develops in the first 6 to 12 months of life. The normal infant eye may have some thinning of the peripheral iris.

Gonioscopy of the eye with primary congenital glaucoma reveals an anterior insertion of the iris directly into the trabecular meshwork (Fig. 42-5). This iris insertion is most commonly flat, although a concave insertion may also be seen. In a concave insertion, the plane of the iris is posterior to the level of the scleral spur, but the anterior stroma of the iris sweeps upward to insert into the trabecular meshwork. The level of the iris insertion may vary at different areas of the angle, with some portions of the iris inserting posterior to the scleral spur and other portions inserting anterior to it. The surface of the trabecular meshwork may have a stippled appearance and the meshwork may appear thicker than normal. There is no pigmented band present, but a thin section of ciliary body can be seen through the thickened trabeculum. The peripheral iris may show a thinning of the anterior stroma.

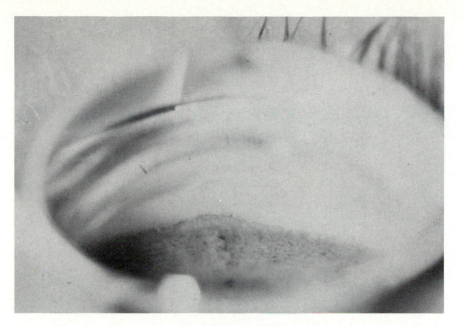

Fig. 42-5   Gonioscopy of an infant with primary congenital glaucoma.

Ophthalmoscopy

Evaluation of the optic disc is an essential part of the examination. A good view can be facilitated by the use of a Koeppe contact lens, which neutralizes irregular corneal reflexes and also improves the view through a small pupil by allowing one to see the entire nerve head in one field. Cupping of the optic nerve is an early sign of increased pressure and occurs much more quickly and at lower pressures than in adults.

In most eyes, the physiologic cupping is bilaterally symmetric, and asymmetry is suggestive evidence of glaucoma. Cup-to-disc ratios greater than 0.3 are rare in normal infants but common in infants with glaucoma and must also be considered suspicious (Table 42-2).

The infant glaucomatous cup usually has a configuration different from adult glaucoma. Although it can be oval, it is more commonly round, steep walled, and central, surrounded by a uniform pink rim (Fig. 42-6). The cup tends to enlarge circumferentially with glaucomatous progression.

A decrease in cupping can occur within hours or days after intraocular pressure control in the very young. This is especially marked in infants below 1 year of age (Table 42-3).

If therapy is successful, the cup will either remain stable or decrease in size. Evidence of increased cup size is indicative of uncontrolled glaucoma in an individual of any age. To provide records for future comparison, it is best to make a careful drawing or take photographs of the optic nerve head.

Axial length measurement

The measurement of axial length by A-scan ultrasonography has been recommended by some investigators for routine use in the diagnosis and follow-up of congenital glaucoma.[8,9] However, there is an overlap of values with normal eyes, which gives the examination a low sensitivity for diagnostic and follow-up purposes.[4] The corneal diameter is a simpler and more specific measurement and does not require special equipment.

Table 42-2   Cup-disc (C/D) ratios at birth to 3 years

Glaucomatous eyes (total 95)		Normal eyes (total 46)	
C/D	Eyes	C/D	Eyes
0.2	1	0-0.1	33
0.3	3	0.2	3
0.4	12	0.3	4
0.5	12	0.4	4
0.6	14	0.5	2
0.7	17	>0.5	0
0.8	18		
0.9	18		

From the New Orleans Academy of Ophthalmology: Symposium on glaucoma, St. Louis, 1981, The CV Mosby Co

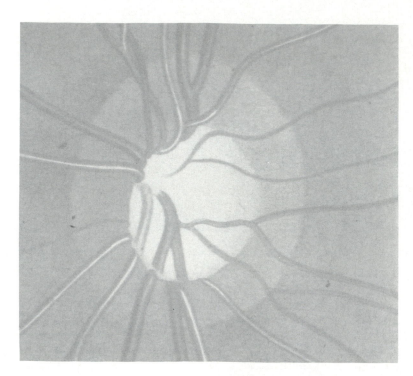

Fig. 42-6 Infant glaucomatous cup: steep walled and centrally located within optic disc. (From Kolker, AE, and Hetherington J, Jr.: Becker-Shaffer's diagnosis and therapy of the glaucomas, ed 5, St Louis, 1983, The CV Mosby Co)

Fig. 42-7 Sclerocornea. (From Grayson, M: Diseases of the cornea, ed 2, St. Louis, 1983, The CV Mosby Co)

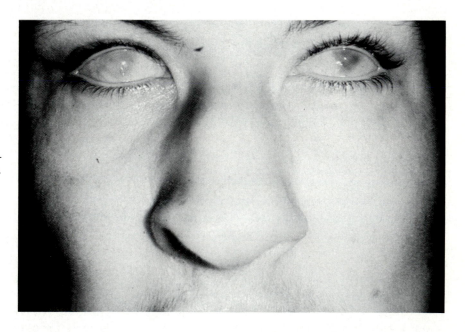

Table 42-3 Changes in the cup-disc ratio (C/D) after control of intraocular pressure

	Under 1 yr	Over 1 yr
No improvement in C/D	28	12
Reduction in C/D of 0.1	15	3
Reduction in C/D of 0.2	15	0
Reduction in C/D of >0.2	28	0
TOTAL EYES	86	15

From the New Orleans Academy of Ophthalmology: Symposium on glaucoma, St. Louis, 1981, The CV Mosby Co

DIFFERENTIAL DIAGNOSIS

Other Glaucomas

Primary congenital glaucoma is diagnosed by the finding of glaucoma in a child with isolated trabeculodysgenesis without other ocular or systemic developmental anomalies and no other ocular diseases that could result in an increased intraocular pressure. A complete general physical examination, as well as a complete ocular examination must be performed. Isolated trabeculodysgenesis can also be found in a variety of systemic syndromes such as Rubinstein-Taybi, Sturge-Weber, trisomy 13-15, Lowe's syndrome, and rubella. One must be able to distinguish the changes in the infant eye that occur as a result of elevated intraocular pressure from the various forms of dysgenesis and disease that cause elevation of the intraocular pressure.

Other Causes of Corneal Enlargement or Clouding

Megalocornea is a condition of marked corneal enlargement often to diameters of 14.0 to 16.0 mm. Other signs of congenital glaucoma, such as elevated intraocular pressure, and abnormal cupping of the optic nerve or tears in Descemet's membrane, are not present. These eyes have deep anterior chambers and may have iridodonesis secondary to stretched zonules and a loose lens. On gonioscopic examination, one may find a normal angle, prominent iris processes, or a broad, dense area of pigmentation. Ninety percent of cases occur in males with sex-linked inheritance evident. Families have been reported in which megalocornea occurs in some children and primary congenital glaucoma in others. Individuals with megalocornea must be followed for the development of glaucoma, as well as cataracts, which can also occur.

In sclerocornea, extensions of opaque scleral

tissue course into the cornea. Vessels usually accompany the tissue in this typically bilateral (90%), nonhereditary disease (Fig. 42-7).

High degrees of axial myopia can present with large eyes, including large corneas. The other symptoms and signs of glaucoma are not present.

Numerous metabolic diseases, such as the infantile form of cystinosis; the mucopolysaccharidoses, including Hurler's syndrome and Maroteaux-Lamy syndrome; and the mucolipidoses, can cause corneal haze.

Posterior polymorphous dystrophy can occasionally present in infancy with corneal edema and without corneal enlargement. It is a dominantly inherited, bilateral disease characterized by peripheral anterior synechiae and polymorphous opacities, typically vesicular, at the level of Descemet's membrane.

Congenital hereditary endothelial dystrophy can present at birth or in the first 1 to 2 years of life as a diffuse, bilaterally symmetric corneal edema with possible tearing and photophobia. Stromal thickness can be three times the normal, and the clouding can vary from a mild haze to a milky, ground glass opacification (Fig. 42-8).

Obstetrical trauma can cause rupture of Descemet's membrane with resultant corneal edema and clouding. These ruptures are usually vertical, but this is not necessarily true as they may run in various directions. There is no corneal enlargement and the optic nerve is normal. The intraocular pressure is typically normal, but in some cases, may be temporarily elevated. The condition is usually unilateral and more commonly affects the left eye caused by the higher incidence of left anterior occiput presentation at birth. The periorbital tissues frequently exhibit signs of trauma as well.

Inflammatory diseases, such as keratitis and iridocyclitis, can cause corneal edema and clouding. Rubella keratitis is particularly suspect in the newborn.

Other Causes of Epiphora or Photophobia

Diseases presented in the previous section on corneal clouding such as inflammation and congenital hereditary endothelial dystrophy, can cause symptoms of tearing and photophobia. Some of the disorders in this section can result in opacification of the cornea, particularly the corneal dystrophies.

The most common cause of epiphora is obstruction of the nasolacrimal duct. Photophobia is not associated with this problem. A chronic mucopurulent discharge may be evident.

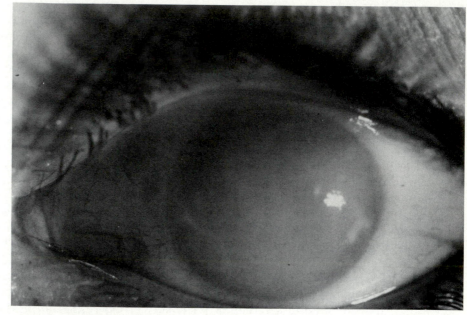

Fig. 42-8   Congenital hereditary endothelial dystrophy.

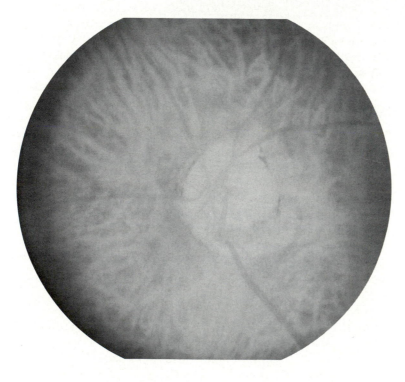

Fig. 42-9   Optic pit located inferiorly.

Any of the several causes of conjunctivitis in the infant can present with redness and tearing. Chemical conjunctivitis secondary to silver nitrate prophylaxis is the most common cause in the newborn. Bacterial, chlamydial, and viral infections are usually associated with a mucoid or mucopurulent discharge and must be ruled out.

Corneal abrasions are frequent causes of acute ocular irritation in children and are diagnosed by history and external examination.

Meesman's corneal dystrophy usually presents in the first several months of life with ocular irritation. Examination reveals multiple clear to gray-white, punctate opacities of the corneal epithelium, which are intraepithelial cysts. The condition is bilateral, dominantly inherited, and is the probable equivalent of Stocker-Holt dystrophy.

Reis-Bückler's dystrophy can present in the first few years of life with ocular pain secondary to recurrent epithelial erosions. Examination reveals irregular patches of opacity in the region of Bowman's layer, with progression to a diffuse reticular pattern associated with an anterior stromal haze.

Other Causes of Optic Nerve Abnormalities

Congenital malformations of the disc must be distinguished from disc changes caused by glaucoma. These would include congenital pits (Fig. 42-9), colobomas (Fig. 42-10), and hypoplasia.

Axial myopia can be associated with a tilted disc and accompanying scleral crescent, which is usually located inferiorly or temporally (Fig. 42-11). This can give the optic nerve a "chopped off" appearance.

Large physiologic cups must also be distinguished from pathological cupping caused by glaucoma (see Chapter 22). This is not a common problem in the infant where accompanying signs and symptoms are evident, but it can be a problem in the child over 3 years of age who is too young for precise visual field testing and in whom the changes secondary to globe elasticity are not as evident. Careful examination of all parameters is essential, and follow-up examinations may be required before a definitive diagnosis can be made. Examination of family members can be helpful as this may reveal similar optic cups in several members.

MANAGEMENT

Overview

Primary congenital glaucoma is essentially a surgical disease, with goniotomy or trabeculotomy recommended in children under 2 to 3 years of age. Trabeculotomy is recommended in children over 2 to 3 years of age and in those of all ages in whom corneal clouding prevents adequate visualization of the angle.

Surgery is preferred for several reasons, in-

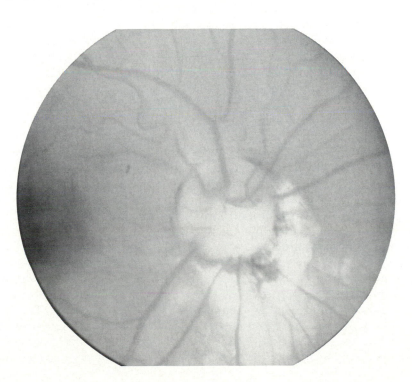

Fig. 42-10   Optic disc coloboma.

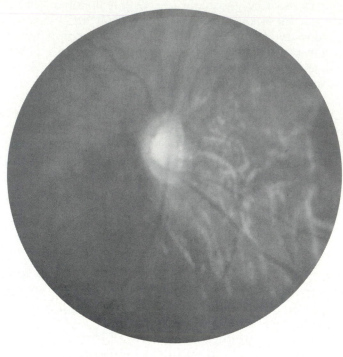

Fig. 42-11 Myopic tilted disc.

cluding problems with compliance with medications, a lack of knowledge concerning the systemic effects of medications in the infant, and a generally poor response of infants to medications. Most important, surgery has a high success rate and a low incidence of complications.

Early surgery is essential in these patients. Damage is increasingly likely the longer the elevated intraocular pressure is maintained. It also appears that prompt surgery may improve the chances for control of intraocular pressure. We will operate on day 2 or 3 of life if the diagnosis is made at birth.

In an infant in whom glaucoma is the presumptive diagnosis, it is best to have the initial examination under anesthesia performed by the ophthalmologist who will be performing the surgery. This minimizes the time to treatment and avoids unnecessary anesthesia.

Neither goniotomy nor trabeculotomy should be performed by surgeons inexperienced with the procedure. Both require exacting technique to achieve success and minimize complications. The first operation, whether goniotomy or trabeculotomy, has the greatest chance of success. If complications occur, such as hemorrhage or flat chamber, then an opportunity to cure this child may be lost forever.

Preoperative Management

Parental reassurance is important, as parents are frequently anxious and may have significant guilt feelings. The parents should be advised that the disease has occurred because of factors beyond their control.

Surgery should not be delayed. Medications are used primarily in the preoperative management of these patients. These can allow a clearing of the corneal edema and improved visualization at the time of diagnostic examination and surgery, as well as help to control any damage that might occur preoperatively.

Timolol 0.25% may be administered one drop every 12 hours. Although it has not yet been approved for use in children, studies have shown a minimum of side effects in short-term use. Parents should be cautioned to discontinue the medication if any side effects, such as asthmatic symptoms, develop. The selective beta$_1$-blockers, such as betaxolol, should have even less pulmonary side effects. Acetazolamide (5 to 10 mg/kg body weight every 6 to 8 hours) may also be administered orally as a suspension, as can pilocarpine 1% to 2% one drop every 6 hours.

A thorough systemic evaluation is indicated preoperatively in all patients, both to ensure the safety of general anesthesia and to search for signs of any syndromes that may have an association with glaucoma.

Initial Surgery

As Shaffer[10] recently reported in a series of 287 eyes, one or two goniotomies cured 94% of patients diagnosed between the ages of 1 month and 24 months. As this is the most common age of occurrence of primary congenital glaucoma, this is an encouraging statistic. Patients with the onset of glaucoma at birth to 1 month showed a less encouraging response, with a success rate of 26%. Some of these patients had significant hypoplasia and increased vascularity of the iris and would now be classified as iridotrabecular dysgenesis rather than isolated trabeculodysgenesis.

Patients with the onset of the disease after 2 years of age show poorer control with goniotomy. Shaffer reported a 38% control rate with one or two goniotomies.[10]

Goniotomy is a very safe procedure when performed skillfully. Analysis of 695 goniotomies revealed only one complication of severe visual loss, an eight ball hemorrhage with blood staining of the cornea. There were no infections and no lens injuries. There were a few small iridodialyses,[4] small cyclodialyses,[2] and shallow anterior chambers of 1 to 2 days' duration,[5] which had no sequelae. The most common complication was a cardiopulmonary event of concern to the anesthesiologist during anesthesia.[6] Although all patients recovered, we advise performing bilateral goniotomies when indicated to avoid the risk of an additional anesthesia. This approach also limits any delay in required surgery.

We prefer goniotomy as the initial surgery in all patients under 2 to 3 years of age in whom corneal clouding does not prevent adequate visualization of the angle. We have found that corneal clouding only rarely prevents performance of the goniotomy, particularly if the cloudy epithelium is removed. In patients under 2 years of age, our preference is to perform two goniotomies before proceeding to trabeculotomy or trabeculectomy.

Some investigators prefer trabeculotomy as the initial surgical procedure, but others indicate no preference between the two procedures.[1,3,6,7] Trabeculotomy also has a high success rate, with most studies citing an 80% to 90% success rate.[1] There

is a low incidence of complications. These include hyphemas, small and transient in most cases but occasionally large and persistent, tears in Descemet's membrane, cyclodialysis, iridodialysis, difficulty locating Schlemm's canal, synechiae, and staphyloma formation.

We prefer goniotomy because of its simplicity; the fact that it does not disturb the conjunctiva, which may be needed for later filtering surgery; and the fact that it is performed with direct visualization of trabecular meshwork and incises only those tissues necessary to cure the disease, the superficial trabecular tissues.

Follow-up Evaluations

If corneal clouding subsides, the patient is reexamined at 4 to 6 weeks postoperatively using the same procedure that was performed initially. Again, one must keep in mind the pressure-lowering effects of general anesthesia. If well controlled, the patient's symptoms of epiphora, photophobia, and blepharospasm will be reduced, but they may persist in some degree for many months. Examination will reveal no increase in the corneal diameters, and there will be no increase, and often a decrease, in disc cupping. The surgical area is inspected gonioscopically to ensure accuracy of placement of the initial procedure and to check for complications.

Reexaminations are then performed in 3 to 4 months, then every 6 months for 1 year, and then yearly. In most children, examinations can be performed in the office beginning at approximately 3 years of age.

Filtering Surgery

If goniotomy and/or trabeculotomy around 360 degrees of the angle fails to control the glaucoma, the prognosis for ultimate success falls dramatically.

Trabeculectomy would be our first choice as a filtering operation in these children. It has a lower incidence of complications, such as flat anterior chamber, cataract formation, bleb complications, and staphyloma formation, than full-thickness filtration. The most common complication of trabeculectomy is its failure to function secondary to scar formation. When trabeculectomy fails, full-thickness filtering surgery could be considered.

Healing inhibitors

Inhibitors of scar formation, such as the antimetabolite 5-fluorouracil, may be useful as a surgical adjunct to filtering surgery in patients in whom initial filtering surgery has failed. At the present time, this treatment requires the cooperation of the patient for subconjunctival injections and thus is applicable only to selected children. Long-acting forms of the drug are being developed that might allow injection only at the time of surgery or topical administration. The long-acting steroid, triamcinolone acetonide, injected subconjunctivally at the site of the filtering surgery, may also prove to be beneficial in the prevention of scar formation.

Synthetic drainage devices

Many synthetic drainage devices have been developed through the years with generally poor results. Recently, the Molteno implant has shown promising results, although the recommended postoperative medical regimen, which includes oral prednisone, indomethacin, and colchicine, has serious side effects. Presently, the insertion of the Molteno implant should be considered in patients in whom filtering surgery has failed. Continuing investigations into the synthetic drainage devices are ongoing and should lead to subsequent improvements.

Cyclodestructive Procedures

Cyclocryotherapy is used when repeated surgery to improve outflow has failed. It often causes severe pain in children and frequently must be repeated.

The therapeutic use of ultrasound is being investigated as a treatment for refractory glaucoma. The results in children, however, have been disappointing.[2]

Long-term Follow-up, Management, and Prognosis

An important feature in the management of these patients is the treatment of amblyopia, which can result from tears of Descemet's membrane involving the visual axis and from anisometropia. Although the amount of myopia, which is induced by the stretching of the infant globe, can be neutralized by the flattening of the cornea, it is often significant. A significant amount of irregular astigmatism is also evident in many cases. A cycloplegic refraction should be performed as soon as possible and should be followed with frequent adjustments in lens power as the anisometropia changes. Appropriate occlusion therapy must be started as soon as amblyopia is recognized. Even brief periods of corneal clouding can cause deprivation amblyopia.

Long-term medical therapy in children can be difficult because of side effects and compliance problems. Medical therapy is used primarily in difficult cases that have not responded well to surgical intervention. Timolol 0.25% has been well tolerated in most patients who do not have asthma or cardiac disease. The selective beta$_1$-blocking agents, such as betaxolol, should decrease the incidence of pulmonary side effects. Miotics can induce visually disabling myopia in the young patient. Either the pilocarpine membrane delivery system (Ocusert) or pilocarpine gel applied only at bedtime may be better tolerated by children. Dipivefrin is well tolerated in the young. Carbonic anhydrase inhibitors should be administered cautiously because of their many systemic effects, including rapid and severe acidosis in infants. Cooperation of a pediatrician is important if their use is to be prolonged.

Patients with primary congenital glaucoma require follow-up examinations for life. Corneal edema can develop in adulthood when aging changes are superimposed on the endothelial damage that occurred in infancy. Most important, increases in intraocular pressure can occur at any time in the life of the patient and must be detected and appropriate therapy instituted.

The long-term prognosis for intraocular pressure control in successfully treated cases of primary congenital glaucoma appears excellent. Although few patients with primary congenital glaucoma successfully treated in infancy have reached the fourth decade of life, the majority have maintained good pressure control with stable optic nerves and stable, usually full, visual fields.

SUMMARY

It appears that surgical prognosis for patients with primary congenital glaucoma is best when onset of the disease occurs between the first and 24th month of life. The reasons for this are uncertain. Earlier cases with onset at birth may represent a more severe developmental disorder. Later there may be changes in the trabecular tissues, such as decreased cellularity or reduced elasticity, that prevent retraction of the trabecular sheets after goniotomy. Possibly, apposition and compression of the trabecular sheets or the walls of Schlemm's canal or impermeability of its inner wall play a role. It is hoped that further study will help clarify these issues.

The most important aspect of this disease concerning the pediatrician and general ophthalmologist is recognition. If glaucoma is promptly recognized and appropriate treatment instituted, the chances for these patients having a lifetime of good vision is greatly increased. It is also very important not to be lulled into a false sense of security by surgical control of the intraocular pressure. The anisometropia and amblyopia must also be aggressively managed to give these children the best chance for good vision in both eyes.

REFERENCES

1. Anderson, DR: Trabeculotomy compared to goniotomy for glaucoma in children, Ophthalmology 90:805, 1983
2. Burgess, SEP, et al: Treatment of glaucoma with high intensity focused ultrasound, Ophthalmology 93:831, 1986
3. Kiffney, GT, Meyers, GW, and McPherson, SD, Jr: The surgical management of congenital glaucoma, South Med J 53:989, 1960
4. Kiskis, AA, Markowitz, SN, and Morin, JD: Corneal diameter and axial length in congenital glaucoma, Can J Ophthalmol 20:93, 1985
5. Litinsky, SM, Shaffer, RN, Hetherington, J, Jr, and Hoskins, HD, Jr: Operative complications of goniotomy, Trans Am Acad Ophthalmol Otolaryngol 83:78, 1977
6. Luntz, MH, and Livingston, DG: Trabeculotomy ab externo and trabeculectomy in congenital and adult onset glaucoma, Am J Ophthalmol 83:174, 1977
7. McPherson, SD, Jr, and Berry, DP: Goniotomy vs external trabeculotomy for developmental glaucoma, Am J Ophthalmol 95:427, 1983
8. Reibaldi, A: Biometric ultrasound in the diagnosis and follow-up of congenital glaucoma, Ann Ophthal 707, 1982
9. Sampaolesi, R, and Caruso, R: Ocular echometry in the diagnosis of congenital glaucoma, Arch Ophthalmol 100:574, 1982
10. Shaffer, RN: Prognosis of goniotomy in primary infantile glaucoma (trabeculodysgenesis), Trans Am Ophthalmol Soc 80:321, 1982

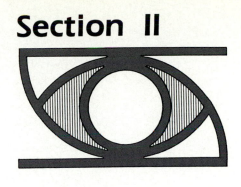

Open-angle Glaucoma

Chapter 43

The Epidemiology of Primary Open-angle Glaucoma and Ocular Hypertension

William M. Hart, Jr.

HISTORICAL BACKGROUND

Although the term glaucoma has its origins in the writings of Greek antiquity, the earliest recognition of an association between elevated intraocular pressure and loss of vision has been found in Arabic manuscripts dating from the tenth and fourteenth centuries.[28] It was first mentioned in the European literature in the seventeenth century, when Banister described a disease characterized by a tetrad of palpably increased hardness of the eye, chronic course, absence of light perception, and a fixed pupil. It was not until the early nineteenth century that Demours clearly associated intraocular pressure with the appearance of rainbow colors around lights and subsequent loss of vision. The concept that increased intraocular pressure produced visual loss became an accepted pathophysiologic sequence of events. Guthrie (1823) was perhaps the first to use the term "glaucoma" for diseases characterized by hardness of the eye.

These earliest clinical observations were evidently made in patients with angle-closure glaucoma with its attendant acute inflammatory syndromes. It was not until the second half of the nineteenth century that Donders recognized a chronic, noninflammatory form of the disease as a member of the same family of disorders. At about the same time, the earliest ophthalmoscopic observations of the optic disc by von Graefe produced the first descriptions of glaucomatous cupping. The phenomenon of cupping was confirmed pathologically by Müller (1856). The clear association of elevated intraocular pressure with cupping of the optic disc and subsequent loss of vision led to the pathogenic theory that elevated intraocular pressure causes damage to the optic nerve.

The most obvious acute congestive glaucomas of the angle-closure type were the first to be recognized, and only more careful observation allowed recognition of the chronic, noninflammatory types of the disease. Gradual refinements in clinical observations, including gonioscopy and improved accuracy of intraocular pressure and visual function measurements, have forced physicians to adopt more rigorous definitions for the clinical diagnosis of open-angle glaucoma. It was not recognized until the midtwentieth century that elevation of intraocular pressure is not always associated with damage to the optic disc and loss of vision. Conversely, some patients with glaucomatous optic nerve and visual field damage can never be shown to have an elevated intraocular pressure. The glaucomas are now best defined as a related group of clinical syndromes characterized by damage to the optic nerve and loss of visual function obeying a characteristic pattern usually associated with a statistically defined elevated intraocular pressure.

OCULAR HYPERTENSION AS A STATISTICALLY DEFINED ENTITY

The earliest attempts to estimate intraocular pressure were crude and were successful only at detecting gross elevations. With technologic advances, investigators improved their understanding of the statistical distribution of intraocular pressures in large populations. The earliest clinical observations of the association between elevated pressure and loss of vision led clinicians to accept tacitly the cause and effect sequence of elevated intraocular pressure leading to optic nerve damage. This reasoning led to the assumption that all people with elevated intraocular pressure by definition were subject to the disease. However, large population studies revealed that elevated intraocular pressure in the absence of visual damage was not uncommon and that patients with optic nerve damage and visual field loss in a pattern characteristic of glaucoma were frequently found to have apparently normal intraocular pressures.

In order to avoid selection bias, population studies of intraocular pressure require that large groups of subjects be recruited in a method that does not preferentially select for those with ocular disease. This has been more difficult than it would seem. Large, representative population samples have been reported in the United States[1,2] and the United Kingdom.[33] Great care had to be taken to avoid technical or procedural errors[57] or variations in findings due to diurnal[33] or seasonal[22,33] factors.

Although at first intraocular pressure was thought to be normally distributed, it became apparent that significant deviations from a gaussian distribution were characteristic of large populations.[2,33,37] This was seen as a skew toward higher pressures, a phenomenon that increases with age.[2,33,37] The skew can be modeled by assuming that the population consists of two mixed groups: one large group of normals and a second, smaller group with higher pressures.[2,37]

The results are markedly similar for different studies. For large, mixed populations there is a mean value of 15.9 mm Hg, with a standard deviation of about 2.89 mm Hg. Abnormally increased intraocular pressure has been arbitrarily defined as two standard deviations above the mean, so that pressures of 21.7 mm Hg or greater have been considered abnormal. However, the clinical relevance of this number to glaucomatous damage is not clear cut. Armaly[1] found glaucomatous visual loss distributed in the population without apparent respect to intraocular pressure. Many of the people with glaucomatous visual field loss had normal intraocular pressures by the statistical definition, whereas the vast majority of those with elevated pressures had normal visual fields. Other studies have focused on patients with glaucomatous damage who have been discovered primarily by visual field examination[17] and/or by ophthalmoscopy and who have "normal" or even "low" intraocular pressures.[27] As a result of these observations, it became apparent that only a minority of persons with elevated intraocular pressure went on to develop glaucomatous damage and that indiscriminate treatment of all patients with elevated pressures was both unnecessary and suboptimal medical care. Ocular hypertension defined those patients with "abnormally high" intraocular pressures but without clinically detectable visual field or optic nerve head damage.

THE PREVALENCE OF OCULAR HYPERTENSION AND GLAUCOMA

Another problem with the statistical definition of elevated intraocular pressure is the very large number of people that fall into this group. Using pressures of 23 mm Hg or greater as abnormal, Armaly[2] found that on an age-corrected basis, approximately 1.25% of those aged 30 to 39, increasing to 10.5% of those aged 70 to 79, would be screened as abnormal. These represent figures for the prevalence of statistically defined ocular hypertension. The total for the United States population in 1965 would have been 3.2 million people.

This should be compared with figures for the estimated prevalence of primary open-angle glaucoma. Estimates have been reported for the population at large of 0.28% to 0.43% in the United States[41] and 0.64% in the United Kingdom.[32] The prevalence of glaucoma increases dramatically with age from about 0.2% of those aged 50 to 54 to about 2.0% of those aged 70 to 74.[60] The prevalence of ocular hypertension also increases with age in a pattern that closely mimics the age-related rise of systemic blood pressure.[18] Thus, for those aged 70 to 75 years, ocular hypertension affects about 10%, whereas glaucoma can be found in at most 2%.

THE INCIDENCE OF NEW CASES OF GLAUCOMA

That the majority of people with ocular hypertension alone do not develop glaucomatous visual loss has been borne out by several studies. In a Swedish report, glaucomatous visual loss developed in only 3 of 192 eyes with ocular hypertension over a 5-year period, approximately a 1.5% incidence.[49] By comparison, of 3936 randomly selected normal individuals from Des Moines, Iowa, followed for 10 years, four developed glaucomatous visual loss (approximately a 0.1% incidence over the 10-year period), and only one had had ocular hypertension at the initial examination.[7] In a large survey of 5941 subjects in Bedford, England, of 124 ocular hypertensives followed for 5 to 7 years, four developed manifest glaucoma, an incidence of 3.23%.[55] In the same survey, an additional 770 subjects initially classified as normal were also followed for 5 to 7 years, and among these, four developed glaucoma, an incidence of 0.62%.[56] Somewhat higher percentages have been reported by the Swedish investigators.[50] Among subjects with ocular hypertension, there was an incidence of 10% after a 10-year follow-up and 34% after 20 years, with 5% after 20 years of follow-up in a normotensive group.

Another Scandinavian study estimated the incidence of glaucoma among normotensive subjects at between 0.25% and 1.0% over a 5-year period.[40] A long-term prospective study in Japan found a 10% incidence over a 9-year period of follow-up in patients with untreated ocular hypertension.[44] Representative epidemiologic estimates are summarized in the box at right.

CONSEQUENCES FOR THE SCREENING OF POPULATIONS

If we accept as approximations (1) that the prevalence of ocular hypertension in the general population over age 30 is 5% and that the prevalence of glaucoma is 1%, and (2) that the incidence of glaucoma among those with ocular hypertension will be 5% over a 5-year period whereas that among people with initially normal intraocular pressures will be 0.5% over the same 5-year period, then examining the entire population would yield the following result. For every 10,000 people examined, 500 would have ocular hypertension with normal visual function, and 100 would have manifest glaucoma. Over the ensuring 5 years, 25 of the ocular hypertensives and 47 of the 9400 people with initially normal pressures and visual fields would develop glaucomatous damage. Clearly, screening people for elevated intraocular pressure at a single point in time is not a very efficient way of identifying those at risk for glaucoma because during follow-up nearly twice as many cases are likely to occur among those classified as "normal" as among those identified as having ocular hypertension. Also, screening for ocular hypertension alone will miss at least half of the people with manifest disease.

REPRESENTATIVE EPIDEMIOLOGIC ESTIMATES

PREVALENCE OF OCULAR HYPERTENSION

Intraocular pressure $\geq$ 23 mm Hg

Population over age 30	1.6%
Age 30 to 39	1.25%
Age 70 to 79	10.5%

PREVALENCE OF OPEN-ANGLE GLAUCOMA

Elevated intraocular pressure with glaucomatous optic disc and visual field damage

Total population	0.5%
Age 50 to 55	0.2%
Age 70 to 75	2.0%

INCIDENCE OF DEVELOPING OPEN-ANGLE GLAUCOMA WITHIN A 5-YEAR INTERVAL

Normotensive population over age 30	0.5% to 1.25%
Ocular hypertensive population over age 30	3% to 5%

ALTERNATIVE SCREENING STRATEGIES FOR DISEASE DETECTION

Because our definition of primary open-angle glaucoma includes three essential components—elevated intraocular pressure, and optic disc and characteristic visual field changes—alternative strategies for disease detection could involve looking for the two components other than elevated intraocular pressure.

Pathologic changes in the optic disc in glaucoma have been well characterized and are usually expressed as the ratio of the diameter of the cup to that of the disc. Increased cupping occurs in a graded fashion, not only in eyes with manifest glaucoma, but even in eyes with ocular hypertension and apparently normal visual fields.[8,11] One clue to the presence of such change is asymmetry in the extent of cupping between the two eyes.[30] However, assessment of disc pathology is not so simple as intraocular pressure measurement, requiring greater skill on the part of the examiner and/or the use of stereophotography.[9,51]

In spite of the greater cost, examination of the optic disc does seem to have greater sensitivity and specificity for disease detection. Drance and Begg[25] reported a sensitivity of 85% for detection of glaucomatous visual field loss when reading a masked series of optic disc stereophotographs. Unfortunately, this degree of sensitivity cannot be attained when screening for glaucoma before the onset of manifest visual field defects. A somewhat greater specificity for ophthalmoscopic detection of glaucoma is possible in a subset of patients who show the presence of disc hemorrhages.[26] Splinter hemorrhages on the disc surface can antedate the onset of visual field defects in some patients.[20,46] Thus, frequent reexamination can reveal telltale hemorrhages that may indicate the presence of disease in evolution and may predict the onset of new areas of visual loss.

The alternative strategy of searching for glaucomatous visual field loss presents another set of problems. Early glaucomatous visual field defects are usually nonspecific and very subtle, and manual kinetic perimetry is often insensitive to such changes.[34,35] Automated static perimetry appears to have significantly greater sensitivity for detecting the subtle, early changes in the visual field that can develop in patients with ocular hypertension.[29]

Limiting the examination to those people with ocular hypertension may result in missing large numbers of people with the disease. This has been borne out by use of automatic perimetry on a population-wide basis in a Scandinavian community.[21] Perimetric screening in a majority (77%) of all people aged 55 to 70 years in the community detected a 1% prevalence of manifest glaucoma.[17] Of interest was that intraocular pressure among those with manifest disease was not markedly elevated, a pattern very similar to that previously reported in a large population study in North America.[1] Pressures were distributed narrowly around a mean value only 5 mm Hg higher than that for the population at large. Repetition of the screening 3 years later found four additional patients, suggesting an incidence of new cases of 0.26%.[19] These figures agree closely with the estimates for incidence and prevalence of glaucoma obtained by the more extensive population studies previously cited.

Although population-wide screening for existing cases of disease is technically possible, it is not a practical strategy. Screening of intraocular pressure does not detect more than about half of existing cases, and follow-up of cases with ocular hypertension has a very low yield. Screening by ophthalmoscopy and/or perimetry has greater sensitivity and specificity for case detection but is excessively time-consuming and expensive. Further, because the 5-year incidence of the disease is about one-tenth that of the prevalence of cases in the population, there is a turnover of about 10% of patients every 5 years, with deaths among those with glaucoma being balanced by the onset of new

cases. Strategies are needed for detection of existing cases, but just as important is the detection of new cases. Clearly, the entire population cannot be rescreened annually or even every 5 years.

THE HEREDITY OF GLAUCOMA AND ITS ASSOCIATED TRAITS

First-degree relatives (siblings and children) of patients with glaucoma have a prevalence of ocular hypertension more than twice that of the general population.[14] The prevalence of glaucoma in these relatives is 6%, about six times that of the general population,[24] and the incidence of new cases of glaucoma was reported as 2.7% over 10 years, a rate about 2.5 times that found in the general population.[54] Others have calculated the incidence of glaucoma among first-degree relatives over the age of 40 to be five times that of the general population.[52]

Virtually all of the ocular characteristics associated with glaucoma are found to occur in familial patterns. These include elevated intraocular pressure,[14,24,48,53] reduced outflow facility,[14,24,53,54] and increased cup-disc ratio.[5] Even ocular dimensions fall into familial patterns,[59] perhaps reflecting the associations of myopia with open-angle glaucoma and hyperopia with angle closure. Whether familial traits are genetically determined or simply artifacts introduced by common environmental factors shared by close relatives still remains open to some question. Bengtsson[16] reported evidence of concordance of tonometric findings among spouses, which would be consistent with the environmental hypothesis, but Armaly[4] did not find this association. In any event, a family history of glaucoma has been identified as a major risk factor for the future development of the disease, independent of any other factors, including elevated intraocular pressure or evidence of disc cupping.[36,38,42]

The familial pattern of glaucoma has led to a search for genetically linked traits in the hope that an easily identifiable trait would allow detection of those at risk, even in the absence of a known family history. Increased intraocular pressure in response to topical cortiocosteroids appears to be inherited as an autosomal dominant trait,[3,6,13,39,58] which is closely linked to the development of glaucoma (see Chapter 64). Other traits possibly linked to glaucoma include the inability to taste phenylthiourea[15] and the presence of diabetes mellitus.[12] However, monogenic inheritance of the topical corticosteroid response trait has not been demonstrable in studies of monozygotic twins,[58] and none of the associated traits show more than a loose linkage. Others have searched without success for genetic markers of glaucoma among histocompatibility antigens[43] and the polymorphic expressions of serologic antigens.[23] Thus, glaucoma and its related traits are not inherited according to simple mendelian predictions. The causes of glaucoma, whether genetic or environmental, seem rather to be multifactorial.

THE MULTIFACTORIAL NATURE OF GLAUCOMA

Recognition of the multifactorial nature of risk distribution and the use of modern biostatistical techniques for assessing the multivariate contributions to risk of multiple, independent factors has markedly improved our ability to identify individuals in need of careful diagnostic evaluation. Early studies of multifactorial risk[31,61] recognized the problem, but the proper statistical tools to approach the solution were not available. Later studies employed the same techniques of multivariate risk analysis that had been used so successfully in analyzing multiple contributions to the risk of ischemic myocardial disease in the Framingham study.[36,42]

The first study to employ this method was a retrospective analysis of 92 well-documented cases of ocular hypertension that showed an extraordinarily high incidence of disease: about 33% over 5 years of follow-up.[36] Four major, independent factors were found to contribute separately and synergistically to the level of risk for glaucoma: optic disc cupping, intraocular pressure, a positive family history of glaucoma, and age. A methodologically similar study was reported on a much larger population sample that had overall a lower level of risk (incidence of disease of 1.7% over 13 years).[10] The findings were largely similar but unfortunately failed to consider family history as a separate risk factor and did not reduce the number of factors to the minimum by collapsing closely correlated phenomena.[10]

EPIDEMIOLOGIC CONTRIBUTIONS TO OUR UNDERSTANDING OF GLAUCOMA

Through epidemiologic methods, such as large scale population surveys and biostatistical analyses of selected population samples, we have gained a great deal of insight into the nature of glaucoma. Before 1960, elevated intraocular pressure was considered to be a specific hallmark of the disease— both a necessary and sufficient condition for the diagnosis. We now understand that patients with primary open-angle glaucoma need not have consistently elevated intraocular pressure and that all patients with an elevated intraocular pressure will not necessarily develop the disease. Low-tension glaucoma presents another perplexing problem. In fact, this realization has led some authors to question the very hypothesis that elevated intraocular pressure is the primary cause of visual loss in the glaucoma syndrome.[45,47]

IMPLICATIONS FOR CLINICAL MANAGEMENT

Independent of the actual pathophysiologic mechanisms of visual loss in glaucoma, intraocular pressure remains one of the four most important risk factors for the onset of the disease in patients with ocular hypertension. The higher the pressure, the greater the risk of developing visual loss. In addition, optic disc cupping, age, and family history contribute a comparable significance. Consequently, a young patient under 30 years old with elevated intraocular pressure who has no family history of glaucoma, cup-disc ratios of 0.3 or less, and normal visual fields may have a very low risk of visual loss over the next 5 years. This person's risk of developing visual loss would be significantly increased if the intraocular pressure was consistently higher than 30 to 35 mm Hg. On the other hand, an ocular hypertensive patient over 65 years old with a positive family history (a first-degree relative, such as a parent, sibling, or child with glaucoma) and cup-disc ratios in excess of 0.4, appears to be at increased risk of developing visual loss over the next 5 years. The clinical management of individual patients should be directly affected by these realizations.

REFERENCES

1. Armaly, MF: The Des Moines population study of glaucoma, Invest Ophthalmol Vis Sci 1:618, 1962
2. Armaly, MF: On the distribution of applanation pressure. I. Statistical features and the effect of age, sex, and family history of glaucoma, Arch Ophthalmol 73:11, 1965
3. Armaly, MF: Statistical attributes of the steroid hypertensive response in the clinically normal eye. I. The demonstration of three levels of response, Invest Ophthalmol Vis Sci 4:187, 1965
4. Armaly, MF: Applanation pressure in husband-wife pairs, Am J Ophthalmol 62:635, 1966
5. Armaly, MF: Genetic determination of cup/disc ratio of the optic nerve, Arch Ophthalmol 78:35, 1967
6. Armaly, MF: Inheritance and dexamethasone hypertension and glaucoma, Arch Ophthalmol 77:747, 1967
7. Armaly, MF: Ocular pressure and visual fields. A ten-year follow-up study, Arch Ophthalmol 81:25, 1969

8. Armaly, MF: Optic cup in normal and glaucomatous eyes, Invest Ophthalmol Vis Sci 9:425, 1970

9. Armaly, MF: Glaucoma, Arch Ophthalmol 90:485, 1973

10. Armaly, MF, et al: Biostatistical analysis of the collaborative glaucoma study. I. Summary report of the risk factors for glaucomatous visual field defects, Arch Ophthalmol 98:2163, 1980

11. Armaly, MF, and Sayegh, RE: The cup/disc ratio, Arch Ophthalmol 82:191, 1969

12. Becker, B: Diabetes mellitus and primary open-angle glaucoma. The XXVII Edward Jackson Memorial Lecture, Am J Ophthalmol 71:1, 1971

13. Becker, B, and Hahn, KA: Topical corticosteroids and heredity in primary open-angle glaucoma, Am J Ophthalmol 57:543, 1964

14. Becker, B, Kolker, AE, and Roth, FD: Glaucoma family study, Am J Ophthalmol 50:557, 1960

15. Becker, B, and Morton, WR: Phenylthiourea taste testing and glaucoma, Arch Ophthalmol 72:323, 1964

16. Bengtsson, B: Resemblance between tonometer readings on relatives and spouses, Acta Ophthalmol [Suppl] 54:27, 1978

17. Bengtsson, B: Findings associated with glaucomatous visual field defects, Acta Ophthalmol 58:20, 1980

18. Bengtsson, B: Aspects of the epidemiology of chronic glaucoma, Acta Ophthalmol [Suppl] 2, 1981

19. Bengtsson, B: Repeated automatic visual field screening in a cohort study, Acta Ophthalmol 63:242, 1985

20. Bengtsson, B, Holmin, C, and Krakau, CET: Disc hemorrhage and glaucoma, Acta Ophthalmol 59:1, 1981

21. Bengtsson, B, and Krakau, CET: Automatic perimetry in a population survey, Acta Ophthalmol 57:929, 1979

22. Blumenthal, M, et al: Seasonal variation in intraocular pressure, Am J Ophthalmol 69:608, 1970

23. David, R, and Jenkins, T: Genetic markers in glaucoma, Br J Ophthalmol 64:227, 1980

24. Davies, TG: Tonographic survey of the close relatives of patients with chronic simple glaucoma, Br J Ophthalmol 52:32, 1968

25. Drance, SM: Doyne Memorial Lecture, 1975. Correlation of optic nerve and visual field defects in simple glaucoma, Trans Ophthalmol Soc UK 95:288, 1975

26. Drance, SM, and Begg, IS: Sector haemorrhage—a probably acute ischaemic disc change in chronic simple glaucoma, Can J Ophthalmol 5:137, 1970

27. Drance, SM, et al: Studies of factors involved in the production of low tension glaucoma, Arch Ophthalmol 89:457, 1973

28. Duke-Elder, S: Section III: Glaucoma and hypotony Chapter VI: Introduction. In System of ophthalmology, vol 11: Diseases of the lens and vitreous; glaucoma and hypotony, St Louis, 1969, The CV Mosby Co

29. Dyster-Aas, K, Heijl, A, and Lundqvist, L: Computerized visual field screening in the management of patients with ocular hypertension, Acta Ophthalmol (Copenh) 58:918, 1980

30. Fishman, RS: Optic disc asymmetry. A sign of ocular hypertension, Arch Ophthalmol 84:590, 1970

31. Graham, PA: The definition of pre-glaucoma. A prospective study, Trans Ophthalmol Soc UK 88:153, 1969

32. Graham, PA: Prevalence of glaucoma. Population surveys, Trans Ophthalmol Soc UK 98:288, 1978

33. Graham, P, and Hollows, FC: Sources of variation in tonometry, Trans Ophthalmol Soc UK 84:597, 1965

34. Hart, WM, Jr, and Becker, B: Visual field changes in ocular hypertension. A computer-based analysis, Arch Ophthalmol 95:1176, 1977

35. Hart, WM, Jr, and Becker, B: The onset and evolution of glaucomatous visual field defects, Ophthalmology 89:268, 1982

36. Hart, WM, et al: Multivariate analysis of the risk of glaucomatous visual field loss, Arch Ophthalmol 97:1455, 1979

37. Hollows, FC, and Graham, PA: Intra-ocular pressure, glaucoma, and glaucoma suspects in a defined population, Br J Ophthalmol 50:570, 1966

38. Hovding, G, and Aasved, H: Prognostic factors in the development of manifest open-angle glaucoma. A long-term follow-up study of hypertensive and normotensive eyes, Acta Ophthalmol (Copenh) 64:601, 1986

39. Jay, B, and Paterson, G: The genetics of simple glaucoma, Trans Ophthalmol Soc UK 90:161, 1971

40. Jensen, JE: Glaucoma screening. A 16-year follow-up of ocular normotensives, Acta Ophthalmol (Copenh) 62:203, 1984

41. Kahn, HA: The prevalence of chronic simple glaucoma in the United States, Am J Ophthalmol 74:355, 1972

42. Kass, MA, et al: Risk factors favoring the development of glaucomatous visual field loss in ocular hypertension, Surv Ophthalmol 25:155, 1980

43. Kass, MA, et al: Histocompatibility antigens and primary open-angle glaucoma. A reassessment, Arch Ophthalmol 96:2207, 1978

44. Kitazawa, Y, et al: Untreated ocular hypertension. A long-term prospective study, Arch Ophthalmol 95:1180, 1977

45. Krakau, CET: Intraocular pressure elevation—cause of effect in chronic glaucoma? Ophthalmologica 182:141, 1981

46. Krakau, CET: Disc haemorrhages—forerunners of chronic glaucoma. In Krieglstein, GK, and Leydhecker, W, editors: Glaucoma update II. Munchen, Bergmann-Verlag

47. Krakau, CET, Bengtsson, B, and Holmin, C: The glaucoma theory updated, Acta Ophthalmol [Suppl] (Copenh) 61:737, 1983

48. Levene, RZ, et al: Heritability of ocular pressure, Arch Ophthalmol 84:730, 1970

49. Linnér, E, and Stromberg, U: Ocular hypertension. A five year study of the total population in a Swedish town, Skovde. In Leydhecker, W, editor: Glaucoma symposium, Tützing Castle, 1966. Basel, Karger

50. Lundberg, L, Wettrell, K, and Linnér, E: Ocular hypertension. A twenty-year follow-up at Skovde, Acta Ophthalmol [Suppl] (Copenh) 63:473, 1985

51. Miller, S: The enigma of glaucoma simplex. Doyne Memorial Lecture, Trans Ophthalmol Soc UK 92:561, 1972

52. Miller, SJH: Genetics of glaucoma and family studies, Trans Ophthalmol Soc UK 98:290, 1978

53. Miller, SJH, and Paterson, GD: Studies on glaucoma relatives, Br J Ophthalmol 46:513, 1962

54. Paterson, G: A nine-year follow-up of studies on first-degree relatives of patients with glaucoma simplex, Trans Ophthalmol Soc UK 90:515, 1971

55. Perkins, ES: The Bedford glaucoma Survey. I. Long-term follow-up of borderline cases, Br J Ophthalmol 57:179, 1973

56. Perkins, ES: The Bedford glaucoma survey. II. Re-screening of normal population, Br J Ophthalmol 57:186, 1973

57. Schwartz, JT: Influence of small systematic errors on the results of tonometric screening, Am J Ophthalmol 60:409, 1965

58. Schwartz, JT, et al: Twin heritability study of the corticosteroid response, Trans Am Acad Ophthalmol Otolaryngol 77:126, 1973

59. Tomlinson, A, and Leighton, DA: Ocular dimensions and the heredity of open-angle glaucoma, Br J Ophthalmol 58:68, 1974

60. Viggosson, G, Bjornsson, G, and Ingvasson, JG: The prevalence of open-angle glaucoma in Iceland, Acta Ophthalmol (Copenh) 64:138, 1986

61. Wilensky, JT, Podos, SM, and Becker, B: Prognostic indicators in ocular hypertension, Arch Ophthalmol 91:200, 1974

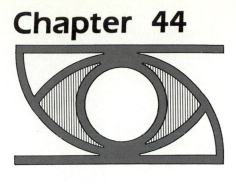

Chapter 44

Low-tension Glaucoma

Elliot B. Werner

HISTORY

When low-tension glaucoma was first described by von Graefe[116,117] in 1857, the concept of glaucoma as a distinct disease characterized by elevated eye pressure had been accepted for about 150 years. There was such vigorous opposition to the concept of glaucoma without pressure, however, that von Graefe[118] renounced his own belief in the existence of the condition.

The introduction of the Schiøtz tonometer in 1905 and its rapid adoption by clinicians were followed by additional reports of low-tension glaucoma.[105] By the middle of the twentieth century, the existence of low-tension glaucoma was firmly established, although it was thought to be uncommon. Many cases were felt to represent ischemic optic neuropathy that had been incorrectly diagnosed.[41]

Since the 1960s a number of population studies on glaucoma and intraocular pressure have shown low-tension glaucoma to be more prevalent than was generally recognized.*

DEFINITION

A number of different definitions of low-tension glaucoma have been proposed. These generally fall into the following two categories: those that are purely descriptive and those that include a statement as to the cause or course of the disease.[75] Von Graefe's original definition[116] was purely descriptive, calling only for the presence of

cupping of the optic nerve in the absence of palpably elevated intraocular pressure. Duke-Elder and Jay[41] included in the definition of low-tension glaucoma some detectable abnormality of aqueous humor dynamics in addition to cupping and visual field loss. They felt that it was a contradiction in terms to call something glaucoma in the presence of normal intraocular pressure and normal aqueous humor outflow facility.

Chandler and Grant[24] and Hoskins[56] included progressive visual field loss or progressive optic nerve cupping in the definition of low-tension glaucoma. As Drance[35] has pointed out, however, this definition requires that the disease cannot be diagnosed until an indefinite period of time has passed. The amount of time one must wait for progression before the diagnosis of low-tension glaucoma may be excluded or confirmed is not specified by those who include progression in their definition. Progression is not required by definition for the diagnosis of chronic primary open-angle glaucoma or for any other of the primary or secondary glaucomas. It seems unreasonable to make low-tension glaucoma the only exception in this regard. Some cases of low-tension glaucoma progress, and some do not.

Spaeth[107] and Kolker and Hetherington[67] imply that the definition of low-tension glaucoma should include optic nerve damage induced by intraocular pressure even though the pressure is always found to be within the range regarded as normal for the population. The role of intraocular pressure is the

---

*References 9, 12, 17, 19, 55, 71, 75, 85, 86, 103, 119.

production of the optic nerve damage in low-tension glaucoma is still controversial, nor is it universally accepted that intraocular pressure is causally related to cupping in all cases. Thus, in light of current knowledge, it seems premature to include a statement about intraocular pressure as the cause of optic nerve damage in the definition of low-tension glaucoma.

Shields[102] defines primary open-angle glaucoma in a strictly descriptive way. Elevated intraocular pressure is noted to be present in the disease, but the definition makes no statement about the cause of the optic nerve damage. Unless the cause of a disease is well established, it seems logical not to include statements about causality in the definition. Levene and others[32,51,75] give a strictly descriptive definition of low-tension glaucoma. This seems the most reasonable approach at the present time.

In view of the above, low-tension glaucoma may be defined as a condition in which there is cupping of the optic nerve head and visual field loss resembling that seen in other forms of chronic glaucoma, in which an intraocular pressure greater than 21 mm Hg without treatment cannot be documented, and in which there is no other obvious or apparent cause for these changes.

Drance[35] has noted that the term low-tension glaucoma is a misnomer in that the intraocular pressure is rarely low in this disease, but rather in the normal range and proposes that the condition be called "glaucoma with normal pressure." Low-tension glaucoma, however, is widely used, and we retain the term in this chapter.

CLINICAL PICTURE

Patients with low-tension glaucoma present in one of two ways. They either complain of loss of vision or other visual difficulties resulting from extensive visual field loss, or the abnormal optic nerve head appearance is noted during an eye examination (Figs. 44-1 and 44-2). Since by definition these patients do not have elevated intraocular pressure, and since they often have good central

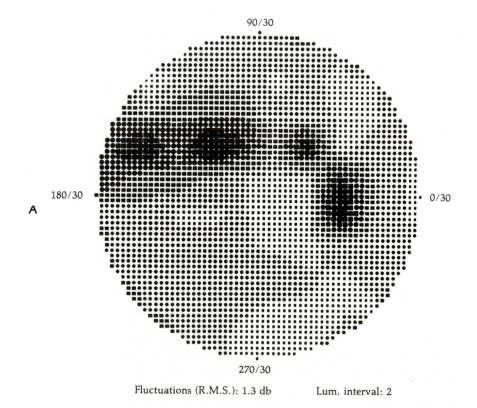

90/30

180/30

A

0/30

270/30

Fluctuations (R.M.S.): 1.3 db   Lum. interval: 2

Fig. 44-1 Low-tension glaucoma. **A** and **B,** Visual field and **C,** right optic disc of 73-year-old woman with acute conjunctivitis. Cupping was noted coincidentally on fundus examination. Disc shows fairly extensive loss of neuroretinal rim and peripapillary atrophy. Visual field shows typical superior nerve fiber bundle defect of arcuate variety. Despite two diurnal tension curves and tonometry on repeated occasions, this patient has never had intraocular pressure greater than 18 mm Hg recorded in either eye.

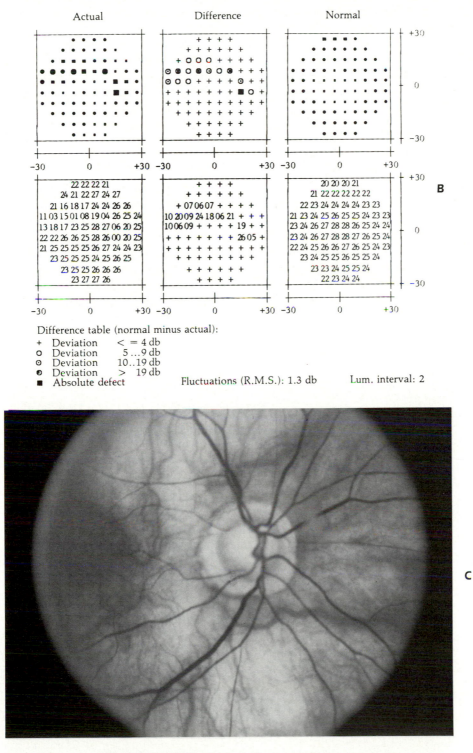

Actual   Difference   Normal

Difference table (normal minus actual):
+ Deviation   < = 4 db
o Deviation   5 ...9 db
⊙ Deviation   10..19 db
◓ Deviation   > 19 db
■ Absolute defect   Fluctuations (R.M.S.): 1.3 db   Lum. interval: 2

B

C

Fig. 44-1, cont'd   For legend see opposite page.

visual acuity, the disease is frequently missed unless a careful optic nerve head evaluation is performed. Routine use of the slit-lamp with the Hruby or hand-held 90 diopter lens to examine the optic nerve head with stereopsis under high magnification will increase the likelihood of detecting cupping, even when glaucoma is not suspected. The features that characterize glaucomatous optic nerve damage are described in detail in Chapter 22.

Optic Disc

Optic disc cupping in low-tension glaucoma (Figs. 44-1, A, and 44-2, A)

There has been some controversy over the appearance of the optic nerve head in low-tension glaucoma and whether or not it differs from that seen in other forms of glaucoma. Older texts such as Duke-Elder and Jay[41] do not generally recognize any difference in the appearance of the optic nerve head in chronic open-angle glaucoma and low-tension glaucoma. Epstein states that the cupping seen in progressive low-tension glaucoma is "just like that induced by elevated intraocular pressure."[44] There have, however, been few studies designed specifically to detect differences in the appearance of the optic nerve head in patients with low-tension glaucoma when compared with patients with chronic open-angle glaucoma.

Levene[75] did not describe any difference in appearance of the optic nerve head between low-tension glaucoma and chronic open-angle glaucoma. He did, however, feel that certain features, such as a disproportion between the amount of cupping and the amount of visual field loss, and the occurrence of a splinter hemorrhage on the optic disc, were more frequent in low-tension glaucoma.

Anderson[5] suggested that peripapillary halos might be more common in patients with low-tension glaucoma, but that they were also seen in patients with chronic open-angle glaucoma and could not be used to differentiate the two conditions.

Greve and Geijssen[49] felt that patients with high intraocular pressures tended to have larger and steeper excavations of the optic nerve head,

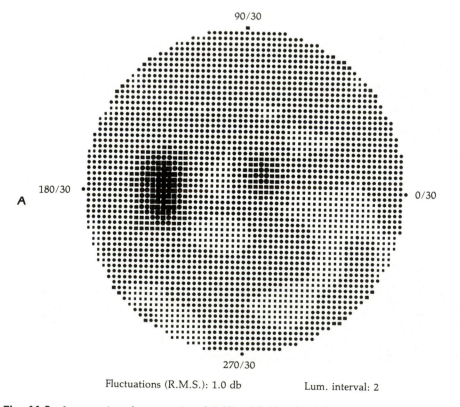

90/30

180/30 •

A

0/30

270/30

Fluctuations (R.M.S.): 1.0 db   Lum. interval: 2

Fig. 44-2 Low-tension glaucoma. **A** and **B,** Visual field and **C,** left optic disc of patient in Fig. 44-1. In addition to cupping and peripapillary atrophy, there is a small hemorrhage just off disc margin at one o'clock position. Visual field shows superior paracentral scotoma.

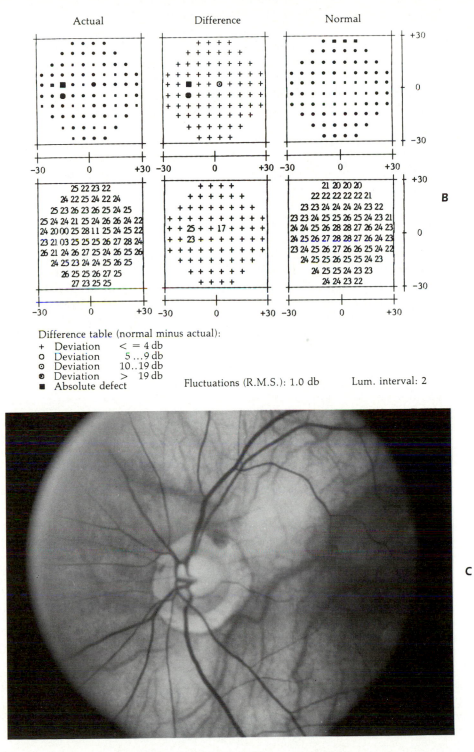

Actual	Difference	Normal

```
                25 22 23 22
               24 22 25 24 22 24
             25 23 26 23 26 25 24 25
           25 24 24 21 25 24 26 26 24 22
           24 20 00 25 28 11 25 24 25 22
           23 21 03 25 25 25 26 27 28 24
           26 21 24 26 27 25 24 26 25 26
             24 25 23 24 24 25 26 25
               26 25 25 26 27 25
                27 23 25 25
```

```
                + + + +
               + + + + + +
             + + + + + + + +
           + + + + + + + + + +
           + + 25 + + 17 + + + +
           + + 23 + + + + + + +
           + + + + + + + + + +
             + + + + + + + +
               + + + + + +
                + + + +
```

```
                21 20 20 20
               22 22 22 22 22 21
             23 23 24 24 24 24 23 22
           23 23 24 25 25 26 25 24 23 21
           24 24 25 26 28 28 27 26 24 23
           24 25 26 27 28 28 27 26 24 23
           23 24 25 26 27 26 26 25 24 22
             24 25 25 26 25 25 24 23
               24 25 25 24 23 23
                24 24 23 22
```

B

Difference table (normal minus actual):

+	Deviation	< = 4 db
o	Deviation	5 ...9 db
⊙	Deviation	10..19 db
⊗	Deviation	> 19 db
■	Absolute defect	

Fluctuations (R.M.S.): 1.0 db   Lum. interval: 2

C

Fig. 44-2, cont'd   For legend see opposite page.

whereas patients with low-tension glaucoma had more pale, sloping, and "moth-eaten" optic nerve heads. There was, however, a marked difference in the ages of the two patient samples in their study. The high intraocular pressure group had a mean age of 52 years, whereas the low-tension glaucoma group had a mean age of 76 years. It is, therefore, possible that the differences in optic nerve head appearance that the authors detected were caused in part by the effects of age as well as intraocular pressure.

Caprioli and Spaeth[23] found that patients with low-tension glaucoma tended to have neural rims that statistically were significantly thinner in the temporal and inferotemporal portions of the disc when compared with patients with glaucomas associated with high intraocular pressure. They also found that the cups of patients with low-tension glaucoma had more sloping margins, whereas the cups of patients with chronic open-angle glaucoma tended to be steeper. These authors also support Levene's impression of disproportionate cupping.

Lewis et al.[77] found that the relationship between the amount of cupping and field loss correlated equally well in low-tension and chronic open-angle glaucoma.

King et al.[62] recently reported no detectable difference in the appearance of the optic nerve head of low-tension glaucoma patients compared to those of patients with chronic open-angle glaucoma when studied with computerized optic disc topography. Although there may be differences in the appearance of the optic nerve head in populations of low-tension glaucoma patients compared with populations of chronic open-angle glaucoma patients, the appearance of the optic nerve head probably cannot be used to distinguish low-tension glaucoma in an individual patient.

Optic disc hemorrhage in low-tension glaucoma

Bjerrum[20] is said to have been the first to describe the hemorrhages on the optic disc in glaucoma and to have regarded them as precursors of other glaucomatous changes. Drance et al.[15,37,68,111,112] have pointed out in the modern literature that optic disc hemorrhages are common in glaucoma and that their presence is a risk factor for future progressive optic nerve damage. Their findings have been confirmed by others.[2,3,18,98]

Few studies specifically relate optic disc hemorrhages to low-tension glaucoma (Table 44-1). In Drance's series[40] 11 of 45 patients were noted to have disc hemorrhage at some point. All of these

patients had an additional systemic vascular abnormality. In the Mayo Clinic series,[25] disc hemorrhages were noted in 8 of 77 eyes, and in Levene's series,[75] in 6 of 53 eyes.

Kitazawa et al.[65] have recently studied optic disc hemorrhages in low-tension glaucoma patients in some detail. In the retrospective portion of their study, they found optic disc hemorrhages in 16 of 78 low-tension glaucoma patients. They prospectively studied 58 of these patients at monthly intervals for 6 months. The overall incidence of hemorrhages in this group was 25 of 58 patients (43.1%) or 28 of 113 eyes (24.8%). They also found that optic disc hemorrhages were significantly more common in patients with low-tension glaucoma than in patients with chronic open-angle glaucoma.

Most investigators have felt that disc hemorrhages in glaucoma are evidence for a role of ischemia in the cause of glaucomatous optic nerve damage. Others have disagreed with this notion and have suggested other interpretations.[81,95,109]

Visual Fields (Figs. 44-1, A and B, and 44-2, A and B)

There has also been controversy as to whether the visual field changes seen in low-tension glaucoma differ from those seen in chronic open-angle glaucoma. Levene[75] stated that a larger proportion of patients with low-tension glaucoma have visual field defects closer to fixation.

Several authors have reported statistically significant differences in the appearance of the visual field in low-tension glaucoma and chronic open-angle glaucoma.[62,22,50] The defects of low-tension glaucoma are said to be closer to fixation, to be deeper, to have steeper slopes, and to be more often found in the superior half of the visual field. Others, however, have failed to find such differences.[83,90,103] In fact, King et al.[63] in a prospective

Table 44-1 Studies relating the presence of optic disc hemorrhage to low-tension glaucoma

Author	Total subjects in study	Total with disc hemorrhage
Drance[40](R)	45*	11* (24.4%)
Chumbley[25](R)	77†	8† (10.4%)
Levene[75](R)	53†	6† (11.3%)
Kitazawa[65](R)	78*	16* (20.5%)
Kitazawa[65](P)	58*	25* (43.1%)

R, retrospective (prevalence) study; P, prospective (incidence) study.
*Subjects.
†Eyes.

study, found that the scotomas of chronic open-angle glaucoma were closer to fixation than those of low-tension glaucoma. The subject of the visual field in low-tension glaucoma continues to inspire polite disagreement.[21,35,91]

It seems that although differences may exist in the visual fields of patients with low-tension glaucoma compared to chronic open-angle glaucoma, there is considerable overlap. When dealing with an individual patient, one cannot use the visual field appearance to determine whether or not the patient has low-pressure or high-pressure glaucoma.

Associated Ocular Findings

Aqueous humor dynamics

It has been traditionally taught that, even though patients with low-tension glaucoma may have intraocular pressures measured in the normal range, there is often some abnormality of aqueous humor dynamics detectable.[41,44,80]

By definition, intraocular pressure in low-tension glaucoma is in the normal range. The range of intraocular pressure in the normal population is generally determined from the mean pressure reading for each individual in the sample.[71] If one wishes to compare the intraocular pressures of a population of low-tension glaucoma with that of normal subjects, the mean pressure readings of the subjects in the low-tension glaucoma group should also be used. It is not correct to compare the highest of many readings in low-tension glaucoma patients with the mean of a few readings in normal subjects. If one intends to evaluate low-tension glaucoma patients in terms of their peak intraocular pressures, then one should compare the data with the peak intraocular pressures found on repeated tonometry in the normal population. Studies of this nature have not been reported.

There are studies reporting the means and ranges of intraocular pressures seen in patients with low-tension glaucoma. Some of these have found that low-tension glaucoma patients do not differ much from normal.[16,43,46,53,100] On the other hand, some studies indicate that low-tension glaucoma patients tend to have intraocular pressures at the high range of normal.[9,47]

Tonography has been used to study aqueous humor dynamics in low-tension glaucoma patients. The ranges reported for outflow facility are quite wide. In general, however, the outflow facilities in low-tension glaucoma patients are somewhat lower than one would expect in a normal population, but not as disturbed as is usually found

in a population of chronic open-angle glaucoma patients.[25,40,53,75,82]

Armaly[7] has reported that low-tension glaucoma patients have a higher than normal intraocular pressure response to topical corticosteroids. Drance,[40] however, could not confirm this finding.

It seems that low-tension glaucoma patients are more likely to have subtle abnormalities of aqueous humor dynamics than the normal population. The implications of this for understanding the cause or management of low-tension glaucoma are not immediately apparent. Most of the studies addressing the question of aqueous humor dynamics in low-tension glaucoma have not yielded clinically useful data.

Family history of glaucoma

A relationship between low-tension glaucoma and chronic open-angle glaucoma is suggested by the frequent report of the occurrence of clusters of cases of both conditions within the same family.* It is fairly conclusive that in many cases, low-tension glaucoma and chronic open-angle glaucoma are really the same disease, and that intraocular pressures are distributed in such a way that the population of patients with chronic open-angle glaucoma includes individuals whose intraocular pressures remain in the normal range each time they are measured.

Refractive error

There is now good evidence that myopia is a risk factor for the development of glaucoma. The same may be true for low-tension glaucoma as well.[27,73,75,88] Leighton and Tomlinson[73] reported a significantly greater prevalence of axial myopia in low-tension glaucoma patients compared with patients with chronic open-angle glaucoma. Neither Drance[40] nor Bengtsson,[16] however, could confirm a higher prevalence of myopia in their series of low-tension glaucoma cases.

Associated Systemic Findings

Age

Low-tension glaucoma is most often a disease of the elderly, the mean reported age in clinical studies generally being in the 60s.[25,40,46,75,103] In an epidemiologic study, Shiose[103] found the majority of low-tension glaucoma patients in the 40- to 60-year-old age group. However, this study included only employed individuals and so did not include

---

*References 25, 40, 46, 75, 80, 84, 87, 105.

many older subjects. The prevalence of low-tension glaucoma, however, was much higher in the older age groups. Low-tension glaucoma is unusual below the age of 50, although it does occur.

Sex

Some studies have suggested that a significant majority of low-tension glaucoma patients are women.[25,46,75,105] This may, however, reflect the fact that there are generally more women than men in the elderly population of western societies. In Drance's series,[40] a majority of the patients were men, whereas Shiose[103] found an equal prevalence in both sexes.

Race

There is now evidence suggesting that black patients are at greater risk for the development of glaucoma[79,120,122] There is also evidence suggesting that the mean size of the optic cup is larger in blacks than in whites.[13] There do not, however, seem to be any studies specifically relating race to low-tension glaucoma.

Blood pressure

The relationship of systemic blood pressure to glaucoma has inspired a large volume of literature and controversy. In low-tension glaucoma there are two aspects to the relationship between systemic blood pressure and optic nerve damage. One is whether there are chronic abnormalities of blood pressure in low-tension glaucoma patients. The other is the possible role of episodes of acute hypotension in patients with low-tension glaucoma.

Sjogren[105] originally suggested that a tendency to low blood pressure was found more often in low-tension glaucoma patients. Several more recent studies have also found that hypotension of one sort or another, including postural hypotension, may be more prevalent in patients with low-tension glaucoma.[28,40,46,47,72]

Systemic hypertension appears prevalent among patients with low-tension glaucoma,[25,75] but systemic hypertension is also generally prevalent in the older population. There do not seem to be any studies specifically relating systemic hypertension to low-tension glaucoma.

Drance[33] has pointed out that low-tension glaucoma patients often have a history of a previous acute hypotensive episode, or "hemodynamic crisis." He subsequently showed that a history of a hemodynamic crisis was significantly more prevalent among low-tension glaucoma patients than ocular hypertensive controls and that patients with such a history were less likely to show progressive visual field loss.[38,40] He also showed that a history of a hemodynamic crisis was a significant risk factor for the presence of glaucomatous visual field loss.[39]

Another study has also found a high prevalence of a history of a hemodynamic crisis in low-tension glaucoma patients.[25] Other studies, however, have not been able to confirm Drance's findings.[28,46,75] In a prospective study of 18 patients in an intensive care unit who survived an episode of shock, Jampol et al.[58] were unable to find a single patient who subsequently developed cupping similar to that seen in low-tension glaucoma.

Vascular disease

The large number of patients with low-tension glaucoma and concomitant systemic vascular disease is quite striking. The clinical impression that low-tension glaucoma is an ocular manifestation of generalized vascular disease is widespread.[102,107] As with most areas of investigation in low-tension glaucoma, a review of the literature on the association with vascular disease reveals contradictory evidence.

Drance[40] did not find a higher prevalence of overt extraocular vascular disease in low-tension glaucoma patients than in ocular hypertensive controls. Goldberg et al.[46] found a higher prevalence of cardiovascular disease and a "sedentary life style" among low-tension glaucoma patients than among ocular hypertensive controls. Others[18,28,47] could not confirm these findings. There has not been a proven association between systemic vascular disease and low-tension glaucoma.[74]

The relationship between carotid artery disease and low-tension glaucoma has occasioned more specific investigation. There are isolated case reports of patients with cupping and carotid disease in whom the association seems more than coincidental.[45] A common association between low-tension glaucoma and significant carotid occlusive disease has not been confirmed.[28,59,75]

Migraine

Phelps et al.[26,89] found migraine to be strikingly more common among patients with low-tension glaucoma than in patients with chronic open-angle glaucoma, patients with ocular hypertension, or normal patients. Drance[36] and Ederer[42] find their data convincing.

EPIDEMIOLOGY

Several authors feel that low-tension glaucoma is quite uncommon, that most cases can be described as "so-called low-tension glaucoma," and that the majority of these cases can be explained one way or another.[45,67,80] This position is becoming increasingly difficult to sustain in the face of mounting epidemiologic evidence that low-tension glaucoma is far more common than generally recognized.

Naturally, the prevalence of any disease depends heavily on the definition of the disease. A very restrictive definition that excludes certain classes of patients will result in a much lower prevalence than a broad, widely inclusive definition.[74]

There is also a relationship between the definition of the upper acceptable limit of intraocular pressure, the frequency with which intraocular pressure is measured, and the prevalence of low-tension glaucoma. The higher the pressure used as the cutoff between low tension glaucoma and chronic open-angle glaucoma, the higher the prevalence of low-tension glaucoma. More frequent measurements of intraocular pressure are more likely to uncover occasional abnormally high pressures in any patient. If frequent diurnal measurements of intraocular pressure or home tonometry are to be used to diagnose low-tension glaucoma, then one must use the same techniques to redefine normal limits of intraocular pressure. The weight of evidence from several independent population studies suggests that low-tension glaucoma is actually a fairly common condition (Table 44-2).

The population study conducted in Wales by Hollows and Graham[55] was the first to indicate the possibility of a high prevalence of low-tension glaucoma. They found 20 cases of glaucomatous visual field loss in a population of 4231 adults over the age of 40. Of this number, 7 were felt to have low-tension glaucoma.

The Bedford glaucoma survey[12] found 45 cases of open-angle glaucoma in a population of 5941. Three of the 45 had low-tension glaucoma. In a follow-up study 5 years later[86] four previously normal individuals developed glaucoma, of whom two had low-tension glaucoma.

In a study in Des Moines, Armaly[8] found that 129 of 189 eyes with glaucomatous visual field loss had normal intraocular pressure. Later, in a large prospective study, Armaly et al.[11] found 98 eyes that developed glaucomatous visual field loss. The mean intraocular pressure in this group during the year preceding the appearance of the field defect was less than 21 mm Hg. The average peak intraocular pressure of the group developing visual field loss was only 23.3 mm Hg, compared with 18.7 mm Hg for the normal group.[10] This would seem

Table 44-2 *Prevalence of glaucoma with apparently normal intraocular pressure relative to all open-angle glaucomas*

Author	Total glaucomas	Total with normal IOP	Percent
Hollows and Graham[55]	20	7	35.0
Bankes et al.[12]	45	3	6.7
Armaly[8]	189	129	68.3
Leibowitz et al.[71]	40	21	52.5
Bengtsson[18]	15	7	46.7
Shiose[103]	151	99	65.6
Smith[106]	400*	120*	30.0

*Total represents eyes, not subjects.

to indicate that a large number of eyes develop glaucoma at what appear to be normal pressures.

The Framingham eye study[71] found 40 patients with definite open-angle glaucoma. Of this number, only 19 had an average intraocular pressure greater than 21 mm Hg, whereas 6 of the 40 had an average pressure less than 16 mm Hg. Regardless of the features used to define glaucoma, low-tension glaucoma was found to represent about 40% of all open-angle glaucoma in this study.[61]

In a study of 1511 subjects in a town in Sweden, Bengtsson[18] found 15 with glaucomatous visual field defects, of whom only 7 had an intraocular pressure greater than 20.5 mm Hg. In a study of a selected population of confirmed and suspected glaucoma patients in Texas, Smith[106] found that fully 30% of patients with visual field loss did not have a pressure over 23 mm Hg.

In a massive study in Japan, Shiose et al.[104] found low-tension glaucoma and high-tension glaucoma to be approximately equally prevalent. In a later study, Shiose[103] screened over 21,000 workers and found 52 cases of glaucoma with elevated intraocular pressure and 99 cases of low-tension glaucoma.

These studies, of course, have not measured diurnal pressure fluctuations or gone to great lengths to rule out other conditions that might simulate low-tension glaucoma. However, unless evidence to the contrary is forthcoming, the studies available to date suggest that low-tension glaucoma is a common condition and may represent anywhere from one fifth to more than one half of all open-angle glaucoma cases. That most clinical practices do not reflect the high prevalence of low-tension glaucoma may be the result of lack of detection.[76,108]

DIAGNOSIS AND EVALUATION

The differential diagnosis of low-tension glaucoma can be thought of either as glaucoma in which elevated intraocular pressure is or has been present but is undetected, or as ersatz glaucoma (i.e., a disease that resembles glaucoma but is not). Undetected high tension glaucoma exists in the following three varieties:

1. Chronic open-angle glaucoma with large diurnal swings of intraocular pressure
2. Intermittent high pressures such as might be seen in intermittent angle-closure or glaucomatocyclitic crisis
3. Resolved glaucoma in which pressure was high in the past for some reason, is no longer present, but has caused optic nerve cupping

Ersatz glaucoma includes a list of congenital or acquired optic nerve diseases that are sometimes associated with changes in the optic nerve or visual field that bear a superficial resemblance to glaucoma (see box at right).

Chronic Open-angle Glaucoma With Large Diurnal Variation

Numerous studies have shown that there is a normal diurnal fluctuation of intraocular pressure, and that this fluctuation tends to be larger in glaucoma patients.* Therefore, the intraocular pressure of suspected low-tension glaucoma patients should be sampled at frequent intervals throughout the day. If peaks of high intraocular pressure are found, a diagnosis of low-tension glaucoma cannot be sustained.

Some authors feel that even occasional peaks of intraocular pressure are important and that these may be missed during a single diurnal tension curve determination. Home tonometry has been advocated and techniques for measuring the pressure at home by the patient or a family member have been developed.[4,60,125] Other authors have suggested that large variation in postural changes of intraocular pressure may be important in low-tension glaucoma.[70,115]

The significance of an occasional abnormal intraocular pressure reading in a low-tension glaucoma patient is unclear. In a series of patients with glaucoma of all types who were referred for evaluation, Smith[106] found no difference in the diurnal variation of patients with or without visual field defects. The problems and logical fallacies involved

---

*References 29, 31, 52, 64, 92, 93, 123.

> **DIFFERENTIAL DIAGNOSIS OF LOW-TENSION GLAUCOMA**
>
> I. Undetected high-pressure glaucoma
>   A. Chronic open-angle glaucoma with large diurnal intraocular pressure variation
>   B. Intermittent elevation of intraocular pressure caused by another type of glaucoma
>   1. Intermittent angle-closure
>   2. Glaucomatocyclitic crisis
>   C. Previous episode of elevated intraocular pressure
>   1. Old secondary glaucoma (e.g., pigmentary glaucoma)
>   2. Burned-out glaucoma
> II. Nonglaucomatous optic nerve disease resembling glaucoma
>   A. Congenital anomalies
>   B. Compressive lesions of the optic nerve and chiasm
>   C. Ischemic optic neuropathy

in the analysis of the relationship between intraocular pressure and glaucomatous optic nerve damage have been well reviewed by Krakau.[69]

Intermittent Elevation of Intraocular Pressure Caused by Another Type of Glaucoma

This situation will usually be confirmed or ruled out by a careful history and ocular examination. Occasionally a patient may have a condition that produces temporary elevations of intraocular pressure and may not leave any physical signs behind other than cupping and visual field loss. Intermittent angle-closure glaucoma and the glaucomatocyclitic crisis are two such conditions.

Previous Episode of Elevated Pressure

A patient may have a secondary glaucoma caused by uveitis or the use of topical steriods in which a high intraocular pressure for a period of time has produced cupping and visual field loss. If the original problem resolves, the patient may have low-tension glaucoma years later. Here again, a careful history and examination will usually uncover such a problem.

A more troublesome concept is that of burned-out glaucoma. Burned-out glaucoma is usually described as a condition seen in an older individual with extensive cupping and visual field loss, normal intraocular pressures, and a very low outflow facility. Such patients are thought to have had chronic open-angle glaucoma with high pressures in the past, but because of ciliary body atrophy and hyposecretion, they now have intraocular pressures in the normal range and low-tension glaucoma.

Several authors assert that burned-out glaucoma exists and is an important consideration in the differential diagnosis of low-tension glaucoma.[45,67,107,121] There do not appear, however, to be any documented cases in the literature of chronic open-angle glaucoma actually progressing to a burned-out state. There are cases of low-tension glaucoma associated with a low facility of outflow,[75] and cases associated with pigment dispersion syndrome.[99] It is presumed that these patients had high intraocular pressure sometime in the past, although there is no direct evidence. Studies on patients with very advanced visual loss caused by long-standing, chronic open-angle glaucoma have not yielded many cases where intraocular pressure was normal without treatment,[48,66] indicating that progression of chronic open-angle glaucoma to a burned-out state may actually be fairly uncommon.

Nonglaucomatous Optic Nerve Disease Resembling Low-tension Glaucoma

Congenital anomalies of the optic disc

A variety of congenital anomalies of the optic nerve may simulate glaucomatous cupping and be associated with nerve fiber bundle–type visual field loss. Colobomas, optic pits, large physiologic cups, tilted discs, myopia, and optic nerve head drusen are among the lesions said to mimic glaucoma.[107,121,124] A careful history and examination will usually allow a correct diagnosis to be made, although some of these cases can present difficulties in diagnosis.

Compressive lesions of the chiasm and optic nerve

Optic atrophy caused by compressive lesions of the optic nerve or chiasm does not generally resemble glaucomatous cupping. Glaucomatous and nonglaucomatous optic atrophy can usually be distinguished by clinical examination.[97,113,114] Occasionally, however, the optic nerve in a patient with nonglaucomatous optic atrophy may appear to be cupped to such a degree that low-tension glaucoma is suspected.*

In one study, 6% of unselected eyes with optic atrophy were misdiagnosed as being glaucoma-

tous.[113] When the eyes with an appearance of pathologic cupping caused by nonglaucomatous atrophy were selected out, 44% of these were misdiagnosed by at least one expert[114] as having glaucoma. In another study, 8 of 141 subjects suspected of having glaucoma by optic disc screening were found to have intracranial lesions.[104] Visual field defects similar to those of glaucoma may also be seen resulting from intracranial compressive lesions.[57] The possibility of a compressive lesion must always be kept in mind when evaluating a patient suspected of having low-tension glaucoma.

Ischemic optic neuropathy

The relationship of low-tension glaucoma and ischemic optic neuropathy has been a subject of considerable discussion. Cupping resembling that seen in low-tension glaucoma sometimes follows acute ischemic insults to the optic nerve.[54,75,82,96] Lichter and Henderson[78] have described a syndrome of acute optic nerve infarction followed by cupping that closely resembles that of glaucoma, but it is not progressive. In their series of 45 low-tension glaucoma cases, Chumbley and Brubaker[25] found 10 with a history of sudden visual loss that would suggest a diagnosis of ischemic optic neuropathy.

Despite the evidence cited above, some authors have presented data indicating that glaucomatous-like cupping is quite uncommon in patients with ischemic optic neuropathies, but may be seen mostly in the patients with giant cell arteritis.[14,30,97] In any case, a previous episode of ischemic optic neuropathy must be considered in the differential diagnosis of any patient with low-tension glaucoma.

Diagnostic Evaluation of Patients With Low-tension Glaucoma

In light of the information presented above, it is possible to develop a rational approach to the diagnostic evaluation of a patient presenting with cupping of the optic nerve, visual field loss, and normal intraocular pressure (see the box on p. 808).

Ocular evaluation

History and ophthalmologic examination. A careful ophthalmologic and general medical history, including a past medical and surgical history, combined with a meticulous and thorough ocular examination will usually uncover any obvious cause or associated illnesses.

---

*References 44, 45, 75, 81, 94, 121.

DIAGNOSTIC EVALUATION OF PATIENTS WITH LOW-TENSION GLAUCOMA

I. Ocular evaluation
  A. Complete history and careful ophthalmologic examination including perimetry and gonioscopy
  B. Diurnal tension curve (24 hours)
II. General medical evaluation
  A. Physical examination by general medical practitioner familiar with cardiovascular and neurologic disorders
  B. Blood tests
    1. Complete blood count
    2. Serum chemistries
    3. Erythrocyte sedimentation rate
  C. Carotid blood flow evaluation
  D. Computed tomography (CT scan)

Diurnal tension curve. To assess the diurnal variation of the intraocular pressure, the patient should be available for tonometric measurement every 2 hours during the course of a day. Ideally, the diurnal tension curve should include an early morning as well as a late evening measurement and should be performed more than once, but this is not always practical. Tonography may be performed to look for low outflow facility, but it is rarely helpful in the diagnostic evaluation of low-tension glaucoma.

General medical evaluation

Physical examination. The patient should be examined by a general medical practitioner to look for important systemic illnesses. Vascular disease, neurologic abnormalities, and blood pressure findings should be especially emphasized.

Blood tests. A complete blood count should be performed to rule out anemia or hyperviscosity. Blood chemistry tests should be performed to rule out hyperlipidemias that are often associated with vascular disease. A sedimentation rate should be performed to screen for giant cell arteritis in older patients.

Carotid blood flow evaluation

The patient may be referred to a vascular laboratory to rule out significant carotid occlusive disease. Alternatively, the general practitioner should be alerted to the possibility of carotid disease and allow him or her to decide the extent of work-up.

Computed tomography

Routine computed tomography (CT scanning) of the skull and orbits is controversial. Certainly the yield of abnormalities in low-tension glaucoma

patients is very low. Useful guidelines for obtaining a CT scan might be the following:
1. Patient under 65 or 70 years of age
2. Patient whose visual field loss is progressing rapidly
3. Patient with unusual visual fields or whose optic discs show excessive pallor relative to the amount of cupping

TREATMENT

There are no good, controlled studies showing that treatment is of any benefit in low-tension glaucoma. Furthermore, many patients with low-tension glaucoma do not show progressive visual loss.[25,40] Conservativism and patience should be exercised in managing these patients. In most cases there is little reason to panic or rush to give the patient potentially harmful medications or to risk the complications of therapeutic procedures.

Most of the written material on the treatment of low-tension glaucoma consists of the personal approach taken by an authority in the field, based on his or her own clinical experience.* In general, what is advocated is to lower the intraocular pressure as much as possible using medications, laser techniques, or surgery. There is, however, no good scientific evidence in these reports that pressure-lowering therapy actually alters the course of the disease. The risks of using medications such as beta-blockers, epinephrine, or carbonic anhydrase inhibitors in an elderly population are well known and not inconsiderable. Filtering surgery also has its risks. There is, therefore, no information available to use in formulating a rational approach to the treatment of low-tension glaucoma. The real risks of a treatment must always be considered in light of the uncertain benefits.

Although a rational basis for making treatment decisions is lacking, the following scheme for managing patients with low-tension glaucoma may be considered.

Determine the Severity of the Disease

If the cupping and visual field loss are very far advanced, vigorous application of treatment to lower the intraocular pressure is more likely. If the cupping and visual field loss are only moderate or minimal, much more caution can be used.

Determine Whether the Disease Is Progressive

Many patients with low-tension glaucoma do not show progressive loss. In these cases, treat-

---

*References 1, 34, 44, 47, 101, 107, 110, 121.

ment is probably not necessary. If there is something that suggests that progression is unlikely, such as a history of a major hemodynamic crisis or a sudden visual loss, treatment can be deferred. In any case, vigorous treatment should probably wait until progressive change of the optic disc or visual field can be documented over time.

Start With Medical Therapy

Pilocarpine is probably the safest drug and the one most likely to lower pressure in a normotensive eye. If the medication is well tolerated and the pressure is significantly lowered, it should be continued; otherwise there is no reason to continue. The use of epinephrine and beta-blockers in low-tension glaucoma is controversial because of their systemic cardiovascular effects and possible adverse effect on optic nerve perfusion pressure. Most authorities, however, would advocate their use if well tolerated and if the pressure is significantly lowered. Carbonic anhydrase inhibitors can be very useful in treating low-tension glaucoma if the side effects are not too great a problem.

In any circumstance, however, therapy should not be continued unless a significant decrease in intraocular pressure is obtained. One way to decide if medical therapy is effective in the normotensive eye is the uniocular trial of therapy to compare the response to the untreated eye. Nonmedical forms of therapy should probably not be considered unless progression has been well documented or unless the disease is already very far advanced.

Laser Trabeculoplasty

Laser trabeculoplasty has been used in low-tension glaucoma and is sometimes effective in lowering the intraocular pressure,[101] but may not halt the progression of the disease. In general, the pressure-lowering effect of laser trabeculoplasty is less impressive in normotensive eyes. Therefore, the low-tension glaucoma patient must be approached with a much more guarded prognosis when contemplating laser therapy.

Filtering Surgery

Filtering surgery should not be considered unless progressive visual field loss or progressive optic nerve cupping has been demonstrated beyond doubt. Many authors recommend full-thickness filtering procedures such as thermal sclerostomy, scleral trephine, or sclerectomy in low-tension glaucoma. It is felt that these procedures are likely to result in a lower postoperative intraocular pressure than guarded procedures such as trabeculectomy.

SUMMARY

Low-tension glaucoma is a syndrome in which cupping and visual field loss similar to other forms of glaucoma are present in the absence of elevated intraocular pressure. There is still considerable disagreement about the definition of this disease, its true nature, and its relationship to chronic open-angle glaucoma.

Low-tension glaucoma appears to be much more common than was generally recognized in the past. Low-tension glaucoma patients comprise a heterogeneous group in which certain ocular, systemic, vascular, and neurologic features may be unusually common. Patients presenting with low-tension glaucoma need to be investigated to rule out other forms of glaucoma or nonglaucomatous optic nerve disease.

Treatment is similar to that for chronic open-angle glaucoma and is aimed at lowering intraocular pressure. It is uncertain, however, that treatment is of any benefit in low-tension glaucoma, and potentially harmful therapies should only be applied in the presence of well-documented progression.

REFERENCES

1. Abedin, S, Simmons, RJ, and Grant, WM: Progressive low-tension glaucoma treatment to stop glaucomatous cupping and field loss when these progress despite normal intraocular pressure, Ophthalmology 89:1, 1982
2. Airaksinen, PF: Are optic disc hemorrhages a common finding in all glaucoma patients? Acta Ophthalmol 62:193, 1984
3. Airaksinen, PJ, and Tuulonen, A: Early glaucoma changes in patients with and without an optic disc hemorrhage, Acta Ophthalmol 62:197, 1984
4. Alpar, JJ: The use of home tonometry in the diagnosis and treatment of glaucoma, Glaucoma 5:130, 1983
5. Anderson, DR: Correlation of peripapillary anatomy with the disc damage and field abnormalities in glaucoma, Doc Ophthalmol Proc Ser 35:1, 1983
6. Anderson, S, and Hitchings, RA: A comparative study of visual fields of patients with low-tension glaucoma and those with chronic simple glaucoma, Doc Ophthalmol Proc Ser 35:97, 1983
7. Armaly, MF: Effect of corticosteroids on intraocular pressure. II. The effect of dexamethasone on the glaucoma eye, Arch Ophthalmol 70:492, 1963
8. Armaly, MF: On the distribution of applanation pressure and arcuate scotoma. In Paterson, G, Miller, SJH, and Paterson, GD, editors: Drug mechanisms in glaucoma, Boston, 1966, Little, Brown & Co
9. Armaly, MF: Ocular pressure and visual fields: a ten year follow-up study, Arch Ophthalmol 81:25, 1969

10. Armaly, MF: Lessons to be learned from the collaborative glaucoma study, Surv Ophthalmol 25:139, 1980

11. Armaly, MF, et al: Biostatistical analysis of the collaborative glaucoma study, Arch Ophthalmol 98:2163, 1980

12. Bankes, JLK, Perkins, ES, Tsolakis, S, and Wright, JE: Bedford glaucoma survey, Br Med J 1:791, 1968

13. Beck, RM, et al: Is there a racial difference in physiologic cup size? Ophthalmology 92:873, 1985

14. Beck, RW, et al: Optic disc structure in anterior ischemic optic neuropathy, Ophthalmology 91:1334, 1984

15. Begg, IS, Drance, SM, and Sweeney, VP: Ischemic optic neuropathy in chronic simple glaucoma, Br J Ophthalmol 55:73, 1971

16. Bengtsson, B: Findings associated with glaucomatous visual field defects, Acta Ophthalmol 58:20, 1980

17. Bengtsson, B: Manifest glaucoma in the aged. II. Cases detected by ophthalmoscopy, Acta Ophthalmol 59:1, 1981

18. Bengtsson, B: Aspects of the epidemiology of chronic glaucoma, Acta Ophthalmol Suppl 146:1, 1981

19. Bengtsson, B, and Krakau, CET: Automatic perimetry in a population survey, Acta Ophthalmol 57:929, 1979

20. Bjerrum, J: Cited in Krakau, CET: Intraocular pressure elevation—cause or effect in chronic glaucoma? Ophthalmologica 182:141, 1981

21. Caprioli, J, Sears, M, and Spaeth, GL: Comparison of visual field defects in normal-tension glaucoma and high-tension glaucoma, Am J Ophthalmol 102:402, 1986

22. Caprioli, J, and Spaeth, GL: Comparison of visual field defects in the low-tension glaucomas with those in the high-tension glaucomas, Am J Ophthalmol 97:730, 1984

23. Caprioli, J, and Spaeth, GL: Comparison of the optic nerve head in high- and low-tension glaucoma, Arch Ophthalmol 103:1145, 1985

24. Chandler, PA, and Grant, WM: Glaucoma, ed 2, Philadelphia, 1979, Lea & Febiger

25. Chumbley, LC, and Brubaker, RF: Low-tension glaucoma, Am J Ophthalmol 81:761, 1976

26. Corbett, JJ, Phelps, CD, Eslinger, P, and Montague, PR: The neurologic evaluation of patients with low-tension glaucoma, Invest Ophthalmol Vis Sci 26:1101, 1985

27. Daubs, JG, and Crick, RP: Effect of refractive error on the risk of ocular hypertension and open-angle glaucoma, Trans Ophthalmol Soc UK 101:121, 1981

28. Demailly, P, et al: Do patients with low-tension glaucoma have particular cardiovascular characteristics? Ophthalmologica 188:65, 1984

29. de Venecia, G, and Davis, MD: Diurnal variation of intraocular pressure in the normal eye, Arch Ophthalmol 69:752, 1963

30. Doro, S, and Lessel, S: Cup-disc ratio and ischemic optic neuropathy, Arch Ophthalmol 103:1143, 1985

31. Drance, SM: The significance of the diurnal tension variations in normal and glaucomatous eyes, Arch Ophthalmol 64:494, 1960

32. Drance, SM: Some factors involved in the production of low tension glaucoma. In Cant, JS, editor: The optic nerve, London, 1972, Henry Kimpton

33. Drance, SM: Some factors in the production of low-tension glaucoma, Br J Ophthalmol 56:229, 1972

34. Drance, SM: Low-tension glaucoma and its management. In Transactions of the New Orleans Academy of Ophthalmology: Symposium on glaucoma, St Louis, 1975, The CV Mosby Co

35. Drance, SM: Low-tension glaucoma, enigma and opportunity, Arch Ophthalmol 103:1131, 1985

36. Drance, SM: The neurologic evaluation of patients with low-tension glaucoma, Surv Ophthalmol 31:74, 1986

37. Drance, SM, Fairclough, M, Butler, DM, and Kottler, MS: The importance of disc hemorrhage in the prognosis of chronic open-angle glaucoma, Arch Ophthalmol 95:226, 1977

38. Drance, SM, Morgan, RW, and Sweeney, VP: Shock-induced optic neuropathy: a cause of nonprogressive glaucoma, New Engl J Med 288:392, 1973

39. Drance, SM, Schulzer, M, Douglas, GR, and Sweeney, VP: Use of discriminant analysis. II. Identification of persons with glaucomatous visual field defects, Arch Ophthalmol 96:1571, 1978

40. Drance, SM, Sweeney, VP, Morgan, RW, and Feldman, F: Studies of factors involved in the production of low-tension glaucoma, Arch Ophthalmol 89:457, 1973

41. Duke-Elder, S, and Jay, B: Diseases of the lens and vitreous: glaucoma and hypotony, London, 1969, Henry Kimpton

42. Ederer, F: Migraine and low-tension glaucoma, letter to the editor, Invest Ophthalmol Vis Sci 27:632, 1986

43. Ehlers, N, and Hansen, FK: Central corneal thickness in low tension glaucoma, Acta Ophthalmol 52:740, 1974

44. Epstein, DL: Chandler and Grant's glaucoma, ed 3, Philadelphia, 1986, Lea and Febiger

45. Gittinger, JW, Miller, NR, Keltner, JL, and Burde, RM: Glaucomatous cupping—sine glaucoma, Surv Ophthalmol 25:383, 1981

46. Goldberg, I, Hollows, FC, Kass, MA, and Becker, B: Systemic factors in patients with low-tension glaucoma, Br J Ophthalmol 65:56, 1981

47. Gramer, E, and Leydhecker, W: Glaukom ohne Hochdruck: eine klinische Studie, Klin Mbl Augenheilkd 186:262, 1985

48. Grant, WM, and Burke, JF: Why do some people go blind from glaucoma? Ophthalmology 89:991, 1982

49. Greve, EL, and Geijssen, HC: The relationship between excavation and visual field in patients with high and low intraocular pressures, Doc Ophthalmol Proc Ser 35:35, 1983

50. Greve, EL, and Geijssen, HC: Comparison of visual fields in patients with high and with low intraocular pressures, Doc Ophthalmol Proc Ser 35:101, 1983

51. Hayreh, SS: Pathogenesis of optic nerve damage and visual field defects. In Heilmann, K, and Richardson, KT, editors: Glaucoma: conceptions of a disease, Philadelphia, 1978, WB Saunders Co

52. Henkind, P, Leitman, M, and Weitzman, E: the diurnal curve in man: new observations, Invest Ophthalmol Vis Sci 9:705, 1973

53. Hiatt, RL, Deutsche, AR, and Ringer, G: Low-tension glaucoma, Ann Ophthalmol 3:85, 1971

54. Hitchings, RA: The optic disc in glaucoma. III. Diffuse optic disc pallor with raised intraocular pressure, Br J Ophthalmol 62:670, 1978

55. Hollows, FC, and Graham, PA: Intraocular pressure, glaucoma and glaucoma suspects in a defined population, Br J Ophthalmol 50:570, 1966

56. Hoskins, HD: Definition, classification, and management of the glaucoma suspect. In Transactions of the New Orleans Academy of Ophthalmology: Symposium on glaucoma, St Louis, 1981, The CV Mosby Co

57. Hupp, SL, et al: Nerve fiber bundle visual field defects and intracranial mass lesions, Can J Ophthalmol 21:231, 1986

58. Jampol, LM, Board, RJ, and Maumenee, AE: Systemic hypotension and glaucomatous changes, Am J Ophthalmol 85:154, 1978

59. Jampol, LM, and Miller, NR: Carotid artery disease and glaucoma, Br J Ophthalmol 62:324, 1978

60. Jensen, AD, and Maumenee, AE: Home tonometry, Am J Ophthalmol 76:929, 1973

61. Kahn, HA, and Milton, RC: Alternative definitions of open-angle glaucoma: effect on prevalence and associations in the Framingham eye study, Arch Ophthalmol 98:2172, 1980

62. King, D, Douglas, GR, Drance, SM, and Wijsman, K: Optic nerve analysis in low-tension glaucoma versus high pressure glaucoma, Invest Ophthalmol Vis Sci Suppl 27:41, 1986

63. King, D, et al: Comparison of visual field defects in normal-tension glaucoma and high-tension glaucoma, Am J Ophthalmol 101:204, 1986

64. Kitazawa, Y, and Horie, T: Diurnal variation of intraocular pressure in primary open-angle glaucoma, Am J Ophthalmol 79:557, 1975

65. Kitazawa, Y, Shirato, S, and Yamamoto, T: Optic disc hemorrhage in low-tension glaucoma, Ophthalmology 93:853, 1986

66. Kolker, AE: Visual prognosis in advanced glaucoma: a comparison of medical and surgical therapy for retention of vison in 101 eyes with advanced glaucoma, Trans Am Ophthalmol Soc 75:539, 1977

67. Kolker, AE, and Hetherington, J, Jr.: Becker-Shaffer's diagnosis and therapy of the glaucomas, ed 5, St Louis, 1983, The CV Mosby Co

68. Kottler, MS, and Drance, SM: Studies of hemorrhage on the optic disc, Can J Ophthalmol 11:102, 1976

69. Krakau, CET: Intraocular pressure elevation—cause or effect in chronic glaucoma? Ophthalmologica 182:141, 1981

70. Krieglstein, GK, and Langham, ME: Glaukom ohne Hochdruck: ein Beitrag zur Ätiologie, Klin Mbl Augenheilkd 166:18, 1975

71. Leibowitz, HM, et al: The Framingham eye study monograph, Surv Ophthalmol 24(suppl):335, 1980

72. Leighton, DA, and Phillips, CI: Systemic blood pressure in open-angle gluacoma, low-tension glaucoma, and the normal eye, Br J Ophthalmol 56:447, 1972

73. Leighton, DA, and Tomlinson, A: Ocular tension and axial length of the eyeball if open-angle glaucoma and low-tension glaucoma, Br J Ophthalmol 57:499, 1973

74. Leske, MC: The epidemiology of open-angle glaucoma: a review, Am J Epidemiol 118:166, 1983

75. Levene, RZ: Low-tension glaucoma: a critical review and new material, Surv Ophthalmol 24:621, 1980

76. Levene, RZ: Low tension glaucoma. In Cairns, JE, editor: Glaucoma, London, 1986, Grune and Stratton

77. Lewis, RA, Hayreh, SS, and Phelps, CD: Optic disk and visual field correlations in primary open-angle glaucoma and low-tension glaucoma, Am J Ophthalmol 96:148, 1983

78. Lichter, PR, and Henderson, JW: Optic nerve infarction, Am J Ophthalmol 85:302, 1978

79. Martin, MJ, Sommer, A, Gold, EB, and Diamond, EL: Race and primary open-angle glaucoma, Am J Ophthalmol 99:383, 1985

80. Maumenee, AE: Visual loss in glaucoma. In Transactions of the New Orleans Academy of Ophthalmology: St Louis, 1981, The CV Mosby Co

81. Maumenee, AE: Causes of optic nerve damage in glaucoma, Ophthalmology 90:741, 1983

82. Miller, S: The enigma of glaucoma simplex, Trans Ophthalmol Soc UK 92:561, 1972

83. Motolko, M, Drance, SM, and Douglas, GR: The visual field defects of low-tension glaucoma, Arch Ophthalmol 100:1074, 1982

84. Paterson, G: A nine-year follow-up on first-degree relatives of patients with glaucoma simplex, Trans Ophthalmol Soc UK 90:515, 1970

85. Perkins, ES: The Bedford glaucoma survey. I. Long-term follow-up of borderline cases, Br J Ophthalmol 57:179, 1973

86. Perkins, ES: The Bedford glaucoma survey. II. Rescreening the normal population, Br J Ophthalmol 57:186, 1973

87. Perkins, ES: Family studies in glaucoma, Br J Ophthalmol 58:529, 1974

88. Perkins, ES, and Phelps, CD: Open-angle glaucoma, ocular hypertension, low-tension glaucoma and refraction, Arch Ophthalmol 100:1464, 1982

89. Phelps, CD, and Corbett, JJ: Migraine and low-tension glaucoma, Invest Ophthalmol Vis Sci 26:1105, 1985

90. Phelps, CD, Hayreh, SS, and Montague, PR: Visual fields in low-tension glaucoma, primary open-angle glaucoma and anterior ischemic optic neuropathy, Doc Ophthalmol Proc Ser 35:113, 1983

91. Phelps, CD, Hayreh, SS, and Montague, PR: Comparison of visual fields in the low-tension glaucomas with those in high-tension glaucomas, letter, Am J Ophthalmol 98:823, 1984

92. Phelps CD, Woolson, RF, Kolker, AE, and Becker, B: Diurnal variation in intraocular pressure, Am J Ophthalmol 77:367, 1974

93. Piltz, JR, Starita, R, Miron, M, and Henkind, P: Momentary fluctuation of intraocular pressure in normal and glaucomatous eyes, Ophthalmology 99:333, 1985

94. Portney, GL, and Roth, AM: Optic cupping caused by an intracranial aneurysm, Am J Ophthalmol 84:98, 1977

95. Quigley, HA: Pathophysiology of the optic nerve in glaucoma. In McAllister, JA, and Wilson, RP, editors: Glaucoma, London, 1986, Butterworth

96. Quigley HA, and Anderson, DR: Cupping of the optic disc in ischemic optic neuropathy, Trans Amer Acad Ophthalmol Otol 83:755, 1977

97. Radius, RL, and Maumenee, AE: Optic atrophy and glaucomatous cupping, Am J Ophthalmol 85:145, 1978

98. Richler, M, Werner, EB, and Thomas, D: Risk factors for progression of visual field defects in medically treated patients with glaucoma, Can J Ophthalmol 17:245, 1982

99. Ritch, R: Nonprogressive low-tension glaucoma with pigmentary dispersion, Am J Ophthalmol 94:190, 1982

100. Sandvig, K: Pseudoglaucoma of autosomal dominant inheritance: a report of three families, Acta Ophthalmol 39:33, 1961

101. Schwartz, AL, Perman, KI, and Whitten, M: Argon laser trabeculoplasty in progressive low-tension glaucoma, Ann Ophthalmol 16:560, 1984

102. Shields, MB: Textbook of glaucoma, ed 2, Baltimore, 1986, Williams & Wilkens

103. Shiose, Y: Prevalence and clinical aspects of low-tension glaucoma. In Paul Henkind, editor: Acta 24th International Congress of Ophthalmology, Philadelphia, 1983, JB Lippincott

104. Shiose, Y, et al: New system for mass screening of glaucoma, as part of automated multiphasic health testing services, Jpn J Ophthalmol 25:160, 1981

105. Sjogren, H: A study of pseudoglaucoma, Acta Ophthalmol 24:239, 1946

106. Smith J: Diurnal intraocular pressure: correlation to automated perimetry, Ophthalmology 92:858, 1985

107. Spaeth, GL: Low-tension glaucoma: its diagnosis and management, Doc Ophthalmol Proc Ser 22:263, 1980

108. Spaeth, GL: The pansy picking phenomenon, Ophthalmic Surg 10:625, 1986

109. Spaeth, GL: Discussion of optic disc hemorrhage in glaucoma, Ophthalmology 93:857, 1986

110. Sugar, HS: Low-tension glaucoma: a practical approach, Ann Ophthalmol 11:1155, 1979

111. Susanna, R, and Drance, SM: Use of discriminant analysis. I. Prediction of visual field defects from features of the optic disc, Arch Ophthalmol 96:1568, 1978

112. Susanna, R, Drance, SM, and Douglas, GR: Disc hemorrhages in patients with elevated intraocular pressure, occurrence with and without field changes, Arch Ophthalmol 97:284, 1979

113. Trobe, JD, Glaser, JS, and Cassady, JC: Optic atrophy differential diagnosis by fundus observation alone, Arch Ophthalmol 98:1041, 1980

114. Trobe, JD, et al: Nonglaucomatous excavation of the optic disc, Arch Ophthalmol 98:1046, 1980

115. Tsukahara, S, and Sasaki, T: Postural changes of IOP in normal persons and in patients with primary wide open-angle glaucoma and low-tension glaucoma, Br J Ophthalmol 68:389, 1984

116. von Graefe, A: Amaurose mit Sehnervenexcavation, Archiv f Ophthalmol 3(II):484, 1857

117. von Graefe, A: Die Iridectomie bei Amauros mit Sehnervenexcavation, Archiv f Ophthalmol 3(II):546, 1857

118. von Graefe, A: Ueber die glaucomatose Natur de Amaurosen mit Sehnervenexcavation und ueber das Wesen und die Classification des Glaucoms, Archiv f Ophthalmol 8(II):271, 1861

119. Wallace, J, and Lovell, HG: Glaucoma and intraocular pressure in Jamaica, Am J Ophthalmol 67:93, 1969

120. Wilensky, JT, Gandhi, N, and Pan, T: Racial influences in open-angle glaucoma, Ann Ophthalmol 10:1398, 1978

121. Wilensky, JT, and Gieser, DK: Low-tension glaucoma. In Weinstein, GW, editor: Open-angle glaucoma, New York, 1986, Churchill Livingstone

122. Wilson, R, Richardson, TM, Hertzmark, E, and Grant, WM: Race as a risk factor for progressive glaucomatous damage, Ann Ophthalmol 17:653, 1985

123. Worthen, DM: Intraocular pressure and its diurnal variation. In Heilmann, K, and Richardson KT, editors: Glaucoma conceptions of a disease, Philadelphia, 1978, WB Saunders Co

124. Yanoff, M, and Fine, B: Ocular pathology: a text and atlas, ed 2, Philadelphia, 1982, Harper & Row, Publishers

125. Zeimer, RC, et al: Application of a self-tonometer to home tonometry, Arch Ophthalmol 104:49, 1986

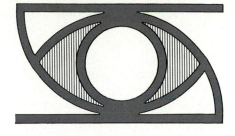

Chapter 45

Primary Open-angle Glaucoma

Murray A. Johnstone

A therapeutic overview

For purposes of clinical research and epidemiologic studies, primary open-angle glaucoma is defined as elevated intraocular pressure accompanied by glaucomatous disc damage and/or visual field loss. The iridocorneal angle must be open and any secondary etiology absent. Adherence to this definition often creates a conceptual dilemma when the physician is faced with the decision of instituting or increasing therapy. If the disease process does not fit the complete definition of "glaucoma," should it be treated with glaucoma medications?

The strict definition of primary open-angle glaucoma obviously excludes many patients who require treatment. It is often possible to identify patients who do not fulfill all of the above criteria but in whom treatment is appropriate. Examples include patients with very high intraocular pressure without disc damage, those with high intraocular pressure and disc damage without field loss, and those with disc damage and field loss without elevated pressure. Each of these situations is recognizable as a part of the spectrum of primary open-angle glaucoma.

For therapeutic purposes, therefore, glaucoma may be more satisfactorily defined as the presence of an intraocular pressure that is high enough to eventually cause loss of vision. Such a definition includes patients with a sufficient number of risk factors for glaucomatous damage to justify treatment.

The widespread consensus that reduction of intraocular pressure is effective in arresting the progress of glaucomatous damage is supported by at least one long-term study.[31] Instances of unilateral secondary glaucoma illustrate that elevated intraocular pressure alone may cause damage to the healthy optic nerve. Although the concept certainly seems logical, it remains to be proven in a prospective clinical trial that lowering intraocular pressure actually prevents the onset of glaucomatous changes in ocular hypertensives.

In addition to intraocular pressure elevation, less well-defined pathogenetic factors involving the optic nerve head must be implicated to explain the increased vulnerability to pressure in some patients. This is well illustrated by the dilemma of low-tension glaucoma (see Chapter 44).

The goal of therapy in all cases is to prevent visual loss. To minimize complications, one should attempt to achieve the goal with the minimum number and strength of medications necessary. When elevated intraocular pressure exists without evidence of other damage, the therapeutic goal may at times be realized by careful monitoring of the optic nerve head and visual field rather than by initiating treatment.

Diagnostic and monitoring techniques are discussed in Section II and include tonometry, tonography, diurnal curves, gonioscopy, optic disc and nerve fiber evaluation, visual field tests, and possibly psychophysical measurements. Definitional boundaries of the normal are blurred in relation to intraocular pressure, disc cupping, and early visual field changes. Intraocular pressure and visual field findings vary considerably as a result of physiologic variations. These limitations underscore the value of periodic observation and serial testing to detect the presence or progression of an abnormality.

WHEN TO INITIATE THERAPY

Treatment is initiated whenever intraocular pressure is high enough to cause eventual loss of vision. No specific pressure level can be defined that will avoid visual loss in all patients. In each case, one must attempt to decide what level is required to avoid progression of functional visual loss. This decision is based on a number of interrelated factors.

Primary considerations are the current intraocular pressure, appearance of the optic disc, and status of the visual field. Other risk factors to be considered include age, race, myopia, and a family history of glaucoma, which may suggest a greater susceptibility to damage. Systemic factors, such as hypertension, diabetes, and arteriosclerotic cardiovascular disease, increase the risk of damage from glaucoma and should also be considered (see Chapter 63).[2,6] An intraocular pressure up to 30 mm Hg may at times be monitored carefully without treatment in the absence of disc damage, visual field loss, or additional significant risk factors. Monitoring is necessary because many patients are not aware of early visual field damage.[3] These patients are spared the psychological impact of being treated for a chronic, incurable disease, as well as avoiding the cost, inconvenience and potential side effects of treatment. Such patients need to be clearly advised of the potential risk for glaucomatous visual field loss and the need for careful monitoring. Intraocular pressure above 30 mm Hg is generally an indication for treatment.

Optic nerve damage, particularly when progressive in the presence of elevated intraocular pressure, warrants treatment. Optic nerve damage can be difficult to assess in high myopes and patients with large physiologic cups. When evaluation is difficult and intraocular pressure is elevated, treatment is generally advisable.

When there is elevated intraocular pressure, disc damage and visual field loss, treatment is clearly indicated. Low-tension glaucoma consists of optic disc damage and visual field loss in the presence of normal intraocular pressure (see Chapter 44). If causes other than glaucoma of optic nerve damage have been excluded, treatment is initiated to reduce intraocular pressure to a level below that which has been demonstrated to cause damage.

GUIDELINES FOR ACCEPTABLE PRESSURE CONTROL

As a general rule, the greater the existing amount of damage to the optic nerve head and visual field, the lower the intraocular pressure should be to avoid further visual loss. The small safety margin present in eyes already severely damaged from glaucoma requires a more aggressive approach in achieving a low intraocular pressure, especially when the damage threatens fixation. Although degrees of glaucomatous damage may be thought of as a continuum along which any single patient lies, functional groupings may be defined for therapeutic purposes. One such schema has been outlined by Richardson.[32]

It is desirable to assign an "ideal" target pressure in each patient. If we are able to achieve the "ideal" or "acceptable" pressure and our estimate of such a pressure level is correct, we may reasonably hope to avoid progressive glaucomatous damage.

A distinction may be made between the "ideal" pressure, an "acceptable" pressure, and a "borderline" pressure. For example, when optic discs are normal and there is no detectable visual field loss, an ideal intraocular pressure might be regarded as under 21 mm Hg, one in the high 20s acceptable, and a pressure of 30 mm Hg borderline. The latter usually warrants initiation or escalation of therapy.

In a patient with total cupping and pallor of the disc with visual field loss involving fixation, 8 mm Hg might represent an ideal pressure. This is a pressure at which there would be very little risk of further loss. An acceptable pressure might be 12 mm Hg, since the risk of further loss remains low, and further escalation of therapy might expose the patient to questionably acceptable morbidity. A pressure of 16 mm in the same patient may be "borderline" in that the risk of further damage is significantly increased and the prospect of escalation of therapy, even to the point of surgery, may be entertained. These stated absolute levels of intraocular pressure are somewhat arbitrary and based on clinical impressions. Unfortunately, there are currently no methods to determine for any given optic nerve what pressure level is required to prevent the onset or progression of damage.

If the ideal pressure is easily reached with medications with minimal side effects, treatment has been optimized. Much more commonly, acceptable but less than ideal pressure levels are achieved. We are hindered in pursuing therapy to attain the ideal pressure by the fact that benefits begin to be outweighed by unacceptable side effects and risks.

The target for an optimal level of intraocular pressure may be adjusted upward under certain conditions. Pretreatment pressures may be compared with current ones. If moderate optic nerve damage has occurred at an intraocular pressure in the 40s, then pressure reduction to the low 20s may be acceptable. On the other hand, if the same damage occurred as a result of pretreatment pressures in the 20s, then reduction of pressure to the teens may be considered appropriate.

If it is obvious that longevity is limited and that glaucomatous damage will not progress significantly within the patient's lifespan, it may be appropriate to avoid initiating or escalating therapy. The target level for optimal intraocular pressure must be adjusted downward if added risk factors are present or if previous damage occurred at low pressures.

INDICATIONS FOR ESCALATION OF THERAPY

As with initiation of therapy, the first step in determining the need for an increase in therapy is to assess what constitutes an acceptable pressure in the involved eye. Primary factors to consider remain the appearance of the optic disc and visual field appearance, along with other predisposing risk factors and systemic conditions. A compelling indication for escalation of therapy is progression of disc damage with visual field loss under the current treatment regimen. Other indications for escalation are elevation of intraocular pressure to a level that has previously caused damage or to a level judged likely to cause eventual visual damage.

LIFESTYLE ISSUES

Restrictions of use of the eyes has not been shown to improve intraocular pressure; in fact, accommodation acts to reduce intraocular pressure.[4] Stress effects have been studied by creating a stresslike syndrome with stimulants and the converse with sedatives.[30] Clinically meaningful changes in intraocular pressure do not result, and there is no clear evidence to support the idea that stress increases the difficulty of maintaining intraocular pressure control in patients with open angles. Exercise does not make intraocular pressure

more difficult to control and it actually decreases transiently.[24,39]

The effect of caffeine on intraocular pressure is modest and is little different from that experienced in drinking a comparable amount of fluid without caffeine.[26] Ethanol ingestion significantly reduces intraocular pressure and alcohol restriction is not necessary to control glaucoma.[29]

Systemic drugs are frequently a source of concern in patients with open-angle glaucoma, particularly drugs with anticholinergic (atropinelike) action. These include preanesthetic agents, psychotropic medications, antiparkinsonism drugs, antihistamines, and antispasmodic drugs for gastrointestinal problems. As a rule, these agents do not represent a concern in open-angle glaucoma patients.[17] The risks of use of such agents in patients with narrow angles is a separate issue and is discussed in Chapter 65.

MEDICAL THERAPY ALTERNATIVES

Options include topical beta-adrenergic blocking agents, adrenergics, miotics, and systemic carbonic anhydrase inhibitors. Detailed discussion of these agents may be found in Section III. Hyperosmotic agents are valuable for temporary control of acute pressure elevations but are not useful for chronic therapy.

Beta Blockers

These agents represent a valuable advance in the management of open-angle glaucoma. The efficacy and minimal ocular side effects of timolol coupled with the need for only once or twice daily use rapidly led to its widespread acceptance. Recently, levobunolol[44] and betaxolol[9] have become available.

Of considerable concern is the potential for respiratory problems in predisposed individuals due to the beta$_2$-blocking action of the nonspecific beta-blocking agents. Respiratory difficulties appear to be generally circumvented with a beta$_1$-specific agent, such as betaxolol.[43]

Adrenergic Agents

Advantages of using adrenergic agents include the convenience of once or twice daily usage and the lack of significant effects on accommodation. Topical allergic reactions are often the limiting factor in their use. Both a follicular conjunctivitis and an unsightly red eye resulting from reactive hyperemia are common problems. Of special concern is the potential for epinephrine maculopathy in the aphakic and pseudophakic population,[22] limiting the clinical use of adrenergics after cataract surgery. This complication occurs in approximately 20% of such patients and is almost always reversible when the drug is discontinued.

Dipivefrin, a prodrug of epinephrine, has better corneal penetration than epinephrine. As a result, the drug is effective in a much lower topical concentration than epinephrine. Dipivefrin is often better tolerated topically with a lower incidence of allergic reactions.[48] It also causes fewer systemic side effects than other epinephrine compounds.

Miotics

These agents may be divided into short-acting and long-acting groups. Pilocarpine is the mainstay among the short-acting drugs and echothiophate has been the most commonly used of the long-acting ones.

The popularity of pilocarpine drops over a period of many years has resulted from their efficacy, their limited potential for producing topical allergy, and relative lack of systemic side effects.

Major limitations in the use of short-acting miotics relate to the need for a frequent dosage; this represents a significant inconvenience to patients, and in addition greatly increases the potential for poor compliance. Younger patients experience fluctuating myopia and ciliary spasm. Elderly patients with lens opacities may experience reduced vision associated with miosis. Such effects can be incapacitating and as a result, these two groups of patients are often unable to tolerate short-acting miotics.

In an effort to circumvent the need for frequent dosage, a pilocarpine gel (Pilopine) has been developed that may be used daily at bedtime. For 18 hours or more after instillation, the efficacy of the drug is similar to that of 4% pilocarpine drops while providing the convenience of once daily dosage.[14] Limitations of the gel include blurred vision at night and occasionally in the morning. This may be due to both the use of an ointment and intense miosis and myopia, which may persist into the morning hours of activity. There is some uncertainty about 24-hour effectiveness, leading to the suggestion that pressures should be measured just before nighttime administration.[27] Superficial corneal opacities are common but rarely interfere with vision.

Ocusert, a membrane-controlled delivery system placed in the cul-de-sac, releases pilocarpine continuously by diffusion at a predetermined dosage rate. Advantages include better compliance (with the need to change only weekly), less miosis,

less induced myopia, and theoretically better diurnal intraocular pressure control than drops.[36] Although this is an excellent alternative when tolerated, insertion and removal difficulties, as well as retention problems, have tended to limit its use to prepresbyopic patients who are unable to tolerate drops.

Despite greater efficacy and convenience, long-acting miotics are infrequently used because of their cataractogenic effect in phakic patients and their potential to cause retinal detachment, a significant concern in the aphakic population. However, these drugs can be very effective and useful in glaucoma in aphakia or pseudophakia.

Carbonic Anhydrase Inhibitors

Commonly used preparations are acetazolamide tablets and slow-release capsules, and methazolamide tablets. Carbonic anhydrase inhibitors are often administered before consideration of laser trabeculoplasty or filtration surgery. Their use should be tempered by the realization that side effects are frequent, at times severe, and may not be recognized by the patient as being drug-related.

A common symptom complex includes depression with associated personality changes, fatigue, lethargy, malaise, anorexia, weight loss, and loss of libido. Paresthesias and gastrointestinal disturbances are also frequent. Kidney stones are an additional concern. An especially troublesome problem is the propensity of carbonic anhydrase inhibitors to cause blood dyscrasias.[13] These medications should not be used in patients with known allergy to sulfa drugs. With the noninvasive alternative of laser trabeculoplasty, ophthalmologists now are less likely to press their patients to continue with carbonic anhydrase inhibitors when they are poorly tolerated.

THE INITIAL THERAPEUTIC AGENT

Beta-blockers are often selected as the agent with which to initiate treatment. Although it is controversial whether they represent the best alternative, their relatively high efficacy combined with minimal ocular side effects make them an attractive choice.

Adrenergic agents, especially dipivefrin with its somewhat reduced tendency for topical allergy, also represent a valuable initial treatment alternative. Miotics are less often used as the initial drug of choice. The combination of increased ocular side effects and the need for a more frequent dosage schedule leads to relatively poor patient acceptance and reduced compliance. Nonetheless, miotics are very effective and often represent a mainstay of therapy, especially where the other agents alone are inadequate to control pressure. Carbonic anhydrase inhibitors are seldom chosen as the initial drug when considering long-term glaucoma therapy because of their frequent and troublesome side effects.

UNILATERAL TRIALS

Efficacy may be assessed by a therapeutic trial involving treatment of one eye while monitoring the other eye as a control. Such trials permit assessment of the efficacy of individual drugs; allow discontinuation of ineffective agents; and thus avoid unnecessary side effects, inconvenience, and cost.[35] Unilateral trials may also prevent the abandonment of a drug thought to be ineffective, when in reality it is not; for example, where diurnal swings in pressure mask the actual pressure-lowering benefit.

Unilateral trials require that both eyes have a similar initial intraocular pressure or a consistent ratio between the two eyes. It is also assumed that both eyes have similar diurnal and long-term fluctuations. This is often not the case, especially when one eye has developed progressive difficulty with control of intraocular pressure over a short period of time. Pilocarpine is an ideal drug for unilateral testing, having a direct effect on the eye in which it is instilled, with no measurable crossover effect on pressure in the fellow eye. Extra visits are at times required with unilateral trials because there is a need to verify that the previously untreated control eye is also controlled after medication has been added.

Patients should be taught to occlude the nasolacrimal duct or, at least, to keep the eyelids closed gently after each drop instillation. These maneuvers have each been shown to markedly increase ocular absorption and decrease systemic absorption of eye drops.[49] Five or more minutes between drop instillations is recommended to avoid immediate dilution effects that are proportional to the volume of each drug added.[34] In addition, the cul-de-sac is capable of retaining less than the actual volume of one drop.

MULTIPLE DRUG THERAPY

When therapy with a single agent is inadequate to control intraocular pressure, combined treatment is indicated. Generally, a second agent is not fully additive to the first when the reductions of intraocular pressure provided by each agent separately are compared. The additive benefit of two agents depends to some extent on whether they have a similar mechanism of action in reducing intraocular pressure. A unilateral therapeutic trial is recommended when additional topical agents are required for glaucoma control.

Beta-blockers and adrenergics are attractive to consider when initiating combined therapy because they have limited topical side effects. Unfortunately, adrenergic agents may have only a modest effect when added to beta-blocker therapy.[11,42] In fact, it has been questioned whether there is any clinically significant added benefit of the addition of an adrenergic agent to a nonselective beta-blocker.[40] If a large reduction in intraocular pressure will obviously be necessary to control pressure, then miotics or carbonic anhydrase inhibitors are more appropriate. On the other hand, if only a slight additional reduction in pressure appears to be required, adrenergics may prove satisfactory. The effect of the two drugs is the same whether they are administered 10 minutes or 4 hours apart.[42]

Because of the generally small incremental decrease in intraocular pressure in relation to spontaneous intraocular pressure variations, it becomes difficult to assess clinically whether the addition of adrenergics to beta-blockers has provided any benefit. Recent evidence suggests that adrenergics in conjunction with betaxolol, a relatively specific beta$_1$-blocker, may have a greater additive effect than that seen in conjunction with nonspecific beta-blockers.[1,46]

Beta-blockers and miotics are quite useful in combination for reducing intraocular pressure despite the fact that their effects are not fully additive.[20] They represent a rational combination since beta-blockers reduce aqueous inflow and miotics improve outflow.

Beta-blockers and carbonic anhydrase inhibitors are used effectively together to reduce intraocular pressure but their effects are only partially additive,[8] as may be expected, since both drugs reduce aqueous secretion. Miotics and adrenergics in combination may provide a partially additive effect.[15] Miotics and carbonic anhydrase inhibitors in combination may be useful,[16] probably because miotics increase aqueous outflow, whereas carbonic anhydrase inhibitors reduce inflow.

A typical sequence of drug additions is as follows. Initial treatment with a beta-blocker may be followed by the addition of an adrenergic agent if only a small additional pressure reduction is required. If a large intraocular pressure reduction is required, miotics are a more effective second class of agents. If control remains inadequate with the use of beta-blockers and miotics, adrenergics may then be added. If intraocular pressure control is still inadequate, carbonic anhydrase inhibitors can be added to maximize medical therapy. The additive effect of each additional agent can become difficult to assess when multiple agents are used. This assessment may be facilitated by a unilateral therapeutic trial when topical agents are introduced.

MAXIMAL MEDICAL THERAPY

The term "maximal medical therapy" is used to indicate that no further escalation of medical treatment is available or appropriate. Because the next step in escalation of therapy involves tissue damage with laser or an invasive surgical alternative, considerable significance is attached to the term.

Maximal medical therapy should not be interpreted to mean that every patient must be on a combination of the strongest strength of beta-blockers, miotics, adrenergics, and carbonic anhydrase inhibitors before considering a nonmedical approach to treatment. Many factors must be considered for any given patient when establishing what constitutes maximal medical therapy.

Lack of efficacy of a drug indicates that it should be discontinued and its inclusion as part of the regimen not be necessary to regard the patient as being maximally treated. An effort should be made, therefore, to determine whether an added medication is truly lowering intraocular pressure.

Lack of tolerance is another factor altering the criteria of maximal medical therapy. Medical contraindications may preclude the use of various agents; a common example is the use of nonselective beta-blockers in asthmatics. Ocular side effects may also make a drug intolerable, an especially frequent problem with miotics in young people. At times, systemic side effects so alter the quality of life that continued drug usage is inappropriate, a problem commonly encountered with carbonic anhydrase inhibitors.

Lack of compliance is also an important factor. When the necessary routine for administration of drops is imposed on a busy or overly casual lifestyle, drops may be taken so infrequently that for practical purposes their usage is meaningless. This is a common problem with pilocarpine. Under such circumstances, maximal therapy must be defined as the maximum that will be taken in a meaningful way. For example, the ophthalmologist might need to regard the intraocular pressure measured in the absence of pilocarpine as the clinically significant one, despite an apparently "good" pressure measured soon after the patient has used it, if compliance with it is admittedly poor. Often, poorly compliant patients will use their prescribed medications diligently before an office appointment, and they should be questioned carefully about this if glaucomatous damage progresses despite an apparently controlled intraocular pressure.

Lack of attendance must also be considered when defining maximal medical therapy. At times patients are unwilling or unable to keep appointments to permit assessment of the efficacy of therapy. Not uncommonly, poor attendance is combined with poor compliance. Such behavior requires more serious consideration of laser and surgical therapeutic options, which are less reliant on consistent patient cooperation.

LASER TRABECULOPLASTY

Noninvasive laser therapy has filled an important gap between maximal medical therapy and filtration surgery (see Chapter 31).[47] Because of the morbidity associated with filtration surgery, many patients were previously maintained on maximal medical therapy despite poorly tolerated side effects. For the same reason, patients with borderline pressures and the associated increased risk of further field loss were also maintained on medical therapy. Laser trabeculoplasty permits an escalation of therapy in these difficult situations without exposure to the risks of invasive surgery.[41]

Laser trabeculoplasty should be considered as an alternative in an open-angle glaucoma patient before proceeding to filtration surgery because of its more favorable risk-benefit ratio. Although its place is well defined in patients who would otherwise undergo filtration surgery, its role in replacing medical therapy is less clear. The issue is currently controversial, but a case may be made for using it in place of long-term carbonic anhydrase inhibitor therapy when the latter is poorly tolerated. When miotics limit useful vision to such an extent that they severely alter the quality of life, laser trabeculoplasty may again be considered as a reasonable treatment alternative.

CONVENTIONAL SURGICAL THERAPY

Invasive filtration surgery can ideally provide lifelong control of glaucoma, with unchanged visual acuity and no glaucoma medications. On the other hand, complications or failure of surgery may result in further decrease in vision, visual field loss, or blindness. Because of the potential for major ocular complications, invasive and destructive surgical procedures are currently reserved for patients who have had laser trabeculoplasty and continue to have inadequate pressure control and progressive glaucomatous optic nerve or visual field damage despite maximally tolerated medical therapy.

Filtration surgery involves potential complications that represent a major threat to visual function. The risks of endophthalmitis, vitreous hemorrhage, suprachoroidal hemorrhage, persistent hypotony leading to chronic macular edema, and late bleb infections, illustrate the seriousness of the decision to operate. Cataract development or progression is a common risk in filtration surgery. Whereas the cataract does not represent a permanent threat to vision, cataract removal in these complicated eyes does create new risks and may lead to failure of previously successful filtration surgery.

Among the surgical alternatives, filtering operations are currently regarded as the initial procedure (see Chapter 35). Trabeculectomy is the most frequently chosen procedure.[45] Because it is a guarded procedure done under a scleral flap, complications associated with postoperative flat chambers and cataracts are reduced.[38] On the other hand, long-term postoperative intraocular pressure tends to be higher than in the full-thickness procedures.[25]

Full-thickness procedures, such as trephination, thermal sclerostomy, and posterior lip sclerectomy, are generally reserved for patients with advanced damage, in whom a very low intraocular pressure is desired. Full-thickness procedures also represent an alternative when trabeculectomy has failed. The use of setons is typically limited to the difficult secondary glaucomas,[23] although they are occasionally used in open-angle glaucoma after repeated failure of conventional filtration surgery.[28]

Cyclodestructive procedures, which destroy healthy ocular tissue, are not routinely employed as the initial surgical procedure but are generally considered as a last resort after other surgical measures have failed. Cyclocryotherapy has proven effective in control of intraocular pressure. Severe pain following the procedure, the tendency to cause a persistent smoldering iritis, as well as the risks of macular edema and phthisis bulbi all contribute to the limitation of cyclocryotherapy to eyes that have proven recalcitrant to control by filtration surgery.[7]

Therapeutic ultrasound and transscleral cyclophotocoagulation are currently being evaluated as alternatives to cyclocryotherapy. Their relative roles in this regard should become more clear with long-term experience. Transpupillary argon laser cyclophotocoagulation can be effective, but its use is typically restricted to those few eyes with large sector iridectomies, permitting exposure of enough ciliary processes to provide a meaningful area of treatment.

Cyclodialysis creates a cleft between the scleral spur and ciliary body providing a communication between the anterior chamber and the suprachoroidal space. The risks of hyphema and persistent hypotony have significantly limited enthusiasm for the procedure.[10,33]

MONITORING LIMITATIONS

Therapeutic decisions are based on information obtained from our diagnostic and monitoring techniques. Inherent inadequacies in these techniques limit the quality of our decisions.

Diurnal pressure variations may be as great as 6 mm Hg in the normal population and as high as 30 mm Hg in those with open-angle glaucoma,[21] illustrating the limitations of random office pressure measurements. Due to time constraints and financial limitations, patients are often reluctant to submit to office diurnal curves on a sufficiently regular basis to permit their use as a routine monitoring tool.

For practical purposes, pressures are rarely assessed at times other than office hours, but attempts should at least be made to schedule measurements at different times of the day at different appointments to obtain a partial profile of diurnal variation. Intraocular pressure measurements toward the end of a dosage schedule, just before the administration of the next dose, provide a better measure of medical control than pressures taken shortly after a drug is given.

We are generally left with random daytime pressure measurements as the basis for making decisions about changes in therapy. Our therapeutic decisions are necessarily compromised because they are based on such limited information relative to pressure.

The presence of optic disc damage, as well as its progression, can be difficult to identify in two groups of patients. In myopic patients, it is difficult to identify and monitor glaucomatous changes because of physiologically large cups, tilting of the disc, myopic conus, and peripapillary atrophy. In cases of advanced glaucoma where extensive disc damage has occurred, it may not be possible to document alterations in the thin, atrophic or absent rim of glial tissue. Because progressive changes in disc appearance in these patients are difficult to identify or interpret, the value of the optic nerve as a parameter to follow in making therapeutic decisions may be limited. Assessment of the optic nerve is improved by using stereophotography to document the appearance of the disc. However, recent advances in computerized optic disc topography (see Chapter 23) may provide useful and important measurements for assessment of optic nerve damage or progression. The clinical usefulness of these techniques requires greater experience.

Visual fields, as a subjective psychophysical test, have several inadequacies for making therapeutic decisions. The value of field testing is limited in some patients because of difficulty with cooperation. A major additional problem involves the spontaneous short-term and long-term fluctuation innate in field testing.[12] This fluctuation sets limits on our ability to identify visual field changes. Fluctuation is typically greater in disturbed areas in glaucoma fields, further limiting the value of visual fields as a means of determining the need for escalation of therapy.[5]

With extensive visual field loss approaching or splitting fixation, monitoring for progressive field loss becomes an inadequate and possibly inappropriate tool for making therapeutic decisions. Under such circumstances, the monitoring method may only provide the answer to a need for increase in therapy after additional critical damage has occurred. For the same reason, the monitoring of small islands of residual vision is of limited value in making therapeutic decisions. Attempts are being made to circumvent this problem with static threshold perimetry using fine grid patterns to evaluate the central visual field. However, the major difficulty in these patients with extensive damage is the variability in visual field testing and the lack of functional visual reserve to prevent progression and loss of central fixation.

Intraocular pressure at times may be the only meaningful parameter to follow. Often, this occurs in advanced glaucoma with badly damaged discs and advanced field loss. Further damage to the optic nerve or visual field becomes either too subtle to identify or, if identified, represents a devastating progression of loss. It becomes especially important in the therapy of such patients to maintain as low an intraocular pressure as feasible to provide insurance against further loss.

COMPLIANCE

Patients will often volunteer that they do not comply with the prescribed medical regimen. At the same time they will freely admit that they are careful to take their drops before their visit to the ophthalmologist's office. When such patients can be clearly identified and the behavior is not amenable to correction, some other form of therapy such as laser trabeculoplasty or filtering surgery can be recommended.

A troublesome situation arises in the group of patients who do not admit to substantial defaulting; such a situation arises in a disturbingly large number of patients.[19] One study, using a pilocarpine eye drop monitor, demonstrated that subjects took a mean of 76% of their eyedrops, but at the same time the subjects reported that they took 97% of the prescribed doses.[18] Ophthalmologists are often not able to distinguish adequately patients with a low rate of compliance. These findings may explain why some patients develop progressive visual field loss in spite of apparently good intraocular pressure control under therapy. Compliance is somewhat enhanced in such patients when they are made fully aware of the nature of the glaucomatous process and the ramifications of lack of compliance.[37]

REFERENCES

1. Allen, RC, and Epstein, DL: Additive effect of betaxolol and epinephrine in primary open-angle glaucoma, Arch Ophthalmol 104:1178, 1986
2. Armaly, MF: The Des Moines population study of glaucoma, Invest Ophthalmol Vis Sci 1:618, 1962
3. Armaly, MF: Ocular pressure and visual fields, Arch Ophthalmol 81:25, 1969
4. Armaly, MF, and Burian, HM: Changes in the tonogram during accommodation, Arch Ophthalmol 60:60, 1958
5. Bebie, H, Fankhauser, F, and Spahr, J: Static perimetry: accuracy and fluctuation, Acta Ophthalmol 54:339, 1976
6. Becker, DB: Diabetes mellitus and primary open-angle glaucoma, Am J Ophthalmol 71:1, 1971
7. Bellows, AR, and Grant, WM: Cyclocryotherapy in advanced inadequately controlled glaucoma, Am J Ophthalmol 75:679, 1973
8. Berson, FG, and Epstein, DL: Additive effect of timolol and acetazolamide in the treatment of open-angle glaucoma, Am J Ophthalmol 92:788, 1981
9. Boger, WP III, Puliafito, CA, Steinert, RF, and Langston, DP: Long-term experience with timolol ophthalmic solution in patients with open-angle glaucoma, Ophthalmology 85:259, 1978
10. Chandler, PA, and Maumenee, AE: A major cause of hypotony, Trans Am Acad Ophthalmol Otolaryngol 65:563, 1961
11. Cyrlin, MN, Thomas, JV, and Epstein, DL: Additive effect of epinephrine to timolol therapy in primary open-angle glaucoma, Arch Ophthalmol 100:414, 1982

12. Fankhauser, F, and Bebie, H: Threshold fluctuations, interpolations and spatial resolution in perimetry, Doc Ophthalmol Proc Series 19, 295, 1979

13. Fraunfelder, FT, Meyer, SM, Bagby, GC, Jr, and Dries, MW: Hematologic reactions to carbonic anhydrase inhibitors, Am J Ophthalmol 100:79, 1985

14. Goldberg, I, et al: Efficacy and patient acceptance of pilocarpine gel, Am J Ophthalmol 88:843, 1979

15. Harris, LS, Mittag, TW, and Galin, MS: Aqueous dynamics of pilocarpine-treated eyes. The influence of topically applied epinephrine, Arch Ophthalmol 86:1, 1971

16. Havener, WH: Ocular pharmacology, ed 5, St. Louis, 1983, The CV Mosby Co

17. Hiatt, RL, et al: Systemically administered anticholinergic drugs and intraocular pressure, Arch Ophthalmol 84:735, 1970

18. Kass, MA, Gordon, M, and Meltzer, SW: Can ophthalmologists correctly identify patients defaulting from pilocarpine therapy? Am J Ophthalmol 101:524, 1986

19. Kass, MA, et al: Compliance with topical pilocarpine treatment, Am J Ophthalmol 5:515, 1986

20. Keates, EU: Evaluation of timolol maleate combination therapy in chronic open-angle glaucoma, Am J Ophthalmol 88:565, 1979

21. Kitazawa, Y, and Horie, T: Diurnal variation of intraocular pressure in primary open-angle glaucoma, Am J Ophthalmol 79:557, 1975

22. Kolker, AE, and Becker, B: Epinephrine maculopathy, Arch Ophthalmol 79:552, 1968

23. Krupin, T, et al: Filtering valve implant surgery for eyes with neovascular glaucoma, Am J Ophthalmol 89:338, 1980

24. Lempert, P, Cooper, K, Culver, JF, and Tredici, TJ: The effect of exercise on intraocular pressure, Am J Ophthalmol 63:1673, 1967

25. Lewis, RA, and Phelps, CD: Trabeculectomy vs. thermosclerostomy, a five-year follow-up, Arch Ophthalmol 102:533, 1984

26. Leydhecker, W: Influence of coffee upon ocular tension, Am J Ophthalmol 39:700, 1955

27. March, WF, Stewart, RM, Mandell, AI, and Bruce, LA: Duration of effect of pilocarpine gel, Arch Ophthalmol 100:1270, 1982

28. Molteno, ACB: New implant for drainage in glaucoma, clinical trial, Br J Ophthalmol 53:606, 1969

29. Pecson, JD, and Grant, WM: Glaucoma, alcohol, and intraocular pressure, Arch Ophthalmol 73:495, 1965

30. Pecson, JD, and Grant, WM: Sedatives, stimulants, and intraocular pressure in glaucoma, Arch Ophthalmol 72:178, 1964

31. Quigley, HA, and Maumenee, E: Long-term followup of treated open-angle glaucoma, Am J Ophthalmol 87:519, 1979

32. Richardson, KT: Evaluation of medical therapy in chronic glaucoma. In New Orleans Academy of Ophthalmology: Symposium on glaucoma, St. Louis, 1981, The CV Mosby Co

33. Shaffer, RN, and Weiss, DL: Concerning cyclodialysis and hypotony, Arch Ophthalmol 68:25, 1962

34. Shell, JW: The pharmacokinetics of topical glaucoma medications. In Glaucoma: Applied pharmacology in medical treatment, Orlando, FL, 1984, Grune & Stratten

35. Smith, J, and Wandel, T: Rationale for the one-eye therapeutic trial, Ann Ophthalmol 18:8, 1986

36. Smith, SE, Smith, SA, Friedman, AI, and Chaston, JM: Comparison of the pupillary, refractive, and hypotensive effects of Ocusert-40 and pilocarpine eyedrops in the treatment of chronic simple glaucoma, Br J Ophthalmol 63:228, 1979

37. Spaeth, GL: Visual loss in a glaucoma clinic, Invest Ophthalmol Vis Sci 9:73, 1970

38. Spaeth, GL: A prospective, controlled study to compare the Scheie procedure with Watson's trabeculectomy, Ophthalmic Surg 11:688, 1980

39. Stewart, RH, Leblanc, R, and Becker, B: Effects of exercise on aqueous dynamics, Am J Ophthalmol 69:245, 1970

40. Thomas, JV, and Epstein, DL: Timolol and epinephrine in primary open-angle glaucoma, Arch Ophthalmol 99:91, 1981

41. Thomas, JV, Simmons, RJ, and Belcher, CD: Argon laser trabeculoplasty in the management of the surgical glaucoma patient, Ophthalmology 89:187, 1982

42. Tsoy, EA, Meekins, BB, and Shields, MB: Comparison of two treatment schedules for combined timolol and dipivefrin therapy, Am J Ophthalmol 102:320, 1986

43. Van Buskirk, EM, et al: Betaxolol in patients with glaucoma and asthma, Am J Ophthalmol 101:531, 1986

44. Wandel, T, et al: Glaucoma treatment with once-daily levobunolol, Am J Ophthalmol 101:298, 1986

45. Watson, PG, and Grierson, I: The place of trabeculectomy in the treatment of glaucoma, Ophthalmology 88:175, 1981

46. Weinreb, RN, Ritch, R, and Kushner, FH: Effect of adding betaxolol to dipivefrin therapy, Am J Ophthalmol 101:196, 1986

47. Wise, JB: Long-term control of adult open-angle glaucoma by argon laser treatment, Ophthalmology 88:197, 1981

48. Yablonski, ME, et al: Depivefrin in use in patients with intolerance to topically applied epinephrine, Arch Ophthalmol 95:2157, 1977

49. Zimmerman, TJ: Timolol: systemic absorption for different methods of application, Invest Ophthalmol Vis Sci (Suppl)24:90, 1983

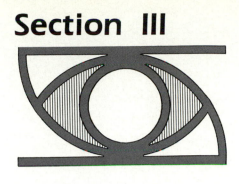

Angle-closure Glaucoma

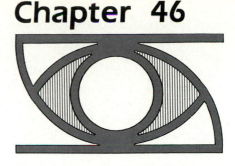

Chapter 46

Angle-closure Glaucoma

Ronald F. Lowe
Robert Ritch

Mechanisms and epidemiology

HISTORICAL INTRODUCTION

The term "acute glaucoma" was first used by Lawrence[48] in 1829 in describing severe ocular inflammation. Mackenzie[65] (1830) emphasized firmness of the eye to touch. The beneficial effect of iridectomy and the observation of progressive optic disc cupping with the newly introduced ophthalmoscope led von Graefe[93] to stress the importance of elevated intraocular pressure, which later became synonymous with glaucoma. Miotic therapy was shown to be valuable soon after the introduction of pilocarpine by Laquer in 1876.

The awareness of angle-closure as a distinct form of glaucoma was slow to develop. Even in 1922, Elliot[33] wrote that acute and chronic glaucoma were merely phases of the same disease. Raeder[77] (1923) classified two main types: one with a shallow anterior chamber and the other with a normal or deep chamber. Curran[26] (1920) and Banziger[15] (1922) introduced the concept of physiologic obstruction of aqueous humor flow through the pupil from the posterior chamber to the anterior chamber (pupillary block). Curran[27] (1931) reported peripheral iridotomy to be successful in eyes with shallow chambers, but not in eyes with normal depths.

The introduction of gonioscopy and the recognition of synechial angle-closure provided the basis for the differentiation of open-angle and angle-closure glaucomas. Barkan[16] described the

opening of closed angles by peripheral iridectomy. Chandler[23] further advanced the understanding of the anatomic relationships underlying the physiologic changes involved in pupillary block. Biometry of eyes with angle-closure glaucoma was investigated by Lowe[61] and by Delmarcelle et al.,[29] while the concept of polygenic inheritance was introduced by Lowe[58,60] and refined by François.[36]

Until Becker[17] introduced acetazolamide, eyes with acute angle-closure glaucoma were prepared for surgery by intensive miotic therapy, purges, and the application of leeches. The use of hyperosmotic agents to withdraw fluid from the eye began with intravenous urea, then intravenous mannitol, and finally oral agents. In the past decade, the development of the argon and Nd:YAG lasers has revolutionized the surgical treatment of angle-closure glaucoma.

ANATOMIC FEATURES

Biometry

Several anatomic features or parameters of the structures of the anterior segment are amenable to measurement, or *biometry*. Taken independently, each of these parameters follows a Gaussian frequency distribution in the general population.[63] If they were combined randomly, there would be a very high incidence of refractive errors. The predominance of emmetropia in the population suggests the existence of compensatory mechanisms. For example, eyes with greater axial lengths usually have flatter corneal curvatures, deeper anterior chambers, and flatter lenses, all of which help to minimize the myopia. Similarly, eyes with shorter axial lengths usually have steeper corneal curvatures, more shallow anterior chambers, steeper lens curvatures, and thicker lenses, which diminish the degree of hyperopia.[82] Failure of compensation leads to refractive errors.

Eyes with primary angle-closure glaucoma have significant biometric differences from normal eyes. Compared to the "average" normal eye, the "average" eye with angle-closure glaucoma has the following characteristics:

1. Smaller corneal diameter[29,87]
2. Smaller radius of anterior corneal curvature (steeper corneal curvature)[29,61,87]
3. Smaller radius of posterior corneal curvature[63]
4. More shallow anterior chamber[29,49,61]
5. Thicker lens[29,61,87]
6. Smaller radius of anterior lens curvature (steeper lens surface)[61,62]
7. More anterior lens position[61,87]
8. Shorter axial length[29,61,87]

These characteristics of eyes with angle-closure glaucoma are also present in many eyes that do not develop angle-closure. The latter function normally and have a normal distribution of refractive errors, although there is a tendency toward hyperopia, which is commonly associated with a shallow anterior chamber and angle-closure glaucoma.[85] The most important biometric feature predisposing to primary angle-closure glaucoma is the relatively forward position of the anterior lens surface in relation to the root of the iris (shallow anterior chamber).[57] In this situation, the iris, particularly the sphincter, is apposed to the lens and impedes aqueous humor flow through the pupil from the posterior to the anterior chamber (relative pupillary block). The ciliary body also tends to be larger when the lens position is more forward and may extend more anteriorly in some eyes with angle-closure glaucoma. The angle is narrower and shallower superiorly and nasally than inferiorly and temporally.

Other anatomic features of eyes with angle-closure glaucoma are less amenable to biometric measurement. Especially important are the width and depth of the anterior chamber angle. The *width* of the angle depends on the convexity of the iris and the length and thickness of the iris root and its site of insertion (that is, posterior or anterior ciliary face or scleral spur). The *depth* of the angle recess depends on the distance between the scleral spur and the junction of the anterior surface of the iris root with the ciliary body. In eyes with crowded anterior segments predisposed to primary angle-closure glaucoma, the angle is characteristically narrow and the recess shallow, whereas in large myopic eyes, the angle is wide and the recess deep.

Anterior Chamber Depth

Central anterior chamber depth is determined primarily by the position of the anterior lens surface, which depends on the lens position along the optical axis and on lens thickness. The depth of the anterior chamber follows a normal distribution curve in the general population.[88] The mean anterior chamber depth of eyes with angle-closure glaucoma is 1.0 mm shallower than the mean anterior chamber depth of "normal" eyes (Table 46-1). Increased lens thickness accounts for 0.35 mm of this, and a more forward lens position accounts for 0.65 mm.[89] The anterior chamber depth of patients with angle-closure glaucoma is distributed about a mean of 1.8 mm. Relative pupillary block is rare when the anterior chamber depth is greater than 2.5 mm.

Anterior chamber depth is not a static dimension but can undergo rapid, transient change.[69] The anterior chamber depth and volume are significantly less in the evening than in the morning in normal eyes, especially peripherally.[71] Mapstone[72] thought that individual differences in diurnal variation may explain why certain eyes develop acute angle-closure and other eyes, anatomically similar, do not.

Significant asymmetry of anterior chamber depths between the two eyes occasionally occurs (Table 46-2). Slight symmetry, however, is common. The greater the difference, the less is the risk of angle-closure glaucoma in the fellow eye. Considerable inequality also suggests the possibility of a change in the position of the lens. Lee et al.[49] found that the anterior chamber volume in eyes with acute angle-closure glaucoma and in eyes with subacute or chronic angle-closure was less than in normal controls.

Lens Position and Thickness

The lens position and thickness are determined primarily by genetic factors influencing the overall shape of the eye. Thicker lenses tend to be situated more anteriorly.[55,82] A very small anterior movement of the lens also occurs with age.[56] Continued growth of the lens during adult life (about 50 years)

Table 46-1 Mean values (with standard deviations) for various ocular dimensions of eyes with primary angle-closure glaucoma (ACG) compared with normal controls

Parameter	Normal	ACG	Authors
Corneal diameter (mm)	11.76 (0.42) 11.05	10.85 (0.37) 10.72	Delmarcelle et al.[29] Tomlinson and Leighton[87]
Anterior corneal radius (mm)	7.67 (0.24) 7.92 (0.29) 7.65	7.61 (0.29) 7.64 (0.25) 7.55	Lowe[61] Delmarcelle et al.[29] Tomlinson and Leighton[87]
Posterior corneal radius (mm)	6.46 (0.26)	6.23 (0.34)	Loe and Clark[63]
True anterior chamber depth (mm)	2.8 (0.36) 2.91 (0.40)	1.8 (0.25) 1.72 (0.22)	Lowe[61] Delmarcelle et al.[29]
Lens thickness (mm)	4.50 (0.34) 4.46 (0.42) 4.67	5.09 (0.34) 5.43 (0.46) 5.23	Lowe[61] Delmarcelle et al.[29] Tomlinson and Leighton[87]
Anterior lens radius (mm)	10.29 (1.78)	7.96 (0.99)	Lowe[59,62]
Axial length (mm)	23.10 (0.82) 22.58	22.01 (1.06) 22.06	Lowe[61] Tomlinson and Leighton[87]
Lens thickness/axial length	1.91 (0.44)	2.27 (0.29)	Markowitz and Morin[72]

Table 46-2 Asymmetry in anterior chamber depth (mm) in 107 cases of primary angle-closure glaucoma

Differences	Percent
0.0-0.1	54
0.2	17
0.3	17
0.4	3
0.5	4
0.6	5

results in about 0.75 to 1.1 mm increased thickness and about 0.4 to 0.6 mm forward movement of the anterior lens surface.[29,61,87] The ratio of lens thickness to axial length of the globe increases with age and is greater in patients with angle-closure glaucoma.[72]

Anterior Lens Curvature

The radius of curvature of the anterior lens surface decreases (the lens surface steepens) as the lens increases in thickness (thicker and more anteriorly situated lenses have a steeper anterior curvature).[59,62] The radius of curvature (mean 10.29 mm; range 7.50 to 15.38 mm) is large compared with the radius of curvature of the anterior corneal surface (range 7.13 to 8.54 mm) and correlates with the anterior chamber depth (Fig. 46-1). The mean radius of anterior lens curvature was 7.96 mm in one series of eyes with angle-closure.[62]

PHYSIOLOGY

Pupillary Block

The fundamental cause of primary angle-closure glaucoma is relative pupillary block, an impedance to the flow of aqueous humor from the posterior to the anterior chamber between the anterior surface of the lens and the posterior surface of the iris. If the anterior lens surface is positioned sufficiently forward, the impeded aqueous humor flow causes pressure in the posterior chamber to become higher than that in the anterior chamber. The peripheral iris is pushed forward, but as long as there is sufficient aqueous humor flow through the pupil, the angle stays open.

Relative pupillary block usually causes no symptoms. However, if it is sufficient to cause appositional closure of a portion of the angle without elevating intraocular pressure, peripheral anterior synechiae may gradually form and lead to chronic angle-closure. If the pupillary block becomes absolute, the pressure in the posterior chamber increases and pushes the peripheral iris farther forward to cover the trabecular meshwork and close the angle with an ensuing rise of intraocular pressure (acute angle-closure glaucoma) (Fig. 46-2).

Several features of the lens, zonules, iris stroma, and musculature play an important role in the development of angle-closure and in determining whether it will become acute or chronic. The ways in which these features interact are complex and still incompletely understood.

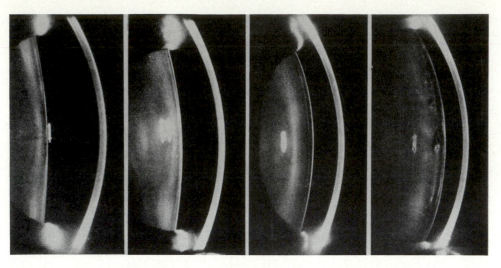

Fig. 46-1 Slit-lamp photographs of series of eyes showing correlation between anterior chamber depth and curvature of anterior lens surface.

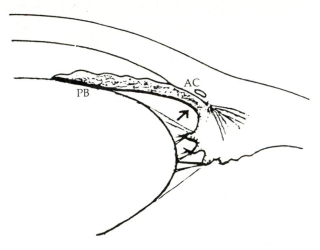

Fig. 46-2 Pupillary block glaucoma. Functional block between lens and iris *(PB)* leads to increased pressure in posterior chamber *(arrow)* with forward shift of peripheral iris and closure of anterior chamber angle *(AC)*.

Role of the Lens and Zonules

Anterior lens surface

In an eye with a shallow anterior chamber, the lens surface is situated more anteriorly than normal and is very steep.[59,62] The lens is usually large, so that the chamber is shallow peripherally and the surface of the lens is close to the peripheral cornea (see Fig. 46-1). The lens pushes the iris forward and increases the resistance to aqueous humor flow between the posterior and anterior chambers.

As the pupil dilates in an eye with this configuration, the lens appears to protrude into or even beyond the pupillary margin. Apposition between the iris and the lens can be readily observed with the slit-lamp. Wide dilation can cause the iris to clear the lens and overcome pupillary block in some eyes with deeper anterior chambers, but in more shallow ones, the sphincter region remains closely applied to the lens.

Stability of the lens

The lens usually maintains a relatively stable position. Anterior movement of the surface caused by lens subluxation or swelling increases pupillary block. Anterior lens movement may occur in some eyes in the prone position, of possible importance in provocative testing and in the etiology of some attacks of angle-closure glaucoma. Miotic-induced ciliary muscle constriction relaxes the zonules, producing anterior lens movement and increased lens thickness and curvature, all of which augment pupillary block.

Role of the Iris

In Europeans, no differences in the susceptibility of blue, hazel, and brown irides to primary angle-closure glaucoma have been reported, but iris texture and thickness must have some influence.[46] A flaccid iris can become more convex than a rigid one. The thickness and rigidity of the iris of Asians and blacks may account for their tendency toward gradual angle-closure.

Pupillary dilation causes the peripheral iris to be thrown into circumferential folds. Chandler[23] postulated that the musculature of the iris exerts a backward pressure against the lens. Early in dilation, the dilator muscle and pigment epithelium move faster than the bulk of the stroma and drag the sphincter more posteriorly to the stroma around the pupil (Figs. 46-3 and 46-4). The folding

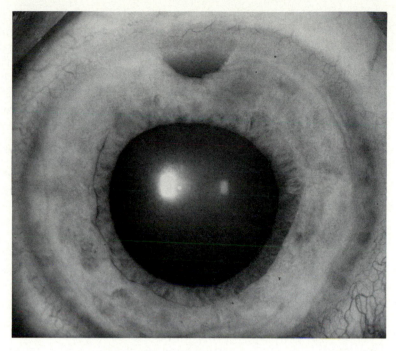

Fig. 46-3 With pupillary dilation the dilator muscle and pigment epithelium move faster than the stroma. Collarette appears closer to pupil.

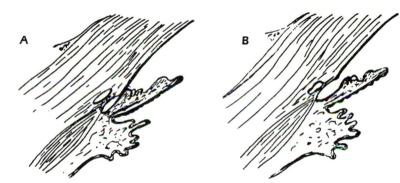

Fig. 46-4 Mydriasis. **A,** Iris folds peripherally and occludes narrow angle. **B,** Iris folds to ridges away from angle and in absence of increased pupillary block angle widens.

of the iris increases its thickness, and in the presence of a narrow angle and iris convexity, contact between the outer and inner walls of the angle, which leads to closure, is more likely.

The folding of the iris in relation to the angle may vary. In some eyes with a short iris root and shallow angle, the iris may fold into the angle and occlude it (plateau iris). In others, the iris folds toward ridges away from the angle, widening it (see Fig. 46-4). These effects may be readily seen after pupillary block and iris convexity have been eliminated by iridectomy, and they account for some of the unexpected results occasionally noted after mydriasis.

Elasticity of the iris determines the degree of convexity induced by pupillary block. Increased tautness caused by pupillary constriction can un-

fold the peripheral iris, reducing angle crowding and relieving angle-closure. However, the iris remains convex while the pupillary block persists.

The dilator and sphincter muscles exert forces in two direction: parallel to the plane of the iris and posteriorly. The resultant directionality of these forces is an important determinant of the degree of pupillary block.

Dilator muscle

The dilator muscle extends beneath the sphincter and is attached to it by cell processes. Dilator muscle activity can be a potent force in pupillary block.[66] With active pupillary dilation, the dilator may move faster than the adjacent stroma, pulling the sphincter backward against the lens. If the anterior chamber is shallow and the iris is pushed forward by the lens, then the posteriorly directed force of the dilator muscle is greater and enhances the apposition of the iris to the lens.

Sphincter muscle

When the pupil is maximally constricted, relative pupillary block is increased, but the posteriorly directed force of the sphincter is minimal. With increasing pupillary dilation, a larger component of the sphincter force is directed posteriorly.[66] After dilation, as the pupil is constricting, the sphincter increases appositional pressure of the iris against the lens. Angle-closure glaucoma may occur as the pupil is constricting, particularly if miotics have been given to reverse dilation.

Miotics may ameliorate or exacerbate angle-closure. By constricting the pupil and drawing the peripheral iris away from the angle, a closed angle may be opened. However, sphincter activity can also increase pupillary block.

Pupillary block is especially likely to occur when the dilator and the sphincter are both stimulated to contract, placing the pupil in a semidilated position.[67] This maximizes the force of contact between the iris and the lens and, at the same time, increases crowding of the angle by the peripheral iris. This has been used as a basis for provocative testing,[68] and explains the occurrence of angle-closure glaucoma when topical epinephrine is added to pilocarpine for the treatment of open-angle glaucoma in eyes with shallow anterior chambers.

The physiologic abnormalities which convert a relative pupillary block to an absolute block are unknown. Although predisposing factors have been repeatedly described (for example, fatigue, anxiety, excitement, close work, or upper respiratory illness), the actual mechanisms, which may include a neural component affecting the iris muscles or vessels, still require elucidation. Mapstone[70] has suggested increased autonomic sensitivity of the sphincter and dilator muscles. Pharmacologically induced cocontraction of the sphincter and dilator muscles provides a potent pupillary blocking force, but spontaneous cocontraction has not been demonstrated in angle-closure glaucoma.

SPECIAL METHODS OF EXAMINATION
Anterior Chamber Depth

Central anterior chamber depth is related primarily to the position of the anterior lens surface. Peripheral anterior chamber depth is also dependent on iris convexity caused by pupillary block.

If a penlight beam is aimed from the temporal side close to the eye at the level of the iris, the entire iris will be illuminated if it is flat and the anterior chamber is deep. If the iris-lens diaphragm is forward and the chamber is shallow centrally, the temporal iris will be illuminated, whereas the nasal iris will be in shadow[92] (Fig. 46-5). This test is useful for nonophthalmologists.

Central anterior chamber depth may be measured with the Haag-Streit slit-lamp.[81] The eyepieces are set for viewing the eye along its optical axis. The slit-beam is turned horizontally and the housing set at 60 degrees temporally. The nasal end of the slit beam is focused on the midpoint of the corneal endothelium. Behind it will be another out-of-focus slit on the lens. The length of the beam is adjusted until the nasal end on the corneal endothelium is in line with the temporal end of the beam on the lens. The length of the slit in millimeters is read from the scale, multiplied by 1.1, and then 0.5 is added. The method is sufficiently accurate for anterior chamber depths between 1.4 and 3.0 mm. Another simple and clinically effective method

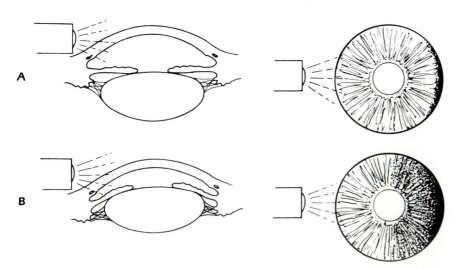

Fig. 46-5 Oblique flashlight illumination for estimating anterior chamber depth. **A,** With deep chamber, nearly entire iris is illuminated. **B,** When iris is bowed forward, only temporal portion is illuminated, and shadow is seen in nasal half.

matches the height of the corneal slit beam to anterior chamber depth.[44]

Pachymetry with the Haag-Streit pachymeter is a quick and accurate method of measurement.[54] The vertical slit beam is split into mobile and stationary halves. When the anterior surface of the cornea is aligned with the anterior lens surface, the scale shows the distance between them. The corneal thickness must be subtracted from this measurement. Direct measurement from posterior cornea to anterior lens is inaccurate. A-scan ultrasonographic measurements of anterior chamber depth are not as accurate as pachymetry. Anterior chamber volume may be measured photogrammetrically by the method of Johnson et al.[45]

More important diagnostically is the depth of the peripheral anterior chamber.[22] The peripheral anterior chamber is shallower in hyperopes and decreases with age.[34] It can be assessed clinically by the method of van Herick et al.[91] (Figs. 46-6 and

46-7). A narrow slit beam is aligned vertically to the peripheral cornea either temporally or nasally. The distance between the corneal endothelium and the surface of the iris is compared with the thickness of the corneal optical section. When the peripheral anterior chamber depth exceeds one-half corneal thickness, the angle is unlikely to close; one-fourth corneal thickness or less suggests a narrow, occludable angle. This is a useful method for population screening.[12]

Gonioscopy

Accurate assessment of the narrow or closed iridocorneal angle demands precise four-mirror indentation gonioscopy.[35,39] Gonioscopy is a dynamic examination, and the Goldmann lens is much less accurate than four-mirror indentation gonioscopy. Pressure on the cornea forces aqueous humor into the angle, widening it to permit viewing over the iris convexity. The presence and extent of synechial

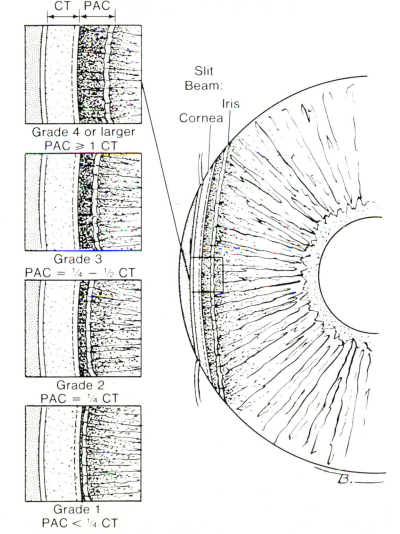

CT   PAC

Grade 4 or larger
PAC ≥ 1 CT

Grade 3
PAC = ¼ − ½ CT

Grade 2
PAC = ¼ CT

Grade 1
PAC < ¼ CT

Slit
Beam:
Iris
Cornea

Fig. 46-6   Method of van Herick et al. for estimating depth of peripheral anterior chamber *(PAC)* by comparing it to adjacent corneal thickness *(CT)*. (From Shields, MB: Textbook of glaucoma, ed 2, Baltimore, 1987, Williams & Wilkins)

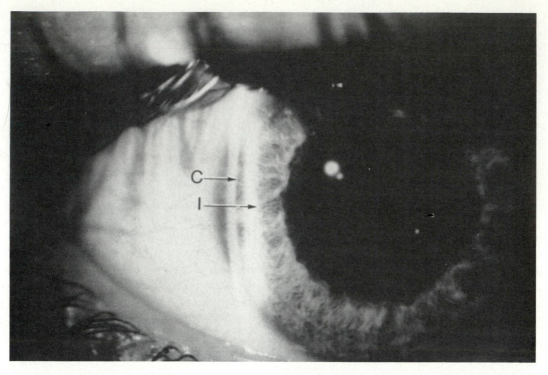

Fig. 46-7 Slit-lamp photograph of van Herick technique for estimation of peripheral anterior chamber depth showing slit beam on cornea *(C)* and iris *(I)*. (From Shields, MB: Textbook of glaucoma, ed 2, Baltimore, 1987, Williams & Wilkins)

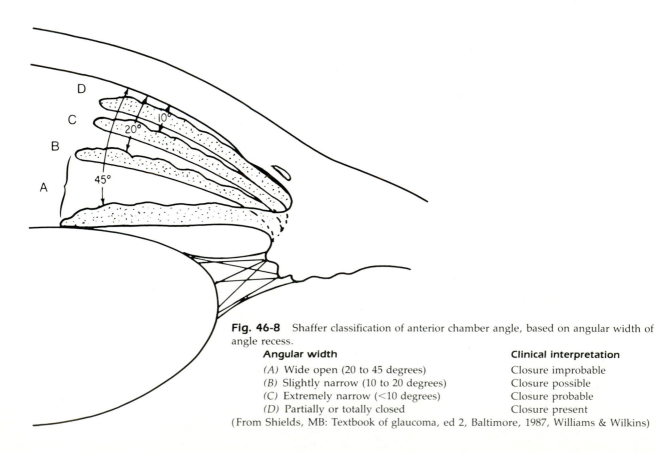

Fig. 46-8 Shaffer classification of anterior chamber angle, based on angular width of angle recess.

Angular width	Clinical interpretation
(A) Wide open (20 to 45 degrees)	Closure improbable
(B) Slightly narrow (10 to 20 degrees)	Closure possible
(C) Extremely narrow (<10 degrees)	Closure probable
(D) Partially or totally closed	Closure present

(From Shields, MB: Textbook of glaucoma, ed 2, Baltimore, 1987, Williams & Wilkins)

closure and the depth of the angle can be determined. The angle should be assessed with respect to iris convexity, width, depth, and the dimensions of peripheral anterior synechiae or the presence of other pathology.

The degree of iris convexity is determined by the degree of pupillary block and the flaccidity of the peripheral iris. In general, the more shallow the anterior chamber, the greater the iris convexity.

The last roll of the iris forms the medial edge of the angle. From this edge the angle recess extends posteriorly and laterally across the iris root to the anteromedial face of the ciliary body, over which it extends forward, past the scleral spur, to its anterolateral border above the trabecular meshwork.

Width of the angle is determined both by iris convexity and the extent to which the iris is pushed forward by the anterior lens surface and by the insertion of the iris root. A completely closed angle may be mistaken for a wide open angle. The slit-lamp beam on the back of the cornea meets the beam running across the iris without a break when the angle is closed. If the beams on the iris and the cornea do not meet directly, but one is displaced alongside the other, at least the entrance to the angle is open.

The depth of the angle depends on the site of insertion of the iris root into the ciliary body or the scleral spur.

Peripheral anterior synechiae may be deep in the angle and hidden from view. Then they usually occupy large arcs of the circumference and form particularly when the angle is narrow and shallow.[19] They may be difficult to see when the angle is very narrow and the iris is very convex. Both appositional closure and, later, peripheral anterior synechiae most commonly form initially in the superior angle.[19] Irregular, more narrow, or tented synechiae may form elsewhere around the angle and must be differentiated from prominent iris processes, which are more common in brown irides.

The amount of pigment deposited on the meshwork should be noted. With subacute and acute attacks, pigment characteristically collects in the inferior angle, but where angle-closure is limited to the superior angle (as with appositional closure), maximum pigmentation may be in that region.[30] This pigment is characteristically blotchy and scattered over the trabecular meshwork. Pigment may also be greater in the superior angle in regressing pigmentary dispersion syndrome, but in this case the pigment is homogenous and localized to the pigmented portion of the trabecular meshwork.

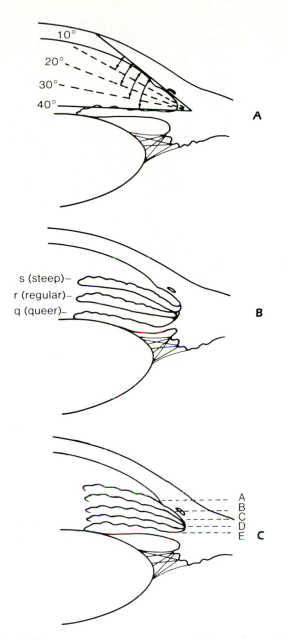

Fig. 46-9 Spaeth's gonioscopic classification of anterior chamber angle. **A,** Angular width of angle recess. **B,** Configuration of peripheral iris. **C,** Apparent insertion of iris root. (From Shields, MB: Textbook of glaucoma, ed 2, Baltimore, 1987, Williams & Wilkins)

The most commonly used grading system is that of Shaffer,[79,80] in which the width of the angle is graded from 0 (closed) to 4 (wide open) (Fig. 46-8). Scheie[78] had earlier proposed a system based on the extent of angle structures visible, a grade 4 angle being closed and a grade 0 angle being wide open. These classifications do not assess angle depth or peripheral iris configuration, which are included in the more detailed descriptive classification proposed by Spaeth[83,84] (Fig. 46-9). Although more difficult to learn initially, it provides a more accurate representation of the anatomic features in angle-closure.

EPIDEMIOLOGY

Inheritance

A more forward position of the lens and a greater-than-average lens thickness are apparently determined by polygenic inheritance.[60] Shallow anterior chambers are commonly observed in close relatives of patients with angle-closure glaucoma.[53,89] In one study, 20% of 95 such relatives were thought to have potentially occludable angles.[84] However, only about 10% of such angles actually develop closure. The reported frequency of angle-closure glaucoma in relatives of probands varies between 1% and 12%.* François[36] calculated that the risk for first-degree relatives developing acute angle-closure is about 2% to 5% and for second-degree relatives from 1% to 2.5%, suggesting a multifactorial cause.

Race

The incidence of acute angle-closure glaucoma varies in different ethnic groups. Narrow angles are found in approximately 2% of whites,[91] whereas the frequency of acute angle-closure glaucoma in whites is somewhat less than 0.1%,[43] being about one fifth as common as open-angle glaucoma. In Australia, it is more common among persons of northern European ancestry than among Italians or Greeks.[52] Chronic angle-closure, however, is much more common than previously believed, because many patients with this disorder are never diagnosed as such unless intraocular pressure rises.

The highest known incidence of angle-closure glaucoma occurs in Eskimos, in whom the frequency is 40 times that of nearby Europeans.[5,10,24,31] Arkell et al.[14] found 2.65% of Eskimos over the age of 40 to have angle-closure glaucoma and 17% over the age of 50 were thought to have occludable angles. Anterior chamber shallowing and narrowing of the angle are age-related.[7,32] Women are affected 3 to 4 times as commonly as men[9,14] and have significantly shallower anterior chambers.[6] In Greenland Eskimos, relatives of probands had an increased incidence of shallow anterior chambers and angle-closure glaucoma.[8] Interestingly, Eskimos living in Denmark had deeper anterior chambers and a lower incidence of angle-closure without a shift in refraction toward myopia, suggestive of environmental influences.[11]

*References 8, 50, 53, 60, 75, 76.

A high prevalence was also found in a tribe of Amazonian Indians.[3] Angle-closure is less common among blacks, who tend to develop chronic angle-closure when they do get the disease.[4,25,94] Although anterior chambers less than 2.5 mm deep occur in Australian aborigines,[74] angle-closure glaucoma was not found in mass screenings of these people.

In Asians, the incidence of acute angle-closure appears to be intermediate between that in whites and blacks. It is more common among Chinese than Malays in Singapore, where its prevalence is greater than that of primary open-angle glaucoma.[51] However, chronic angle-closure is extremely common, and severe damage is often present by the time the patient is initially seen.[37] Blindness resulting from chronic angle-closure is common. More information from different areas and races would enhance our knowledge of the epidemiology of angle-closure glaucoma.

Sex

In Europeans with acute angle-closure glaucoma, women are affected 3 to 4 times as often as men. Women have slightly shallower anterior chambers than men, but the absolute difference is small in comparison to the range of measurements found in primary angle-closure glaucoma. In South African Bantu, about twice as many women as men are affected,[64] whereas among American blacks, the incidence in either sex is reported to be equal.[4]

Age

The anterior chamber decreases in depth and volume with age.[34] The prevalence of primary angle-closure glaucoma also increases with age, peaking between the ages of 55 and 70 years and then declining. The incidence of acute angle-closure glaucoma increases to its maximum between the ages of 55 and 65 years, but onset may occur very late in life. Women are affected 3 times as often as men. In older patients, angle-crowding caused by lens intumescence is a common predisposing factor.

Attacks of primary angle-closure glaucoma are rare before age 45. Angle-closure glaucoma has been reported, however, in children and young adults.[13,20,21,41] In younger patients, one should think of plateau iris or angle-crowding related to the shape or position of the lens (see Chapter 58), and ciliary block (malignant glaucoma) (see Chapter 70). We have seen angle-closure caused by retinopathy of prematurity in a 2-year-old girl, in whom the mechanism was thought to be forward lens movement.

Table 46-3 Mean spectacle refraction of 127 eyes with primary angle-closure glaucoma

| | Diopters | | | | | | | | | |
	0 to 1.0	1.25 to 2.0	2.25 to 3.0	3.25 to 4.0	4.25 to 5.0	5.25 to 6.0	6.25 to 7.0	7.25 to 8.0	8.25 to 9.0	Over 9.0
Hyperopia (+)	42	31	19	14	6	6	—	—	2	—
Myopia (−)	4	1	—	—	—	—	1	1	—	—

Refraction

Angle-closure glaucoma is typically associated with hyperopia, although it may occur in eyes with any type of refractive error. The anterior chamber depth and volume are smaller in hyperopes.[34] In cases of acute angle-closure glaucoma, we have noted that the refractive error in the eye with the attack is very often less than that in the fellow eye, reflecting cataract progression and/or a slight forward shift in the position of the lens.

Chronic angle-closure was reported in members of a family of myopes.[40] We have seen this in 5 patients with myopia as high as 12.0 diopters. All of these patients were black and had circumferential synechial shortening of the angle (creeping angle-closure). Table 46-3 illustrates the spherical equivalents of the refraction of 127 eyes with primary angle-closure glaucoma.

Other Factors

Reports have correlated the frequency of angle-closure attacks with sunspot activity,[42] meteorologic conditions,[90] and seasonal variation in the weather.[28] In Finland, Teikari[86] found a higher incidence of acute angle-closure glaucoma in the autumn and winter than in the spring and summer, an inverse correlation with the mean hours of sunshine daily. There is no correlation of angle-closure with HLA antigens.[38] In contrast to primary open-angle glaucoma, topical steroid testing produces a distribution of intraocular pressures similar to that produced in the general population,[18,47,73] although exceptions have been noted.[1,2]

REFERENCES

1. Akingbehin, AO: Corticosteroid-induced ocular hypertension. I. Prevalence in closed-angle glaucoma, Br J Ophthalmol 66:536, 1982
2. Akingbehin, AO: Corticosteroid-induced ocular hypertension. II. An acquired form, Br J Ophthalmol 66:541, 1982
3. Allen, HF: Amazonian ophthalmology, Am J Ophthalmol 77:426, 1971
4. Alper, MG, and Laubach, JL: Primary angle-closure glaucoma in the American Negro, Arch Ophthalmol 79:663, 1968
5. Alsbirk, PH: Angle-closure glaucoma surveys in Greenland Eskimos, Can J Ophthalmol 8:260, 1973
6. Alsbirk, PH: Anterior chamber depth in Greenland Eskimos. I. A population study of variation with age and sex, Acta Ophthalmol 52:551, 1974
7. Alsbirk, PH: Anterior chamber depth and primary angle-closure glaucoma. I. An epidemiologic study in Greenland Eskimos, Acta Ophthalmol 53:89, 1975
8. Alsbirk, PH: Anterior chamber depth and primary angle-closure glaucoma. II. A genetic study, Acta Ophthalmol 53:436, 1975
9. Alsbirk, PH: Corneal diameter in Greenland Eskimos: anthropometric and genetic studies with special reference to primary angle-closure glaucoma, Acta Ophthalmol 53:635, 1975
10. Alsbirk, PH: Primary angle-closure glaucoma: oculometry, epidemiology, and genetics in a high risk population, Acta Ophthalmol Suppl 54:5, 1976
11. Alsbirk, PH: Anterior chamber depth, genes, and environment: a population study among long-term Greenland Eskimo immigrants in Copenhagen, Acta Ophthalmol 60:223, 1982
12. Alsbirk, PH: Limbal and axial chamber depth variations: a population study in Eskimos, Acta Ophthalmol 64:593, 1987
13. Appleby, RSL, and Kinder, RSL: Bilateral angle-closure glaucoma in a 14-year-old boy, Arch Ophthalmol 86:449, 1971
14. Arkell, SM, et al: The prevalence of glaucoma among Eskimos of northwest Alaska, Arch Ophthalmol 105:482, 1987
15. Banziger, TH: The mechanism of acute glaucoma and the explanation for the effectiveness of iridectomy for the same, Ber Dtsch Ophthalmol Ges 43:43, 1922
16. Barkan, O: Glaucoma: classification, causes and surgical control, Am J Ophthalmol 21:1099, 1938
17. Becker, B: Decrease in intraocular pressure in man by a carbonic anhydrase inhibitor, Diamox, Am J Ophthalmol 37:13, 1954
18. Becker, B, and Kolker, AE: Topical corticosteroid testing in conditions related to glaucoma, Int Ophthalmol Clin 6:1005, 1966
19. Bhargava, SK, Leighton, DA, and Phillips, CI: Early angle-closure glaucoma: distribution of iridotra-

becular contact and response to pilocarpine, Arch Ophthalmol 89:369, 1973

20. Boase, AJ: Acute glaucoma in an adolescent, Am J Ophthalmol 31:997, 1948
21. Brosnan, JD: Primary chronic angle-closure glaucoma in a young woman of 19 years: a case report, Tr Asia-Pac Acad Ophthalmol 4:130, 1973
22. Chan, RY, Smith, J, and Richardson, K: Anterior segment configuration correlated with Shaffer's grading of anterior chamber angle, Arch Ophthalmol 99:104, 1981
23. Chandler, PA: Narrow-angle glaucoma, Arch Ophthalmol 47:695, 1952
24. Clemmeson, V, and Alsbirk, PH: Primary angle-closure glaucoma in Greenland, Acta Ophthalmol 49:47, 1971
25. Clemmesen, V, and Luntz, MH: Lens thickness and angle-closure glaucoma: a comparative oculometric study in South African Negroes and Danes, Acta Ophthalmol 54:193, 1976
26. Curran, EJ: A new operation for glaucoma involving a new principle in the aetiology and treatment of chronic primary glaucoma, Arch Ophthalmol 49:131, 1920
27. Curran, EJ: Peripheral iridotomy in acute and chronic glaucoma: some results after ten years' duration: anatomical classification of glaucoma, Trans Ophthalmol Soc UK 51:520, 1931
28. David, R, Tessler, Z, and Yassur, Y: Epidemiology of acute angle-closure glaucoma: incidence and seasonal variations, Ophthalmologica 191:4, 1985
29. Delmarcelle, Y, et al: Biometrie oculaire clinique (oculometrie), Bull Soc Belge Ophthalmol 172 (fascicule 1), 1976
30. Desjardins, and Parrish: Inversion of anterior chamber pigment as a possible prognostic sign in narrow angles (corresp), Am J Ophthalmol 100:480, 1985
31. Drance, SM: Angle-closure glaucoma among Canadian Eskimos, Can J Ophthalmol 8:252, 1973
32. Drance, SM, et al: Anterior chamber depth and gonioscopic findings among the Eskimos and Indians in the Canadian Arctic, Can J Ophthalmol 8:255, 1973
33. Elliot, RH: A treatise on glaucoma, ed 2, London, 1922, Henry Froude
34. Fontana, SC, and Brubaker, RF: Volume and depth of the anterior chamber in the normal aging human eye, Arch Ophthalmol 98:1803, 1980
35. Forbes, M: Gonioscopy with corneal indentation: a method for distinguishing between appositional closure and synechial closure, Arch Ophthalmol 76:488, 1966
36. François, J: Multifactorial or polygenic inheritance in ophthalmology. In Henkind, P, editor: ACTA: XXIV Intl Cong Ophthalmol. I., Philadelphia, 1985, Lippincott
37. Fujita, K, et al: Epidemiology of acute angle-closure glaucoma, Jpn J Clin Ophthalmol 37:625, 1983
38. Gieser, DK, Wilensky, JT: HLA antigens and acute angle-closure glaucoma, Am J Ophthalmol 88:232, 1979

39. Gorin, G: Re-evaluation of gonioscopic findings in angle-closure glaucoma: static versus manipulative gonioscopy, Am J Ophthalmol 71:894, 1971
40. Hagan, JC, and Lederer, CM, Jr: Primary angle-closure glaucoma in a myopic kinship, Arch Ophthalmol 103:353, 1985
41. Hallett, M: Acute angle-closure glaucoma in a young Negro boy, JAMA 215:293, 1971
42. Hillman, JS, and Turner, JDC: Association between acute glaucoma and weather and sunspot activity, Br J Ophthalmol 61:512, 1977
43. Hollows, FC, and Graham, PA: Intraocular pressure, glaucoma, and glaucoma suspects in a defined population, Br J Ophthalmol 50:570, 1966
44. Jacobs, IH: Anterior chamber depth measurement using the slit-lamp microscope, Am J Ophthalmol 88:236, 1979
45. Johnson, SB, Coakes, RL, and Brubaker, RF: A simple photogrammetric method of measuring anterior chamber volume, Am J Ophthalmol 85:469, 1978
46. Kessler, J: The resistance to deformation of the tissue of the peripheral iris and the space of the angle of the anterior chamber, Am J Ophthalmol 42:734, 1956
47. Kitazawa, Y: Primary angle-closure glaucoma: corticosteroid responsiveness, Arch Ophthalmol 87:724, 1970
48. Lawrence, W: Lectures on surgery: medical and operative, lectures 70-72, Lancet 705, 1829
49. Lee, DA, Brubaker, RF, and Illstrup, DM: Anterior chamber dimensions in patients with narrow angles and angle-closure glaucoma, Arch Ophthalmol 102:46, 1984
50. Leighton, DA: Survey of the first degree relatives of glaucoma patients, Trans Ophthalmol Soc UK 96:28, 1976
51. Loh, RCK: The problems of glaucoma in Singapore, Singapore Med J 9:76, 1968
52. Lowe, RF: Comparative incidence of angle-closure glaucoma among different national groups in Victoria, Australia, Br J Ophthalmol 47:721, 1963
53. Lowe, RF: Primary angle-closure glaucoma: family histories and anterior chamber depths, Br J Ophthalmol 48:191, 1964
54. Lowe, RF: New instruments for measuring anterior chamber depth and corneal thickness, Am J Ophthalmol 62:7, 1966
55. Lowe, RF: Causes of shallow anterior chamber in primary angle-closure glaucoma: ultrasonic biometry of normal and angle-closure glaucoma eyes, Am J Ophthalmol 67:87, 1969
56. Lowe, RF: Anterior lens displacement with age, Br J Ophthalmol 54:117, 1970
57. Lowe, RF: Aetiology of the anatomical basis for primary angle-closure glaucoma: biometrical comparisons between normal eyes and eyes with primary angle-closure glaucoma, Br J Ophthalmol 54:161, 1970
58. Lowe, RF: Primary angle-closure glaucoma: changing concepts of inheritance and environment, Trans Aust Coll Ophthalmol 9:3, 1971

59. Lowe, RF: Anterior lens curvature: comparisons between normal eyes and those with angle-closure glaucoma, Br J Ophthalmol 56:409, 1972

60. Lowe, RF: Primary angle-closure glaucoma: inheritance and environment, Br J Ophthalmol 56:13, 1972

61. Lowe, RF: Primary angle-closure glaucoma: a review of ocular biometry, Aust J Ophthalmol 5:9, 1977

62. Lowe, RF, and Clark, BAJ: Radius of curvature of the anterior lens surface: correlations in normal eyes and eyes involved with primary angle-closure glaucoma, Br J Ophthalmol 57:471, 1973

63. Lowe, RF, and Clark, BAJ: Posterior corneal curvature: correlations in normal eyes and in eyes involved with primary angle-closure glaucoma, Br J Ophthalmol 57:475, 1973

64. Luntz, MH: Primary angle-closure glaucoma in caucasoid and negroid communities, Br J Ophthalmol 57:445, 1973

65. Mackenzie, W: A practical treatise on diseases of the eye, London, 1830, Longman, Rees, Orm, Brown & Green

66. Mapstone, R: Mechanics of pupil block, Br J Ophthalmol 52:19, 1968

67. Mapstone, R: Closed-angle glaucoma: theoretical considerations, Br J Ophthalmol 58:36, 1974

68. Mapstone, R: Provocative tests in closed-angle glaucoma, Br J Ophthalmol 60:115, 1976

69. Mapstone, R: Acute shallowing of the anterior chamber, Br J Ophthalmol 65:446, 1981

70. Mapstone, R: Angle-closure mechanisms in glaucoma, Seminars in Ophthalmology 1:35, 1986

71. Mapstone, R, and Clark, CV: Diurnal variation in the dimensions of the anterior chamber, Arch Ophthalmol 103:1485, 1985

72. Markowitz, SN, and Morin, JD: Ratio of lens thickness to axial length for biometric standardization of angle-closure glaucoma, Am J Ophthalmol 99:400, 1985

73. Masuda, H: The steroid ocular pressure response in the glaucomatous eye, Acta Soc Ophthalmol Jpn 73:2060, 1969

74. Murchland, JB: Anterior chamber depth of eyes of full blood aborigines at a reserve in South Australia, Aust J Ophthalmol 3:56, 1975

75. Paterson, G: Studies on siblings of patients with both angle-closure and chronic simple glaucoma, Trans Ophthalmol Soc UK 81:561, 1961

76. Perkins, ES: Family studies in glaucoma, Br J Ophthalmol 58:529, 1974

77. Raeder, JG: Untersuchungen der Lage und Dicke der Linse im menschlichen Augen bei physiologischen und pathologischen Zustanden nach einer neuen Methode gemessen, Arch f Ophthalmol 112:44, 1923

78. Scheie, HG: Width and pigmentation of the angle of the anterior chamber: a system of grading by gonioscopy, Arch Ophthalmol 58:510, 1957

79. Shaffer, RN: Gonioscopy, ophthalmoscopy, and perimetry, Trans Am Acad Ophthalmol Otolaryngol 64:112, 1960

80. Shaffer, RN: A suggested anatomic classification to define the pupillary block glaucomas, Invest Ophthalmol 12:540, 1973

81. Smith, RJH: A new method of estimating the depth of the anterior chamber, Br J Ophthalmol 63:215, 1979

82. Sorsby, A, et al: Emmetropia and its aberrations, Med Res Council Spec Rep Ser 193, London, 1956, HMSO

83. Spaeth, GL: The normal development of the human chamber angle: a new system of descriptive grading, Trans Ophthalmol Soc UK 91:709, 1971

84. Spaeth, GL: Gonioscopy: uses old and new: the inheritance of occludable angles, Ophthalmology 85:222, 1978

85. Sugar, HS: The mechanical factors in the etiology of acute glaucoma, Am J Ophthalmol 24:851, 1941

86. Teikari, J, Raivio, I, and Nurminen, M: Incidence of acute glaucoma in Finland from 1973 to 1982, v Graefe Arch Klin Exp Ophthalmol 225:357, 1987

87. Tomlinson, A, and Leighton, DA: Ocular dimensions in the heredity of angle-closure glaucoma, Br J Ophthalmol 57:475, 1973

88. Tornquist, R: Shallow anterior chamber in acute glaucoma: a clinical and genetic study, Acta Ophthalmol (Suppl) 39:1, 1953

89. Tornquist, R: Chamber depth in primary acute glaucoma, Br J Ophthalmol 40:421, 1956

90. Tupling, MR, and Junet, EJ: Meteorological triggering of acute glaucoma attacks, Trans Ophthalmol Soc UK 97:185, 1977

91. van Herick, W, Shaffer, RN, and Schwartz, A: Estimation of width of angle of anterior chamber: incidence and significance of the narrow angle, Am J Ophthalmol 68:626, 1969

92. Vargas, E, and Drance, SM: Anterior chamber depth in angle-closure glaucoma: clinical methods of depth determination in people with and without the disease, Arch Ophthalmol 90:438, 1973

93. von Graefe, A: Three memoirs on iridectomy. In Selected monographs, London, 1861, The New Sydenham Society

94. Wilensky, J: Racial influences in glaucoma, Ann Ophthalmol 9:1545, 1977

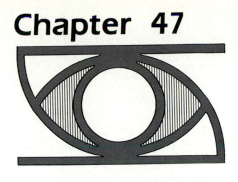

Chapter 47

Angle-closure Glaucoma

Ronald F. Lowe
Robert Ritch

Clinical types

The nomenclature for the various clinically distinct types of primary angle-closure glaucoma used by different investigators has created some confusion, particularly between the European and American literature. This pertains in particular to the terms intermittent, prodromal, subacute, chronic, and creeping.

There are three basic types of primary angle-closure glaucoma: (1) mild forms of angle-closure—intermittent and subacute angle-closure; (2) acute angle-closure; and (3) chronic angle-closure and its variant, creeping angle-closure. In addition, acute or subacute angle-closure can develop with time into chronic angle-closure (Fig. 47-1). Pupillary block is the underlying mechanism in all of these types.

PRIMARY GLAUCOMAS

Intermittent and Subacute Angle-closure Glaucomas

Intermittent angle-closure glaucoma

Intermittent angle-closure defines repeated, brief episodes of angle-closure with mild symptoms and elevated intraocular pressure caused by pupillary block, which resolve spontaneously. Ocular function is normal between attacks. Intermittent angle-closure is often a prelude to acute angle-closure and is probably more frequently partial than complete, affecting particularly the narrower superior part of the angle.[22] Intermittent attacks are most commonly associated with fatigue,

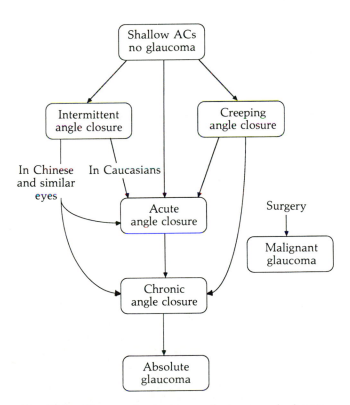

Fig. 47-1 Diagram of various types of primary angle-closure glaucoma and their potential progression.

Table 47-1 *Intermittent angle-closure glaucoma: precipitating factors in 70 patients*

Activity	Number of patients
Near work (reading, sewing, etc.)	20
Cinema and television	13
Fatigue	12
Excitement, anxiety, stress, illness	8
Other activity	8
No cause known	9

Table 47-2 *Relief of symptoms of intermittent angle-closure glaucoma in 45 patients*

Factor providing relief	Number of patients
Sleep	21
Rest	6
Cessation of activity	7
Mild analgesics	5
Other	6

dim light, and using the eyes for near work (Table 47-1).

The symptoms of an intermittent attack are a dull ache in or around one eye and mildly blurred vision. Halos around lights are often not seen unless the patient is outdoors. They are thought to represent stretching of the corneal lamellae, causing the cornea to act as a diffraction grating, producing a blue-green central and yellow-red peripheral halo.[21] Halos that are seen every night are caused by cataracts, corneal disease, or persistently high intraocular pressure. Transient monocular visual loss has also been noted.[37]

The attacks tend to recur under similar circumstances and at about the same time of day or evening. The patient may recognize the cause and avoid or reduce the activity, such as watching television or reading. The attacks last for about half an hour after cessation of the inciting activity. Sleep is so often recognized as beneficial that many patients go to bed early or take a nap to obtain relief (Table 47-2). Amelioration of the attack is attributed to sleep-induced miosis and possibly to decreased intraocular pressure resulting from decreased aqueous humor secretion.[38] If the symptoms persist into the next day, a true attack has developed, and the symptoms are not caused by intermittent angle-closure glaucoma.

Initially, intermittent attacks occur at intervals of weeks or months, but eventually may occur almost nightly. They may continue uneventfully for months or years. Usually only one eye is involved, but bilateral attacks can occur. Because the eyes appear normal between attacks, the diagnosis is frequently missed, and even ophthalmologists may be misled by the patient's self-diagnosis of migraine, sinusitis, anxiety or eyestrain.

Examination reveals shallow anterior chambers, iris bombé, narrow angles, and sometimes an enlarged or oval pupil. Provocative testing (see Chapter 48) may result in angle-closure, elevated intraocular pressure, and reproduction of the patient's symptoms.

The end result of intermittent angle-closure glaucoma usually differs between whites and races with thick, heavily pigmented irides. In whites the attacks are essentially benign and may recur for years without causing damage, but the danger lies in the possibility of the attacks suddenly changing into acute angle-closure glaucoma. Attacks may be accompanied by progressive formation of peripheral anterior synechiae (PAS), leading to chronic angle-closure glaucoma. Laser iridectomy usually cures the glaucoma if the eye is otherwise normal.

In Asians the history may be consistent with intermittent angle-closure glaucoma, but the intraocular pressure will usually be raised and the angle closed by peripheral anterior synechiae to a variable extent, depending on the frequency and severity of the attacks. Asian eyes are more prone to "creeping" angle-closure (see below) and PAS formation. Iridectomy alone may be insufficient to cure the glaucoma.

In the United States black patients also have a greater tendency to develop chronic angle-closure glaucoma, but it is our impression that the anterior chambers are often deeper than those of Asians and have much less iris bombé. Both intermittent and acute attacks are less common in blacks than in Asians. Comparative biometric studies would greatly help to increase our understanding of angle-closure in these groups.

Subacute angle-closure glaucoma

Subacute angle-closure describes a stage in which attacks may be more frequent and prolonged than in intermittent angle-closure, but less so than in acute angle-closure. At least in some cases, this is caused by less than total closure of the angle.[6] Symptoms of blurred vision, pain, and halos may be more marked than in intermittent angle-closure. Attacks may occur over months or years, finally leading to an acute attack. Subacute attacks are much more common in Asians than in whites.

Subacute attacks can cause severe damage without much inflammation. They tend to produce a chronically dilated pupil, mild iris atrophy, PAS, and pigment on the iris close to the inferior angle. Intraocular pressure levels and glaucomatous disc and visual field damage vary according to the severity and duration of the attacks.

Acute Angle-closure Glaucoma

Precipitating events

Various stimuli may trigger the onset of acute angle-closure glaucoma. The response of any one particular eye to these stimuli is highly variable. The physiological factors that convert relative pupillary block to absolute pupillary block remain poorly understood, as are those that determine whether an eye will develop acute or chronic angle-closure. Although pupillary block is the common underlying mechanism, the course of the disease depends on the degree and suddenness of the block, the flaccidity and physiologic responses of the iris, and the width and depth of the anterior chamber angle.

An acute attack of angle-closure glaucoma can lead to irreversible damage. Absolute pupillary block is most commonly triggered when the pupil is middilated, about 3.5 to 6 mm in diameter.[5] In this position, the combination of pupillary block and relaxation of the peripheral iris, allowing its forward displacement into the anterior chamber, are maximal. Mapstone[29] concluded that the posteriorly directed forces of the dilator and sphincter muscles and the stretching force of the sphincter during contraction are greatest when the pupil is middilated.

The most common precipitating events include illness, emotional stress, trauma, intense concentration, and pharmacologic pupillary dilation. The role of emotional stress in inducing acute angle-closure should not be underestimated.[8,10,18] Our most illustrative example was a patient who, after narrowly missing being injured by a grenade thrown into his house during civil strife, immediately developed bilateral attacks. Patients under stress often become depressed, and the initiation of antidepressant therapy, which produces pupillary dilation, is a common trigger (see Chapter 65). However, the warnings in drug package inserts concerning the contraindications of these drugs in patients with "glaucoma" are least recognized as pertaining to those patients for whom they really apply—those patients with unsuspected occludable angles.

Attacks rarely begin simultaneously in both eyes. Minor differences in anterior chamber depth almost invariably result in the eye with the shallower chamber being involved first. Most attacks occur during the evening, beginning mildly and rapidly increasing in severity. Approximately one-third of patients describe episodes of intermittent or subacute angle-closure having occurred before the acute attack. Patients who have had previous intermittent attacks often go to sleep expecting relief, but instead, either the symptoms become worse during the night or the patient awakens with a full-blown attack.

Symptoms and signs

The symptoms of an acute attack result from the sudden, marked elevation of intraocular pressure to as high as 80 mm Hg. Corneal edema results in blurred vision and intense pain and, secondarily, in lacrimation and lid edema. These, in combination with anxiety and fatigue, lead to nausea and vomiting, whereas vasovagal responses cause bradycardia and diaphoresis. Systemic symptoms may be so severe as to mislead the nonophthalmologist, and some patients have actually undergone unwarranted exploratory laparotomies. We saw one patient whose ataxia, blurred vision, and diagnosis of multiple sclerosis disappeared after laser iridectomy.

The diagnosis is usually straightforward (Fig. 47-2). Central visual acuity is reduced and the intraocular pressure is markedly elevated. The lids are swollen and there is conjunctival hyperemia and circumcorneal injection. The cornea is edematous and the pupil usually middilated and vertically oval because of iris sphincter ischemia. The anterior chamber is shallow but usually formed centrally, whereas the midperipheral iris is bowed anteriorly and may touch the cornea peripherally. An inflammatory reaction is present in the anterior chamber.

Corneal edema may initially limit gonioscopic and posterior segment examination, even after the topical application of glycerin. Inability to open the angle with indentation gonioscopy at this stage does not mean that the angle will remain sealed after iridectomy, nor does it accurately reflect the presence or extent of peripheral anterior synechiae (PAS). Examination of the opposite eye is particularly useful in differentiating acute angle-closure glaucoma from neovascular, uveitic or phacolytic glaucoma and usually reveals a shallow anterior chamber and narrow angle.

The optic nerve head may be hyperemic and

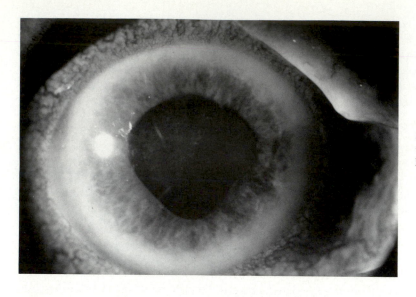

Fig. 47-2 Acute angle-closure glaucoma: intense conjunctival injection, corneal edema, shallow anterior chamber, dilated pupil.

| Number of questions: | 424 | Number of repetitions: | 0 | Date of printout: 4.07.1987 |
| False positive answers (%): | 10 (1/10) | False negative answers (%): | 0 (0/10) | |

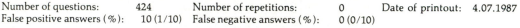

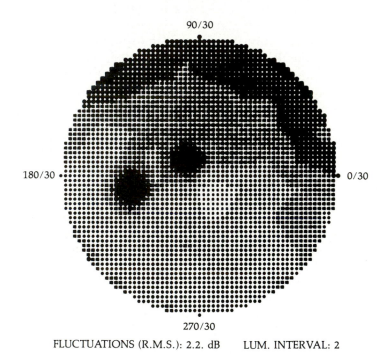

Fig. 47-3 Visual field after prolonged (5 days) acute angle-closure glaucoma showing paracentral scotoma extending into fixation.

FLUCTUATIONS (R.M.S.): 2.2. dB   LUM. INTERVAL: 2

edematous early in the attack. With prolonged attacks or cases in which unrecognized chronic angle-closure glaucoma precedes an acute attack, pallor and cupping, along with visual field damage, may be present. Central retinal vein occlusion may occur as a result of an acute attack[45] or may precipitate one.[4,15,17,33,48]

Visual field changes associated with acute pressure elevation usually show nonspecific constriction or constriction of the upper field.[32] Early loss of central vision, enlargement of the blind spot, and nerve fiber bundle defects may be found (Fig. 47-3).[9,16] After normalization of intraocular pressure, the visual fields may also normalize, or patients may be left with reduced color vision, generalized decreased sensitivity, or specific defects. These may be exaggerated by cataract formation or progression.

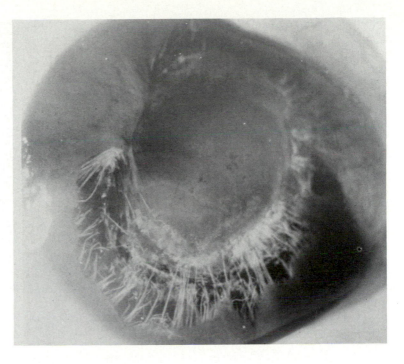

Fig. 47-4 Segmental iris atrophy after severe acute angle-closure glaucoma.

An attack may terminate spontaneously if iris atrophy from tissue necrosis allows aqueous humor to percolate through the iris stroma, equivalent functionally to a spontaneous iridectomy (Fig. 47-4) but more frequently occurs as a result of suppression of aqueous secretion by the high intraocular pressure. Spontaneous termination may also be facilitated by a change in the position of the lens-iris contact, or segmental iris constriction with peaking of the pupil.[36]

Chronic Angle-closure Glaucoma

Chronic angle-closure refers to an eye in which portions of the anterior chamber angle are permanently closed by PAS. Variable and sometimes conflicting terminology has been used to describe somewhat differently appearing forms. The approach to therapy is similar in all of them. The terminology used in this section is an attempt to differentiate the two pathways by which chronic angle-closure can develop.

In the first, iris bombé from relative pupillary block may appositionally close the angle. Prolonged apposition or repeated subacute attacks lead to gradual PAS formation. These usually begin in the superior angle, which is narrower than the inferior angle,[2,30] as pinpoint synechiae reaching to the midtrabecular meshwork and then gradually expanding in width. In early cases, in which appositional closure is present but PAS have not yet formed, we prefer the term *chronic appositional clo-*

sure. This condition can lead to elevated intraocular pressure and glaucomatous disc and visual field damage without PAS formation.[11]

Eyes with progressive PAS formation may eventually develop an acute attack of angle-closure when pupillary block results in closure of the remaining portions of the angle unaffected by PAS. Many cases, however, develop elevated intraocular pressure and glaucomatous damage in the absence of symptoms. The presentation is similar to that of open-angle glaucoma, with progression of glaucomatous cupping and visual field loss. This is the situation most commonly associated in the United States with chronic angle-closure glaucoma. However, eyes with the same appearance but normal intraocular pressure merely constitute an earlier stage.

PAS may also form during an acute attack, remaining after iridectomy has opened the unaffected portions of the angle. These PAS are usually high and broad. When first observed at this stage, it is impossible to determine whether the PAS formed before or during the attack or at both times.

In eyes with darker irides a second mechanism of progressive angle-closure is more common. The closure is circumferential and begins in the deepest portion of the angle. Closure occurs more evenly in all quadrants, so that the angle progressively becomes more shallow. The appearance over time is of a progressively more anterior iris insertion. The PAS gradually creep up the ciliary face to the

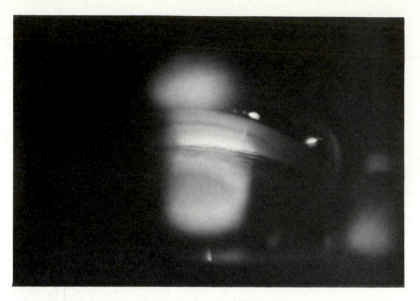

Fig. 47-5 Open angle after laser iridectomy and iridoplasty in patient with plateau iris syndrome. Note dense, blotchy pigment on trabecular meshwork.

scleral spur and then to the trabecular meshwork. Gorin[13] referred to this form as shortening of the angle, although Lowe[24] has termed it *creeping* angle-closure.

Insertion of the iris at or anterior to the scleral spur is rare in young individuals, and in many eyes with angle-closure glaucoma that have such an insertion, creeping angle-closure is the underlying reason for this. Creeping angle-closure is uncommon in whites but much more prevalent in Asians, in whom it ranks high as a cause of blindness. Black patients with angle-closure also tend to have this form. It occurs in eyes with slightly deeper, though still shallow, anterior chambers than are found in acute angle-closure. The gradual shortening of the angle in the presence of iris bombé brings the peripheral iris close to the external angle wall more and more anteriorly, narrowing the gap between the iris and the trabecular meshwork. Eventually, an acute attack may supervene (more commonly in Asians), or the PAS may permanently occlude the trabecular meshwork and lead to elevated intraocular pressure and glaucomatous damage (more commonly in black patients).

The intraocular pressure in eyes with chronic angle-closure may be normal or elevated. As PAS formation progresses in the absence of intermittent attacks, the pressure rises gradually as less and less functional trabecular meshwork becomes available. In eyes with intermittent attacks, the pressure rises more rapidly relative to the extent of PAS formation caused by recurrent damage to the trabecular meshwork by the transient angle-closure.

Dispersed pigment granules collect in the iridocorneal angle where the peripheral iris is in contact with the cornea. Dense blotches of pigment on the meshwork, particularly in the superior angle, or deposits of black pigment in the angle of a lightly pigmented iris are highly suggestive of previous appositional closure (Fig. 47-5). If the angle opens, this deposited line of pigment shows the extent of previous angle closure and can sometimes be a helpful diagnostic feature.

The anterior chamber is quiet and usually deeper than in eyes with primary acute angle-closure glaucoma. The pupil is normal. The gradual elevation of intraocular pressure allows corneal endothelial compensation, and edema is rare. The intraocular pressure is usually less than 40 mm Hg and does not reach the levels found in acute angle-closure glaucoma. Symptoms are absent until the pressure rises high enough to affect the cornea or until extensive visual field damage has occurred. Although iridectomy will eliminate the pupillary block, intraocular pressure often remains elevated, and further medical treatment or surgery is required.

Absolute Glaucoma

Absolute glaucoma refers to an eye with no light perception and a persistently elevated intraocular pressure. The angle initially may be open or closed, but in phakic eyes an intumescent cataract often develops and leads to secondary angle-closure. The time required for a neglected angle-closure attack to cause total blindness is variable and depends on the severity of the acute attack, but appears to be an average of 1 to 2 years.

Treatment is palliative and intraocular surgery is unwarranted. If corneal edema and pain are not relieved by topical beta-adrenergic blocking agents, steroids, and cycloplegics, noninvasive cycloabla-

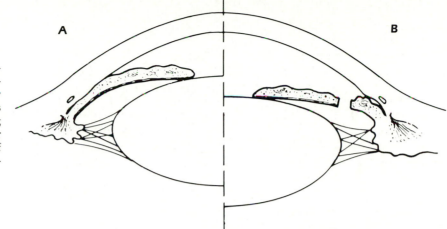

Fig. 47-6 **A,** Pupillary block glaucoma contrasted with **B,** plateau iris syndrome. In latter situation, note relatively deeper central anterior chamber, flat iris plane, patent iridectomy, and bunching up of peripheral iris in anterior chamber angle. (From Shields, MB: Textbook of glaucoma, ed 2, Baltimore, 1987, Williams & Wilkins)

tion may be performed. If this is insufficient or if complications such as phacolytic glaucoma develop, evisceration or enucleation may be necessary. Phthisis bulbi is not an uncommon outcome.

Plateau Iris

Plateau iris *configuration* refers to the anatomic structure in which the iris root angulates forward and then centrally.[45] In many cases the iris root is short and is inserted anteriorly on the ciliary face, so that the angle is shallow and narrow, with a sharp drop-off of the peripheral iris at the inner aspect of the angle. The iris surface appears flat and the anterior chamber is not unusually shallow on slit-lamp examination.

Plateau iris syndrome refers to the development of angle-closure in such an eye even after iridectomy has been performed. Either spontaneously or after dilation, the angle closes because of folding of the peripheral iris into a shortened angle, and some patients may develop acute angle-closure glaucoma[12,26,28,47] (Fig. 47-6). The risk of postoperative pupillary dilation after iridectomy is infrequently realized.

Some element of pupillary block is present before iridectomy in most patients with plateau iris who develop angle-closure glaucoma. As in primary angle-closure, the development of relative pupillary block is caused by increased iris-lens contact. However, because of the nature of the anatomic relationships of the iridocorneal angle structures, the degree of relative pupillary block necessary to induce angle-closure is less than that in primary angle-closure glaucoma; this seems to account for the deeper anterior chamber and flatter iris surface in eyes with angle-closure and plateau iris. Patients with plateau iris who develop angle-closure glaucoma are also somewhat younger than those with primary angle-closure glaucoma.

The last roll of the iris does not necessarily appear clinically as a true plateau, this appearance being more distinctive of the affected eyes of younger patients with normal anterior chamber depth. As a general rule, the older the patient the less prominent the angulation of the peripheral iris and the greater the element of pupillary block. The important diagnostic criterion is the presence of an occludable angle after iridectomy on the basis of the configuration of the iris.

If plateau iris was not diagnosed before iridectomy and intraocular pressure is elevated postlaser, careful gonioscopy should be performed. If the angle is open, secondary damage to the trabecular meshwork or pigment liberation with dilation are the most likely causes. If the angle is closed, the differential diagnosis, besides plateau iris, should include malignant glaucoma, in which the anterior chamber is extremely shallow; PAS, which can be ruled out by indentation goniscopy; or incomplete iridectomy.

Most patients with plateau iris configuration who develop angle-closure glaucoma are cured by iridectomy and elimination of pupillary block and do not develop plateau iris syndrome. In some eyes, however, the angle remains appositionally closed even after iridectomy, whereas in others, it is open but closes when the pupil is dilated. The term "plateau iris syndrome" is used to describe those patients in whom the angle remains capable of closure by angle crowding even after pupillary block has been eliminated by iridectomy.

We have recently differentiated two subtypes of plateau iris syndrome. In the complete syndrome, which comprises the classic situation, intraocular pressure rises when the angle closes with pupillary dilation. In the incomplete syndrome, intraocular pressure does not change. The important factor differentiating the complete and incomplete

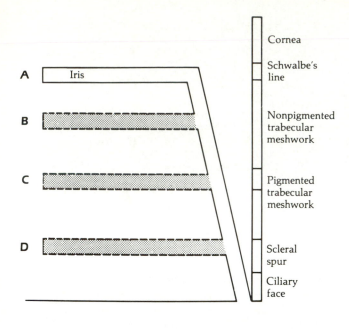

Fig. 47-7 Schematic representation of plateau iris. Angle is occludable when pupil is dilated, but it is height of plateau (extent to which iris stroma protrudes anteriorly), which determines level of lateral iridocorneal angle wall that will be occluded and thus whether intraocular pressure will rise. **A,** Complete plateau iris syndrome. Iris will occlude trabecular meshwork up to Schwalbe's line and intraocular pressure will rise. **B** and **C,** Incomplete plateau iris syndrome. Iris will occlude angle to level of midmeshwork. The lower on the trabecular meshwork that the iris reaches, the less likely a rise in intraocular pressure. **D,** Low plateau. Angle will close only to top of scleral spur.

syndromes is the level of the iris stroma with respect to the angle structures, or the "height" to which the plateau rises (Fig. 47-7). If the angle closes to the upper trabecular meshwork or Schwalbe's line, intraocular pressure rises, whereas if the angle closes only the lower portion of the angle, the pressure remains unchanged.

Although plateau iris syndrome is usually recognized in the postoperative period, it may develop years later. Patients with plateau iris configuration should not be assumed to be permanently cured, even though plateau iris syndrome does not develop immediately.

SECONDARY ANGLE-CLOSURE GLAUCOMAS
Miotic-induced Angle-closure Glaucoma

Prolonged miotic treatment in eyes with open-angle glaucoma and narrow angles may lead to pupillary block and secondary angle-closure glaucoma. We have seen chronic angle-closure develop after several years of miotic therapy in eyes that initially had wide open angles. In some eyes, zonular relaxation occurs more readily than in others, so that anterior lens movement and an increase in axial lens thickness may facilitate pupillary block and angle-closure. In other eyes, there is little change in the lens, but progressively increasing pressure in the posterior chamber gradually pushes the peripheral iris against the trabecular meshwork.

Less commonly, miotic therapy can have a pronounced effect on lens position and trigger malignant glaucoma.[14,23,34,39] Unequal anterior chamber depths, a progressive increase in myopia, or progressive shallowing of the anterior chamber are clues to the correct diagnosis.

Combined Mechanism Glaucoma

Combined mechanism glaucoma refers to situations in which both open-angle and angle-closure components are present. A patient may have open-angle glaucoma and either narrow angles with superimposed intermittent angle-closure glaucoma or miotic-induced angle-closure. More commonly, the diagnosis is made when elevated intraocular pressure persists after elimination of angle-closure, either acute or chronic. The residual open-angle component is treated as open-angle glaucoma.

Lens-related Angle-closure Glaucoma

Swelling of the lens may convert an anterior chamber of medium depth into one that is markedly shallow and precipitate acute angle-closure glaucoma. In countries in which cataracts are prevalent and operations not readily available, acute angle-closure glaucoma from swollen hypermature lenses is common. This topic is discussed further in Chapter 58.

Slight lens subluxation in eyes of elderly patients, formerly termed senile subluxation of the lens, is most commonly associated with exfoliation syndrome. Mild iridodonesis may be seen. In some cases, anterior lens movement may be sufficient to cause angle-closure glaucoma, usually chronic.

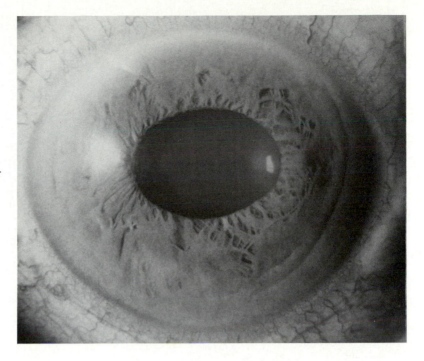

Fig. 47-8   Horizontally dilated pupil after acute angle-closure glaucoma.

These eyes are more susceptible to the development of miotic-induced angle-closure during treatment for open-angle glaucoma. Iridectomy usually suffices to eliminate the angle-closure component.

In younger patients anterior lens movement is often associated with secondary causes or ciliary block. After iridectomy, iridoplasty may be necessary to eliminate continued appositional closure if cycloplegics are unsuccessful at maintaining a more posterior lens position and an open angle. This topic is discussed more fully in Chapter 58.

Malignant Glaucoma

Malignant (ciliary block) glaucoma[23,41,42,49] is a multifactorial disease in which the following components may play varying roles: (1) previous acute or chronic angle-closure glaucoma, (2) shallowness of the anterior chamber, (3) forward movement of the lens, (4) pupillary block by the lens or vitreous, (5) slackness of the zonules, (6) anterior rotation and/or swelling of the ciliary body, (7) thickening of the anterior hyaloid membrane, (8) expansion of the vitreous, and (9) posterior aqueous displacement into or behind the vitreous. This topic is covered more fully in Chapter 70.

Swelling or anterior rotation of the ciliary body with forward rotation of the lens-iris diaphragm and relaxation of the zonular apparatus causes anterior lens displacement favoring direct angle-closure.[35] Accurate diagnosis and treatment are often more difficult when the initiating event is posterior to the lens-iris diaphragm. Some of the disorders that can lead to this picture are listed below and are covered in other chapters.

1. Drug sensitivity, such as the sulfonamides
2. Uveal effusion from adjacent inflammation such as scleritis, AIDS, and other viral disorders
3. Cyclocryotherapy
4. Panretinal photocoagulation
5. After scleral buckling surgery
6. Central retinal vein occlusion
7. Ciliary body swelling, inflammation, or cysts
8. Corneal disease
9. Nanophthalmos
10. Posterior segment tumors
11. Contracting retrolental tissue
12. Trauma

CLINICAL PATHOLOGY OF ANGLE-CLOSURE GLAUCOMA

When the angle totally occludes, aqueous humor outflow is blocked, and intraocular pressure rises markedly. The effect of the elevated pressure depends on the magnitude and rapidity of its rise. At the same time the pupillary reaction to direct light decreases. The pupil becomes partly dilated and tends to assume a vertically oval shape, but may be oblique or even horizontal (Fig. 47-8).

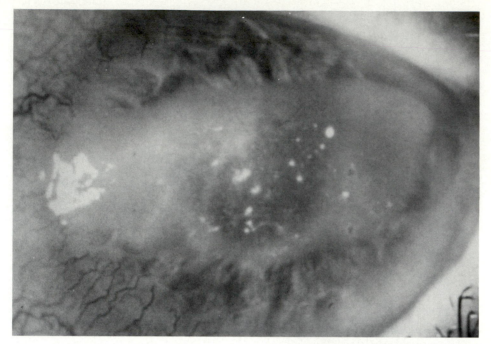

Fig. 47-9   Chronic corneal edema with band-shaped lipoid degeneration.

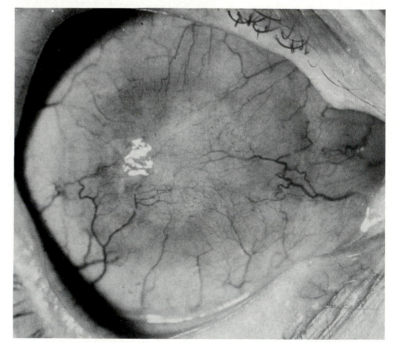

Fig. 47-10   Fibrosis and vascularization of cornea in long-standing untreated angle-closure glaucoma.

Cornea

With very high intraocular pressure, corneal edema is severe. The cornea is cloudy and may be twice its usual thickness. Endothelial cell loss becomes significant if the elevated pressure persists more than 24 hours.[3,31] When the pressure is lowered, the edema clears first at the periphery. Folds in Descemet's membrane form. Following prolonged high pressure, corneal edema and striate keratopathy may persist for some days. With severe damage, chronic edema may persist, lipid is deposited (Fig. 47-9), and the cornea may become fibrosed and vascularized (Fig. 47-10).

Iris

Partial necrosis of the iris stroma is the first sign of damage from elevated intraocular pressure experimentally.[1] At intraocular pressures over 60

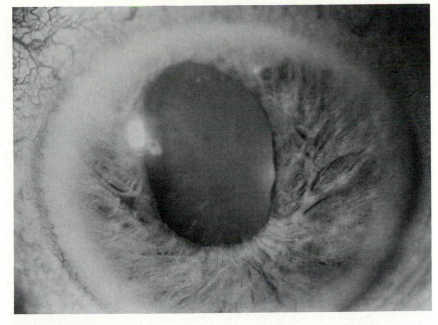

Fig. 47-11   Patches of iris atrophy and whorled stretching of stroma after acute angle-closure glaucoma.

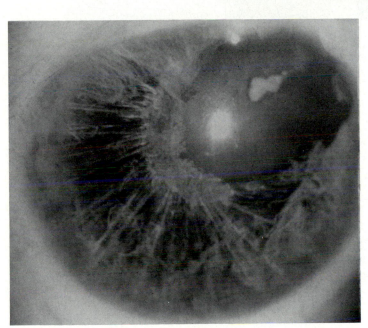

Fig. 47-12   Iris atrophy after acute angle-closure glaucoma may simulate iridoschisis.

mm Hg, the pupil becomes increasingly resistant to miotics, probably caused by direct pressure on the sphincter muscle.[7] The sphincter may respond to miotics after the pressure has been lowered, but when intraocular pressure exceeds the diastolic blood pressure, the iris around the pupil becomes ischemic.[7] The sphincter muscle then loses its ability to contract even if intraocular pressure is lowered, and patchy atrophy of the iris occurs. The dilator muscle is less affected than the sphincter, so that the instillation of 10% phenylephrine usually causes increased pupillary dilation.

In the segments in which the stroma is not obviously atrophic, the pupillary margin is thick, rolled, and bunched with radial folds. At the margins of the atrophic area, the stromal fibers run obliquely to the periphery behind the edges of the atrophic area, thus producing a twisting of this border zone of the stroma[50] (Fig. 47-11). In severe and prolonged attacks, diffuse iris atrophy occurs.

Sometimes a sector of the iris stroma will be disrupted and look like iridoschisis[40] (Fig. 47-12). This may occur with slow progressive atrophy months or years after the acute attack. The pigment

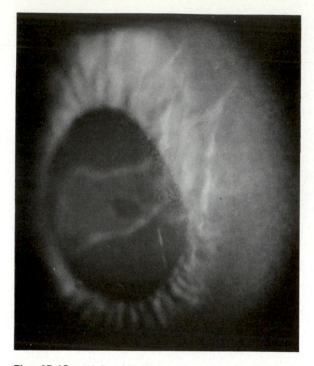

Fig. 47-13 Holes developing in sheet of glaukomflecken. Folds in Descemet's membrane indicate recent fall in intraocular pressure.

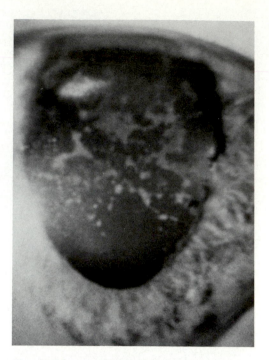

Fig. 47-14 Netlike stage of glaukomflecken.

epithelium and dilator muscle can be patchily affected and areas may transilluminate. Posterior synechiae may be minimal or extensive. After iridectomy aqueous humor flowing into the anterior chamber can bypass the pupil, favoring formation of postoperative posterior synechiae.

Ciliary Body

Ciliary processes may be inserted more anteriorly than normal and extend to the peripheral posterior iris.[20] It is possible that in some cases of angle-closure, such processes facilitate angle-closure by maintaining the peripheral iris in greater proximity to the trabecular meshwork.

Lens

Lens damage can occur as: (1) glaukomflecken, (2) anterior capsular cataract, (3) pigment deposition, posterior synechiae, and fibrosis, (4) cortical cataracts, and (5) nuclear sclerosis.

Glaukomflecken ("glaucoma flakes"), or disseminated anterior subcapsular cataracts of acute glaucoma, are the most characteristic signs of lens damage from sudden severe rises of intraocular pressure. They are thought to be caused by pressure necrosis of anterior lens fibers and do not occur at the posterior pole.

When intraocular pressure is very high, the lens damage simulates a thin, grey deposit of exudate on the lens surface.[19] With a fall in pressure, the sheet becomes thinner in some places and more condensed in others. Holes develop within it, so it may appear as a coarse, irregular, white net (Fig. 47-13).[25] Later these flakes become more discrete and appear as small, irregular, blue-white plaques (Fig. 47-14). They tend to follow suture lines of the lens, suggesting necrosis of the tips of the lens fibers.

Gradually, the flakes diminish and usually become relatively sparse (Fig. 47-15). As new lens fibers grow in from the equator, they overlie the flecks, which sink deeper into the lens and persist as permanent evidence. Glaukomflecken occur almost entirely within the pupil according to its size at the time of the attack.[44]

Glaukomflecken are rare apart from primary angle-closure glaucoma, but have been seen after contusion and chemical burns and also when the anterior chamber has remained flat postoperatively with the cornea and lens in contact for some days.

Occasionally, small white plaques resembling glaukomflecken may persist in the anterior surface of the lens. These are anterior capsular cataracts. Anterior cortical lens opacities commonly follow

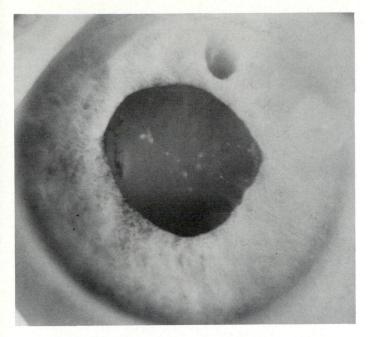

Fig. 47-15   Absorbing glaukomflecken appear as irregular white dots.

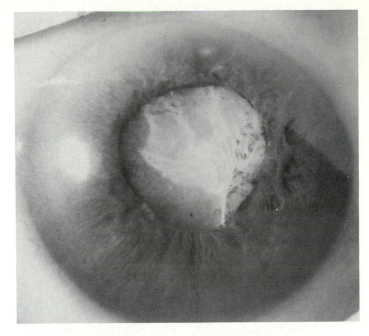

Fig. 47-16   Fibrotic membrane covering lens after acute angle-closure glaucoma.

severe attacks of angle-closure glaucoma and may persist as faint irregular streaks that almost invariably progress.

The first sign of nuclear sclerosis is a myopic refractive change, which may stabilize or progress. Following severe glaucomatous iritis with extensive posterior synechiae, fibrosis may extend from the iris onto the anterior lens surface (Fig. 47-16).

Zonules

The zonules can be damaged, so with surgery the lens may move forward with the development of malignant (ciliary block) glaucoma. Occasionally, the opaque lens may slowly dislocate over the years and sink below the pupil (Fig. 47-17).

Retina and Optic Nerve

In intermittent angle-closure glaucoma, even after many attacks, the optic disc is typically unaffected.

During the initial states of an acute attack, the disc may appear normal, congested, or edematous with retinal venous congestion and retinal hemorrhages near the disc. When intraocular pressure is acutely elevated in owl monkeys, damage to the nerve fiber layer and ganglion cells precedes damage to most other tissues except the iris.[1] Douglas et al.[9] found pallor without cupping following acute attacks, and pallor and cupping in patients

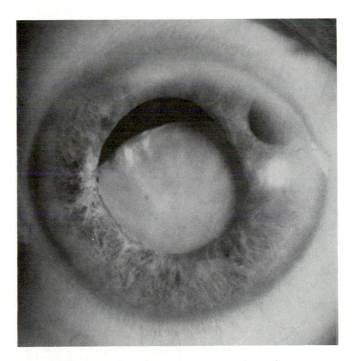

Fig. 47-17   Late dislocation of cataractous lens after acute angle-closure glaucoma.

with chronic angle-closure. Acutely elevated intra-ocular pressure in monkeys leads to optic disc congestion lasting several days before pallor and cupping develop.[51] Large retinal hemorrhages near the disc can occur with sudden lowering of intra-ocular pressure as after hyperosmotic or carbonic anhydrase inhibitor therapy. Retinal function is depressed with raised intraocular pressure.[46]

The final effects will depend on severity and duration of the attack. Recovery may be complete or there may be contraction of isopters and nerve fiber bundle defects.[9,27] Pallor without cupping was found to be characteristic of discs after acute angle-closure glaucoma, whereas both pallor and cupping occurred in chronic angle-closure.[9] In prolonged attacks, when treatment is delayed, glaucomatous damage may progress to the point at which vision is reduced to perception of hand movements or light. In chronic angle-closure glaucoma, the visual field defects and optic disc cupping progress similarly to those of open-angle glaucoma.

REFERENCES

1. Anderson, DR, and Davis, EB: Sensitivities of ocular tissues to acute pressure-induced ischemia, Arch Ophthalmol 93:267, 1975
2. Bhargava, SK, Leighton, DA, and Phillips, CI: Early angle-closure glaucoma: distribution of iridotrabecular contact and response to pilocarpine, Arch Ophthalmol 89:369, 1973
3. Bigar, F, and Witmer, R: Corneal endothelial changes in primary acute angle-closure glaucoma, Ophthalmology 89:596, 1982
4. Bloome, MA: Transient angle-closure glaucoma in central retinal vein occlusion, Ann Ophthalmol 9:44, 1977
5. Chandler, PA: Narrow-angle glaucoma, Arch Ophthalmol 47:695, 1952
6. Chandler, PA, and Trotter, RR: Angle-closure glaucoma: subacute types, Arch Ophthalmol 53:305, 1955
7. Charles, ST, and Hamasaki, DI: The effect of intra-ocular pressure on the pupil size, Arch Ophthalmol 83:729, 1970
8. Cross, M, and Croll, LJ: Emotional glaucoma, Am J Ophthalmol 49:297, 1960
9. Douglas, GR, Drance, SM, and Schulzer, M: The visual field and nerve head in angle-closure glaucoma: a comparison of the effects of acute and chronic angle closure, Arch Ophthalmol 93:409, 1975
10. Egan, JA: Shock glaucoma, Am J Ophthalmol 40:227, 1955
11. Foulds, WS, and Phillips, CI: Some observations on chronic closed-angle glaucoma, Br J Ophthalmol 41:208, 1957
12. Godel, V, Stein, R, and Feiler-Ofry, V: Angle-closure glaucoma following peripheral iridectomy and mydriasis, Am J Ophthalmol 65:555, 1968
13. Gorin, G: Shortening of the angle of the anterior chamber in angle-closure glaucoma, Am J Ophthalmol 49:141, 1960
14. Gorin, G: Angle-closure glaucoma induced by miotics, Am J Ophthalmol 62:1063, 1966
15. Grant, WM: Shallowing of the anterior chamber following occlusion of the central retinal vein, Am J Ophthalmol 75:384, 1973
16. Horie, T, Kitazawa, Y, and Nose, H: Visual field changes in primary angle-closure glaucoma, Jpn J Ophthalmol 1:108, 1975
17. Hyams, SW, and Neumann, E: Transient angle-closure glaucoma after retinal vein occlusion, Br J Ophthalmol 56:353, 1972
18. Inman, WS: Emotion and acute glaucoma, Lancet 2:1188, 1929
19. Jones, BR: Cataracta glaucomatosa and its role in the diagnosis of the acute glaucomas, Trans Ophthalmol Soc UK 59:753, 1959
20. Kerman, BM, Christensen, RE, and Foos, RY: Angle-closure glaucoma: a clinicopathologic correlation, Am J Ophthalmol 76:887, 1973
21. Kolker, AE, and Hetherington, J, Jr: Becker-Shaffer's diagnosis and therapy of the glaucomas, ed 5, St Louis, 1985, The CV Mosby Co
22. Leighton, DA, Phillips, CI, and Tsukahara, S: Profile of presenting states of eyes in angle-closure glaucoma, Br J Ophthalmol 55:577, 1971
23. Levene, RZ: A new concept of malignant glaucoma, Arch Ophthalmol 87:497, 1972
24. Lowe, RF: Primary creeping angle-closure glaucoma, Br J Ophthalmol 48:544, 1964
25. Lowe, RF: Primary acute angle-closure glaucoma: damage to cornea and lens, Br J Ophthalmol 49:460, 1965
26. Lowe, RF: Primary angle-closure glaucoma: postoperative acute glaucoma after phenylephrine eyedrops, Am J Ophthalmol 65:552, 1968
27. Lowe, RF: Primary angle-closure glaucoma: a review 5 years after bilateral surgery, Br J Ophthalmol 57:457, 1973
28. Lowe, RF: Plateau iris, Austral J Ophthalmol 9:71, 1981
29. Mapstone, R: Mechanics of pupil block, Br J Ophthalmol 52:19, 1968
30. Mapstone, R: Partial angle closure, Br J Ophthalmol 61:525, 1977
31. Markowitz, and Morin: The endothelium in primary angle-closure glaucoma, Am J Ophthalmol 98:103, 1984
32. McNaught, EI, Rennie, A, McClure, E, and Chisholm, IA: Pattern of visual damage after acute angle-closure glaucoma, Trans Ophthalmol Soc UK 94:406, 1974

33. Mendelsohn, AD, Jampol, LM, and Schoch, D: Secondary angle-closure glaucoma after central retinal vein occlusion, Am J Ophthalmol 100:581, 1985

34. Merritt, JC: Malignant glaucoma induced by miotics postoperatively in open-angle glaucoma, Arch Ophthalmol 95:1988, 1977

35. Phelps, CD: Angle-closure glaucoma secondary to ciliary body swelling, Arch Ophthalmol 92:287, 1974

36. Phillips, CI, and Woodhouse, DF: Self-limiting closed-angle glaucoma with segmental iris shortening, Br J Ophthalmol 47:547, 1963

37. Ravitz, J, and Seybold, ME: Transient monocular visual loss from narrow-angle glaucoma, Arch Neurol 41:991, 1984

38. Reiss, AR, Lee, DA, Topper, JF, and Brubaker, RF: Aqueous humor flow during sleep, Invest Ophthalmol Vis Sci 25:776, 1984

39. Rieser, JC, and Schwartz, B: Miotic induced malignant glaucoma, Arch Ophthalmol 87:706, 1972

40. Romano, A, Treister, G, Barishak, R, and Stein, R: Iridoschisis and angle-closure glaucoma, Ophthalmologica 164:199, 1972

41. Shaffer, RN, and Hoskins, HD, Jr: Ciliary block (malignant) glaucoma, Trans Am Acad Ophthalmol Otolaryngol 85:215, 1978

42. Simmons, RJ: Malignant glaucoma, Br J Ophthalmol 56:273, 1972

43. Sonty, S, and Schwartz, B: Vascular accidents in acute angle-closure glaucoma, Ophthalmology 88:225, 1981

44. Sugar, HS: Cataracta glaucomatosa acuta, Am J Ophthalmol 29:1396, 1946

45. Tornquist, R: Angle-closure glaucoma in an eye with a plateau type of iris, Acta Ophthalmol 36:413, 1958

46. Uenoyama, K, McDonald, JB, and Drance, SM: The effect of intraocular pressure on visual electrical responses, Arch Ophthalmol 81:722, 1969

47. Wand, M, Grant, WM, Simmons, RJ, and Hutchinson, BT: Plateau iris syndrome, Trans Am Acad Ophthalmol Otolaryngol 83:122, 1977

48. Weber, PA, Cohen, JS, and Baker, D: Central retinal vein occlusion and malignant glaucoma, Arch Ophthalmol 105:635, 1987

49. Weiss, DI, and Shaffer, RN: Ciliary block (malignant) glaucoma, Trans Am Acad Ophthalmol Otolaryngol 76:450, 1972

50. Winstanley, J: Iris atrophy in primary glaucoma, Trans Ophthalmol Soc UK 81:23, 1961

51. Zimmerman, LE, de Venecia, G, and Hamasaki, DI: Pathology of the optic nerve in experimental acute glaucoma, Invest Ophthalmol 6:109, 1967

Chapter 48

Therapeutic Overview of Angle-closure Glaucoma

Robert Ritch
Ronald F. Lowe
Alexander Reyes

The goals of treatment in angle-closure glaucoma are (1) to eliminate pupillary block, (2) to reopen the filtration angle, and (3) to prevent further damage to the optic nerve by lowering intraocular pressure. Iridectomy is the definitive treatment. Medical therapy is necessary before iridectomy to lower intraocular pressure and after iridectomy, if necessary, to control it. Filtration surgery may be required if these measures are insufficient.

ACUTE ANGLE-CLOSURE GLAUCOMA

Acute angle-closure glaucoma (see Chapter 47) should be regarded as a medical emergency. Therapy should be directed at rapidly reducing intraocular pressure and opening the angle. Both medical and laser treatment play a role in opening the angle and in eliminating pupillary block.

Medical Therapy

Hyperosmotic agents

Hyperosmotic agents raise serum osmotic pressure and withdraw fluid from the eye, especially from the vitreous humor (see Chapter 25). In addition to lowering intraocular pressure, vitreous dehydration allows the lens to move posteriorly, deepening the anterior chamber and facilitating opening of the angle.

Intraocular pressure decreases within 30 to 60 minutes after administration, the effect lasting about 5 to 6 hours. Patients should limit fluid intake for maximum benefit. Oral 50% glycerol, 1 to 1.5 g/kg, has been used most commonly. Isosorbide, 1.5 to 2.0 g/kg, is more palatable and causes less nausea and vomiting. It is not metabolized, an advantage particularly in diabetics, and is our preferred agent. A solution of 20% mannitol, 1 to 2 g/kg, given intravenously over 45 minutes has a greater hypotensive effect and may be given when severe nausea and vomiting are present.

Administration of hyperosmotic agents is commonly accompanied by thirst and headache. Hyperosmolar coma can be a serious complication caused by severe CNS dehydration. Patients with renal or cardiovascular disease or those already dehydrated by vomiting are at risk.

Inhibitors of aqueous humor secretion

Carbonic anhydrase inhibitors. Acetazolamide is highly effective in treating acute angle-closure glaucoma. It can open some closed angles even in the presence of ischemic iris atrophy and paralysis of the pupil. The aim is to give a large dose quickly. Rapid reduction of intraocular pressure is most reliably achieved by giving 500 mg intravenously plus 500 mg orally. Intravenous administration is advantageous when vomiting is present and has a more rapid onset of action. Adverse reactions are uncommon. If vomiting prevents the oral dose, it should be given later. Following oral therapy, the maximum effect occurs at 2 hours and high plasma levels persist for 4 to 6 hours, but then drop rapidly because of excretion in the urine. Because acetazolamide is a sulfonamide, there is a remote chance of sensitivity, but we have seen no complications after several hundred injections.

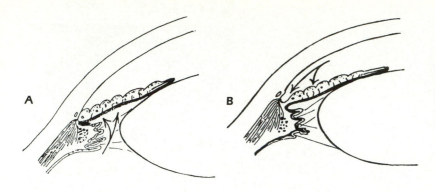

Fig. 48-1 **A,** Pupillary block caused by higher pressure in posterior chamber. **B,** Reversed pupillary block. Pressure in anterior chamber is momentarily higher and pushes iris back to open the angle.

Carbonic anhydrase inhibitors can open the angle by reversing pupillary block.[44] The rapid decrease of inflow produced by intravenous acetazolamide reduces pressure in the posterior chamber. At the same time the hyperosmotic agents may increase absorption of aqueous humor from the posterior chamber through the ciliary body into the choroid (uveoscleral outflow). If pressure in the posterior chamber is lowered rapidly, pressure in the anterior chamber will be transiently higher, the iris will be forced back, and in the absence of PAS, the angle will open[45] (Fig. 48-1).

Beta-blockers. Beta-adrenergic antagonists are additive with acetazolamide but have a more prolonged onset of action in acute angle-closure glaucoma. They are more useful in later stages of treatment and in maintaining reduced intraocular pressure before laser iridectomy.

Miotics

The use of miotics to constrict the pupil and draw the peripheral iris away from the trabecular meshwork was formerly the main approach to treatment of acute angle-closure glaucoma. The more severe and prolonged the attack, the more frequently miotics were applied. A typical recommended regimen was 4% pilocarpine every 5 minutes for four doses, every 15 minutes for four doses, then every hour for four doses or until the attack was broken.

When the intraocular pressure is over 60 mm Hg, the pupil becomes unresponsive to miotics because of ischemia and paralysis of the iris sphincter.

Pilocarpine may be not only ineffective; it may paradoxically worsen the situation.[25,46,56,58] Pilocarpine decreases anterior chamber depth and increases the axial length of the lens, even in elderly patients.[1-3,51,54,74] Although the miotic effect of pilocarpine is blocked when intraocular pressure is extremely high, ciliary muscle contraction and anterior movement of the lens-iris diaphragm are not.

Miotics may increase the pupillary block by causing forward motion of the lens-iris diaphragm, and overtreatment with pilocarpine can severely exacerbate attacks of angle-closure glaucoma that are unresponsive to initial medical treatment.

Pilocarpine may also contribute to maintaining elevated intraocular pressure by reducing uveoscleral outflow.[9] High doses of pilocarpine may produce cholinergic toxicity, which may not be noticed because of the nausea and vomiting associated with the acute angle-closure attack. Strong miotics, such as echothiophate, should not be used because they can increase both the pupillary block and vascular congestion.

Ganias and Mapstone[20] found that immediate treatment with intravenous acetazolamide and repeated instillation of 2% pilocarpine was not more successful in breaking attacks of angle-closure than treatment with acetazolamide and a single drop of pilocarpine given 3 hours later. Similar results were obtained with topically administered timolol in place of acetazolamide.[4]

Most attacks of acute angle-closure glaucoma respond to medical treatment because of the fortunate situation that some degree of pupillary block is present in most eyes presenting with acute angle-closure glaucoma. In this case, the "positive" effect of pilocarpine on the iris is greater than the "negative" effect on the lens. However, eyes in which angle-closure is caused by forward lens movement, ciliary block, or an intumescent lens are frequently made worse by miotics.

In addition, many eyes have what could be called *multimechanism* angle-closure glaucoma (Fig. 48-2), in the sense that some element of pupillary block contributes to the angle-closure in eyes with lens-related glaucoma, malignant glaucoma, and plateau iris. The pupillary block must be eliminated as well as the other mechanisms. When the contribution by pupillary block is small compared with that of direct pressure by the lens, the amount

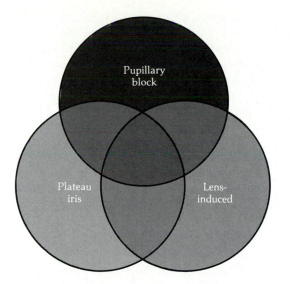

Fig. 48-2 More than one mechanism of angle-closure may be present in an eye. As illustrated in this Venn diagram, combinations of two or even three mechanisms may be present in some patients. Overall approach is to define and treat each separately.

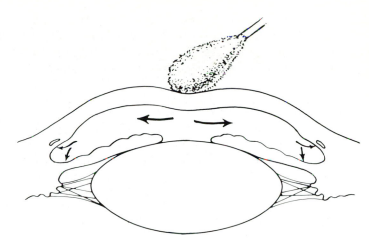

Fig. 48-3 Corneal indentation with cotton-tipped applicator may lower intraocular pressure during attack of angle-closure glaucoma by forcing aqueous humor from central to peripheral anterior chamber *(arrows)*, thereby temporarily opening angle and reestablishing aqueous humor outflow. (From Shields, MB: Textbook of glaucoma, ed 2, Baltimore, 1987, Williams & Wilkins)

of pilocarpine used in attempting to break the attack may well tip the balance between success and failure of medical therapy. Cautious use of pilocarpine may open the angle, whereas the effect of copious pilocarpine on the lens may increase the direct block and make it impossible to open the angle.

Thymoxamine

Thymoxamine is an alpha-adrenergic antagonist that paralyzes the dilator muscle but depends on an active sphincter muscle to produce miosis. It produces miosis without affecting lens position and thickness or intraocular pressure and outflow facility.[26,61,71] In the face of an ischemic sphincter, neither thymoxamine nor pilocarpine will constrict the pupil.

When the iris is damaged, thymoxamine alone has not been found useful in treating acute angle-closure glaucoma,[71] but it can reverse positive provocative tests and break some attacks.[61] It is valuable in neutralizing phenylephrine-induced mydriasis and in differentiating true angle-closure from open-angle glaucoma in the presence of very narrow angles.[72] However, the drug is not available in the United States.

Mydriatics

Wide pupillary dilation by cycloplegics or mydriatics can eliminate sphincter contact with the lens and open the angle. The effect of mydriatics and cycloplegics may be different in any one particular eye. Mydriatics, such as phenylephrine, do not affect the lens position, although cycloplegics may cause the lens to move backward in addition to allowing the pupil to dilate by abolishing sphincter muscle tone. However, in acute angle-closure glaucoma the lens is usually large, anterior, and steep, so that this approach is likely to be unsuccessful and make the condition worse unless the angle-closure is primarily caused by forward lens movement. Dilation may increase crowding of the angle by the iris without eliminating pupillary block and may make laser iridectomy more difficult to perform. Mydriatics and cycloplegics are not recommended for routine first-line use.

Cycloplegics are appropriate when the angle remains closed after laser iridectomy but openable by indentation. If a test dose of cyclopentolate deepens the anterior chamber and further widens the angle, cycloplegics may be used for maintenance therapy (see Chapters 58 and 70). These eyes are prone to develop malignant glaucoma.

Other Treatment

Physical methods have been reported to be successful in breaking an attack of acute angle-closure. Indentation of the central part of the cornea with a Zeiss gonioscopy lens, cotton tip applicator, or muscle hook, forcing aqueous humor peripherally, may open the angle temporarily (Fig. 48-3). Repeated cycles of 30 seconds of indentation followed by release of pressure for 30 seconds may allow enough aqueous humor to flow out of the angle to lower the intraocular pressure and allow miotics to be effective.[5]

Angle-closure glaucoma is associated with a marked inflammatory reaction. The instillation of 1% prednisolone or 0.1% dexamethasone is desirable from the start to reduce inflammation before laser or surgery. Severe pain may be treated with analgesics, and vomiting may be treated with antiemetics.

Approach to Acute Angle-closure Glaucoma

The following is our approach to a patient with acute angle-closure[37]:

1. Compile careful history of symptoms relating to intermittent angle-closure attacks, attacks in the fellow eye, prescription or non-prescription medications that may precipitate attacks, and type of activity preceding the attack.
2. Examine the affected eye and fellow eye with attention to both the central and peripheral anterior chamber depth and the shape of the peripheral iris.
3. Administer oral isosorbide and a topical beta-blocker. Intravenous acetazolamide may may be given simultaneously.
4. Have the patient lie supine to permit the lens to fall backward with vitreous dehydration.
5. Reassess ocular findings after 1 hour. Intraocular pressure is usually decreased, but the angle usually remains appositionally closed. Give 1 drop of 2% or 4% pilocarpine and reexamine the patient 30 minutes later.
   a. If intraocular pressure is reduced and the angle is open, the patient may be treated medically with topical low-dose pilocarpine, beta-blockers and steroids, and oral acetazolamide, if necessary, until the eye quiets and laser iridectomy can be performed.
   b. If intraocular pressure is unchanged or elevated and the angle remains closed, lens-related angle-closure should be suspected, further pilocarpine withheld, and the attack broken by argon laser peripheral iridoplasty[58,59,64] (see Chapter 30).

We have performed peripheral iridoplasty in over 50 attacks of angle-closure unresponsive to medical therapy, even after several days. All eyes but one, which was totally synechially closed, responded with normalization of intraocular pressure and opening of the angle. Peripheral iridoplasty does not eliminate pupillary block and is not a substitute for laser iridectomy, which must be performed as soon as the eye is quiet. However, even in eyes with extensive synechial closure, intraocular pressure is lowered sufficiently for a few days, allowing the eye to quiet. Ciliary hyposecretion may help the situation.

Peripheral iridoplasty is much safer than attempting surgical iridectomy on an inflamed eye with an elevated intraocular pressure. The risks of intraoperative surgery are avoided and, even if malignant glaucoma is present, the angle remains open long enough for the eye to quiet. The alternative of waiting and prolonging medical therapy for several days seriously increases the possibility of irreversible damage to the iris, lens, drainage pathways, and optic nerve head.[14]

Iridectomy

The definitive management of primary angle-closure glaucoma is relief of the pupillary block by an iridectomy (see Chapter 30), which opens the angle unless extensive synechial closure has occurred. With its ease, low complication rate, and ready patient acceptability, laser iridectomy has become the primary procedure of choice in virtually all cases, rendering the earlier arguments of iridectomy versus a filtering operation irrelevant.

Approach to the Patient after Iridectomy

Once the pupillary block component has been eliminated by iridectomy, the status of the iridocorneal angle should be assessed by gonioscopy. Presuming that peripheral iridoplasty was not used to break the attack, the angle may be open, partially open, or closed.

As many as one third of angles without PAS remain narrow after iridectomy, and approximately half of these are capable of closure with mydriasis.[41] When conventional surgical iridectomy was the routine procedure for angle-closure glaucoma, eyes were routinely dilated postoperatively for several days and gonioscopy was much less routinely performed than it is now. Many eyes capable of closure after iridectomy developed peripheral anterior synechiae during this time, and when gonioscopy was performed, a diagnosis of chronic angle-closure was made.

One additional benefit of laser iridectomy is its

lack of effect on the anatomic relationships of the anterior segment apart from the iris. The depth of the anterior chamber and the position of the lens are not altered, permitting for the first time the possibility of accurate assessment of the contributions of other mechanisms besides pupillary block to the development of angle-closure.

Indentation gonioscopy should be performed immediately after laser iridectomy to assess the status of the angle. If the angle is open without PAS or if there are PAS but no residual element of appositional closure, the eye should be maintained on antiglaucoma medications and topical corticosteroids until inflammation has disappeared. At this point, the pupil should be dilated and intraocular pressure measured and indentation gonioscopy performed. The angle may close either in the presence of plateau iris or if the lens is large and the iris stroma crowds the angle. Intraocular pressure may or may not rise. If neosynephrine alone is used, intraocular pressure may rise in the absence of angle-closure if diffuse pigment liberation occurs.[38,68] If cycloplegics are used, intraocular pressure may also rise if there has been damage to the trabecular meshwork. Previous miotic therapy predisposes the eye to a pressure rise.[63] Gonioscopy is essential to differentiate the mechanism of the postdilation pressure rise.

If the angle remains appositionally closed after iridectomy, the mechanism may be plateau iris, a large lens, forward lens movement, or malignant glaucoma. If the closure encompasses more than half the angle, we prefer to perform peripheral iridoplasty and then proceed as below, because cycloplegia at this point may be detrimental. If the closure is partial, our approach is to discontinue miotic therapy after measuring anterior chamber depth by pachymetry and reexamine the patient 2 days later.

At this next examination, if the angle remains appositionally closed, peripheral iridoplasty should be performed. A few days later, when any inflammation has cleared, the eye is tested with a drop of cyclopentolate. If the anterior chamber deepens and the angle opens, the patient is maintained on cyclopentolate or a longer-acting cycloplegic if this does not adversely affect intraocular pressure. If the angle closes, the mechanism is angle-crowding, usually caused by plateau iris or a large lens, and no further cycloplegics are given.

If, after discontinuation of pilocarpine, the angle is open, the appositional closure was caused by the effect of pilocarpine on the lens, and repeat pachymetry usually reveals a deeper anterior

chamber. If intraocular pressure is normal, the patient should be maintained off miotic therapy. If intraocular pressure is elevated and cannot be controlled without miotics, peripheral iridoplasty should be performed.

Although it appears difficult initially, this mechanistic approach to angle-closure allows the ophthalmologist to tailor optimal therapy for the individual eye in complicated cases in which factors in addition to pupillary block are present. These factors are much more common than has been previously realized.

Long-term Follow-up

If intraocular pressure remains elevated after iridectomy, continued medical treatment may be necessary. If intraocular pressure remains uncontrolled and glaucomatous damage develops, filtration surgery is indicated. An increased chance of developing malignant glaucoma during filtration surgery exists in patients who have had angle-closure glaucoma.[16] Campbell and Vela[11] have reported successful results with goniosynechialysis, a procedure designed to strip PAS from the meshwork and restore trabecular function. The procedure is apparently successful only if the synechiae have been present for less than 1 year.

Eyes that have had acute angle-closure glaucoma have higher intraocular pressures and lower outflow facility than uninvolved fellow eyes, even in the absence of PAS.[50] Approximately 25% of eyes that have been successfully treated for angle-closure glaucoma with normalization of intraocular pressure may develop elevated pressure in subsequent years.[31,38] These cases should be treated similarly to open-angle glaucoma if the angle is not appositionally closed. Some investigators have reported lack of success with laser trabeculoplasty in eyes with narrow angles and angle-closure glaucoma.[75] Our experience has suggested that argon laser trabeculoplasty is quite successful in eyes with residual open-angle glaucoma when performed after opening of the angle for acute or chronic angle-closure glaucoma if PAS are present for less than 180 degrees, or if circumferential, do not extend above the scleral spur.

Repeated gonioscopy is essential for proper management. Some patients may develop secondary angle-closure glaucoma, most commonly caused by closure of the iridectomy, plateau iris syndrome, or lens-related glaucoma with continued progression of PAS (see Chapter 58). Cataracts may develop or progress, requiring extraction, or corneal decompensation may develop.

INTERMITTENT AND SUBACUTE ANGLE-CLOSURE GLAUCOMA

Laser iridectomy is also indicated for eyes with intermittent or subacute angle-closure glaucoma. Maintenance on miotic therapy is no longer warranted and does not prevent the development of either acute or chronic angle-closure glaucoma.

FELLOW EYE

A prophylactic iridectomy is indicated for the fellow eye following an acute attack of primary angle-closure glaucoma. Before laser iridectomy, a number of investigators compared the advantages and disadvantages of prophylactic surgical iridectomy in the fellow eye.[30,33,34,52] The chance of angle-closure glaucoma developing in the fellow eye may be as high as 75% over 5 to 10 years, even with prophylactic miotic therapy.[7,8,40,65,76] After iridectomy such an event is unusual and is usually caused by plateau iris syndrome or malignant glaucoma.[34,45,76] Surgical iridectomy was concluded to be safer overall than miotic treatment. With laser iridectomy, there is no argument.

A high proportion of acute attacks in fellow eyes develop within 1 year of the attack in the first eye[15,40,52] and may develop within days. Prophylactic iridectomy should be performed as soon as possible, preferably while the first eye is quieting from the attack.

Provocative tests are of limited value since a negative test does not rule out angle-closure in the future. Dark room testing has been negative in eyes that have had previous attacks.[36] Laser iridectomy, with its greater safety and acceptance over surgical iridectomy, has greatly facilitated the treatment of the fellow eye.

If for any reason the patient refuses iridectomy in the fellow eye, pilocarpine may be given in an attempt to maintain an open angle. Even if the intraocular pressure is normal with pilocarpine treatment, we would consider adding a topical beta-blocker to reduce aqueous humor inflow and reduce the volume of the posterior chamber, minimizing the chance of pupillary block. Epinephrine compounds should be avoided. Gonioscopy should be performed frequently.

CHRONIC ANGLE-CLOSURE GLAUCOMA

It is important to recognize early stages of appositional angle-closure in the absence of PAS and to recognize deep, circumferential angle-closure.[41] This is best accomplished with careful indentation gonioscopy.[17] A false angle may be recognized by applying light pressure on the cornea with the four-mirror prism, which may open up small spaces between broad synechiae. If intraocular pressure is elevated, pressure on the lens may be ineffective in opening areas of appositional closure, leading to overestimation of the proportion of the angle closed by synechiae.

Laser iridectomy is indicated for all stages of chronic angle-closure glaucoma.[22,57] Iridectomy will open these areas of the angle not involved by synechiae and prevent further synechial closure. Miotic treatment may enhance the development of chronic angle-closure in the absence of an iridectomy.

In earlier times the extent of synechial closure of the angle was evaluated to determine whether conventional surgical iridectomy or trabeculectomy should be performed.[12,17] Some considered glaucomatous damage an indication for filtration surgery.[21] Laser iridectomy has retired this argument. If laser iridectomy plus medical treatment is insufficient to control the disease, one can proceed with a filtration procedure.

The need for continued medical treatment after iridectomy is determined by the level of intraocular pressure and the extent of glaucomatous damage. Treatment is similar to that of open-angle glaucoma. Repeated gonioscopy is necessary. The need for further surgery cannot be predicted from the level of initial intraocular pressure or the gonioscopic changes.

MIOTIC-INDUCED ANGLE-CLOSURE GLAUCOMA

Miotic treatment may exacerbate relative pupillary block. In eyes with open-angle glaucoma and narrow angles, pupillary constriction may lead to increased iris bombé and progressive narrowing of the angle. Appositional closure and the development of chronic angle-closure glaucoma is not infrequent, whereas acute angle-closure is rare. Epinephrine compounds, by stimulating the dilator muscle, facilitate the process. Routine gonioscopy helps to avoid this situation.

When miotic-induced angle-closure occurs, the approach to treatment should be determined by assessing the medications necessary to control the glaucoma. If a patient is taking epinephrine or dipivefrin, discontinuation of the drug may be sufficient to open the angle and allow the patient to remain on miotics, presuming intraocular pressure remains under control. If the patient has been treated with miotics alone, substitution of a beta-blocker often suffices. If discontinuation of miotics opens the angle, but the patient requires both miotics and beta-blockers for control of intraocular pressure, then laser iridectomy is warranted.

PLATEAU IRIS

If the angle remains appositionally closed or spontaneously occludable after laser iridectomy, further treatment is necessary to prevent progressive damage to or closure of the angle. Low-dose pilocarpine may open the angle and, if tolerated well by the patient (these patients are frequently under 50 years old), may be used for maintenance. Either 1% pilocarpine or an Ocusert is usually sufficient to maintain an open angle. The alternate choice is to perform peripheral iridoplasty. If miotics are needed for control of intraocular pressure after iridectomy, then iridoplasty is indicated only if the angle remains appositionally closed on miotics.

If the angle is open after iridectomy but closes appositionally with pupillary dilation, we feel that treatment is indicated if intraocular pressure rises with closure. If incomplete plateau iris syndrome is present and intraocular pressure remains normal, we prefer observation.

If plateau iris configuration is diagnosed incidentally in an eye with an open angle, caution should be exercised in dilation, and the patient should be followed gonioscopically at routine intervals for signs of spontaneous angle-closure.

COMBINED MECHANISM GLAUCOMA

In some instances of apparent open-angle glaucoma with narrow angles without definite PAS, it may be difficult to decide whether an angle-closure mechanism is superimposed, or even primarily responsible for the increased intraocular pressure. This may be suspected especially when large fluctuations of intraocular pressure occur.[42] The pressure may be aggravated by miotics, epinephrine, or both. Differentiation between this and pure open-angle glaucoma may be clinically impossible. In these cases, iridectomy eliminates any element of angle-closure caused by pupillary block. It may make the intraocular pressure easier to control and prevent pressure spikes, further angle damage, or closure with the use of strong miotics or epinephrine compounds.[55]

NARROW ANGLES

Before the advent of laser iridectomy, the question of whether to perform prophylactic conventional surgical iridectomy in eyes with normal vision and asymptomatic narrow angles presented a more difficult choice than does laser iridectomy today. Elimination of the potential complications of intraocular surgery, particularly cataract formation, has created a de facto liberalization of criteria for performing iridectomy.[60]

To perform laser iridectomy in all eyes with narrow angles, however, would certainly be an overapplication of the procedure. Some 1.5% of the general population and 4.5% of those aged over 60 years have occludable angles. In a survey of 947 eyes of patients of all ages, Spaeth[66] thought as many as 6% of angles were capable of occlusion. Nevertheless, only about 5% to 10% of these will develop angle-closure glaucoma. Furthermore, gonioscopy does not guarantee that one will be able to determine whether an angle is occludable. Gonioscopy with a Koeppe gonioscopy lens generally gives the impression of a wider angle than that obtained with the Zeiss or Goldmann lenses, probably because of posterior lens movement in the supine position. Even glaucomatologists have disagreed about whether a particular angle is or is not occludable when judged gonioscopically with any of these lenses.[73]

A variety of tests have been developed to attempt to determine whether a narrow angle is actually occludable. The earlier literature on this topic has been reviewed previously.[24,35,43] These tests have been designed to more or less reproduce the conditions that might lead to spontaneous angle-closure with the rationale that it is better for this to occur in a setting in which it can be treated definitively than in one in which it might go unrecognized or where medical attention might not be readily available.

Nonpharmacologic tests have been regarded as more accurately reproducing natural conditions than those that involve stimulating the sphincter and dilator muscles. However, the prognostic value of provocative tests remains unknown, and both presumed false positives and false negatives occur.[70] Because of this, some feel that occludability under any reasonable circumstances warrants laser iridectomy and that pharmacologic tests are justified. Intensive provocative testing using multiple tests on a periodic basis has become less routine since the advent of laser iridectomy.

Dark Room Test

Some surgeons consider the dark room test the most physiologic provocative test.[28,67] The patient is placed in a dark room for 1 to 2 hours. It is useful for the patient to have company or a radio in the room during both this and the prone provocative test to prevent the patient's falling asleep. Exposure to light should be minimized while performing intraocular pressure measurements and gonioscopy after the test to avoid reversing the pressure-inducing mechanism.[23]

A rise in intraocular pressure of 8 to 10 mm Hg

is considered positive when verified by noting closure of the angle on gonioscopy. Mydriasis alone may lead to an elevated intraocular pressure, most commonly through liberation of pigment from the iris into the anterior chamber in patients with pigment dispersion syndrome or exfoliation syndrome. Gonioscopy should be performed with the minimum amount of light necessary. The vertical height of the beam should be shortened as much as possible to avoid causing inadvertent pupillary constriction and opening of the angle. Positive dark room tests are accompanied by a tonographically decreased outflow coefficient.[18]

Prone Provocative Test

In the prone provocative test the subject lies face down with forehead on the back of the hands or on a firm pillow for 1 hour (often in a darkened room) without sleeping.[31] A rise of 8 mm Hg with gonioscopic confirmation of angle-closure is considered positive.

The mechanism of angle-closure is apparently unrelated to mydriasis.[27] It is possible that pupillary block associated with a slight forward movement of the lens is responsible, but one study showed no significant shallowing of the anterior chamber.[53] After peripheral iridectomy, about 7.5% of the tests are still positive, suggesting some role for the lens in these patients.[19,29]

Prone Dark Room Provocative Test

Performing the prone provocative test in a darkened room significantly increases the yield of positive tests.[27] This test is the most popular of the nonpharmacologic tests.

Mydriatics

Dilation in eyes with shallow anterior chambers and narrow angles is a calculated risk. When eyes with narrow angles are dilated, the patient should be observed until the pupil has constricted, since the angle may be open when the pupil is dilated, but may be closed while it is constricting. The intraocular pressure may be normal in the presence of a closed angle only to rise 1 or 2 hours later. Alpha-adrenergic agonists, especially 10% phenylephrine, carry greater risk than mydriatics which paralyze the sphincter. Tropicamide 0.5% is weakly cycloplegic, of short duration, and can be reversed with pilocarpine.[10,48] Phenylephrine can overcome the action of miotics, and pharmacologic constriction of the pupil with miotics after dilation with phenylephrine enhances the forces leading to pupillary block.[48] With pupillary dilation and an open angle, the risk of pupillary block with spontaneous recovery for the mydriasis is small. If pilocarpine is used, the pupil should be well constricted before the patient is discharged.

Mydriatic test

In the mydriatic test the pupil is semidilated with a weak cycloplegic, and intraocular pressure is measured after 1 to 2 hours. A rise of 8 to 10 mm Hg is considered positive. Gonioscopic confirmation of angle-closure is essential, since cycloplegics can also cause intraocular pressure rises in eyes with open angles, even in the absence of pigment liberation.[69]

Phenylephrine-Pilocarpine Test

The phenylephrine-pilocarpine test involves instilling 2% pilocarpine and 10% phenylephrine after initial measurement of intraocular pressure.[47] The phenylephrine is repeated half-hourly unless the intraocular pressure rises 8 mm Hg. If no rise occurs by 2.5 hours, the test is terminated by 0.5% thymoxamine. Positive tests of 8 mm Hg or more are terminated by thymoxamine and intravenous acetazolamide 500 mg. This powerful pupillary blocking test can be difficult to control, and acute angle-closure glaucoma may be precipitated. Decreased aqueous humor outflow has been documented during positive tests.[49]

REFERENCES

1. Abramson, DH, et al: Pilocarpine-induced lens changes: an ultrasonic biometric evaluation of dose response, Arch Ophthalmol 92:464, 1974
2. Abramson, DH, Coleman, DJ, Forbes, M, and Franzen, LA: Pilocarpine: effect on the anterior chamber and lens thickness, Arch Ophthalmol 87:615, 1972
3. Abramson, DH, Franzen, LA, and Coleman, DJ: Pilocarpine in the presbyope: demonstration of an effect on the anterior chamber and lens thickness, Arch Ophthalmol 89:100, 1973
4. Airaksinen, PJ, et al: Management of acute closed-angle glaucoma with miotics and timolol, Br J Ophthalmol 63:822, 1979
5. Anderson, DR: Corneal indentation to relieve acute angle-closure glaucoma, Am J Ophthalmol 88:1091, 1979
6. Anderson, DR, and Davis, EB: Sensitivities of ocular tissue to acute pressure-induced ischemia, Arch Ophthalmol 93:267, 1975
7. Bain, W: The fellow eye in acute closed angle glaucoma, Br J Ophthalmol 41:193, 1957
8. Benedikt, O: Prophylactic iridectomy in the fellow eye after angle-closure glaucoma, Klin Monatsbl Augenheilkd 156:80, 1970

9. Bleiman, B, and Schwartz, AL: Paradoxical response to pilocarpine, Arch Ophthalmol 97:1305, 1979

10. Brooks, AMV, West, RH, and Gillies, WE: The risk of precipitating acute angle-closure glaucoma with the clinical use of mydriatic agents, Med J Austral 145:36, 1986

11. Campbell, DG, and Vela, A: Modern goniosynechialysis for the treatment of synechial angle-closure glaucoma, Ophthalmology 91:1052, 1984

12. Chandler, PA: Narrow-angle glaucoma, Arch Ophthalmol 47:695, 1952

13. Charles, ST, and Hamasaki, DI: The effect of intraocular pressure on the pupil size, Arch Ophthalmol 83:729, 1970

14. David, R, Tessler, Z, and Yassur, Y: Long-term outcome of primary acute angle-closure glaucoma, Br J Ophthalmol 69:261, 1985

15. Edwards, RS: Behavior of the fellow eye in acute angle-closure glaucoma, Br J Ophthalmol 66:576, 1982

16. Eltz, H, and Gloor, B: Trabeculectomy in cases of angle-closure glaucoma: successes and failures, Klin Monatsbl Augenheilkd 177:556, 1980

17. Forbes, M: Gonioscopy with corneal indentation: a method for distinguishing between appositional closure and synechial closure, Arch Ophthalmol 76:488, 1966

18. Foulds, WS: Observations on the facility of aqueous outflow in closed-angle glaucoma, Br J Ophthalmol 43:613, 1959

19. Friedman, Z, and Neumann, E: Comparison of prone position, dark room and mydriatic tests for angle-closure glaucoma before and after peripheral iridectomy, Am J Ophthalmol 74:24, 1976

20. Ganias, F, and Mapstone, R: Miotics in closed-angle glaucoma, Br J Ophthalmol 59:205, 1975

21. Gelber, EC, and Anderson, DR: Surgical decisions in chronic angle-closure glaucoma, Arch Ophthalmol 94:1481, 1976

22. Gieser, D, and Wilensky, J: Laser iridectomy in the management of chronic angle-closure glaucoma, Am J Ophthalmol 98:446, 1984

23. Gloster, J, and Poinoosawmy, D: Changes in intraocular pressure during and after the dark-room test, Br J Ophthalmol 57:170, 1973

24. Gorin, G: Provocative tests in angle-closure glaucoma, Am J Ophthalmol 60:235, 1965

25. Gorin, G: Angle-closure glaucoma induced by miotics, Am J Ophthalmol 62:1063, 1966

26. Halasa, AH, and Rutkowski, PC: Thymoxamine therapy for angle-closure glaucoma, Arch Ophthalmol 90:177, 1973

27. Harris, LS, and Galin, MA: Prone provocative testing for narrow angle glaucoma, Arch Ophthalmol 87:493, 1972

28. Higgit, AC: The dark-room test, Br J Ophthalmol 38:242, 1954

29. Hung, PT, and Chou, LH: Provocation and mechanism of angle-closure glaucoma after iridectomy, Arch Ophthalmol 97:1862, 1979

30. Hyams, SW, Friedman, Z, and Keroub, C: Fellow eye in angle-closure glaucoma, Br J Ophthalmol 59:207, 1975

31. Hyams, SW, Friedman, Z, and Neumann, E: Elevated intraocular pressure in the prone position: a new provocative test for angle-closure glaucoma, Am J Ophthalmol 66:661, 1968

32. Hyams, SW, Keroub, C, and Pokotilo, E: Mixed glaucoma, Br J Ophthalmol 61:105, 1977

33. Imre, G, and Bogi, J: The fellow eye in acute angle-closure glaucoma, Klin Monatsbl Augenheilkd 169:264, 1976

34. Imre, G, and Bogi, J: The results of prophylactic iridectomy, Klin Monatsbl Augenheilkd 181:409, 1982

35. Kirsch, RE: A study of provocative tests for angle-closure glaucoma, Arch Ophthalmol 74:770, 1965

36. Kolker, AE, and Hetherington, J, Jr: Becker-Shaffer's diagnosis and therapy of the glaucomas, ed 5, St Louis, 1985, The CV Mosby Co

37. Kramer, P, and Ritch, R: The treatment of angle-closure glaucoma revisited (editorial), Ann Ophthalmol 16:1101, 1984

38. Kristensen, P: Mydriasis-induced pigment liberation in the anterior chamber associated with acute rise in intraocular pressure in open-angle glaucoma, Acta Ophthalmol 43:714, 1965

39. Krupin, T, Mitchell, KB, Johnson, MF, and Becker, B: The long term effects of iridectomy for primary acute angle-closure glaucoma, Am J Ophthalmol 86:506, 1978

40. Lowe, RF: Acute angle-closure glaucoma—the second eye: an analysis of 200 cases, Br J Ophthalmol 46:641, 1962

41. Lowe, RF: Primary angle-closure glaucoma investigations after surgery for pupillary block, Am J Ophthalmol 57:931, 1964

42. Lowe, RF: The natural history and principles of treatment of primary angle-closure glaucoma, Am J Ophthalmol 61:642, 1966

43. Lowe, RF: Primary angle-closure glaucoma: a review of provocative tests, Br J Ophthalmol 51:727, 1967

44. Lowe, RF: Acute angle-closure glaucoma: acetazolamide therapy, Aust J Ophthalmol 1:24, 1973

45. Lowe, RF: Primary angle-closure glaucoma: a review 5 years after bilateral surgery, Br J Ophthalmol 57:457, 1973

46. Mapstone, R: Closed angle glaucoma: theoretical considerations, Br J Ophthalmol 58:36, 1974

47. Mapstone, R: Provocative tests in closed-angle glaucoma, Br J Ophthalmol 60:115, 1976

48. Mapstone, R: Normal response to pilocarpine and phenylephrine, Br J Ophthalmol 61:510, 1977

49. Mapstone, R: Outflow changes in positive provocative tests, Br J Ophthalmol 61:634, 1977

50. Mapstone, R: Outflow changes in normal eyes after closed-angle glaucoma, Br J Ophthalmol 61:637, 1977

51. Mapstone, R: Acute shallowing of the anterior chamber, Br J Ophthalmol 65:446, 1981

52. Mapstone, R: The fellow eye, Br J Ophthalmol 65:410, 1981

53. Neumann, E, and Hyams, SW: Gonioscopy and anterior chamber depth in the prone-position provocative test for angle-closure glaucoma, Ophthalmologica 167:9, 1973

54. Poinoosawmy, D, Nagasubramanian, S, and Brown, NP: Effect of pilocarpine on visual acuity and on the dimensions of the cornea and anterior chamber, Br J Ophthalmol 60:676, 1976

55. Pollack, IP: Chronic angle-closure glaucoma: diagnosis and treatment in patients with angles that appear open, Arch Ophthalmol 85:676, 1971

56. Rieser, JC, and Schwartz, B: Miotic induced malignant glaucoma, Arch Ophthalmol 87:706, 1972

57. Ritch, R: The treatment of chronic angle-closure glaucoma, Ann Ophthalmol 13:21, 1981

58. Ritch, R: Argon laser treatment for medically unresponsive attacks of angle-closure glaucoma, Am J Ophthalmol 94:197, 1982

59. Ritch, R, and Solomon, IS: Glaucoma surgery. In L'Esperance, FA, Jr, editor: Ophthalmic lasers, St Louis, The CV Mosby Co (In press)

60. Rivera, AH, Brown, RH, and Anderson, DR: Laser iridotomy vs surgical iridectomy: have the indications changed? Arch Ophthalmol 103:1350, 1985

61. Rutkowski, PC, Fernandes, JL, Galin, MA, and Halasa, AM: Alpha adrenergic receptor blockade in the treatment of angle-closure glaucoma, Trans Am Acad Ophthalmol Otolaryngol 77:137, 1973

62. Rutkowski, PC, and Thompson, HS: Mydriasis and increased intraocular pressure. I. Pupillographic studies, Arch Ophthalmol 87:21, 1972

63. Shaw, BR, and Lewis, RA: Intraocular pressure elevation after pupilary dilation in open angle glaucoma, Arch Ophthalmol 104:1185, 1986

64. Shin, DH: Argon laser treatment for relief of medically unresponsive angle-closure glaucoma attacks, Am J Ophthalmol 94:821, 1982

65. Snow, JT: Value of prophylactic peripheral iridectomy on the second eye in angle-closure glaucoma, Trans Ophthalmol Soc UK 97:189, 1977

66. Spaeth, GL: The normal development of the human chamber angle: a new system of descriptive grading, Trans Ophthalmol Soc UK 91:709, 1971

67. Tornquist, R: Dark-room test on eyes with a shallow anterior chamber, Acta Ophthalmol 36:664, 1958

68. Valle, O: The cyclopentolate provocative test in suspected or untreated open-angle glaucoma. III. The significance of pigment for the result of the cyclopentolate provocative test in suspected or untreated open-angle glaucoma, Acta Ophthalmol 54:654, 1976

69. Valle, O: Effect of cyclopentolate on the aqueous dynamics in incipient or suspected open-angle glaucoma, Acta Ophthalmol 123(Suppl):52, 1973

70. Wand, M: Provocative tests in angle-closure glaucoma: a brief review with commentary, Ophthalmic Surg 5:32, 1974

71. Wand, M, and Grant, WM: Thymoxamine hydrochloride: effects on the facility of outflow and intraocular pressure, Invest Ophthalmol 15:400, 1976

72. Wand, M, and Grant, WM: Thymoxamine test, Arch Ophthalmol 96:1009, 1978

73. Wilensky, J, et al: Gonioscopy, Invest Ophthalmol Vis Sci 17(Suppl):144, 1978

74. Wilkie, J, Drance, SM, and Schulzer, M: The effect of miotics on the anterior chamber depth, Am J Ophthalmol 68:78, 1969

75. Wishart, PK, Nagasubramanian, S, and Hitchings, RA: Argon laser trabeculoplasty in narrow angle glaucoma, Eye 1:567, 1987

76. Wollensak, J, and Ehrhorn, J: Angle block glaucoma and prophylactic iridectomy in the eye without symptoms, Klin Monatsbl Augenheilkd 167:791, 1975

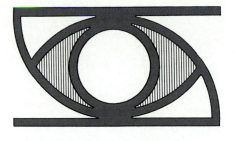

PART EIGHT

THE SECONDARY GLAUCOMAS

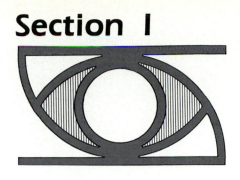

Section 1

Glaucomas Associated With Developmental Disorders

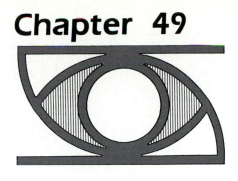

Chapter 49

Aniridia

Helen Mintz Hittner

Aniridia, which was first described in 1818 by Barratta,[3] is a rare, bilateral developmental disorder, occurring in 1.8 per 100,000 live births. It can be subdivided into at least three genetically identifiable types. Furthermore, there has been considerable diagnostic confusion with other anterior segment developmental disorders that may be phenotypically similar (Fig. 49-1 and see box, p. 870), especially with Axenfeld-Reiger syndrome (Chapter 50) and Peters' anomaly (Chapter 51).

CLASSIFICATION OF ANIRIDIA

It is not possible to accurately classify aniridia within the spectrum of anterior segment developmental anomalies until we unravel the complexities of the human genome and the pathogenic mechanisms of disorders of differentiation. Any classification based on our current concepts of ocular differentiation will need major revision as new information becomes available. The diseases of the anterior segment have a variety of presentations, but it is possible to suggest the following classification based on the major embryologic layer experiencing damage:
1. Neuroectoderm (aniridia)
2. First neural crest mesenchymal wave
    a. Peters' anomaly
    b. Anterior segment mesenchymal dysgenesis (ASMD)
    c. Congenital hereditary endothelial dystrophy (CHED)
3. Second neural crest mesenchymal wave
    a. Congenital hereditary stromal dystrophy (CHSD)
4. Third neural crest mesenchymal wave
    a. Axenfeld-Rieger syndrome

The following three genetic types of aniridia are given in order of decreasing prevalence (see Fig. 44-1):
1. Isolated autosomal dominant aniridia (AN1) with complete penetrance and variable expressivity (approximately 85%)
2. Autosomal dominant aniridia (AN2) associated with Wilms' tumor, genitourinary anomalies, and mental retardation (approximately 13%)
3. Autosomal recessive aniridia (AN3) with cerebellar ataxia and mental retardation (approximately 2%)

Isolated Autosomal Dominant Aniridia (AN1) With Complete Penetrance and Variable Expressivity

Since the first pedigree was reported in 1837 by Gutbier,[35] numerous families have been described to document the existence of an autosomal dominant mode of inheritance for isolated aniridia. The gene has a mutation rate of 4×10^{-6} mutations/locus/generation per 100,000 live births.[76] Two thirds of the cases have an affected parent (familial); the remaining one-third are new mutations (sporadic). Although aniridia was reported classically with complete penetrance,[69,76] aspects of variable expressivity have been stressed repeatedly.[17,36,38,58,80] Linkage has been reported for isolated autosomal dominant aniridia on chromosomes 1,[79] 2,[19] and 9.[43] The autosomal dominant mode of inheritance may be linked to more than

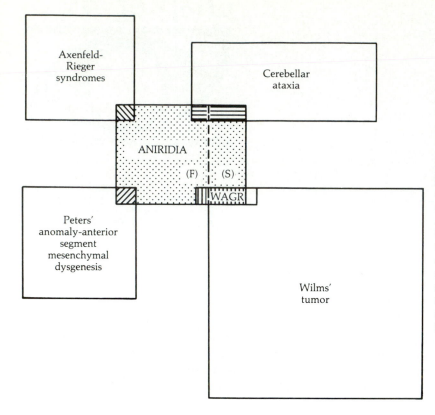

Fig. 49-1 Schematic representation of relationship between three types of aniridia, Wilms' tumor, cerebellar ataxia, Axenfeld-Rieger syndromes, and Peters' anomaly–anterior segment mesenchymal dysgenesis. ⠒⠒, AN1, isolated autosomal dominant aniridia with complete penetrance and variable expressivity. ‖‖ AN2, autosomal dominant aniridia associated with Wilms' tumor, genitourinary anomalies, and mental retardation (WAGR). ≡ AN3, autosomal recessive aniridia with cerebellar ataxia and mental retardation. ⧄, Anterior segment abnormalities (Rieger's syndrome) with ambiguous genitalia and mental retardation—XXXXY; and anterior segment abnormalities (Rieger's syndrome) with mental retardation—del 6q22. ⧄, Anterior segment mesenchymal dysgenesis-1—autosomal dominant linkage to 4p. *F*, familial; *S*, sporadic.

CHROMOSOMAL FINDINGS IN SYNDROMES WITH ANTERIOR SEGMENT DEVELOPMENTAL DISORDERS

I. Neuroectoderm: iris pigment epithelium and pupillary musculature
  A. Aniridia (AN)
    1. AN1: 2p25 (AD) isolated[19]
    2. AN2: 11p13 (AD) isolated,[59,78] or more commonly, associated with Wilms' tumor, genitourinary anomalies, and mental retardation[73]
    3. AN3: chromosome undetermined (AR) with cerebellar ataxia and mental retardation[29]
II. First neural crest mesenchymal wave: corneal endothelium and trabecular meshwork
  A. Peters' anomaly (PT)
    1. PT1: chromosome undetermined (AR)
    2. Subtype: 9 trisomy[30]
  B. Anterior segment mesenchymal dysgenesis (ASMD)
    1. ASMD1: 4p (AD)[21]
  C. Congenital hereditary endothelial dystrophy (CHED)
    1. CHED1: chromosome undetermined (AD)
III. Second neural crest mesenchymal wave: corneal stroma
  A. Congenital hereditary stromal dystrophy (CHSD)
    1. CHSD1: chromosome undetermined (AD)
IV. Third neural crest mesenchymal wave: iris stroma
  A. Axenfeld-Rieger syndrome (AXRG)
    1. AXRG1: chromosome undetermined (AD) with dental anomalies and protruding umbilicus
    2. Subtype: XXXXY Rieger's syndrome with ambiguous genitalia and mental retardation[64]
    3. Subtype: 21 trisomy[22]
    4. Subtype: dup 3p[54]
    5. Subtype: del 4p16[87]
    6. Subtype: del 4q[50]
    7. Subtype: del 6q22 Rieger's syndrome with mental retardation[49]

one chromosomal site. Only the linkage with chromosome 2, however, has been substantiated by an isolated short arm terminal deletion[1] and by studies on additional members of the originally reported family (lod score linkage to acid phosphatase 1 has increased from 1.8 in 1980[19] to 3.1 in 1987 [Robert E. Ferrell, personal communication]). Study of this family has made possible ordering of two enzymes on the short arm of chromosome 2 (Fig. 49-2).

The differential diagnosis of this type of aniridia includes other anterior segment developmental disorders that are associated with minor or no systemic abnormalities: Axenfeld-Rieger syndrome (facial, dental, genital, umbilical, and inguinal ab-

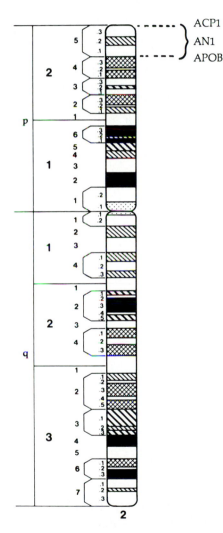

Fig. 49-2 Genetic map of chromosome 2; isolated autosomal dominant aniridia (AN1) has been tentatively assigned to region 2p25. Two markers have been studied that also have been assigned to region 2p25: apolipoprotein B (APOB) is distal to AN1; and acid phosphatase 1, soluble (ACP1) is proximal to AN1.

normalities), Peters' anomaly, and anterior segment mesenchymal dysgenesis (see Fig. 49-1 and see box on p. 870).

Autosomal Dominant Aniridia (AN2) Associated with Wilms' Tumor, Genitourinary Anomalies, and Mental Retardation

The association of aniridia with Wilms' tumor was first reported in 1953.[12] According to several large series, the frequency of occurrence in association with Wilms' tumor is: 1:43,[75] 1:64,[48] 1:73,[57] 1:87,[74] and 1:91.[65] Conversely, the frequency with which Wilms' tumor occurs in cases of sporadic aniridia has been reported to be 1:3[26,66] and 1:7.[23] This association is part of a constellation of findings including Wilms' tumor, Aniridia, Genitourinary anomalies, and mental Retardation (WAGR). In 1974, the initial report of a chromosome deletion in a WAGR patient erroneously placed the deletion on chromosome 8.[45] This patient was found on reanalysis to have a translocation involving chromosomes 8 and 11 with an 11p13 deletion.[24] An 11p13 deletion was reported initially in 1978.[73] The 11p13 segment and Wilms' tumor is highly comparable to the 13q14 segment and retinoblastoma, and both fit the Knudson two-hit hypothesis (Table 49-1). According to this hypothesis, retinoblastoma results from two separate gene alterations. The first is either germinal (stem cell) or somatic (retinal); the second is always somatic (retinal). In heritable cases, the first mutation is germinal and the second is retinal. In nonheritable cases, both mutations are retinal. For this reason, the heritable cases generally are multifocal and occur at an early age; the nonheritable cases are unifocal and occur at a later age.

The 11p13 segment has been extensively studied, and two markers have been identified within this band (Fig. 49-3). In 1980, catalase (CAT) was assigned to this segment.[41] A decrease in CAT may be useful to identify patients with sporadic aniridia at risk for Wilms' tumor, who have undetectable deletions.[20] However, a report of a patient with WAGR with normal CAT demonstrates that CAT is not within the WAGR region, i.e., between WT1 and AN2.[67] Furthermore, the report of a family with AN2 and a translocation 4/11(q22;p13) without Wilms' tumor and with normal CAT,[78] and the report of a patient with Wilms' tumor and a deletion of 11p13 without aniridia but with decreased CAT have been used to map CAT closer to WT1 than to AN2.[82] In 1986, the beta-subunit of follicle-stimulating hormone (FSHB) was assigned to this

Table 49-1 Comparison of retinoblastoma and Wilms' tumor

	Retinoblastoma	Wilms' tumor
Incidence	3/million/year	7.8/million/year[88]
Mortality	Low	High
Second tumors	Common	Uncommon[84]
ONE-HIT CASES		
Maternal age at conception	Older	Older[75]
Patient age at diagnosis	Younger	Younger[75]
Sex predilection	None	Males[75] (2:1)[56,82]
Bilateral/unilateral (common)	3:1	2:1;[75] 5:1[55]
Tumor: chromosomal abnormalities	13q14	11p13
Lymphocyte		
Chromosomal deletions	13q14	11p13 all cases with aniridia except in cases in reference 82
Chromosomal rearrangements		
Translocations	Numerous	t(1;2)(p13;p13 del(11)(p13)[85]
		t(2;17)(q23;q25) del(11)(p13)[61]
		t(4;7;15)(q21.2;p14;q26) del(11)(p13p14)[41,83]
		inv(7)(q21.2q31) del(11)(p13.05p14.05)[71]
		t(8;11)(p21.2q14.4) del (11)(p14.7p13.4)[24,45]
		t(8;11)(q13;p14) del(11)(p14p12)[32]
		t(9;11)(q21.2;p11.2—qter) del(11)(p11.2—qter)[20]
		t(11;22)(p13;q12) del(11)(p13)[27]
Insertions	Numerous	ins(2;11)(q32;p13p14.1)*[89]
		ins(11)(q22;p11.3p14)*[39]
		ins(11;12)(p12p14.2;p11.2)[60]
		ins(11;16)(p13;p11.3p14)*[44]
Markers near these sites	Esterase D	Catalase[41]
		Aniridia[73]
		Follicle stimulating hormone (beta)[31]
Other chromosomes		Cases without aniridia:
		t(Bq+"−)[28]
		t(7;13)(q36;q13)[8]
Trisomy	XXX	XX/XY[15]
	XXY	8[63]
	21	18[42]
TWO-HIT CASES		
Maternal age at conception	Younger	Younger[75]
Patient age at diagnosis	Older	Older[75]
Sex predilection	None	None[75,82]
Bilateral/unilateral	Rarely bilateral	1:7;[10] 1:25;[68] 1:50[75]
Tumor		
Chromosomal abnormalities	13q14; N-myc; isochromosome 6p21; trisomy 1q25-q32; and many others	11p13; c-Ha-ras1 oncogene;[70] and many others
Lymphocyte (autosomal dominant)	Normal	Normal

*Familial.

segment after studying four patients with 11p13 deletions.[31] The identification of a partial androgen receptor defect in a patient with 11p13 deletion supports this assignment.[52] Most WAGR patients who were reported to be without deletions can now be found to have deletions +/−CAT and +/−FSHB. For example, monozygous twins (discordant for Wilms' tumor) reported as 46XX in 1978,[13] were restudied and found to have an 11p13 deletion in 1978.[73] WAGR patients who were reported to be without microscopic deletions and without CAT deficiency [72] should have FSHB determinations. Thus, studies of WAGR patients with varying deletions have been used to map the sequence of 11p13 from the centromere as follows: CAT, WT1, AN2, and FSHB (see Fig. 49-3). Further

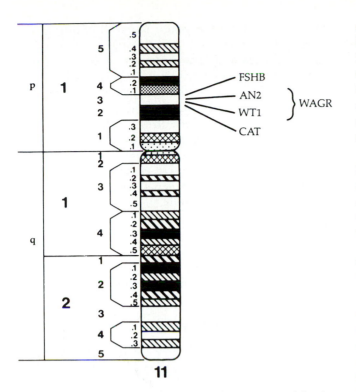

Fig. 49-3 Genetic map of chromosome 11; autosomal dominant aniridia (*AN2*) associated with Wilms' tumor (*WT1*), genitourinary anomalies, and mental retardation (*WAGR*). Three markers have been studied that are assigned to region 11p13: follicle-stimulating hormone, beta polypeptide (*FSHB*); and catalase (*CAT*).

work will be required to sequence and clone the 11p13 region in humans as has been done for the 13q14 region (retinoblastoma).[47] The ultimate goal is to control tumorigenic expression of Wilms' tumor in children, as has been done in mice.[86]

Other syndromes reported with WAGR appear to be caused by difficulties in identifying small chromosome 11p13 deletions. Whenever possible, these cases should be restudied with current techniques. For example, one apparent case of WAGR was reported in 1976 as Smith-Lemli-Opitz syndrome with 46XY.[33] Similarly, multiple cases of WAGR have been reported to have ocular findings other than "aniridia": Peters' anomaly,[16] and anterior segment dysgenesis.[5] These cases only attest to the diverse appearance of this form of aniridia.

Patients with aniridia have been reported to have translocations with and without deletions. When translocations occur without deletions, that is, with one break, aniridia can occur as an autosomal dominant (AN2) without Wilms' tumor, without CAT deficiency, and presumably without FSHB deficiency. This indicates that AN2 is a separate locus.[59,78] When translocations occur with

deletions, that is, with two breaks, two-thirds have Wilms' tumor.[59] When single breaks occur, the 11p13 site is always involved. When two breaks occur, the sites are highly variable, but always encompass the 11p13 site. Similarly, there are reports of patients with Wilms' tumor who do not have aniridia, indicating that WT1 is also a separate locus.[82]

The differential diagnosis of this type of aniridia includes the chromosome pattern XXXXY with aniridia—Rieger's syndrome, ambiguous genitalia, and mental retardation;[64] and complex deletions at 66q22 with aniridia—Rieger's syndrome and mental retardation.[49]

Autosomal Recessive Aniridia (AN3) with Cerebellar Ataxia and Mental Retardation

Autosomal recessive aniridia (AN3) with cerebellar ataxia and mental retardation was first described in 1965.[29] A cerebellar lesion can often be documented by CT scanning. This association can be sporadic or can occur in siblings, and it is felt to represent an autosomal recessive mode of inheritance.[25] No chromosomal location has been suggested for this rare syndrome.

The differential diagnosis of this form of aniridia (also known as Gillespie's syndrome) includes the following multiple syndromes with cerebellar ataxia:

1. Cerebellar ataxia, congenital cataracts, and mental subnormality (Marinesco-Sjögren syndrome)
2. Infantile cerebellar ataxia with progressive external ophthalmoplegia
3. Pyramidal and cerebellar dysfunction with optic atrophy (Behr's disease)
4. Spinocerebellar ataxia with pupillary paralysis
5. Congenital nonprogressive cerebellar ataxia associated with mental retardation and retinal colobomas
6. Cerebellar ataxia with chronic hypertrophic polyneuritis and atypical progressive pigmentary degeneration of the retina (Refsum's disease).

CLINICAL MANIFESTATIONS

The most common clinical manifestations of aniridia are photophobia, nystagmus, decreased vision, amblyopia, and strabismus. Photophobia occurs primarily in patients with virtually complete absence of the iris or very large colobomas. Pendular nystagmus is present in most patients with aniridia regardless of visual acuity. Decreased vision, 20/100 or less in the better eye, has been found in approximately 86% of affected individuals. Progressive visual loss ensues because of secondary ocular complications that have a poor surgical prognosis, including corneal opacities, cataract formation, and angle-closure glaucoma. There are isolated AN1 families with variable iris abnormalities with good visual acuity (greater than 50% of the individuals with 20/40 or better vision).[17,38] In these AN1 families and in AN2 patients with minimal iris abnormalities, corneal opacification is uncommon, the response to cataract surgery is favorable, and development of angle-closure glaucoma is infrequent. High refractive errors and absence of stereoacuity are common. Thus, amblyopia and strabismus occur frequently.

CLINICAL FINDINGS

Iris Anomalies

Typically, the iris appears as a small rudimentary stump (Fig. 49-4, *A*). However, extreme variability in the iris can occur within isolated AN1 families.[38] In such families, irides may vary from rudimentary stumps to mild iris hypoplasia with round pupils (Fig. 49-4, *A* to *E*). In those patients who are minimally affected, iris fluorescein angiography demonstrates vascular abnormalities (Fig. 49-4, *F*). Persistent iris strands,[6] persistent tunica vasculosa lentis,[36] and pupillary displacements[58] are additional iris abnormalities in AN1 families. The same spectrum of iris variability (Fig. 49-5, *A* to *C*) can occur in patients with AN2 associated with Wilms' tumor, genitourinary anomalies, and mental retardation.[72] A fluorescein angiogram will document minimal iris abnormalities in AN2 patients (Fig. 49-5, *D*). Some iris variability (Fig. 49-6, *A* to *B*) also exists in patients with AN3 with cerebellar ataxia and mental retardation, as well as a large spectrum of CT abnormalities (Fig. 49-6, *C* to *D*).

Glaucoma

The glaucoma associated with aniridia appears to have two closely related mechanisms.[53] In patients with AN2, developmental anomalies of the angle can obstruct the trabecular meshwork. In patients with AN1 (and probably in patients with AN3), angle-closure glaucoma can develop by progressive apposition of the rudimentary stump of the iris to the trabecular meshwork.

Aniridia with congenital glaucoma is a rare occurrence (Fig. 49-7, *A*). Infantile glaucoma is also uncommon in patients with aniridia. Usually, glaucoma develops in aniridic patients in the preadolescent or early adult years. Thus, the findings of congenital glaucoma, including buphthalmus with megalocornea and Haab's striae, are rare. Routine gonioscopic evaluation (Fig. 49-7, *B*) of patients with a rudimentary stump of iris reveals sequential anatomic changes in the angle that are consistent with progressive closure of the trabecular meshwork during the first two decades of life.[34] The incidence of glaucoma in aniridia is highly variable (from 6% to 75%).[62] This variance relates to the absence of angle-closure glaucoma in those aniridic patients with round pupils or small colobomas.

Ptosis

Ptosis is known to occur in aniridic patients. A protective ptosis in response to photophobia is often noted; however, a true developmental ptosis is less common.[77]

Corneal Abnormalities

Microcornea is associated with aniridia.[14] Other corneal changes rarely occur congenitally or in the neonatal period. However, sometimes a cellular infiltrate may develop between the epithelium and Bowman's layer as early as 2 years of age. This is seen clinically as a gray opacification involving the superficial layers of the peripheral cornea. Subsequently, fine radial vessels invade this cellular infiltrate and ultimately may cover the entire cornea. This is seen clinically as pannus formation in these superficial corneal layers. Progressive corneal changes mimic a "dystrophy" (Fig. 49-8).[51]

Lens Abnormalities

Congenital lens abnormalities include cataracts (Fig. 49-9, *A*), microphakia (Fig. 49-9, *B*), and lens subluxation (Fig. 49-9,*B*). Those patients with AN2 may have optically significant nuclear cataracts requiring surgery in the neonatal period (see Fig. 49-5, *B*) Patients with AN1 generally have optically insignificant cortical cataracts at birth (see Fig. 49-4, *A* to *D*). These cataracts may progress and compromise vision sufficiently to require surgical intervention by the second or third decade of life. No significant cataracts have been reported in cases of AN3 (see Fig. 49-5, *A* to *B*). The reported incidence of cataracts is between 50% and 85%.[62] This variance probably reflects the failure to report optically insignificant cataracts. Microphakia is an unusual occurrence and often is associated with lens dislocation. Lens dislocation has been reported repeatedly, and the incidence varies from 0% to 56%.[62] This wide variance probably reflects the failure to recognize small degrees of lens subluxation.

Text continued on p. 879.

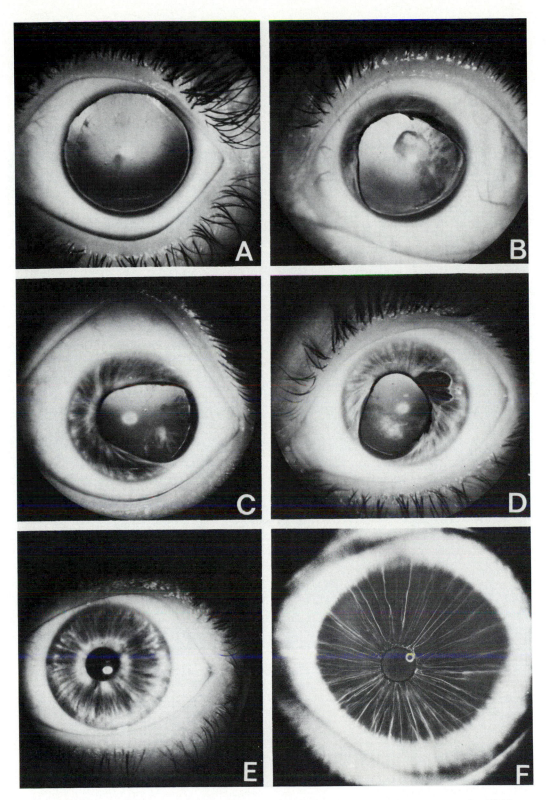

Fig. 49-4   Spectrum of iris abnormalities found in isolated autosomal dominant aniridia (AN1).
A, Virtually total aniridia. **B,** Remnant of iris visible. **C,** Atypical coloboma of iris. **D,** Typical coloboma
of iris. **E,** Iris thinning with round pupil. **F,** Fluorescein angiogram of iris shown in **E,** demonstrating
vascular loops.

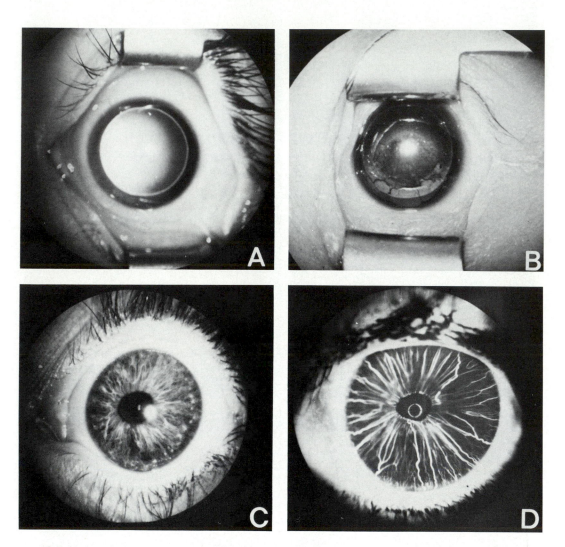

Fig. 49-5 Spectrum of iris abnormalities found in autosomal dominant aniridia (AN2) associated with Wilms' tumor, genitourinary anomalies, and mental retardation. **A,** Virtually total aniridia. **B,** Remnant of iris visible. **C,** Iris thinning with round pupil. **D,** Fluorescein angiogram of iris shown in **C,** demonstrating vascular loops.

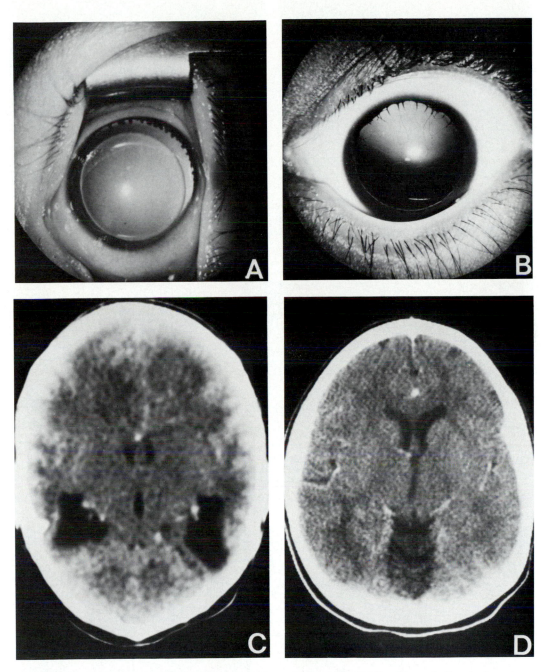

Fig. 49-6 Iris anomalies found in autosomal recessive aniridia (AN3) with cerebellar ataxia and mental retardation. **A,** Virtually total aniridia. **B,** Remnant of iris visible. **C,** CT scan of patient in **A** with dilated lateral ventricles, failure of complete lobulation and diverticulation of brain, and a small posterior fossa. **D,** CT scan of patient in **B** with normal ventricles but dysgenesis of midline structures of cerebellum.

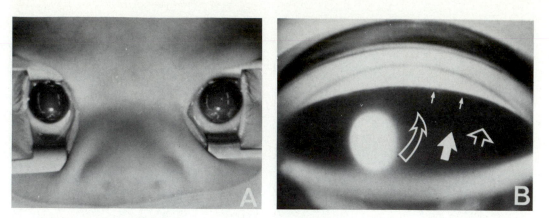

Fig. 49-7   Glaucoma associated with aniridia. **A,** Congenital glaucoma (AN3). **B,** Appearance of angle (AN1) that has not yet developed progressive angle-closure glaucoma. ➡, Edge of lens; ⬆, ciliary processes; ⤴, edge of iris; ⬆, points of iris adherence across trabecular meshwork.

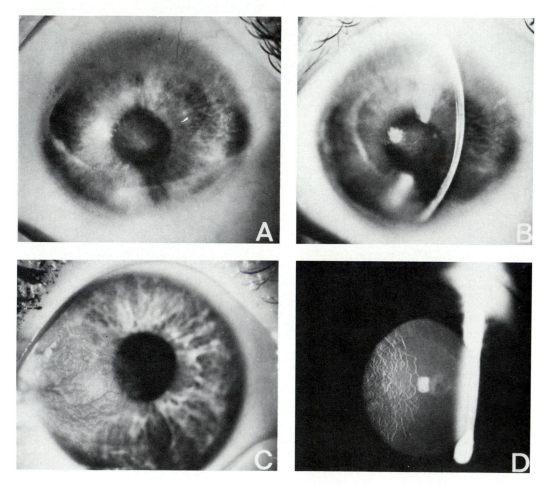

Fig. 49-8   Corneal opacities associated with aniridia. **A,** Small opacity (AN2). **B,** Retroillumination photograph of patient in **A. C,** Hazy cornea (AN1). **D,** Slit-lamp photograph of patient in **C.**

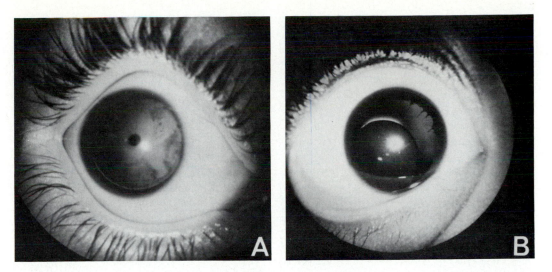

Fig. 49-9 Lens abnormalities associated with aniridia. **A,** Congenital cataract (undetermined type of AN). **B,** Microphakia and lens subluxation (undetermined type of AN).

Posterior Segment Abnormalities

Posterior segment abnormalities include macular (and/or retinal) hypoplasia and optic nerve hypoplasia in AN1 and AN2. In AN3, the macula and optic nerve are usually normal. Macular hypoplasia, and not the iris abnormality, is apparently responsible for the visual reduction and nystagmus of aniridic patients.[17,36,38,58,80] There is no correlation between small amounts of iris and profound macular hypoplasia (Fig. 49-10, *A*), nor between large amounts of iris and minimal macular hypoplasia (Fig. 49-10, *C*) which may be documented only by the presence of vascularization of the macular region by fluorescein angiography (Fig. 49-10, *D*).[38] Thus, there is little support for the former theory that prolonged exposure to light is related to the failure of macular development.

Optic nerve hypoplasia probably occurs in 75% of aniridic patients and is a result of poor macular (and/or retinal) development.[46] This diagnosis is made by calculations of the width of the superior or inferior retinal arterioles before their first bifurcation and the diameter of the optic disc (Fig. 49-10, *B*). The normal ratio for adult disc to arteriole is 14.6 ± 2.4. In hypoplastic discs, this ratio varies from 6.1 to 12.2.[11]

HISTOPATHOLOGY

The pathogenesis of glaucoma associated with aniridia is confused in the literature by the following four important factors:

1. Many case reports describe eyes that have been altered by surgery
2. Isolated case reports of eyes at different stages of glaucoma (from none to severe) make a unified pathogenesis difficult to perceive
3. Case reports of eyes with severe glaucoma confuse the primary cause by secondary changes
4. Case reports with insufficient clinical history obscure the genetic type of aniridia being described

The most comprehensive histopathologic series of aniridic patients is a retrospective review of seven patients from the AFIP files, of whom four had isolated AN1 (three with a positive family history for aniridia), and three had AN2 associated with Wilms' tumor, genitourinary anomalies, and mental retardation.[53] No cases of AN3 with cerebellar ataxia and mental retardation have been studied pathologically.

From this series, the following can be deduced regarding isolated AN1:

1. The iris stroma is hypoplastic, indicating an altered third neural crest wave of mesenchyme
2. The angle may demonstrate a primary abnormality of incomplete cleavage, implying an altered first neural crest wave of mesenchyme, or the angle may demonstrate a secondary abnormality of angle-closure by the formation of peripheral anterior synechiae
3. The cornea reveals a thinning of Bowman's layer with secondary vascular pannus for-

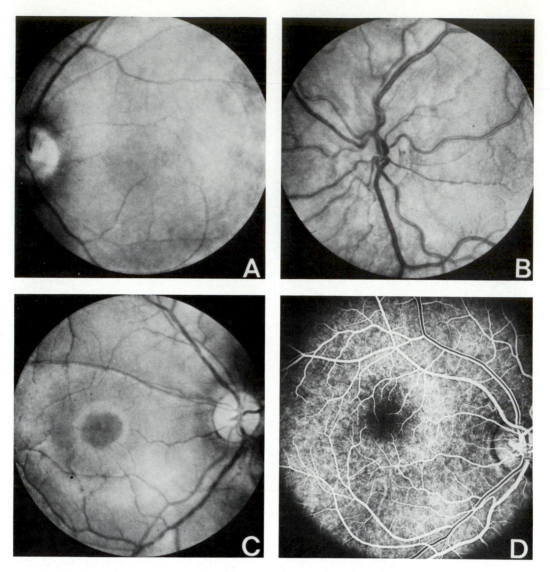

Fig. 49-10 Posterior segment abnormalities associated with aniridia. **A,** Macular hypoplasia (AN1). **B,** Optic nerve hypoplasia (AN1). **C,** Normal macular reflex (AN1). **D,** Fluorescein angiogram of patient in **C** demonstrating an absence of normal macular avascular zone.

mation, suggesting an altered second neural crest wave of mesenchyme

4. The lens is opacified as a secondary phenomenon, revealing the interaction between the lens and cornea during embryogenesis

From the same series, the following differences can be noted in AN2 associated with Wilms' tumor, genitourinary anomalies, and mental retardation:

1. The iris stroma is hypoplastic but with hyperplasia of the vasculature, implying a more severely altered third neural crest wave of mesenchyme and *de novo* vasoformation from the mesenchyme proper

2. The angle contains no trabecular meshwork

or Schlemm's canal, implying a more severely altered first neural crest wave of mesenchyme

Despite these pathologic alterations of mesenchyme,[53] extreme variability in iris appearance,[38] persistence of iris strands,[6] and persistence of the tunica vasculosa lentis,[36] the following four clinical manifestations, listed from the anterior to the posterior aspect of the eye, suggest that aniridia is primarily a disorder of the neuroectoderm:

1. The hypoplasia of iris pigment epithelium and pupillary musculature in aniridia[53]

2. The presence of typical colobomas in members of AN1 families[38]

3. The frequent occurrence of macular hypoplasia in AN1 and AN2[38]

4. The frequent perception of optic nerve hypoplasia in AN1 and AN2[46]

Thus, the pathogenesis of aniridia (AN1 and AN2) is currently attributed to a primary developmental arrest of neuroectoderm and a secondary alteration of all three neural crest waves of mesenchyme. The functional development of the anterior segment is a complex interrelationship between neuroectoderm and neural crest mesenchymal waves. Multiple cellular events, such as cell division, migration, differentiation, and death, are involved in the final appearance of the anterior segment. Multiple biochemical factors essential for these cellular events, such as inducers, cell-surface characteristics, and the extracellular matrix, influence the final functional integrity of the anterior segment. Thus, pathogenesis may involve defective formation or excessive regression of various layers of the anterior segment caused by cellular or biochemical aberrations. This explains the combined anterior and posterior segment neuroectodermal and mesenchymal defects (see the box on p. 870). Because typical colobomas have not been associated with AN3, and because all reported cases of AN3 have no significant cataracts, normal maculae, and normal optic nerves, AN3 may not be primarily a disorder of the neuroectoderm. However, because of the absence of any pathologic reports of AN3 to suggest an alternative primary defect, it has been classified as an aniridia for the present.

MANAGEMENT

Genetic Counseling

It is desirable to assign a specific genetic type to each aniridic patient. Thus, each of the following may be indicated in specific cases (see the box on p. 49-6 for differential diagnosis of aniridia):

1. A thorough family history with specific inquiry regarding any ocular abnormality and/or low vision, dental anomaly, protruding umbilicus, genitourinary anomaly (including Wilms' tumor), or mental retardation

2. Examination of the patient systemically, including teeth, umbilicus, genitalia, urinary system (including ultrasound), and central nervous system (including CT scan)

3. Banded chromosome analysis and quantitative determination of CAT and FSHB on the patient and both parents, and linkage analysis when large families are available for study (see Fig. 49-2)

4. A thorough ocular examination of the patient, both parents, and other relatives (with anterior and/or posterior segment fluorescein angiography)

Treatment of Photophobia and Nystagmus

To establish comfort, photophobia can be treated by tinted or iris contact lenses, or tinted spectacle lenses at any age. In the 1960s, it was reported that the reduction of nystagmus is greatest when tinted or iris contact lenses are fitted in infancy.[18,37] However, the final visual acuity is unaffected by the use of tinted or iris contact lenses. In all pendular nystagmus of early infancy, the initial nystagmus has a large amplitude with a low frequency; with maturation, the amplitude decreases and the frequency increases. Thus, the observation of reduction of nystagmus with the early fitting of tinted contact lenses is simply a reflection of a normal developmental event.

Treatment of Refractive Errors

With lens abnormalities, especially dislocation, large refractive errors may be present. Thus, a careful refraction and complete correction of all refractive errors is mandatory.

Treatment of Amblyopia and Strabismus

In all cases of aniridia, the same vision in both eyes should be achieved when possible, since the potential visual acuity is usually symmetric. Thus, any differences in visual acuity, without structural differences, should be treated by vigorous occlusion of the favored eye in children under 10 years of age. Binocularity can be achieved when macular hypoplasia is not severe. Thus, strabismus surgery is indicated at an early age.

Medical Therapy of Glaucoma

Medical therapy is the safest approach to the treatment of glaucoma in the aniridic patient,[4] although this usually proves inadequate ultimately.[7] Miotics (cholinergics and anticholinesterases) are used for their effect on outflow facility, since in relatively complete aniridia there is no iris pupillary sphincter present. The nonoccluded trabecular meshwork may benefit from this treatment, although the induced myopia may interfere with vision. Usually, patients become refractory to topical sympathomimetics and beta-blockers, and carbonic anhydrase inhibitors.

Surgical Therapy of Glaucoma

Goniotomy

Goniotomy has been suggested as an early surgical therapy[2] or as a prophylactic procedure[34] for aniridia in an attempt to halt progressive angle closure. However, the danger of this procedure, which utilizes an anterior approach, cannot be overemphasized because of the necessity of passing instruments over the vulnerable lens and zonules in the anterior chamber. Further, the appropriate surgical site of dissection is more difficult to achieve in some cases.

Trabeculotomy

Trabeculotomy may be preferable for aniridic patients because of the ab externo approach. This is considered to be both more effective, since the appropriate surgical plane of dissection is more readily achieved, and safer, since instruments are not passed completely across the anterior segment.[40] Nonetheless, this procedure is also associated with risks, failures, and the necessity of repeated intraocular surgery.

Filtering procedures

After a few initial attempts of goniotomy or trabeculotomy, many surgeons prefer to use filtering procedures. Because the iris is not present to prevent the inadvertent damage to the lens, cataract formation or progression may occur. Further, there is a significant increase in the possibility of vitreous loss when filtering procedures are performed in aniridic patients.[7] These, however, have been reported to be successful.[9]

Laser therapy to angle abnormalities

Laser therapy to angle abnormalities is reported to induce an initial pressure decrease that is followed by substantial increase.[81] Thus, although the laser can certainly be used to dissect the early attachments of the iris stump to the trabecular meshwork, extensive synechiae tend to form in the treated areas. Although it is preferable to avoid invasive procedures in aniridic patients, laser therapy to the angle abnormalities does not appear to be of prolonged value.[90]

Cyclocryotherapy

Cyclocryotherapy is designed to destroy part of the ciliary body and may be the safest surgical approach to the patient with aniridia. However, even this may produce complications, such as acceleration of peripheral corneal opacification or cataract formation. When cyclocryotherapy is used, it is imperative that multiple treatments be planned (with a maximum of four applications), using a 3.5 mm glaucoma probe at -90° C for 45 seconds. A single heavy treatment can lead to extreme uveitis, uveal effusion, and phthisis. Even with multiple staged surgeries, vitreous hemorrhage and prolonged hypotony can occur.

Summary

Genetic counseling is the most significant means to prevent this developmental disorder of the anterior segment. Treatment of the associated glaucoma with conservative medical and noninvasive surgical procedures usually fails with time. Invasive surgical procedures usually give only temporary relief and are often disasterous in the treatment of this glaucoma secondary to a developmentally obstructed angle (AN2) or to a progressively closed angle (AN1). When glaucoma develops in the second and third decades of life, the rate of surgical success appears to improve. Cases of congenital and infantile glaucoma respond poorly or only transiently to surgical intervention.

REFERENCES

1. Arias, S, Rolo, M, and Gonzalez, N: Terminal deletion of the short arm of chromosome 2, informative for acid phosphatase (ACP1), malate dehydrogenase (MDH1), and coloboma of iris loci, Cytogenet Cell Genet 37:401, 1984
2. Barkan, O: Goniotomy for glaucoma associated with aniridia, Arch Ophthalmol 49:1, 1953
3. Barratta, G: Observazioni pratiche sulle principali malattie degli orchi, Tomo 2 s. 349, 1818, Cited by Jungken, C: J der Chirurgie Augen-Heilkunde, 2:677, 1821
4. Barsoum-Homsy, M, and Chevrette, L: Incidence and prognosis of childhood glaucoma: a study of 63 cases, Ophthalmology 93:1323, 1986
5. Beauchamp, GR: Anterior segment dysgenesis: keratolenticular adhesion and aniridia, J Pediatr Ophthalmol Strab 17:55, 1980
6. Beauchamp, GR, and Meisler, DM: An alternative hypothesis for iris maldevelopment (aniridia), J Pediatr Ophthalmol Strab 23:281, 1986
7. Berlin, HS, and Ritch, R: The treatment of glaucoma secondary to aniridia, Mount Sinai J Med 48:111, 1981
8. Bernard JL, et al: Wilms' tumor, malformative syndrome, mental retardation and de novo constitutional translocation, t(7;13)(q36;q13), Eur J Pediatr 141:175, 1984
9. Blake, EM: The surgical treatment of glaucoma complicating congenital aniridia, Am J Ophthalmol 36:907, 1953
10. Bond, JV: Bilateral Wilms' tumour: age at diagnosis, associated congenital anomalies, and possible pattern of inheritance, Lancet 2:482, 1975
11. Brown, GC, and Tasman, WS: Congenital anomalies of the optic disc, New York, 1983, Grune & Stratton, Inc
12. Brusa, P, and Torricelli, C: Nefroblastoma di Wilms e affezioni renali congenite nella casistica dell'

I.P.P.A.I. di Milano, Minerva Pediatr 5:457, 1953

13. Cotlier, E, Rose, M, and Moel, SA: Aniridia, cataracts, and Wilms' tumor in monozygous twins, Am J Ophthalmol 86:129, 1978

14. David, R, MacBeath, L, and Jenkins, T: Aniridia associated with microcornea and subluxated lenses, Br J Ophthalmol 62:118, 1978

15. Denys, P, et al: Association d'un syndrome anatomopathologique de pseudohermaphrodisme masculin, d'une tumeur de Wilms, d'une nephropathie parenchymateuse et d'un mosaicisme XX/XY, Arch F Pediatr 24:729, 1967

16. Eiferman, RA: Association of Wilms' tumor with Peters' anomaly, Ann Ophthalmol 16:933, 1984

17. Elsas, FJ, Maumenee, IH, Kenyon, KR, and Yoder, F: Familial aniridia with preserved ocular function, Am J Ophthalmol 83:718, 1977

18. Enoch, JM, and Windsor, CE: Remission of nystagmus following fitting contact lenses to an infant with aniridia, Am J Ophthalmol 66:333, 1968

19. Ferrell, RE, Chakravarti, A, Hittner, HM, and Riccardi, VM: Autosomal dominant aniridia: probable linkage to acid phosphatase-1 locus on chromosome 2, Proc Natl Acad Sci 77:1580, 1980

20. Ferrell, RE, and Riccardi, VM: Catalase levels in patients with aniridia and/or Wilms' tumor: utility and limitations, Cytogenet Cell Genet 31:120, 1981

21. Ferrell, RE, Hittner, HM, Kretzer, FL, and Antoszyk, JH: Anterior segment mesenchymal dysgenesis: probable linkage to the MNS blood group on chromosome 4, Am J Hum Genet 34:345, 1982

22. Finlay, RD: Mesodermal dysgenesis of the anterior segment in a mongoloid child, J Pediatr Ophthalmol 11:148, 1974

23. Flanagan, JC, and DiGeorge, AM: Sporadic aniridia and Wilms' tumor, Am J Ophthalmol 67:558, 1969

24. Francke, U, Holmes, LB, Atkins, L, and Riccardi, VM: Aniridia–Wilms' tumor association: evidence for specific deletion of 11p13, Cytogenet Cell Genet 24:185, 1979

25. François, J, and Lentini, F: Gillespie-Syndrom (inkomplette Aniridie, zerebellare Ataxie und Oligophrenie), Klin Mbl Augenheilk 184:313, 1984

26. Fraumeni, JF, Jr, and Glass, AG: Wilms' tumor and congenital aniridia, JAMA 206:825, 1968

27. Gardner, RJM, Grindley, RM, Chewings, WE, and Holdaway, MDH: Wilms' tumour with somatic rearrangement of chromosome 11 at band p13, Proc University of Otago Medical School 61:32, 1983

28. Giangiacomo, J, Penchausky, L, Monteleone, PL, and Thompson, J: Bilateral neonatal Wilms' tumor with B-C chromosomal translocation, J Pediatr 86:98, 1975

29. Gillespie, FD: Aniridia, cerebellar ataxia, and oligophrenia in siblings, Arch Ophthalmol 73:338, 1965

30. Ginsberg, J, Soukup, S, and Ballard, ET: Pathologic features of the eye in trisomy 9, J Pediatr Ophthalmol Strab 19:37, 1982

31. Glaser, T, et al: The beta-subunit of follicle-stimulating hormone is deleted in patients with aniridia and Wilms' tumour, allowing a further definition of the WAGR locus, Nature 321:882, 1986

32. Godde-Salz, E, and Behnke H: Aniridia, mental retardation and an unbalanced reciprocal translocation of chromosomes 8 and 11 with an interstitial deletion of 11p, Eur J Pediatr 136:93, 1981

33. Gracia, R, et al: Asociacion de aniridia con tumor enbrionario no renal (gonadoblastoma) en nino con sindrome de Smith-Lemli-Opitz, Ann Esp Pediatr 8(suppl):19, 1976

34. Grant, WM, and Walton, DS: Progressive changes in the angle in congenital aniridia, with development of glaucoma, Am J Ophthalmol 78:842, 1974

35. Gutbier, S: Irideremia seu defectu iridis congenito. Dissert inaug Wirceb def Gothae, 1834, p. 14, Cited by Berger: Beitrage zur Lehre von der Irideremia von Carron du Villards, und Gutbier, Ammon's z Oph 5:78, 1837

36. Hamming, NA, Miller, MT, and Rabb, M: Unusual variant of familial aniridia, J Pediatr Ophthalmol Strab 23:195, 1986

37. Hermann, JS, and Koverman, JJ: Prophylaxis of amblyopia in aniridia: the role of pinhole contact lenses, J Pediatr Ophthalmol 5:48, 1968

38. Hittner, HM, et al: Variable expressivity in autosomal dominant aniridia by clinical, electrophysiologic, and angiographic criteria, Am J Ophthalmol 89:531, 1980

39. Hittner, HM, Riccardi, VM, and Francke, U: Aniridia caused by a heritable chromosome 11 deletion, Ophthalmology 86:1173, 1979

40. Hoskins, HD, Shaffer, RN, and Hetherington, J: Goniotomy vs. trabeculotomy, J Pediatr Ophthalmol Strab 21:153, 1984

41. Junien, C, et al: Regional assignment of catalase (CAT) gene to band 11p13: association with the aniridia–Wilms' tumor-gonadoblastoma (WAGR) complex, Ann Genet 23:165, 1980

42. Karayalcin, G, Shanske, A, and Honigman, R: Wilms' tumor in a 13-year-old girl with trisomy 18, Am J Dis Child 35:665, 1981

43. Karmon, G, Savir, H, and Shabtal, F: Chromosome 9 pericentric inversion in familial aniridia, Metabolic Ophthalmol 2:213, 1978

44. Kousseff, BG: Maternal translocation 46,XX,t(11;16) with aniridia–Wilms' tumor association in the offspring, Clin Res 28:99A, 1980

45. Ladda, R, Atkins, L, and Littlefield, J: Computer-assisted analysis of chromosomal abnormalities: detection of a deletion in aniridia/Wilms' tumor syndrome, Science 185:784, 1974

46. Layman, PR, Anderson, DR, and Flynn, JT: Frequent occurrence of hypoplastic optic disks in patients with aniridia, Am J Ophthalmol 77:513, 1974

47. Lee, WH, et al: Human retinoblastoma susceptibility gene: cloning, identification, and sequence, Science 235:1394, 1987

48. Lemerle, J, et al: Wilms' tumor: natural history and prognostic factors, Cancer 37:2557, 1976

49. Levin, H, et al: Aniridia, congenital glaucoma, and hydrocephalus in a male infant with ring chromosome 6, Am J Med Genet 25:281, 1986

50. Ligutic, I, et al: Interstitial deletion 4q and Rieger syndrome, Clin Genet 20:323, 1981

51. Mackman, G, Brightbill, FS, and Opitz, JM: Corneal changes in aniridia, Am J Ophthalmol 87:497, 1979

52. Malpuech, G, et al: Male pseudohermaphroditism, partial androgen receptors defect, 11p13 deletion: indication of gene localization, Am J Med Genet 24:679, 1986

53. Margo, CE: Congenital aniridia: a histopathologic study of the anterior segment in children, J Pediatr Ophthalmol Strab 20:192, 1983

54. Martin, NJ, and Steinberg, BG: The dup(3) (p25—pter) syndrome: a case with holoprosencephaly, Am J Med Genet 14:767, 1983

55. Matsunaga, E: Genetics of Wilms' tumor, Hum Genet 57:231, 1981

56. Miller, RW: Relation between cancer and congenital defects in man, N Engl J Med 275:87, 1966

57. Miller, RW, Fraumeni, JF, Jr, and Manning, MD: Association of Wilms' tumor with aniridia, hemihypertrophy, and other congenital malformations, N Engl J Med 270:922, 1964

58. Mondino, BJ, and Cohn, HC: Corectopia with nystagmus, absent foveal reflexes and corneal changes, Acta Ophthalmol 59:85, 1981

59. Moore, JW, et al: Familial isolated aniridia associated with a translocation involving chromosomes 11 and 22 [t(11;22)(p13;q12.2)], Hum Genet 72:297, 1986

60. Nakagome, Y, et al: High-resolution studies in patients with aniridia–Wilms' tumor association, Wilms' tumor or related congenital abnormalities, Hum Genet 67:245, 1984

61. Narahara, K, et al: Regional mapping of catalase and Wilms' tumor—aniridia, genitourinary abnormalities, and mental retardation triad loci to the chromosome segment 11p1305—p1306, Hum Genet 66:181, 1984

62. Nelson, LB, et al: Aniridia: a review, Surv Ophthalmol 28:621, 1984

63. Niss, R, and Passarge, E: Trisomy 8 restricted to cultured fibroblasts, J Med Genet 13:229, 1976

64. Pashayan, H, Dallaire, L, and MacLeod, P: Bilateral aniridia, multiple webs and severe mental retardation in a 47,XXY/48,XXXY mosaic, Clin Genet 4:125, 1973

65. Pendergrass, TW: Congenital anomalies in children with Wilms' tumor: a new survey, Cancer 37:403, 1976

66. Pilling, GP: Wilms' tumor in seven children with congenital aniridia, J Pediatr Surg 10:87, 1975

67. Punnett, HH, et al: Deletion 11p13 with normal catalase activity, Pediatr Res 17(suppl):217A, 1983

68. Ragab, AH, et al: Bilateral Wilms' tumor: a review, Cancer 30:983, 1972

69. Reed, TE, and Falls, HF: A pedigree of aniridia with a discussion of germinal mosaicism in man, Am J Hum Genet 7:28, 1955

70. Reeve, AE, et al: Loss of a Harvey *ras* allele in sporadic Wilms' tumour, Nature 309:174, 1984

71. Riccardi, VM, et al: The aniridia–Wilms' tumor association: the critical role of chromosome band 11p13, Cancer Genet Cytogenet 2:131, 1980

72. Riccardi, VM, et al: Wilms' tumor with aniridia/iris dysplasia and apparently normal chromosomes, J Pediatr 100:574, 1982

73. Riccardi, VM, Sujansky, E, Smith, AC, and Francke, U: Chromosomal imbalance in the aniridia–Wilms' tumor association: 11p interstitial deletion, Pediatrics 61:604, 1978

74. Schweisguth, O, Campinchi, R, Pivoteau, B, and Lemerle, J: Le risque de tumeur du rein chez l'enfant aniridique, Arch Ophthalmol (Paris) 28:65, 1968

75. Shannon, RS, et al: Wilms' tumor and aniridia: clinical and cytogenetic features, Arch Dis Child 57:685, 1982

76. Shaw, MW, Falls, HF, and Neel, JV: Congenital aniridia, Am J Hum Genet 12:389, 1960

77. Shields, MB, and Reed, JW: Aniridia and congenital ptosis, Ann Ophthalmol 7:203, 1975

78. Simola, KOJ, et al: Familial aniridia and translocation t(4;11)(q22;p13) without Wilms' tumor, Hum Genet 63:158, 1983

79. Sloderbeck, JD, et al: Linkage assignment of aniridia to chromosome 1, Am J Hum Genet 27:83A, 1975

80. Soong, HK, and Raizman, MB: Corneal changes in familial iris coloboma, Ophthalmology 93:335, 1986

81. Strasser, G: Unsuccessful laser cyclophotocoagulation for glaucoma in aniridia, Arch Ophthalmol 103:890, 1985

82. Turleau, C, et al: Del 11p13/nephroblastoma without aniridia, Hum Genet 67:455, 1984

83. Turleau, C, et al: Aniridia, male pseudohermaphroditism, gonadoblastoma, mental retardation, and del 11p13, Hum Genet 57:300, 1981

84. Valdes-Dapena, M, and Arey, JB: Multiple (4) primary neoplasms in a child with aniridia, Am J Pathol 62:22a, 1971

85. Waziri, M, Patil, SR, and Hanson, JW: Chromosomal and clinical findings in aniridia patients, Am J Hum Genet 33:125A, 1981

86. Weissman, BE, et al: Introduction of a normal human chromosome 11 into a Wilms' tumor cell line controls its tumorigenic expression, Science 236:175, 1987

87. Wilcox, LM, Jr, and Bercovitch, L: Ophthalmic features of chromosome deletion 4p- (Wolf-Hirschhorn syndrome), Am J Ophthalmol 86:834, 1978

88. Young, JL, and Miller, RW: Incidence of malignant tumors in U.S. children, J Pediatr 86:254, 1975

89. Yunis, JJ, and Ramsay, NKC: Familial occurrence of the aniridia-Wilms' tumor syndrome with deletion 11p13-14.1, J Pediatr 96:1027, 1980

90. Zinn, KM, and Ritch, R: Spontaneous massive vitreous hemorrhage in a patient with aniridia and glaucoma: a pars plana surgical approach, J Ocul Ther Surg p. 182, May-June, 1982

Chapter 50

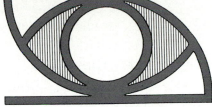

Axenfeld-Rieger Syndrome

M. Bruce Shields

HISTORY AND TERMINOLOGY

In 1920 Axenfeld[4] described a patient who had a white line on the posterior aspect of the cornea near the limbus and tissue strands extending from the peripheral iris to this prominent line. He termed this "posterior embryotoxon of the cornea." Beginning in the mid-1930s Rieger[30,31,32] reported cases with similar anterior segment anomalies, but with additional changes in the iris, including corectopia, atrophy, and hole formation. He referred to this as "mesodermal dysgenesis of the cornea and iris." It was also discovered that some of these patients had associated extraocular developmental defects, especially of the teeth and facial bones.[26,33]

Traditionally, these conditions have been designated by the following three eponyms:

1. *Axenfeld's anomaly:* limited to peripheral anterior segment defects
2. *Rieger's anomaly:* peripheral abnormalities with additional changes in the iris
3. *Rieger's syndrome:* ocular anomalies plus extraocular developmental defects

The similarity of anterior chamber angle abnormalities in these three arbitrary categories has led most investigators to agree that they represent a spectrum of developmental disorders.[1,29,37,38,41] Furthermore, the overlap of ocular and extraocular anomalies is such that the traditional classification is difficult to apply in all cases. Consequently, various collective terms have been applied to this spectrum of disease.

The title "anterior chamber cleavage syndrome" was once proposed,[29] based on a theory of normal anterior chamber angle development in which the angle structures were believed to be formed by a cleavage or separation of two preexisting primordial tissue layers because of differential growth rates.[2] Incomplete cleavage was felt to be responsible for the clinical entities included in this syndrome. However, subsequent study has failed to support this theory of normal anterior chamber angle development. Furthermore, the collective term included the central ocular defects of Peters' anomaly, which is discussed in the following chapter. Although some patients may have the combined defects of Axenfeld's or Rieger's anomaly and Peters' anomaly, the association is rare, and the mechanisms underlying the development of the two disorders are usually different.

Another commonly used collective term is "mesodermal dysgenesis of the cornea and iris," as proposed by Rieger,[32] based on the traditional belief that the involved structures were derived from mesodermal tissue. Further study of ocular development, however, indicates that neural crest cells are the source of these anterior segment structures.[18] Therefore this term is also no longer valid. The term, "iridogoniodysgenesis" is also found in the literature on this spectrum of disorders. However, this term may be too nonspecific, since other conditions exist that also have developmental abnormalities of the iris and anterior chamber angle.

The term "Axenfeld-Rieger (A-R) syndrome" has also been proposed for all clinical variations within this spectrum of developmental disorders.[37,38] This title retains reference to the original eponyms, but does not require arbitrary subclassification of the clinical variations. Furthermore, it is not dependent on any theory of normal ocular development, our understanding of which is still incomplete.

GENERAL FEATURES

The A-R syndrome represents a spectrum of developmental disorders linked by the following common denominators. The ocular component is typically bilateral and is frequently associated with secondary glaucoma. Extraocular defects may also be present. Many, but not all, patients have a family history of the disorder, with an autosomal dominant mode of inheritance. Rare cases may have chromosomal anomalies. No sex predilection has been detected.

The age at which the A-R syndrome is diagnosed ranges from birth to adulthood, although most cases are recognized during infancy or childhood. The diagnosis may result from the discovery of an abnormal iris or other ocular anomaly, signs of congenital glaucoma, reduced vision in older patients, or extraocular anomalies. In other cases, the diagnosis is made during a routine eye examination, which may have been prompted by a family history of the disorder.

OCULAR FEATURES

The ocular structures most commonly involved in the A-R syndrome are the peripheral cornea, anterior chamber angle, and iris.

Cornea

The characteristic abnormality of the cornea in the A-R syndrome is a prominent, anteriorly displaced Schwalbe's line. This can usually be seen on slit-lamp examination as a white line or ring on the posterior cornea near the limbus. In some cases the line is incomplete, usually limited to the temporal quadrant (Fig. 50-1), whereas in other patients it may be seen for 360 degrees (Fig. 50-2). Occasionally, the prominent line can be seen only by gonioscopy, although rare cases with other ocular and extraocular features of the A-R syndrome may have grossly normal Schwalbe's lines.[6]

The presence of a prominent Schwalbe's line is not pathognomonic for the A-R syndrome. It may occur as an isolated defect, which has been referred to as "posterior embryotoxon," the term originally used by Axenfeld.[4] This finding reportedly occurs in 8%[1] to 15%[5] of the general population. It may represent a forme fruste of the A-R syndrome, but it is not traditionally included in the description of this spectrum of anomalies because

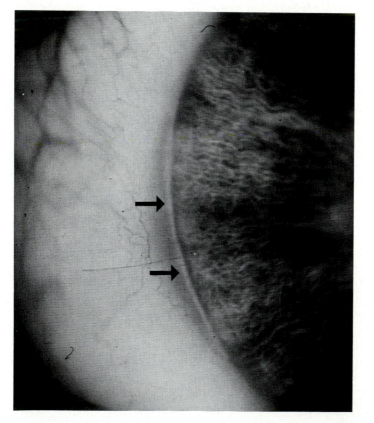

Fig. 50-1   Prominent, anteriorly displaced Schwalbe's line (posterior embryotoxon) in the temporal quadrant (*arrows*).

it is neither associated with an increased incidence of secondary glaucoma nor with extraocular anomalies. Occasionally, a prominent Schwalbe's line may also be associated with other ocular disorders, including primary congenital glaucoma[27] and the iridocorneal endothelial syndrome.[39]

The cornea is otherwise normal in the typical case of A-R syndrome, with the exception of occasional variation in the overall size (megalocornea or, less often, microcornea) or shape of the cornea.[1] Congenital opacities of the central cornea have also been observed in a few cases, although this is not a characteristic feature of the disease spectrum. The corneal endothelium is typically normal. By specular microscopy, the cells have distinct margins and a normal mosaic pattern, although mild to moderate variations in the size and shape of the cells may be observed, especially in older patients and in those with long-standing glaucoma or previous intraocular surgery.[37]

Anterior Chamber Angle

Gonioscopic examination of a patient with the A-R syndrome typically reveals the prominent Schwalbe's line, although there may be considerable variation in the extent of its enlargement and anterior displacement. Occasionally, the line is sus-pended from the cornea in some areas by a thin membrane.[37,43] Tissue strands bridge the anterior chamber angle from the peripheral iris to the prominent ridge (Fig. 50-3). These iridocorneal adhesions are typically similar in color and texture to the adjacent iris. The strands range in size from threadlike structures to broad bands extending for nearly 15 degrees of the angle circumference. In some eyes only one or two tissue strands are seen, whereas others have several per quadrant. Beyond the tissue strands, the anterior chamber angle is open and the trabecular meshwork is visible, but the scleral spur is typically obscured by peripheral iris, which inserts into the posterior portion of the meshwork.[1,5,37]

Iris

Aside from the peripheral abnormalities, the iris is normal in some eyes with the A-R syndrome, which would traditionally be considered as having Axenfeld's anomaly. In other cases, defects of the iris may range from mild stromal thinning to marked atrophy with hole formation, corectopia, and ectropion uveae (the traditional description of Rieger's anomaly) (Fig. 50-4). When corectopia is present, the pupil is usually displaced toward a prominent peripheral tissue strand, which is often

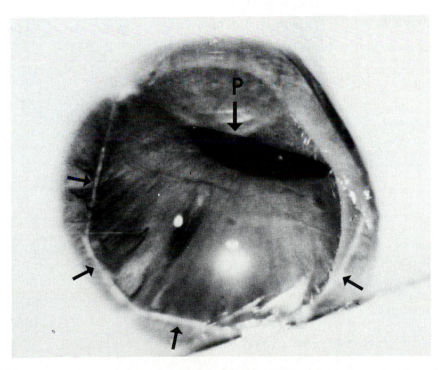

Fig. 50-2   Prominent, anteriorly displaced Schwalbe's line in all quadrants *(arrows)* with pupillary distortion *(P)* in patient with Axenfeld-Rieger syndrome.

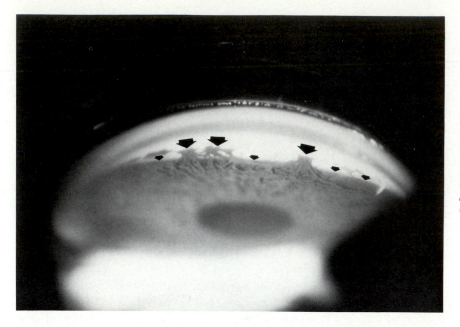

Fig. 50-3 Gonioscopic appearance of patient with Axenfeld-Rieger syndrome showing tissue strands extending from peripheral iris to prominent Schwalbe's line *(large arrows)* and higher insertion of iris into trabecular meshwork *(small arrows)*. (From Shields, MB: Trans Am Ophthal Soc 81:736, 1983)

Fig. 50-4 Advanced iris changes in patient with Axenfeld-Rieger syndrome showing small, markedly displaced pupil *(arrow)* and large iris hole in opposite quadrants. (From Shields, MB: Trans Am Ophthal Soc 81:736, 1983)

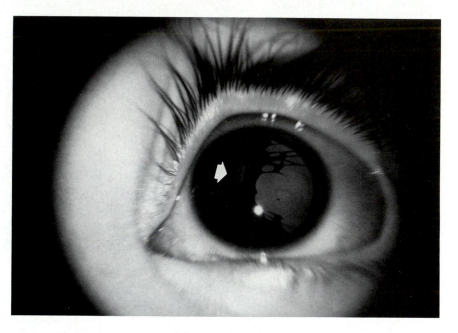

visible by slit-lamp biomicroscopy. The atrophy and hole formation typically occur in the quadrant away from the direction of the corectopia.

In a small number of patients with the A-R syndrome, abnormalities of the central iris have been observed to progress.[8,14,21,37] This is more often seen during the first years of life, but may also occur in older patients. The progressive changes usually consist of displacement or distortion of the pupil and occasional thinning or hole formation of

the iris. Abnormalities of the peripheral iris or anterior chamber angle do not appear to progress after birth, except for occasional thickening of iridocorneal tissue strands.[37]

ADDITIONAL OCULAR ABNORMALITIES

Many additional ocular abnormalities have been reported in one or more cases or pedigrees. Although none of these occur with sufficient frequency to be included as a typical feature of the

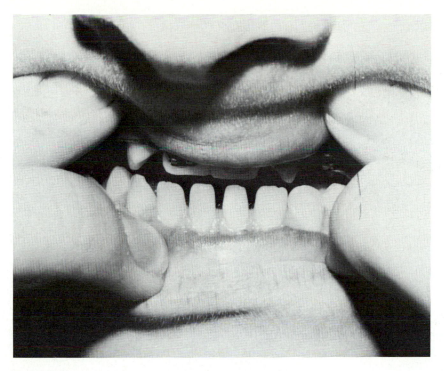

Fig. 50-5   Patient with Axenfeld-Rieger syndrome demonstrating typical dental anomaly of microdontia (reduction in crown size of teeth).

A-R syndrome, there is the impression that these patients are subject to a wide range of ocular anomalies. Reported abnormalities include strabismus, limbal dermoids, cataracts, peripheral spokelike transillumination defects of the iris, retinal detachment, macular degeneration, chorioretinal colobomas, choroidal hypoplasia, and hypoplasia of the optic nerve head.[1,16,37]

GLAUCOMA

Slightly more than half of the patients with the A-R syndrome develop glaucoma. This may become manifest during infancy, although it more commonly appears in childhood or young adulthood. The extent of the iris defects and iridocorneal strands does not correlate precisely with the presence or severity of the glaucoma. However, the high insertion of peripheral iris into the trabecular meshwork, which is present to some degree in all cases, appears to be more pronounced in those eyes with glaucoma.[37]

EXTRAOCULAR FEATURES

The extraocular anomalies most commonly associated with the A-R syndrome are developmental defects of the teeth and facial bones. The dental abnormalities include a reduction in crown size

(microdontia), a decreased but evenly spaced number of teeth (hypodontia), and a focal absence of teeth (oligodontia or anodontia) (Fig. 50-5).[26,33,42] The teeth most commonly missing are anterior maxillary primary and permanent central incisors. Facial anomalies include maxillary hypoplasia with flattening of the midface and a receding upper lip and prominent lower lip, especially in association with dental hypoplasia (Fig. 50-6). Hypertelorism, telecanthus, and a broad flat nose have also been associated with the A-R syndrome.[1]

Anomalies in the region of the pituitary gland are a less common, but more serious finding associated with the A-R syndrome. A primary empty sella syndrome has been documented in several patients,[22,37] and one case of congenital parasellar arachnoid cyst has been reported.[37] Growth hormone deficiency and short stature have also been described in association with the entity.[11,36]

Redundant periumbilical skin and hypospadias may also be seen in some patients with the A-R syndrome.[19] Other associated defects that have been reported include oculocutaneous albinism,[25] heart defects, middle ear deafness, mental deficiency, and a variety of neurologic and dermatologic disorders.[1] As in the case of the less common ocular anomalies, the latter extraocular abnormal-

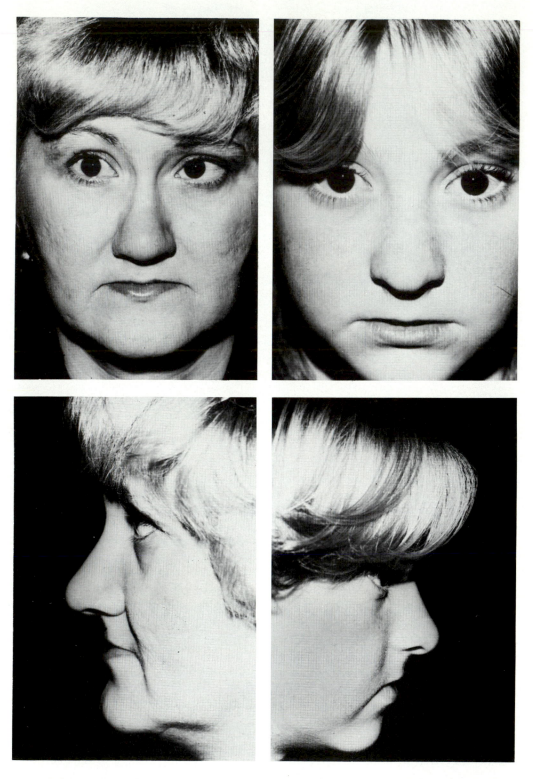

Fig. 50-6 Mother and daughter with Axenfeld-Rieger syndrome demonstrating characteristic facial configuration of midface flattening (upper lip and cheek) and protruding lower lip.

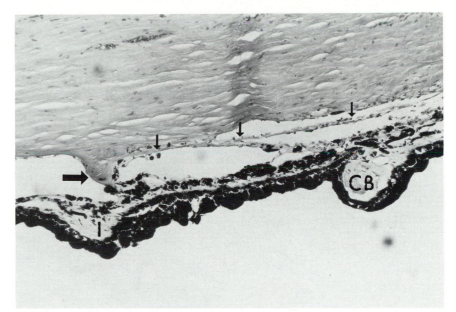

Fig. 50-7 Light microscopic view of eye with Axenfeld-Rieger syndrome showing prominent, anteriorly displaced Schwalbe's line *(large arrow)* attached to iris *(I)* by tissue strand. Scant, attenuated trabecular lamellae *(small arrows)* extend to Schwalbe's line and attach to peripheral iris; anterior portion of ciliary body *(CB)*. (Hematoxylin-eosin, × 150). (From Shields, MB: Trans Am Ophthalmol Soc 81:736, 1983)

ities do not appear with sufficient frequency to be considered typical features of the A-R syndrome. There is the suggestion, however, that these patients are subject to a wide range of both ocular and extraocular developmental defects.

HISTOPATHOLOGIC FEATURES

The histopathologic findings of the central cornea are typically normal, whereas the peripheral cornea has the characteristic prominent, anteriorly displaced Schwalbe's line. The latter structure is composed of dense collagen and ground substance covered by a monolayer of spindle-shaped cells with a basement membrane (Fig. 50-7).[5,37,43] The peripheral iris is attached in some areas to the corneoscleral junction by tissue strands, which usually connect with the prominent Schwalbe's line. Occasionally, however, the adhesions insert either anterior or posterior to Schwalbe's line or on both sides of the ridge.[37] The strands consist of either iris stroma or a membrane composed of a monolayer of spindle-shaped cells and/or a basement membranelike layer. In some areas, the strand is composed of both the iris tissue and the membrane.

A membrane similar to that seen in association with the iridocorneal tissue strands has also been observed on the iris, usually on the portion toward which the pupil is distorted.[1,28,37,40] In the quadrants away from the direction of pupillary displacement, the stroma of the iris is often thin or absent, exposing pigment epithelium that may also contain holes.

The iris peripheral to the iridocorneal adhesions usually inserts into the posterior aspect of the trabecular meshwork (Fig. 50-8). The meshwork may be composed of a scant number of attenuated lamellae, which extend from beneath peripheral iris to the prominent Schwalbe's line. In other specimens, the lamellae are compressed and there is a reduced number of openings in each trabecular layer, especially near Schlemm's canal. Transmission electron microscopy has revealed that the latter changes are caused by incomplete development of the trabecular meshwork. Schlemm's canal may be rudimentary or absent in cases with severe glaucoma.

THEORIES OF MECHANISM

Based on clinical and histopathologic observations and current concepts regarding normal anterior segment development of the eye, it has been postulated that a developmental arrest occurring late in gestation of certain anterior ocular structures derived from neural crest cells leads to the changes seen in eyes of patients with the A-R syndrome[37,38] (Fig. 50-9).

In normal development, at 5 months gestation a continuous layer of endothelium creates a closed cavity to form the anterior chamber.[15] At the same time, the anterior surface of the iris inserts in front of the primordial trabecular meshwork.[3] During the

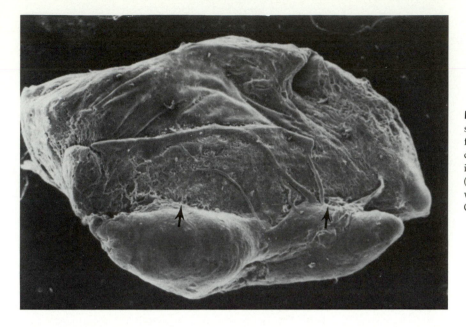

Fig. 50-8 Scanning electron microscopic view of trabeculectomy specimen from patient with Axenfeld-Rieger syndrome showing high insertion of iris into trabecular meshwork *(arrows)*. (From Shields, MB, Buckley, E, Klintworth, GK, and Thresher, R: Surv Ophthalmol 29:387, 1985)

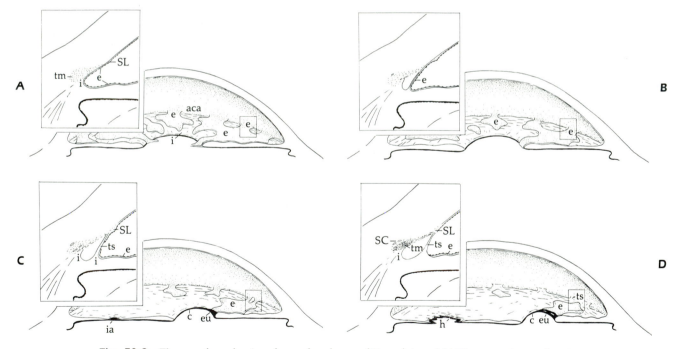

Fig. 50-9 Theory of mechanism for ocular abnormalities of Axenfeld-Rieger syndrome (insets show cross-sectional views of anterior chamber angle corresponding to area within rectangle). **A,** Partial retention of primordial endothelium *(e)* on iris *(i)* and anterior chamber angle *(aca)*; incomplete posterior recession of peripheral uvea from trabecular meshwork *(tm)*; abnormal differentiation between corneal and chamber angle endothelia with a prominent, anteriorly displaced Schwalbe's line *(SL)*. **B,** Development of tissue strands from retained endothelium crossing anterior chamber angle. **C,** Contraction of retained endothelium with iris changes of corectopia *(c)*, ectropion uveae *(eu)*, and iris atrophy *(ia)*, which may continue after birth; tissue strand *(ts)*, **D,** Incomplete development of trabecular meshwork and Schlemm's canal *(SC)*; continued traction on iris, with possible secondary ischemia, may lead to hole formation *(h)*. (From Shields, MB: Trans Am Ophthalmol Soc 81:736, 1983)

third trimester, the endothelial layer progressively disappears from the pupillary membrane and iris surface and cavitates over the anterior chamber angle. It is retained as the corneal endothelium and possibly as the endothelial lining of the trabecular meshwork. During this time, anterior uveal tissue begins to slide posteriorly in relation to chamber angle structures, exposing the underlying meshwork. The development of the trabecular meshwork progresses in a posterior-to-anterior and an inner-to-outer direction toward Schwalbe's line and Schlemm's canal.

In the A-R syndrome, it is postulated that the developmental arrest results in retention of the primordial endothelium over portions of the iris and anterior chamber angle. This leads to the formation of the iridocorneal strands in those portions of the angle in which the endothelial layer, usually with associated iris stromal tissue, extends from peripheral iris to the prominent Schwalbe's line. Contraction of the cellular layer on the iris causes the corectopia and other defects in the central iris, explaining how these changes might continue to progress after birth. The zone of differentiation between the endothelium of the cornea and the anterior chamber angle is abnormally anterior and is associated with excessive basement membrane deposition in most cases, leading to the prominent, anteriorly displaced Schwalbe's line.

The developmental arrest also prevents the complete posterior migration of the anterior uvea, which results in the high insertion of the iris into the posterior trabecular meshwork. The arrest may also lead to the incomplete formation of the trabecular lamellae and Schlemm's canal. The obstruction to aqueous humor outflow in patients with glaucoma associated with the A-R syndrome is believed to be the result of either compression of the trabecular meshwork from tension exerted by the anteriorly inserted uveal tissue or the incomplete development of the meshwork and Schlemm's canal. Patients with severe glaucoma in infancy or early childhood may have a predominance of the latter mechanism, whereas those that develop glaucoma later in life may have prolonged compression of the meshwork by the anterior uveal insertion, eventually leading to chronic changes in the outflow structures.

The neural crest cells give rise to most of the mesenchyme related to the forebrain and pituitary gland, bones and cartilage of the upper face, and dental papillae.[10,18,23] A developmental arrest involving the neural crest, therefore, could also explain the anomalies of the pituitary gland, the facial bones, and the teeth in the A-R syndrome. Other defects, however, such as those of the umbilicus and genitourinary system, are more difficult to associate with a primary defect of cranial neural crest cells, suggesting a broader involvement of the primordial ectodermal plate, of which the neural crest is one portion.

DIFFERENTIAL DIAGNOSIS

Iridocorneal Endothelial (ICE) Syndrome

The iris and anterior chamber angle abnormalities in the iridocorneal endothelial (ICE) syndrome resemble those of the A-R syndrome both clinically and histopathologically. This has led some investigators to suggest that the two syndromes are parts of a common spectrum of disorders.[24,28,40] However, clinical features that distinguish the ICE syndrome include corneal endothelial abnormalities, unilaterality, absence of family history, and onset in young adulthood. Both conditions are characterized histopathologically by a membrane over the anterior chamber angle and iris, the contraction of which leads to many of the alterations in each disorder. However, the membrane in the A-R syndrome represents a primordial remnant, whereas that of the ICE syndrome is caused by a proliferation of the abnormal corneal endothelium (see Chapter 54).

Posterior Polymorphous Dystrophy

Posterior polymorphous dystrophy is a developmental disorder of the corneal endothelium; one variation has changes of the iris and anterior chamber angle similar to those of the A-R syndrome. The differentiation can be made on the basis of the typical corneal endothelial abnormality in posterior polymorphous dystrophy (see Chapter 54).

Peters' Anomaly

Peters' anomaly involves the central portion of the cornea, iris, and lens. Similar changes have been reported in association with the peripheral defects of the A-R syndrome, and the two conditions were once included in a single category of developmental disorders.[29,41] However, this association is rare, and the mechanisms for the two groups of developmental disorders are distinctly different (see Chapter 51).

Aniridia

The rudimentary iris and anterior chamber abnormalities with associated glaucoma in aniridia may, in some cases, lead to confusion with the A-R syndrome (see Chapter 49).

Congenital Iris Hypoplasia

It has been reported that patients may have congenital hypoplasia of the iris without the anterior chamber angle defects of the A-R syndrome or any other ocular abnormality.[35] Iris hypoplasia has also been reported in association with juvenile-onset glaucoma with autosomal dominant inheritance.[17]

Oculodentodigital Dysplasia

The dental anomalies in oculodentodigital dysplasia are similar to those seen in the A-R syndrome. In addition, these patients may occasionally have mild stromal hypoplasia of the iris,[1] anterior chamber angle defects, microphthalmia, and glaucoma.[20]

Ectopia Lentis et Pupillae

Ectopia lentis et pupillae is an autosomal recessive condition characterized by bilateral displacement of the lens and pupil,[7] the two structures typically going in opposite directions. The corectopia in this disorder may resemble that of the A-R syndrome, but the absence of anterior chamber angle defects is a differential feature.

Congenital Ectropion Uveae

Congenital ectropion uveae has been described as a rare, nonprogressive developmental anomaly characterized by the presence of pigmented epithelium on the stroma of the iris.[9,12,13,34] It may be an isolated finding, or appear in association with systemic anomalies, including neurofibromatosis, facial hemihypertrophy, and the Prader-Willi syndrome.[12,34] Glaucoma is present in a high percentage of cases, and the ectropion uveae may be confused clinically with that found in some patients with the A-R syndrome. In addition, similar histopathologic findings include a prominent Schwalbe's line, a high insertion of the iris, and endothelial cells on the iris surface.[9]

Iridoschisis

In iridoschisis there is bilateral separation and dissolution of the stromal layers of the iris, which may be associated with glaucoma.[8] However, it differs from other abnormalities of the iris by an onset in the sixth or seventh decade of life.

MANAGEMENT

The primary concern regarding the management of ocular defects in a patient with the A-R syndrome is detection and control of the associated glaucoma. Intraocular pressure elevation most of-ten develops between childhood and early adulthood, but may appear in infancy or, in rare cases, not until after middle age.[37] Therefore, patients with the A-R syndrome must be followed for suspicion of glaucoma throughout life.

With the exception of infantile cases, medical therapy should usually be tried before surgical intervention is recommended. Pilocarpine and other miotics are often ineffective, but drugs that reduce aqueous humor production, such as beta-blocking agents and carbonic anhydrase inhibitors are most likely to be beneficial. Laser surgery has not been effective in managing the glaucoma in the A-R syndrome. Options for conventional surgery include goniotomy, trabeculotomy, and trabeculectomy. The former two have been utilized in infantile cases with limited success. Trabeculectomy is the surgical procedure of choice for most patients with glaucoma secondary to the A-R syndrome.

REFERENCES

1. Alkemade, PPH: Dysgenesis mesodermalis of the iris and the cornea, Assen, Netherlands, 1969, Charles C Thomas

2. Allen, L, Burian, HM, and Braley, AE: A new concept of the development of the anterior chamber angle: its relationship to developmental glaucoma and other structural anomalies, Arch Ophthalmol 53:783, 1955

3. Anderson, DR: The development of the trabecular meshwork and its abnormality in primary infantile glaucoma, Trans Am Ophthalmol Soc 79:458, 1981

4. Axenfeld, T: Embryotoxon corneae posterius, Ber Deutsch Ophthal Ges 42:301, 1920

5. Burian, HM, Braley, AE, and Allen, L: External and gonioscopic visibility of the ring of Schwalbe and the trabecular zone: an interpretation of the posterior corneal embryotoxon and the so-called congenital hyaline membranes on the posterior corneal surface, Trans Am Ophthalmol Soc 51:389, 1955

6. Chisholm, IA, and Chudley, AE: Autosomal dominant iridogoniodysgenesis with associated somatic anomalies: four-generation family with Rieger's syndrome, Br J Ophthalmol 67:529, 1983

7. Cross, HE: Ectopia lentis et pupillae, Am J Ophthalmol 88:381, 1979

8. Cross, HE, and Maumenee, AE: Progressive spontaneous dissolution of the iris, Surv Ophthalmol 18:186, 1973

9. Dowling, JL, Albert, DM, Nelson, LB, and Walton, DS: Primary glaucoma associated with iridotrabecular dysgenesis and ectropion uveae, Ophthalmology 92:912, 1985

10. Edwards, WC, and Torczynski, E: Neural crest cell behavior and facial anomalies, Pers Ophthalmol 5:47, 1981

11. Feingold, M, Shiere, F, Fogels, HR, and Donaldson, D: Rieger's syndrome, Pediatrics 44:564, 1969
12. Futterweit, W, Ritch, R, Teekhasaenee, C, and Nelson, ES: Coexistence of Prader-Willi syndrome, congenital ectropion uveae with glaucoma, and factor XI deficiency, JAMA 255:3280, 1986
13. Gramer, E, Krieglstein, GK: Infantile glaucoma in unilateral uveal ectropion, v Graefes Arch Klin Exp Ophthalmol 211:215, 1979
14. Gregor, Z, and Hitchings, RA: Rieger's anomaly: a 42-year follow-up, Br J Ophthalmol 64:56, 1980
15. Hansson, HA, and Jerndal, T: Scanning electron microscopic studies on the development of the iridocorneal angle in human eyes, Invest Ophthalmol 10:252, 1971
16. Henkind, P, and Friedman, AH: Iridogoniodysgenesis with cataract, Am J Ophthalmol 72:949, 1971
17. Jerndal, T: Goniodysgenesis and hereditary juvenile glaucoma, Acta Ophthal (Copenh) 107(Suppl):1, 1970
18. Johnston, MC, et al: Origins of avianocular and periocular tissues, Exp Eye Res 29:27, 1979
19. Jorgenson, RJ, et al: The Rieger syndrome, Am J Med Genet 2:307, 1978
20. Judisch, GF, Martin-Casals, A, Hanson, JW, and Olin, WH: Oculodentodigital dysplasia: four new reports and a literature review, Arch Ophthalmol 97:878, 1979
21. Judisch, GF, Phelps, CD, and Hanson, J: Rieger's syndrome: a case report with a 15-year follow-up, Arch Ophthalmol 97:2120, 1979
22. Kleinman, RE, Kazarian, EL, Raptopoulos, V, and Braverman, LE: Primary empty sella and Rieger's anomaly of the anterior chamber of the eye: a familial syndrome, N Eng J Med 304:90, 1981
23. Kupfer, C, and Kaiser-Kupfer, MI: Observations on the development of the anterior chamber angle with reference to the pathogenesis of congenital glaucomas, Am J Ophthalmol 88:424, 1979
24. Kupfer, C, Kaiser-Kupfer, MI, Datiles, M, and McCain, L: The contralateral eye in the iridocorneal endothelial (ICE) syndrome, Ophthalmology 90:1343, 1983
25. Lubin, JR: Oculocutaneous albinism associated with corneal mesodermal dysgenesis, Am J Ophthalmol 91:347, 1981
26. Mathis, H: Zahnunterzahl und Missbildungen der Iris, Z Stomatol 34:895, 1936
27. Maumenee, AE: Further observations on the pathogenesis of congenital glaucoma, Am J Ophthalmol 55:1163, 1963
28. Pau, H: Fortschreitende Atrophie des Irisstromas mit Lochbildung und Proliferation des Hornhautendothels, Klin Monatsbl Augenheilk 147:894, 1965
29. Reese, AB, and Ellsworth, RM: The anterior chamber cleavage syndrome, Arch Ophthalmol 75:307, 1966
30. Rieger, H: Demonstration von zwei Fallen von Verlagerung und Schlitzform der Pupille mit Hypoplasie des Irisvorderblattes an beiden Augen einer 10-und 25-jahrigen Patienten, Z Augenheilk 84:98, 1934
31. Rieger, H: Beitrage zur Kenntnis seltener Missbildungen der Iris. II. Uber Hypoplasie des Irisvorderblattes mit Verlagerung und Entrundung der Pupille, v Graefes Arch Klin Exp Ophthal 133:602, 1935
32. Rieger, H: Dysgenesis mesodermalis Corneae et Iridis, Z Augenheilk 86:333, 1935
33. Rieger, H: Erbfragen in der Augenheilkunde, v Graefes Arch Klin Exp Ophthal 143:277, 1941
34. Ritch, R, et al: Congenital ectropion uveae with glaucoma, Ophthalmology 91:326, 1984
35. Rubel, E: Angeborene Hypoplasie bzw. Aplasie des Irisvorderblattes, Klin Monatsbl Augenheilkd 51:174, 1913
36. Sadeghi-Nejad, A, and Senior, B: Autosomal dominant transmission of isolated growth hormone deficiency in iris-dental dysplasia (Rieger's syndrome), J Ped 85:644, 1974
37. Shields, MB: Axenfeld-Rieger syndrome: a theory of mechanism and distinctions from the iridocorneal endothelial syndrome, Trans Am Ophthalmol Soc 81:736, 1983
38. Shields, MB, Buckley, E, Klintworth, GK, and Thresher, R: Axenfeld-Rieger syndrome: a spectrum of developmental disorders, Surv Ophthalmol 29: 387, 1985
39. Shields, MB, Campbell, DG, and Simmons, RF: The essential iris atrophies, Am J Ophthalmol 85:749, 1978
40. Troeber, R, and Rochels, R: Histological findings in dysgenesis mesodermalis iridis et corneae Rieger, v Graefes Arch Klin Exp Ophthal 213:169, 1980
41. Waring, GO III, Rodrigues, MM, and Laibson, PR: Anterior chamber cleavage syndrome: a stepladder classification, Surv Ophthalmol 20:3, 1975
42. Wesley, RK, Baker, JD, and Golnick, AL: Rieger's syndrome (oligodontia and primary mesodermal dysgenesis of the iris): clinical features and report of an isolated case, J Ped Ophthalmol Strab 15:67, 1978
43. Wolter, JR, Sandall, GS, and Fralick, FB: Mesodermal dysgenesis of anterior eye: with a partially separated posterior embryotoxon, J Ped Ophthalmol 4:41, 1967

Chapter 51

Peters' Anomaly

Edwin M. Schottenstein

CLINICAL FEATURES

Peters' anomaly is characterized by a congenital central corneal leukoma associated with a defect in the corresponding posterior stroma and Descemet's membrane and with synechiae extending from the central iris to the periphery of the corneal opacity. Eighty percent of the cases are bilateral. The cornea may or may not be edematous, and the leukoma may be so dense and extensive as to preclude a view of the anterior chamber, which is often shallow, with the plane of the iris inclined toward the central posterior corneal surface.

Early in the disease, the cornea has a ground-glass appearance with epithelial stippling caused by corneal edema. Initially, increasing corneal edema can give the impression of a progressive course, and glaucoma may exacerbate the situation. However, if intraocular pressure is normal, the edema usually gradually subsides, leaving a more sharply demarcated residual corneal scar with epithelium of normal luster.

The iridocorneal adhesion tends to occur at the iris collarette, usually temporally. The leukoma is localized to the corresponding area with relatively clear cornea elsewhere. The adhesion may also be focal or multiple, extending over 360 degrees of the circumference of the iris collarette.[47]

A central keratolenticular adherence with shallowing of the anterior chamber is sometimes present.[66] Although scleralization of the limbus is common, the peripheral cornea is usually clear, and the affected cornea is rarely vascularized. Other commonly associated anterior segment abnormalities include glaucoma in 50% to 70% of the cases[30,63]

and anterior polar cataract.[30,47] Less commonly, microcornea,[30] microphthalmia[38,40,43,56] cornea plana,[40] sclerocornea,[30] coloboma of the iris,[47] corectopia,[30] aniridia,[6,40] and Axenfeld's anomaly[1,69] have been reported. Other ocular findings that have been noted to occur in association with Peters' anomaly are maldevelopment of the hyaloid system,[47] anterior staphyloma,[44,52] anterior lentiglobus,[40] microphakia,[38] congenital aphakia,[23] persistent hyperplastic primary vitreous,[22,27,38] coloboma of the ciliary body,[43] coloboma of the choroid,[39,49] retinal dysplasia,[1,38,39] and blue sclera.

Systemic abnormalities are rarely associated with Peters' anomaly. Van Schooneveld et al.[60] described 11 patients with Peters' anomaly, short stature, brachymorphia, mental retardation, cheilognathopalatoschisis, and abnormal ears. Other reported associated conditions include mental retardation,[47] cerebral palsy,[47] cleft lip and palate,[26,47] Mongolian spot,[47] anodontia,[10] myotonic dystrophy,[10] syndactylism,[7,29] oligodontia,[12] status dysraphicus,[12] craniofacial dysostosis,[12] Wilms' tumor,[14] holoprosencephaly,[31] hydrocephalus,[17,31] pulmonary hypoplasia,[8,9] Dandy-Walker syndrome,[37] cardiac[48,58,59] and genitourinary[58] malformations, hyaline membrane disease,[58] Lowe's syndrome,[58] and 13-15 trisomy.[36,39,58]

Most cases of Peters' anomaly are sporadic, although reports of parental consanguinity and more than one affected sibling support an autosomal recessive[55] or irregularly dominant mode of inheritance in some cases.[16,25] Peters' anomaly has been associated with a deletion of the short arm of chromosomes 4 and 18,[19] deletion of the long arm of chromosome 11,[5] and ring chromosome 21.[11] Wertelechi et al.[68] reported an abnormal centromere-chromatid apposition, and Mans,[36] Meisner,[39] and Townsend et al.[58] all reported an association with 13-15 trisomy.

HISTOPATHOLOGY AND ELECTRON MICROSCOPY

Histopathologic changes are apparent in all corneal layers. Centrally, the epithelium overlying the posterior defect may appear either edematous and disorganized or normal. Bowman's layer may be replaced by pannus formation or thinned in the midperiphery and absent in the central 3 to 4 mm, but it usually has a normal thickness peripherally. The corresponding stroma usually displays long-standing edema. Abnormally large stromal collagen fibrils and an increased number of stromal cells in the subepithelial zone, where Bowman's layer is absent, may be found. Deeper stromal keratocytes usually appear normal, although a reactive pseudoinflammatory configuration may be evident. Histiocytic cells with residual bodies are common in the developmental forms of Peters' anomaly, but true inflammatory infiltrates with stromal vascularization are rare in those cases that are presumably inflammatory in origin. Usually the stroma is avascular. In some cases a craterlike defect forms in the posterior stroma, whereas in other cases a fibrous scar tissue fills the defect. Like the peripheral corneal epithelium, the peripheral stromal architecture and cells usually appear normal.

The most significant pathology affects the central posterior corneal layers. At the corneal periphery, the endothelium is present in a continuous monolayer, and Descemet's membrane is usually a normal uniform thickness of approximately 5 μm. Centrally, where there are iris synechiae, either the endothelium or Descemet's membrane may terminate abruptly or become attenuated. Ultrastructurally, Descemet's membrane consistently appears as multiple laminations of a basement membrane–like material with interspersed collagen fibrils and fine filaments. At points where iris tissue adheres to the loose connective tissue that has been formed posterior to Descemet's membrane, this connective tissue seems to be continuous with that of the iris stroma. In those cases having keratolenticular adhesions, similar posterior ultrastructural abnormalities may be exhibited, in addition to such variable features as either a stalklike connection between the lens and cornea or close apposition of a morphologically intact lens capsule and cornea.*

Ultrastructural findings vary with the degree of malformation, the time of occurrence, and the pathogenesis. Scanning electron microscopy of one case revealed a central endothelial defect with broad synechiae to the endothelial surface, surrounded by small areas without endothelium.[46] In the areas where there did appear to be endothelium, a double layer of cells covered by a fine retrocorneal fibrous membrane containing many apparent inflammatory cells or macrophages was present. The central cornea revealed no endothelial cells and was covered by large fibroblastic cells posteriorly. The endothelial cells surrounding the central defect were normal.

Transmission electron microscopy reveals normal anterior epithelial cells, except for the presence of fewer tonofilaments.[42,53] The basal portions of the basal cells project deeply and irregularly into the corneal stroma. The epithelium has a well-developed, generally intact basement membrane. The peripheral Bowman's layer appears normal except for its absence immediately posterior to the basement membrane, where it is replaced by fine, closely packed fibrils that are particularly prominent within the infoldings of the basement membrane and basal epithelial cells. In the mid-periphery, the anterior portion of Bowman's layer thins and finally disappears, so that Bowman's layer is absent in the center.

Cytoplasmic processes of keratocytes frequently appear to contact the basal epithelial cells through defects in the basement membrane in the central anterior stroma.[42] In the central posterior stroma, collagen lamellae are disorganized and the cytoplasm of stromal keratocytes is surrounded by an electron-dense, fine filamentous, amorphous material approximately 100 nm in diameter.[42,53]

Peripherally, Descemet's membrane consists of a thin layer of amorphous, nonbanded material contiguous with the endothelial cell membrane. Centrally, this amorphous layer thins and appears similar to the material surrounding the keratocytes in the posterior stroma.[42] The banded portion of Descemet's membrane can be absent.[53] Endothelial cells can either line the posterior surface or be absent centrally.

PATHOGENESIS

The pathogenesis of this condition is not fully understood, but the variations in histopathologic

---

*References 30, 35, 42, 53, 58, 59.

and electron microscopic findings suggest more than one mechanism. Peters' anomaly was first thought to be caused by an intrauterine infection (von Hippel's internal corneal ulcer).[61] This theory postulates that an intrauterine keratitis that is acquired either via the amniotic fluid or transplacentally produces a corneal perforation resulting in forward movement of the lens-iris diaphragm, producing the posterior corneal defect, overlying corneal leukoma, and keratolenticular and iridocorneal adhesions.[24,34] These changes could also result without corneal perforation with the acquisition of a deep corneal abscess that drains into the anterior chamber.[65] Reese and Ellsworth[47] reported that the mothers of 5 of 21 patients with congenital central anterior synechiae and dense central corneal opacities had a viral or specifically, a rubella infection during the first trimester. However, electron microscopic examination of cases with Peters' anomaly have demonstrated that cells in the posterior corneal stroma that by light microscopy appeared to be chronic inflammatory cells, were actually abnormal fibroblastic and histiocytic cells in the disorganized stroma.[67]

In cases with lenticular abnormalities, Peters[43] postulated that the problem was one of incomplete separation of the lens vesicle from the surface ectoderm, suggesting a primary ectodermal abnormality. Stalklike connections between the lens and cornea have been reported, suggesting that primary incomplete separation of the lens vesicle may be responsible for some cases of Peters' anomaly.[21,22] Similarly, Hagedoorn and Velzeboer[20] described an infant in whom both lenses were in contact with the corneas at birth, and then separated after some months, leaving corneal opacities with a posterior keratoconus and anterior lenticonus.

Although incomplete separation of the lens has been described clinically, in pathologic specimens, and in animals,[3,33,45] histopathologic studies of numerous other cases with keratolenticular contact suggest that a well-developed lens was secondarily displaced forward against the cornea, resulting in a secondary loss of Descemet's membrane.[17,53,58,59] Usually, when keratolenticular apposition was observed, there was an intact lens capsule contacting the corneal stroma, indicating that the lens had at some time become separated from the overlying ectoderm.

A variety of mechanisms might be responsible for forward lens displacement, including a retrolenticular mass, such as persistent hyperplastic primary vitreous or a detached and dysplastic retina. Alternatively, pupillary block might result from an altered pupillary membrane or from a swollen lens. In situations such as these, the lens and/or iris would become apposed to the overlying cornea, producing secondary pathologic changes in the endothelium and Descemet's membrane, possibly resulting in permanent adhesions. Subsequent shrinkage of the retrolenticular mass or resolution of the pupillary block would allow the anterior chamber to deepen, leaving iridocorneal or keratolenticular attachments, remnants of the iris or lens on the back of the cornea, or only the isolated posterior corneal defect.[67]

Anoxia has been hypothesized to play a possible role in anteriorly displacing the lens against the cornea.[55] Von Sallmann[62] experimentally induced keratolenticular adhesions with corresponding defects in Descemet's membrane and the endothelium in fetal monkeys by carotid ligation performed as late as mid-gestation, which is long after the separation of the lens vesicle and the formation of Descemet's membrane. Mondino et al.[41] reported bilateral dense corneal opacities and keratolenticular adhesions in one twin whose placenta showed an extensive calcified infarct. Another possible mechanism of anterior lens displacement was suggested by Stone et al.,[53] who reported a case of a central posterior corneal defect in which the zonules were abnormal as indicated by the forward displacement of the lens into the anterior chamber upon pupillary dilation.

Reese and Ellsworth[47] lumped Peters' anomaly with abnormalities of the peripheral cornea and angle such as posterior embryotoxon, Axenfeld's anomaly, and Rieger's anomaly under the name of "the anterior chamber cleavage syndrome." The theory of anterior chamber cleavage has been disproven, however, since embryologically the anterior segment develops from three sequential, axial, migrating waves of mesenchyme from the margin of the optic cup and not from cleavage of the anterior chamber. The first axial migration produces the corneal endothelium and the trabecular meshwork, the second produces the stromal keratocytes, and the third produces the iris stromal components.[25] In addition, development of the central cornea precedes by months that of the angle structures.[2] There have been two proven examples of a combined peripheral and central anomaly.[1,69] One eye had absent Descemet's membrane centrally, a prominent Schwalbe's line, iris adhesions to both the central and peripheral corneal defects, and an anterior chamber angle malformation.[69] The other had adhesions from the peripheral iris to a prominent Schwalbe's ring associated with a central corneal defect that was attached by a strand of connective tissue to the anterior surface of a luxated lens.[1] Similar reports have included a case of unilateral Peters' anomaly with dysgenesis of the iris, anterior chamber angle, and zonules in the fellow eye,[53] and a patient with unilateral Peters' anomaly associated with a prominent Schwalbe's ring.[46]

Initially, it was thought that the corneal mesenchyme was of mesodermal origin, and that incomplete migration centrally left a posterior corneal defect. If the iris, pupillary membrane, and cornea come into contact early in development, iris stands may remain adherent to the cornea with maldifferentiation of the overlying endothelium and Descemet's membrane.[1,12,50,57] This mechanism has been shown to occur in one strain of rats inbred for anterior segment anomalies.[32] However, Johnston et al.[28] have shown that naturally-labeled quail neural crest cells transplanted into the neural crest region of a 35 mm stage chick embryo become incorporated into both corneal endothelium and trabecular endothelial cells. Thus, some cases of Peters' anomaly may represent a failure of differentiation of neural crest cells destined for corneal and trabecular endothelium.[4]

MECHANISM OF GLAUCOMA

In most cases of Peters' anomaly the anterior chamber angle appears to be grossly normal, and the mechanism of obstruction to aqueous humor outflow has not been fully elucidated. Kupfer et al.[35] reported the ultrastructure of a trabeculectomy specimen from the eye of a two-year-old child with Peters' anomaly and glaucoma, and noted that the trabecular meshwork demonstrated senile changes characteristic of an accelerated aging process, including fibrous long-spacing collagen and the presence of phagocytosed pigment granules in the endothelium. They suggested that this might represent a failure in the normal differentiation of the mesenchyme at the rim of the optic cup into typical endothelial cells or failure of differentiation of neural crest cells destined for corneal or trabecular endothelium.

In other cases, the mechanism of aqueous humor outflow obstruction may be secondary to less subtle changes in the anterior chamber angle. Scheie and Yanoff[49] described the histopathology of the eye of an infant with Peters' anomaly and total posterior coloboma of the retinal pigment epithelium and choroid. In this case, there were complete peripheral anterior synechiae, with atrophy of the iris stroma, and no identifiable trabecular meshwork or Schlemm's canal. In other cases,

Peters' anomaly was associated with neural crest cell dysgenesis of the anterior chamber angle, more typical of Axenfeld's anomaly or Reiger's syndrome.[1,69]

DIFFERENTIAL DIAGNOSIS

The main differential problem in Peters' anomaly is distinguishing the central corneal leukoma from other causes of corneal opacification in newborns and infants. These include congenital glaucoma, mucopolysaccharidosis, birth trauma, congenital hereditary endothelial dystrophy, and perforated corneal ulcer with iris incarceration. Although the cornea appears a hazy grey in congenital glaucoma and birth trauma, Descemet's tears develop and remain permanently as curved horizontal or oblique double contoured lines (Haab's striae) in congenital glaucoma or as diagonal and vertical double contoured lines with birth trauma. Other features that differentiate Peters' anomaly from primary congenital glaucoma include normal corneal diameters, generally sharp discontinuity between clear and opaque areas of the cornea, failure of the corneal opacity to clear when the intraocular pressure is lowered, and a shallow anterior chamber in the former condition. The corneal clouding in infants with mucopolysaccharidosis is characteristically diffuse, resulting from the progressive accumulation of fine, punctate, stromal opacities that may be more dense posteriorly than anteriorly. The epithelium and endothelium are spared. Congenital hereditary endothelial dystrophy is not associated with glaucoma and is characterized by a uniform corneal haze, a well-formed anterior chamber, and no evidence of iris involvement. In a perforated corneal ulcer with iris incarceration, the iris is incarcerated in the corneal scar, whereas in Peters' anomaly the iris is apposed to the posterior surface of the cornea.[18] If the corneal opacities are extensive, they may obscure the underlying anterior chamber pathology, making a correct diagnosis difficult.[51]

MANAGEMENT

The management of infants with developmental disorders of the cornea is difficult. A complete examination under anesthesia should be performed as early as possible. Photographs and a careful drawing should be made, including horizontal and vertical measurements of the corneal diameter and size of the corneal opacity. Since the anterior corneal surface may be abnormal, a MacKay-Marg tonometer or pneumatonometer is preferable for measuring the intraocular pressures.

Careful A-scan and B-scan ultrasounds and an ERG should be performed since keratolenticular adhesions, cataracts, and vitreoretinal abnormalities are commonly associated with Peters' anomaly. Specular microscopy discloses an extremely heterogeneous endothelial mosaic with large extracellular spaces, peculiar doughnut-shaped configurations, and patchy areas of reduced total endothelial cell counts.[25]

Elevated intraocular pressures that are unresponsive to topical medications should be treated surgically before penetrating keratoplasty is performed. The mechanism of decreased aqueous humor outflow is not fully understood. Schlemm's canal may be absent. Since goniotomy may be extremely difficult in the presence of a corneal leukoma, a trabeculectomy probably offers the best surgical approach.

If the corneal opacities are dense and bilateral, early penetrating keratoplasties offer the only hope for useful vision before the development of severe deprivation amblyopia. As with bilateral dense, congenital cataracts, surgery within the first 3 months of life is advisable. However, despite improved microsurgical techniques and cooperative, motivated parents, keratoplasty should be approached with caution. A review in 1977 by Waring and Laibson[64] of penetrating grafts for congenital opacities indicated that technically successful grafts were achieved in only approximately 20% of cases, severe complications being common. Stulting et al.[54] reported a 50% 4-year, first-graft survival of penetrating keratoplasties performed on 26 eyes having Peters' anomaly. However, it was also noted that the final visual acuities obtained by the children with this congenital opacity were disappointing, because in most cases surgery had been performed after severe amblyopia had developed. In unilateral cases, even successful keratoplasty and contact lens fitting may not satisfactorily prevent severe amblyopia. On the other hand, weighing against early surgery is the potential for progressive clearing of some of the corneal opacity. Alternatively, if the corneal opacity is well-circumscribed and the periperal cornea is clear, an optical iridectomy may improve vision, avoiding the significant risks associated with keratoplasty.

REFERENCES

1. Alkemade, PPH: Dysgenesis mesodermalis of the iris and the cornea, Assen, 1969, Van Goreum
2. Allen, L, Burian, HM, and Braley, AE: A new concept of the development of the anterior chamber angle, Arch Ophthalmol 53:783, 1955
3. Badtke, G, and Degenhardt, KH: The development of combined malformations of the lens and cornea in the eyes of newborn mice with particular regard to disturbances of separation of the embryonic lens vesicle from the surface ectoderm, Klin Monatsbl Augenheilkd 142:62, 1963
4. Bahn, CF, et al: Classification of corneal endothelial disorders based on neural crest origin, Ophthalmology 91:558, 1984
5. Bateman, JB, Maumenee, IH, and Sparkes, RS: Peters' anomaly associated with partial deletion of the long arm of chromosome 11, Am J. Ophthalmol 97:11, 1984
6. Beauchamp, GR: Anterior segment dysgenesis, keratolenticular adhesion and aniridia, J Pediatr Ophthalmol Strabis 17:55, 1980
7. Berliner, ML: Unilateral microphthalmia with congenital anterior synechiae and syndactyly, Arch Ophthalmol 26:653, 1941
8. Brown, SI: Corneal transplantation in the anterior chamber cleavage syndrome, Am J Ophthalmol 70:942, 1970
9. Bull, MJ, and Baum, JL: Peters' anomaly with pulmonary hypoplasia, Birth Defects 12:181, 1976
10. Busch, G, Weiskopf, J, and Busch, KT: Dysgenesis mesodermalis et ectodermalis: Rieger oder Rieger'sche Krankheit, Klin Monatsbl Augenheilkd 136:512, 1960
11. Cibis, GW, Waeltermann, J, and Harris, D: Peters' anomaly in association with ring 21 chromosomal abnormality, Am J Ophthalmol 100:733, 1985
12. Collier, M: La dysplasie marginale postérieure de la cornée dans le cadre: les anomalies squélettiques et ectodermiques, Ann Oculist 195:512, 1962
13. Collins, ET: Adhesion of a persistent pupillary membrane to the cornea in the eye of a cat, Trans Ophthalmol Soc UK 27:203, 1907
14. Eiferman, RA: Association of Wilms' tumor with Peters' anomaly, Ann Ophthalmol 16:933, 1984
15. Falls, HF: A gene producing various defects of the anterior segment of the eye, Am J Ophthalmol 32:41, 1949
16. Ferrell, RE, Hittner, HM, Kretzer, FL, and Antoszyk, JH: Anterior segment mesenchymal dysgenesis: probable linkage to the MNS blood group and chromosome 4, Am J Hum Genet 34:245, 1982
17. Fogle, JA, et al: Peripheral Peters' anomaly: a histopathologic case report, J Ped Ophthalmol Strab 15:71, 1978
18. Francis, IC, Flynn, F, and Hollows, FC: Deep corneal leukoma adherens in an aboriginal population, Aust J Ophthalmol 9:303, 1981
19. François, J, and Saraux, H: 79th Congress of the French Society of Ophthalmology, Arch Ophthalmol 89:437, 1973
20. Hagedoorn, A, and Velzeboer, CM: Post-natal partial spontaneous correction of a severe congenital anomaly of the anterior segment of the eye, Arch Ophthalmol 62:685, 1959

21. Hamburg, A: Incomplete separation of the lens and related malformations, Am J Ophthalmol 64:729, 1967

22. Harden, AF, and Mooney, DJ: Congenital keratolenticular adhesion, Am J Ophthalmol 70:975, 1970

23. Harris, R, Brownstein, S, and Little, J: Peters' anomaly with congenital aphakia, Am J Ophthalmol 15:91, 1980

24. Heckenlively, J, and Kielar, R: Congenital perforated cornea in Peters' anomaly, Am J Ophthalmol 88:63, 1979

25. Hittner, HM, et al: Variable expressivity of autosomal dominant anterior segment mesenchymal dysgenesis in six generations, Am J Ophthalmol 93:57, 1982

26. Ide, CH, Matta, C, Holt, JE, and Felker, GV: Dysgenesis mesodermalis of the cornea (Peters' anomaly) associated with cleft lip and palate, Ann Ophthalmol 6:841, 1975

27. Jepson, CN: The von Hippel anomaly of the cornea associated with hyperplasia of primary vitreous, Surv Ophthalmol 8:207, 1963

28. Johnston, MC, Bhakdinaronk, A, and Reid, YC: An expanded role of the neural crest in oral and pharyngeal development. In Bosma, JF, editor: Fourth symposium on oral sensation and perception, US Govt Printing Office, Washington, DC, 1973, pp 37-52

29. Karlsberg, RC, et al: Anomalies of iris and anterior-chamber angle: occurrence in a child with multiple congenital anomalies, Arch Ophthalmol 83:287, 1971

30. Kenyon, KR: Mesenchymal dysgenesis in Peters' anomaly, sclerocornea and congenital endothelial dystrophy, Exp Eye Res 21:125, 1975

31. Kenyon, KR: Mesenchymal dysgenesis of the cornea, Metab Ophthalmol 2:173, 1978

32. Kleberger, E: Ueber die Entwicklung der angeborenen zentralen Hornhauttrubung (Peterssche Defektbildung), v Graefes Arch Klin Exp Ophthalmol 175:84, 1968

33. Konyukhov, BV, and Vakhrusheva, MP: Disturbances in eye development in mice of C57BL/6J strain, Folia Biologica 16:3, 1968

34. Krause, U, Koivisto, M, and Rantakallio, P: A case of Peters' syndrome with spontaneous corneal perforation, J Pediatr Ophthalmol 6:145, 1969

35. Kupfer, C, Kuwabara, AT, and Stark, WJ: The histopathology of Peters' anomaly, Am J Ophthalmol 80:653, 1975

36. Mans, R: Die Genese der angeborenen Hornhauttrübungen, v Graefes Arch Klin Exp Ophthalmol 119:77, 1927

37. March, WF, and Chalkley, THF: Sclerocornea associated with Dandy-Walker cyst, Am J Ophthalmol 78:54, 1974

38. Maschimo, M: Ein Beitrag zur Kenntnis der angeborenen Hornhauttrubung, Klin Monatsbl Augenheilkd 71:184, 1923

39. Meisner, W: Ein Kolobom der Aderhaut und Netzhaus mit Aplasie des Sehnerven, v Graefes Arch Klin Exp Ophthalmol 79:308, 1911

40. Mohr, T: Beitrage zur Frage der Entstehung der kongenitalen Hornhauttrübungen, Klin Monatsbl Augenheilkd 48:338, 1910

41. Mondino, BJ, Shahinian, L Jr, Johnson, BL, and Brown, S: Peters' anomaly with the fetal transfusion syndrome, Am J Ophthalmol 82:55, 1976

42. Nakanishi, I, and Brown, SI: The histopathology and ultrastructure of congenital, central corneal opacity (Peters' anomaly), Am J Ophthalmol 72:801, 1971

43. Peters, A: Ueber angeborene Defektbildung der Descemetschen Membran, Klin Monatsbl Augenheilkd 44:27, 105, 1906

44. Peters, A: Weiter Beitrag zur Kenntnis der angeborenen Defektbildung der Descemetschen Membran, Klin Monatsbl Augenheilkd 46:241, 1908

45. Pierro, LJ, and Spiggle, J: Congenital eye defects in the mouse. I. Corneal opacity in C57 black mice, J Exp Zool 166:25, 1967

46. Polack, FM, and Graue, EL: Scanning electron microscopy of congenital corneal leukomas (Peters' anomaly), Am J Ophthalmol 88:169, 1979

47. Reese, AB, and Ellsworth, RM: The anterior chamber cleavage syndrome, Arch Ophthalmol 75:307, 1966

48. Rossetti, D: Su di un caso di "disgenesis mesodermalis iridis et corneae" associata a irizio congenital di cuore, Ann Ottal 78:419, 1952

49. Scheie, HG, and Yanoff, M: Peters' anomaly and total posterior coloboma of retinal pigment epithelium and choroid, Arch Ophthalmol 87:525, 1972

50. Seefelder, R: Pathologisch-anatomische Beitrage zur Frage der angeborenen zentralen Defektbildung der Hornhauthinterflache, Klin Monatsbl Augenheilkd 65:539, 1920

51. Speakman, JS, and Crawford, JS: Congenital opacities of the cornea, Br J Ophthalmol 50:68, 1965

52. Steffan, P: Beitrag zur Erklaerung angeborener Anomalien der Hornhaut, Klin Monatsbl Augenheilkd 5:209, 1867

53. Stone, DL, Kenyon, KR, Green, WR, and Ryan, SJ: Congenital central corneal leukoma (Peters' anomaly): ultrastructure of three cases, Am J Ophthalmol 81:173, 1976

54. Stulting, RD, et al: Penetrating keratoplasty in children, Ophthalmology 91:1222, 1984

55. Tabucki, A, Matsuura, M, and Hirokawa, M: Three siblings with Peters' anomaly, Ophthal Paediat Genet 5:205, 1985

56. Theodore, FH: Congenital opacities of the cornea, Arch Ophthalmol 31:138, 1944

57. Townsend, WM: Congenital corneal leukomas. I. Central defect in Descemet's membrane, Am J Ophthalmol 77:80, 1974

58. Townsend, WM, Font, RL, and Zimmerman, LE: Congenital corneal leukomas. II. Histopathologic findings in 19 eyes with central defect in Descemet's membrane, Am J Ophthalmol 77:192, 1974

59. Townsend, WM, Font, RL, and Zimmerman, LE: Congenital corneal leukomas. III. Histopathologic findings in 13 eyes with non-central defect in Descemet's membrane, Am J Ophthalmol 77:400, 1974

60. Van Schooneveld, MK, Delleman, JW, Beemer, FA, and Bleeker-Wagemakers, EM: Peters'-Plus: a new syndrome, Ophthal Paediat Genet 4:141, 1984

61. von Hippel, E: Über Hydrophthalmos Congenitus nebst Bemerkungen über die ver farbung der Cornea duich Blutfarbstoff, Pathologisch-anatomische Untersuchungen, v Graefes Arch Klin Exp Ophthalmol 4:539, 1897

62. von Sallmann, L: The effect of intrauterine surgical procedure on the development of the primate eye, Invest Ophthalmol 8:51, 1969

63. Waring, GO, Bourne, WM, Edelhauser, HF, and Kenyon, KR: The corneal endothelium, normal and pathologic structure and function, Ophthalmology 89:531, 1982

64. Waring, GO, and Laibson, PR: Keratoplasty in infants and children, Trans Am Acad Ophthalmol Otol 83:283, 1977

65. Waring, GO, Laibson, PR, and Rodrigues, MM: Clinical and pathologic alterations of Descemet's membrane with emphasis on endothelial metaplasia, Surv Ophthalmol 18:325, 1974

66. Waring, GO, and Parks, MM: Successful lens removal in congenital corneolenticular adhesion (Peters' anomaly), Am J Ophthalmol 83:526, 1977

67. Waring, GO, Rodrigues, MN, and Laibson, PR: Anterior chamber cleavage syndrome: a stepladder classification, Surv Ophthalmol 20:3, 1975

68. Wertelecki, W, Dev, VG, and Superneau, DW: Abnormal centromere-chromatid apposition (ACCA) and Peters' anomaly, Ophthal Paediat Genet 5:7, 1985

69. Zimmerman, LE: Keratoconus posticus in Axenfeld's syndrome, Read before the Verhoeff Society meeting, Washington, DC, 1962

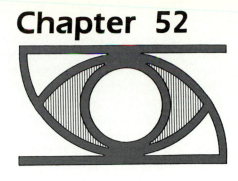
Glaucoma in the Phakomatoses

Jayne S. Weiss
Robert Ritch

The phakomatoses (*phakos,* birthmark), or disseminated hamartomatoses, are a group of ophthalmologically important hereditary disorders exhibiting variable penetrance and expressivity (see outline below). These disorders are characterized by the formation of hamartias and hamartomas in the eye, central nervous system, skin, and viscera. The following are classic features of the phakomatoses:

1. Nontumorous growths on the skin or mucous membranes that arise from cells norally found in the tissue at the involved site (hamartias)
2. Localized tumors arising from cells normally found in the tissue at the site of growth (hamartomas)
3. True neoplasms originating from undifferentiated embryonic cells or dedifferentiated mature cells
4. Other associated congenital abnormalities

Derivatives of all three embryonic layers may be affected. François[51] has listed the following three important stages in pathogenesis of the phakomatoses:

1. The developmental stage at which the abnormal gene functions; estimates have varied from the thirtieth day[78] and the third month[86] to between the third and seventh months of gestation.[33]
2. The phakomatoses may be differentiated embryologically based on the particular germinal layer affected. In neuroectodermal dysplasias, such as neurofibromatosis and tuberous sclerosis, interference with the migration and differentiation of embryonic neural cells results in proliferation. In the mesodermal disorders, such as encephalotrigeminal angiomatosis, angiomatosis retinae, and Klippel-Trenaunay-Weber syndrome, irregularity in the distribution and structure of small vessels results in abnormal proliferation of perivascular cells. Rarely, more than one phakomatosis may occur in a single patient.
3. Multiple malformations may arise from interference with the process of induction.

Glaucoma in the phakomatoses can develop through a number of different mechanisms, even within a single disease entity (see box below).

GLAUCOMA IN THE PHAKOMATOSES

A. Commonly associated with glaucoma
  1. Encephalotrigeminal angiomatosis (Sturge-Weber)
B. Occasionally associated with glaucoma
  1. Neurofibromatosis (von Recklinghausen)
  2. Angiomatosis retinae (von Hippel–Lindau)
  3. Oculodermal melanocytosis (Nevus of Ota)
C. Rarely associated with glaucoma
  1. Basal cell nevus syndrome
  2. Tuberous sclerosis (Bourneville)
  3. Klippel-Trenaunay-Weber (in pure form)
  4. Diffuse congenital hemangiomatosis
D. Unassociated with glaucoma
  1. Ataxia-telangiectasia (Louis-Bar)
  2. Racemose angioma of the retina (Wyburn-Mason) (see Plate III, Fig. 8)

Many different mechanisms have been suggested, but few have been proved. Diagnosis is frequently straightforward, based on the presence of buphthalmos and/or other signs of congenital glaucoma in infancy or early childhood, and on an elevated intraocular pressure in children and adults. Optimal treatment, however, often depends on the determination and analysis of the underlying mechanism of the glaucoma. One should make every effort to do so, both for the patient's benefit and to further elucidate our understanding of these relatively uncommon entities.

Although no universal mechanism to explain the pathogenesis of glaucoma in the phakomatoses exists, there are many similarities among the syndromes. Tissue hypertrophy and developmental abnormalities have been postulated to cause ocular hypertension in both neurofibromatosis and encephalotrigeminal angiomatosis. The anterior chamber angle may be occluded by a neurofibroma in neurofibromatosis, neovascularization in encephalotrigeminal angiomatosis, or melanocytes in oculodermal melanocytosis. A ciliary body or choroidal neurofibroma, or an iris hemangioma may cause the iris root to obstruct the angle. Neovascular glaucoma has been reported in neurofibromatosis, encephalotrigeminal angiomatosis, angiomatosis retinae, and tuberous sclerosis.

NEUROFIBROMATOSIS

Neurofibromatosis is primarily a neuroectodermal dysplasia characterized by tumorlike formations derived from the proliferation of peripheral nerve elements. Von Recklinghausen[144] (1882) first identified the clinical and pathologic complex of neurofibromatosis as a distinct entity. The disease is inherited by means of an autosomal dominant gene with almost complete penetrance but variable expressivity. The mutation rate is 1×10^4, with at least half of these representing new mutations. It is reported to occur in 1 of 2500 to 3300 births.[28] Though congenital, tumors may first present in late childhood or adult life. Mental retardation and seizure disorders may occur, but intelligence is usually normal. It is important to distinguish between classic neurofibromatosis and the central, or acoustic, form. A segmental form, presumably caused by a somatic mutation, also exists.[94]

Systemic Involvement

Neurofibromatosis is considered to be present in a patient with two of the following criteria, provided no other disease accounts for the findings[118]:

1. At least five café au lait macules over 5 mm in greatest diameter, if prepubertal; six café au lait macules over 15 mm in greatest diameter
2. Two or more neurofibromas of any type, or one plexiform neurofibroma
3. Multiple axillary or inguinal freckles
4. Sphenoid wing dysplasia or congenital bowing or thinning of long bone cortex, with or without pseudarthrosis
5. Bilateral optic nerve gliomas
6. Two or more iris Lische nodules on slit-lamp examination
7. A parent, sibling, or offspring with von Recklinghausen neurofibromatosis, by the above criteria

The usual clinical appearance is one of multiple circumscribed areas of hyperpigmentation of the skin accompanied by multiple dermal nodules and neurofibromas. Tumors of the central and peripheral nervous system include neurofibromas, optic nerve and chasmal gliomas, neurinomas, astrocytomas, and meningiomas. The brain, meninges, spinal cord, and peripheral, cranial, or sympathetic nerves may be involved. Acustic neuroma is the most frequent intracranial lesion.

Cutaneous manifestations are common and form the hallmark of the diagnosis. Café au lait spots are regularly circumscribed, brown macules typically found on the trunk (Fig. 52-1). Plexiform neuromas are large, ramifying cords of neurofibromas caused by enlarged nerves and thickened perineural sheaths. Fibroma mollusca are pedunculated, pigmented nodules characterized by an increased number of Schwann's cells, connective tissue elements, and enlarged cutaneous nerves (Fig. 52-2). Regional giantism, or hemihypertrophy of the face or extremities may be caused by diffuse proliferation of mesodermal tissue near a plexiform neuroma. Occasionally a neurofibroma may undergo sarcomatous change and develop into a malignant schwannoma. Skeletal defects occur in 29% of patients, whereas endocrine, vascular, and visceral disturbances are less common.[57]

Evidence has accumulated that elevated nerve growth factor levels exist in patients with neurofibromatosis.[44,129] It has been noted that Schwann cells have many nerve growth factor receptor sites.[116] The decreased binding of epidermal growth factor by fibroblasts of patients with neurofibromatosis suggests that a receptor deficiency or membrane abnormality may play a role in the cause of the disease.[169,170] The recent localization of the gene for neurofibromatosis to chromosome 17 presents

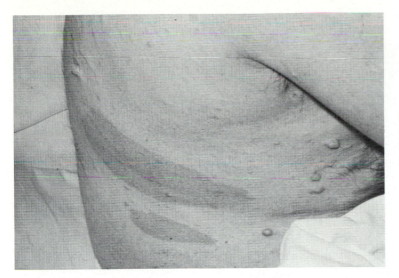

Fig. 52-1 Large café au lait spots on trunk of patient with neurofibromatosis. Cutaneous neurofibromas and slight axillary freckling are also present.

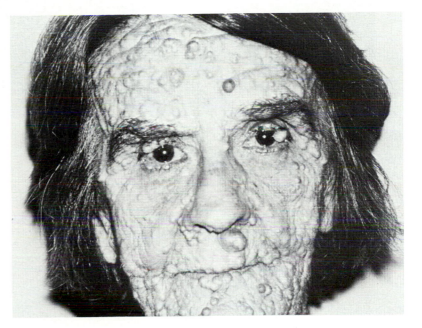

Fig. 52-2 Diffuse cutaneous neurofibromas, or fibroma mollusca, are a hallmark of this disease. (From Gass, JDM: The phakomatoses. In Smith, JL, editor: Neuroophthalmology, vol 2, St Louis, 1965, The CV Mosby Co)

the potential for rapid progress in the elucidation of the underlying genetic and biochemical abnormalities of this disease.[13]

Ocular Involvement

In decreasing order of frequency, neurofibromatosis involves the eyelids, orbit, uvea, optic nerve, retina, cornea, tarsal conjunctiva, and bulbar conjunctiva. Only the lens and vitreous are unaffected.

The lids may be involved by plexiform neuromas with characteristic palapable stringlike swellings (Fig. 52-2 to 52-5). These usually affect

the upper lid unilaterally but rarely may be bilateral[101] or affect primarily the lower lid.[51] In addition to the upper lid, the skin above the orbit and on the adjacent temple may be involved. This lesion is identical histologically to the neurofibroma. The combination of plexiform neuroma of the lid, facial hemihypertrophy, and buphthalmos has been termed François' syndrome.[52] Café au lait spots, pigmented nevi, elephantiasis neuromatosa, fibroma molluscum, and diffuse palpebral neurofibromatosis with absence of cordlike structures may also occur in the lid.

Glial neoplasms or meningoblastomas of the

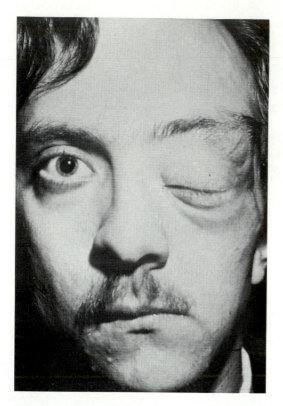

Fig. 52-3 Plexiform neuroma of lids and adjacent temporal region and mild facial hemihypertrophy. When buphthalmos is present, triad is referred to as François' syndrome.

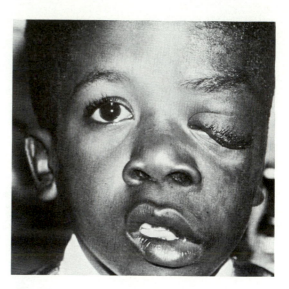

Fig. 52-4 Similar picture in a child (see Fig. 52-3).

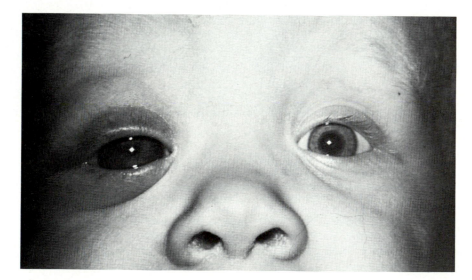

Fig. 52-5 Plexiform neuroma of upper and lower lids in association with congenital glaucoma in an infant. (From Satran, L, et al: Am J Dis Child 134:182, copyright 1980, American Medical Association)

optic nerve may cause loss of vision, proptosis, and optic atrophy. Rarely, neurofibroma of the disc occurs, and glial hamartomas or nerve fiber medullation may involve the retina.[89]

Orbital neurofibroma (Fig. 52-6) or plexiform neurofibromatosis causes displacement of the globe with proptosis. Pulsating exophthalmos unassociated with bruits results from orbital wall defects or meningoceles. Pulsating muscle palsies may be secondary to orbital expansion caused by congenital defects or tumor erosion.

Conjunctival nodules, or diffuse infiltration of the episclera by nerve fibers or small tumors, and scleral melanosis occur rarely. Hyperplasia of nerve fibers or tumor formation may involve the cornea.

Ectropion uveae (Fig. 52-7), Lische nodules (variably pigmented nodules comprising focal collections of spindle cells, which are melanocytic in origin)[105] (Fig. 52-8), or heterochromia may involve the iris. Hyperplastic neurons, Schwann cells, fibroblasts, and/or melanocytes may cause thickening of the choroid and ciliary body. Circumscribed tumors that ophthalmoscopically resemble malignant melanomas may occur in the region of the ciliary nerves. An increased incidence of uveal melanoma has been reported.[58,155,160]

Glaucoma Associated with Neurofibromatosis

Schiess-Gemuseus[123] (1884) first reported the association of neurofibromatosis with congenital glaucoma. There are no reports of the incidence of glaucoma in neurofibromatosis, but despite the frequent mention of the subject in the literature, it appears to be rather rare in proportion to the number of patients with the disease. Of 300 cases of congenital glaucoma in a large series, only one (0.3%) was related to neurofibromatosis.[64] In almost all reported cases, the association of glaucoma with neurofibromatosis occurred at birth or shortly thereafter. Late-onset glaucoma occasionally occurs, however, and patients should be followed routinely if there is any question of orbital or ocular involvement. Open-angle glaucoma appearing in late adulthood should be considered to be primary unless proven otherwise.

Glaucoma associated with neurofibromatosis is almost always unilateral.[83] Neurofibromatous involvement of the upper lid is classically present, especially with buphthalmos (see Fig. 52-5), although exceptions have been reported.[54,64] Glaucoma is present in 50% of all eyes with plexiform neuroma.[83] Patients with plexiform neuroma

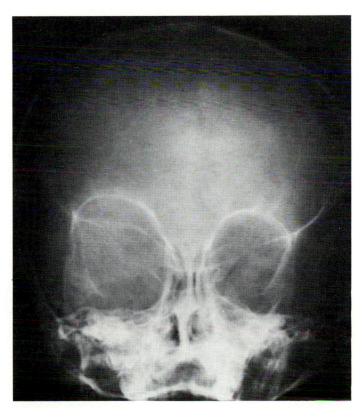

Fig. 52-6 Significant orbital asymmetry caused by extensive orbital plexiform neuroma in same patient as in Fig. 52-5. (From Satran, L, et al: Am J Dis Child 134:182, copyright 1980, American Medical Association)

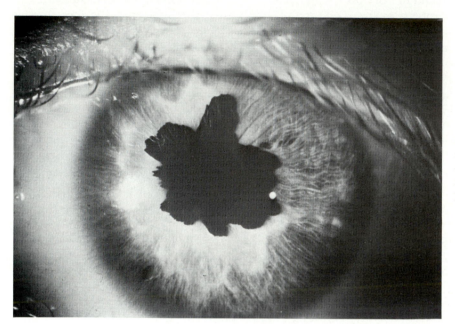

Fig. 52-7 Congenital ectropion uveae in 10-year-old boy with juvenile glaucoma and neurofibromatosis. Plexiform neuroma of lids is not present in this patient.

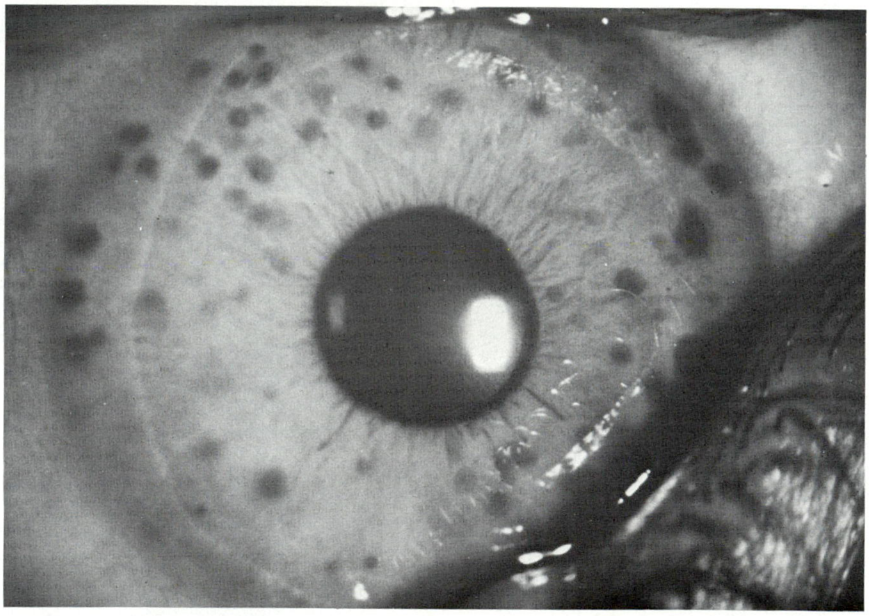

Fig. 52-8 Numerous iris hamartomas (Lische nodules) are characteristically found in neurofibromatosis.

should be followed for the development of glaucoma.

Congenital ectropion uveae is a rare, nonprogressive anomaly characterized by the presence of iris pigment on the anterior surface of the iris stroma (see Plate IV, Fig. 4). Associated iridocorneal angle anomalies and glaucoma may occur. Many of these patients have neurofibromatosis.[113]

Buphthalmos occurring in the absence of documented elevated intraocular pressure has been reported in neurofibromatosis.[9,70,158] This is an important point to consider in the diagnosis to prevent unnecessary surgery. Hoyt and Billson[70] reported an infant with buphthalmos in whom enlargement of the globe continued after the intraocular pressure was controlled. They concluded that the buphthalmos represented an effect of regional giantism similar to the hypertrophy of adjacent structures.

Mechanisms of glaucoma

Many mechanisms have been postulated as causes of glaucoma in neurofibromatosis. Sachsalber[119] (1897) hypothesized that abnormal choroidal innervation led to connective tissue overgrowth and lymphatic (aqueous humor) blockage along the vortex veins, which impeded aqueous humor outflow. Verhoeff[141] described three patients with plexiform neuroma, intraocular nerve involvement, and unilateral buphthalmos. He concluded that a disturbance of the ciliary nerves resulted in buphthalmos, but then later rescinded this theory. Most tenable hypotheses for glaucoma in neurofibromatosis relate to developmental or mechanical abnormalities.

Persistence of embryonic tissue in the filtration angle has been reported.[70,83,157,158] This may block aqueous humor outflow and lead to increased intraocular pressure, but the pressure may also be

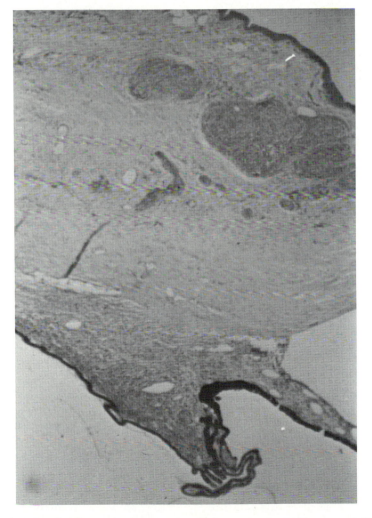

Fig. 52-9 Anterior chamber angle cleavage anomaly in eye exenterated because of diffuse orbital neurofibromatosis and long-standing blindness secondary to congenital glaucoma.

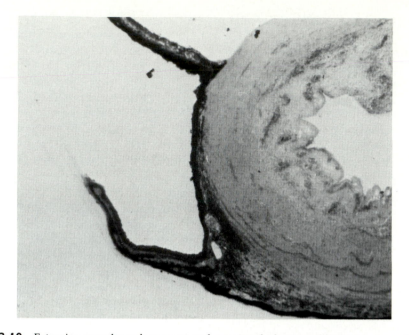

Fig. 52-10   Extensive vascular enlargement and massive thickening of limbus in neurofibromatosis. Angle is sealed by broad peripheral anterior synechiae. Nodular areas of neurofibromatous tissue are present. Angle-closure in this case appears to have been secondary to posterior synechiae between iris sphincter and lens, with resultant peripheral iris bombé, after anterior chamber hemorrhage. (From Friedman, MW, and Ritchey, CL: Arch Ophthalmol 70:294, 1963. Copyright 1963, American Medical Association)

normal.[70] Incomplete development of the iridocorneal angle may give a picture similar to that of primary congenital glaucoma (Fig. 52-9).[59] Malformation[93] or absence of Schlemm's canal* may accompany the anterior chamber angle anomaly as part of the developmental disorder or, in some cases, may be a secondary change caused by long-standing glaucoma and sclerosis or distortion of the angle structures.

The presence of compact iris processes[26,83,96,123] and marked anterior insertion of the iris[83] have been described. However, patients may have increased numbers of iris processes and normal intraocular pressure.[64] The ciliary processes may also be abnormal and extend anteriorly onto the posterior iris surface.

Collins and Batten[26] described adhesions between the iris and the posterior cornea. Neurofibromatous thickening of the ciliary body and choroid might cause anterior displacement of the iris diaphragm, narrowing of the angle, peripheral anterior synechiae, and glaucoma (Fig. 52-10).[32,57,90] The choroid may be as much as six to eight times normal thickness (Fig. 52-11). It is difficult to de-

termine what is primary and what is secondary in these instances, particularly because most eyes coming to enucleation have had previous surgery, which may be responsible for many of the pathologic changes. However, neurofibromatous involvement of the choroid is characteristically present in those cases with glaucoma.

In most cases, patients with the preceding pathologic findings have had buphthalmos.* There have been case reports of adults with choroidal involvement, peripheral anterior synechiae, and glaucoma who did not have buphthalmos.[22,90] Choroidal involvement may also be present without glaucoma.[22,54]

Infiltration of the angle[64] or root of the iris[31] with neurofibromatous tissue may lead to peripheral anterior synechiae formation. Neovascular glaucoma may result from invasion of the chamber angle by fibrovascular tissue with resultant synechial closure of the angle.[162]

A single eye may be affected by more than one mechanism over time. Friedman and Ritchey[57] described a patient with congenital glaucoma and abnormal tissue in the angle on gonioscopy in whom

---

*References 26, 80, 97, 119, 130, 157, 158, 161.

*References 21, 56, 64, 80, 93, 97, 109, 117, 130, 135, 152, 157, 158, 161,163

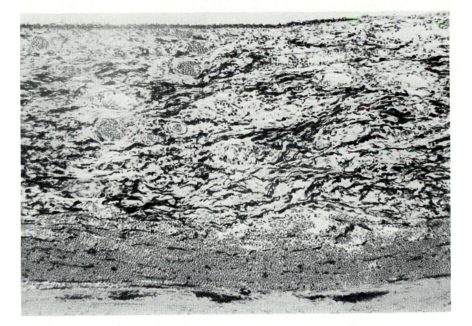

Fig. 52-11   Massive choroidal thickening caused by diffuse neurofibroma in same patient as in Fig. 52-10. Although termed choroidal neurofibroma in the literature, this is really a hyperplasia of Schwannian elements and melanocytes. (From Friedman, MW, and Ritchey, CL: Arch Ophthalmol 70:294, 1963. Copyright 1963, American Medical Association)

intraocular pressure was controlled after goniotomy. Six years later the patient had sudden onset of severe pain with increased pressure. Examination of the enucleated globe revealed total peripheral anterior synechiae, a rudimentary ciliary body, and a markedly thickened choroid. Apparently, thickening of the choroid and ciliary body produced an anterior displacement of the uveal tract and subsequent angle closure.

Management

The choice of treatment depends on the severity of the glaucoma, the patient's age at onset, and the mechanism. Congenital glaucoma should be managed surgically. Medical treatment may be initiated in juvenile or adult-onset glaucoma. A patient with buphthalmos and a clear cornea should not be assumed to have glaucoma without definite evidence of elevated intraocular pressure.

Surgery for glaucoma in neurofibromatosis has reflected the development of glaucoma surgery in general, and goniotomy, goniopuncture, trabeculotomy, trabeculectomy, cyclodiathermy, and cyclocryotherapy have all been reported. The overall rate of success of surgery in the literature, however, is much lower than that for primary congenital glaucoma. Because of the rarity of congenital glaucoma associated with neurofibromatosis, it is difficult to generalize as to the reason. However, it is

possible in some cases that, in addition to anomalies of angle development, abnormalities of the meshwork or sclera retard aqueous humor outflow even after goniotomy. In others, tissue hypertrophy itself may contribute to progressive buphthalmos in the absence of marked elevation of intraocular pressure.

It is important to remember that angle-closure caused by choroidal enlargement may supervene even after successful goniotomy. Therefore, these patients should be followed with repeated gonioscopy even if goniotomy or trabeculotomy is successful. A reasonable approach would be to perform goniotomy or trabeculotomy initially if the angle is open but has the appearance of incomplete cleavage. If the angle is closed at diagnosis or cannot be seen because of corneal edema, trabeculectomy is probably a better choice. Since angle-closure resulting from choroidal enlargement may supervene even after successful goniotomy, patients should be followed with repeated gonioscopy, and trabeculectomy then performed when there is obvious progressive closure of the angle.

ENCEPHALOTRIGEMINAL ANGIOMATOSIS (STURGE-WEBER SYNDROME)

The first case of encephalotrigeminal angiomatosis was probably reported when Schirmer[124] (1860) described a patient with a facial angioma and glaucoma. Sturge[133] described a hemiparetic epileptic girl with a facial angioma and ipsilateral congenital glaucoma and hypothesized that a cerebral angioma resulted in the neurologic defect. Kalischer[74] (1987) confirmed the association between facial and intracranial angiomas at autopsy. Weber[150] and Dimitri[35] independently demonstrated radiologic evidence of intracranial calcification. The disease has little familial tendency and no sexual or racial predisposition. Chromosomal abnormalities have been reported in some patients, and the disorder may be a dominant trait with incomplete penetrance. Ocular manifestations occur in infancy and early childhood.

Systemic Involvement

The hallmark of the disorder is a facial cutaneous angioma (nevus flammeus, port wine stain), which is present at birth, is usually unilateral, and involves the region of distribution of the first and second divisions of the trigeminal nerve[42] (Figs. 52-12 and 52-13). The angioma is a variably sized, burgundy-colored, macular vascular malformation consisting of a loose arrangment of dilated thin-walled capillaries in the dermis and subcutaneous tissue. Bilaterality occurs in 10%[39] to 30%[127] of cases. The supraorbital region is almost always affected, although exceptions have been reported.[36,139] Occasionally, hemangiomas of the oral and nasal cavities occur concomitantly. Facial hypertrophy in the region associated with the angioma is common.

A meningeal racemose hemangioma usually occurs ipsilateral to the facial hemangioma. It is ordinarily confined to the pia mater and develops close to the cerebrum, usually over the occipital lobe. Progressive calcification frequently occurs in the subintimal layer of the meningeal arteries and may obliterate the vascular lumen. Calcification and atrophy of the external layers of the cerebral cortex may result in mental retardation. Approximately 60% of patients have intellectual deficits and 85% have seizures.[14] Focal motor seizures contralateral to the facial nevus may begin at 1 to 2 years of age. The course is characterized by partial or complete remission, followed by increased severity of the attacks. Postepileptic lesions such as hemiparesis, hemiplegia, and homonymous hemianopsia are common.

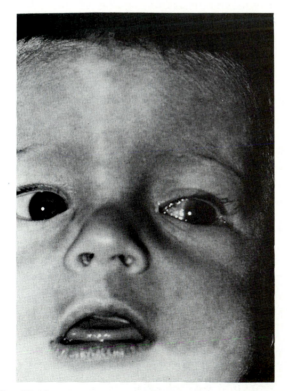

Fig. 52-12 Encephalotrigeminal angiomatosis involving first and second divisions of trigeminal nerve. Congenital glaucoma is present.

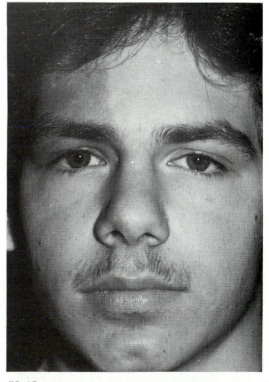

Fig. 52-13 Encephalotrigeminal angiomatosis involving first division of trigeminal nerve. Juvenile-onset glaucoma is present.

Various combinations of involved structures may occur. The trisymptomatic form, classically known as Sturge-Weber syndrome, affects the leptomeninges, eyes, and face. Bisymptomatic forms affect the face and eyes or face and leptomeninges. There are no descriptions of a form involving the leptomeninges and eyes and sparing the face. Monosymptomatic forms also occur.

Skeletal malformations such as hemihypertrophy of the face and body have also been reported. Localized or diffuse visceral angiomas may occur in the kidneys, spleen, intestine, pancreas, lungs and thyroid.

Ocular Involvement

Hemangiomas may affect the lid, episclera conjunctiva, iris, and ciliary body. Anderson's rule[5] states that when the nevus flammeus involves the upper lid, there is ipsilateral intraocular involvement. If the upper lid is spared, the ipsilateral eye is spared. Exceptions may occur.[146] Rarely, orbital involvement results in exophthalmos. Iris hyperchromia occurs in 7% to 8% of cases.[3] Tortuous retinal vessels and scleral melanosis may occur.

Choroidal hemangiomas, which occur in 40% of cases,[39] are the most common abnormality, except perhaps for conjunctival involvement. They are usually diffuse, flat, and involve the posterior pole. The hemangioma is easily overlooked in younger patients and grows slowly. It may appear as an orange-yellow, slightly elevated mass. Pathologically these are cavernous hemangiomas, consisting of thin-walled, blood-filled sinuses, lined by a single layer of endothelium (Fig. 52-14). Exudative retinal detachment may occur after a long period of growth. In some cases diffuse uveal involvement occurs, which has been termed "tomato catsup" fundus.[134] The hemangioma may be so large as to involve nearly the entire choroid, a situation that sets the stage for surgical disaster by predisposing the patient to expulsive choroidal hemorrhage. Exact calculation of the prevalence of hemangiomas at autopsy is difficult, because the lesion may contract artifactitiously during fixation and not be recognized. Of all cases of choroidal hemangiomas noted on examination of enucleation specimens, 50% occur in encephalotrigeminal angiomatosis.[38]

Glaucoma Associated with Encephalotrigeminal Angiomatosis

Elschnig[43] and Nakamura[99] were the first to realize an etiologic relationship between encephalotrigeminal angiomatosis and glaucoma. One third of patients with the syndrome have increased intraocular pressure.[4] Usually this occurs only when the hemangioma involves the lid, tarsus, and conjunctiva.

When the cutaneous angioma is unilateral, the buphthalmos or glaucoma is nearly always unilat-

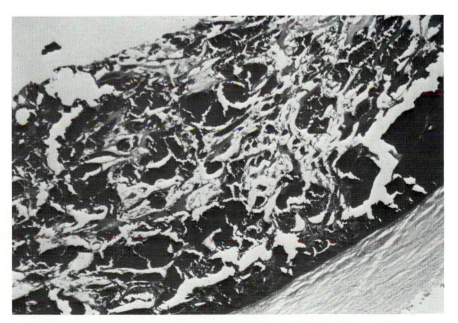

Fig. 52-14 Choroidal hemangioma. (Courtesy R Cordero Moreno, MD)

eral and ipsilateral to it. Contralateral[37,131] and bilateral[43] glaucoma with unilateral cutaneous angioma have been reported. Bilateral angiomas may be accompanied by either unilateral or bilateral glaucoma, although the former is more typical.

In a large series of 174 patients with increased intraocular pressure, 84 had buphthalmos.[30] Alexander and Norman[4] reported that two thirds of their patients had buphthalmos ipsilateral to the nevus and the remaining one third had glaucoma without buphthalmos. Sixty percent of the glaucomas were congenital and 40% were adult onset. Buphthalmos without increased intraocular pressure has been reported.[46,77]

Eighty-eight percent of patients with choroidal hemangiomas develop glaucoma,[48] which may be congenital, adult onset, or secondary to inflammation and uveal reaction, usually following retinal detachment. Some authors have concluded that the presence of a choroidal hemangioma in encephalotrigeminal angiomatosis results in glaucoma. However, patients with choroidal hemangiomas who do not have the Sturge-Weber syndrome rarely develop glaucoma. Furthermore, choroidal hemangiomas are frequently associated with anterior segment structural anomalies, which themselves may result in glaucoma.

Numerous mechanisms have been postulated to explain the pathogenesis of glaucoma in encephalotrigeminal angiomatosis. Hudelo[71] theorized that clinically silent meningeal angiomas obstructed ocular drainage into the cavernous sinus, thereby raising intraocular pressure. In the neural theory,[29,55,117,142] abnormal sympathetic innervation resulted in uveal capillary dilation, stasis, and glaucoma. Cabannes[21] postulated that the choroidal hemangioma provided an increased blood supply, leading to congenital hypertrophy of ocular structures and glaucoma.

These theories are historically interesting, but vascular or mechanical explanations offer more plausible mechnisms. The mechanical theories are based on occlusion of the anterior chamber angle, leading to blockage of aqueous humor outflow, increased intraocular pressure, and glaucoma.

Numerous authors have believed that glaucoma is secondary to developmental anomalies that result in chamber angle malformations. Histology reveals a poorly developed scleral spur, thickened uveal meshwork, and iris root inserted "anteriorly" on the base of the trabecular meshwork* (Figs. 52-

15 and 52-16). In some cases superficial iris stroma appears to cover the meshwork and extend to an insertion on or near Schwalbe's line (see Fig. 52-15). This is similar to the description sometimes reported in neurofibromatosis.[64] Posterior displacement and incomplete development of Schlemm's canal has been described.[23,40,120] Persistent embryonic mesodermal tissue may also be found in the angle.[126,151] Patients who develop glaucoma during adolescence or later may have a milder expression of the angle cleavage anomaly, a forme fruste of the disorder, or unrelated primary open-angle glaucoma. In these patients, gonioscopy usually reveals a normal-looking angle and the glaucoma is generally more easily controlled, although developmental angle abnormalities have been found on pathologic examination. Other authors have reported no abnormalities in the angle, even in the presence of buphthalmos.[25,150,151]

Hemorrhage from the choroidal hemangioma may result in subretinal hemorrhage and retinal detachment with forward displacement of the iris and angle closure secondary to peripheral anterior synechiae formation either on a mechanical basis or secondary to neovascularization.* Most eyes coming under pathologic examination have had this severe outcome.

The vascular theories relate the elevation of intraocular pressure to the presence of vascular malformations that might increase production, decrease outflow, or actually change the components of aqueous fluid or interfere with extrascleral drainage. Tyson[138] noted that fluorescein appeared in the aqueous humor in the glaucomatous eye more quickly than in the normal eye, and hypothesized an increased vascular permeability resulted in blockage of the angle by "plasmoid aqueous." Intravenous injection of 50% dextrose was found not to lower intraocular pressure in the glaucomatous eye, but it did in the opposite eye.[40,72] Dunphy[40] postulated a rapid equalization of osmotic pressure resulting from increased vascular permeability. Others found the protein content of the aqueous humor to be increased in the glaucomatous eye.[72,91] Subsequently, this theory has been experimentally refuted.

Many authors have invoked vascular hypertrophy as the cause for glaucoma.[11,25,43,60,168] Increased number and/or size of choroidal vessels has been postulated to cause choroidal congestion with increased transudation and/or decreased out-

---

*References 5, 12, 17, 23, 48 ,59, 81, 120, 122, 153.

*References 32, 39, 40, 48, 68, 69, 82, 104.

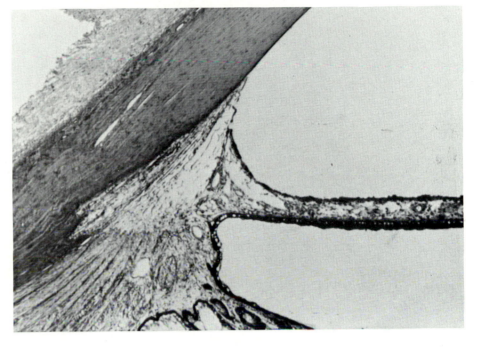

Fig. 52-15 Congenital angle deformity with incomplete cleavage and apparent "anterior insertion of iris" in encephalotrigeminal angiomatosis. (From Weiss, DI: Trans Ophthalmol Soc UK 93:477, 1973)

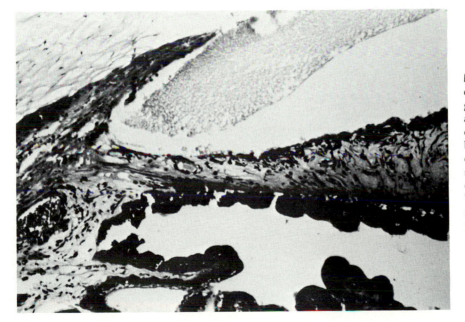

Fig. 52-16 This patient with glaucoma and encephalotrigeminal angiomatosis underwent enucleation at age 16 after hemorrhage from choroidal hemangioma had resulted in a blind, painful eye with elevated intraocular pressure. Angle was partially sealed with peripheral anterior synechiae. In this photograph it is open, but meshwork is compressed and sclerosed. Serosanguinous exudate is present in anterior chamber. (Courtesy R Cordero Moreno, MD)

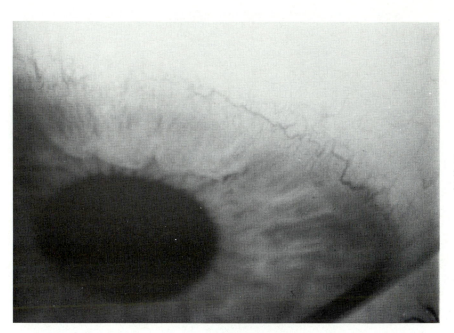

Fig. 52-17 Arteriovenous anastomoses at limbus in same patient as in Fig. 52-13.

Fig. 52-18 Diffuse involvement of conjunctiva and episclera in patient with glaucoma and encephalotrigeminal angiomatosis. (From Shaffer, RN, and Weiss, DI: Congenital and pediatric glaucomas, St Louis, 1970, The CV Mosby Co)

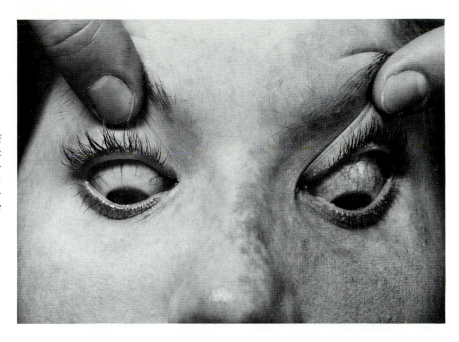

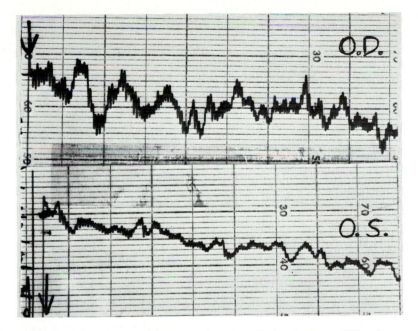

Fig. 52-19 Prominent arterial pulse pressure is present in involved eye *(OD),* whereas outflow coefficient is not significantly reduced. (From Weiss, DI: Trans Ophthalmol Soc UK 93:477, 1973)

flow of aqueous humor.[16,40,60,132] There is no experimental proof for these theories.

Mansheim[87] and Miller[95] found glaucomatous eyes in the Sturge-Weber syndrome to have a normal coefficient of outflow and concluded that elevated intraocular pressure was the result of increased aqueous humor production. In one case, fluorophotometric analysis of aqueous humor production did not document hypersecretion.[6]

More recently Weiss[153] found vascular hamartias of the anterior episclera and conjunctiva in all patients examined (Figs. 52-17 and 52-18). Although in the earlier literature patients without episcleral angiomas were reported, these angiomas may be very subtle and occasionally evident only at surgery. Weiss hypothesized that the increased pulse pressure present on tonography indicated an arteriovenous fistula and that a combination of elevated episcleral venous pressure (indirectly deduced by the presence of engorged vessels) and a congenital angle malformation contributed in variable proportions to elevated intraocular pressure.

Phelps[107] examined 19 patients with encephalo-trigeminal angiomatosis and glaucoma. All had episcleral hemangiomas, the extent of which correlated roughly with the severity of the glaucoma. Elevated episcleral venous pressure was present in 11 of 12 eyes in which this was measured. Two patients without glaucoma had small episcleral hemangiomas. Angle deformities of a congenital nature were seen in only two patients. Phelps concluded that an elevation in episcleral venous pressure caused by arteriovenous shunts was etiologically responsible for the glaucoma. However, no predictable correlation between the episcleral and intraocular pressures in individual eyes was found. Cibis et al.[24] found that trabeculectomy specimens from patients with Sturge-Weber syndrome demonstrated changes in the trabecular meshwork and Schlemm's canal similar to findings in advanced age and primary open-angle glaucoma. They suggested that the primary cause of juvenile glaucoma might be premature aging of the outflow pathway.

The most likely cause for elevated intraocular pressure seems to be a combination of developmental angle anomalies and elevated episcleral venous pressure, which may result in alterations of the meshwork similar to those found with aging. The relative contribution of each is dependent on the individual case. Careful gonioscopy, tonography, and measurement of episcleral venous pressure are useful in the determination of the cause (Fig. 52-19).

Management

Because the glaucoma in encephalotrigeminal angiomatosis is variable in its severity, medical treatment is warranted if buphthalmos is not present and if the pressure can be adequately controlled. If intraocular pressure is high but outflow is normal or nearly so, drugs that decrease aqueous humor production, such as topical beta-blockers or carbonic anhydrase inhibitors, will be most helpful. If outflow is also reduced, miotics and epinephrine compounds may contribute to lowering pressure. In a preliminary report, oral isosorbide dinitrate was found to reduce intraocular pressure in glaucomatous eyes of patients with encephalotrigeminal angiomatosis.[75]

If medical treatment fails, as frequently happens, or if the glaucoma is congenital, surgical intervention is necessary. Argon-laser trabeculoplasty has been found to reduce intraocular pressure in patients with encephalotrigeminal angiomatosis and glaucoma.[115] However, if the pressure-lowering effect is not sufficient, the patient may require conventional surgery. Goniotomy is felt by some to be the treatment of choice in congenital glaucoma when gonioscopy suggests angle abnormalities, and it may be tried if gonioscopy is inconclusive. Nevertheless, this procedure, even when repeated, is frequently unsuccessful.[147] Trabeculectomy may be the best choice if the angle appears clinically normal. Trabeculectomy bypasses any component of the glaucoma caused by elevated episcleral venous pressure, whereas goniotomy does not. Trabeculotomy may reduce the risk of expulsive hemorrhage that occurs with open surgical procedures.[24] Combined trabeculotomy-trabeculectomy does not appear to improve prognosis.[19] If external filtration fails, cyclocryotherapy can be attempted as a last resort. The Krupin-Denver filtering valve[92] has also been tried, but long-term follow-up results are not available.

Two serious complications may result from filtering procedures in this disease. Expulsive choroidal hemorrhage may occur as soon as the globe is entered or immediately thereafter, because of the presence of a choroidal hemangioma.[23,128,136] Precautionary measures should be taken before surgery to reduce intraocular pressure as much as possible, and hyperosmotic agents are strongly recommended. Vitreous loss and bleeding from episcleral vessels are also more common.

The second serious complication is that of sudden onset of choroidal effusion after opening the globe, caused by rapid transudation of fluid from the intravascular to the extravascular space in the face of elevated episcleral (and choroidal) venous pressure when the intraocular pressure is suddenly lowered.[15] Adverse consequences of this may be minimized by performing a posterior sclerotomy before opening the eye.[15,147] Radiotherapy of the choroidal hemangioma[1] might protect against these complications.

Phelps[107] suggested that electrocautery or laser photocoagulation might partially obliterate the anterior episcleral vascular anomaly and result in decreased intraocular pressure. Goniotomy with the Q-switched Nd:YAG laser failed to control the glaucoma in an 8-year-old child with encephalotrigeminal angiomatosis who was previously unsuccessfully treated with goniotomy and trabeculotomy.[167]

Results of therapy for glaucoma in encephalotrigeminal angiomatosis are often disappointing. It is hoped that, with further delineation of the mechanisms responsible for the glaucoma, we may develop more successful modalities of treatment.

KLIPPEL-TRENAUNAY-WEBER SYNDROME

Klippel and Trenaunay[79] (1900) described a syndrome characterized by a triad of cutaneous hemangioma extending over one limb, varicosities in the affected limb, and hypertrophy of bone and soft tissue. Parkes Weber[149] (1907) described a similar triad of findings.

Arteriovenous fistulas, vascular hyperplasia, and osseous hypertrophy occur in both syndromes. In the Klippel-Trenaunay syndrome, the fistulas are small, numerous, and of little consequence, whereas those in the Parkes Weber syndrome are large, few, and may lead to circulatory disturbances.[45] Frequently the two diseases are not differentiated and are included under the heading Klippel-Trenaunay-Weber syndrome.

The disease may be inherited in an irregular dominant pattern.[145] Formes frustes occur, in which one of the three major findings is absent. The congenital hemangioma varies in size, location, and color. Frequently it follows a radicular distribution and may increase in size. Osteohypertrophy is usually present at birth, but may develop afterward. The limbs are most commonly involved and may further increase in size with age (Fig. 52-20).

Although the varices in the Klippel-Trenaunay syndrome are congenital in origin, they may first become evident years after birth. They are unilateral and ipsilateral to the skin lesion. The Parkes Weber syndrome is characterized by the occurrence of large arteriovenous fistulas, cirsoid aneurysms, and telangiectasias.

Neurologic involvement is demonstrated by electroencephalographic (EEG) abnormalities, sei-

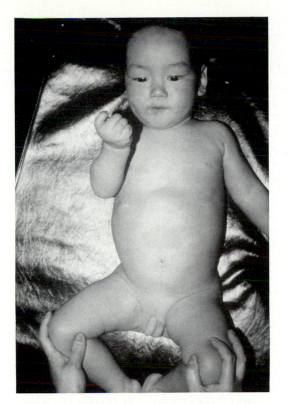

Fig. 52-20 Klippel-Trenauney-Weber syndrome in a 1-year-old Japanese child. (Courtesy Professor Ikuo Azuma, MD, Osaka)

zures, mental retardation, and cerebral hemangiomas.[102]

Ocular findings include enophthalmos, conjunctival telangiectasis, heterochromia iridis, iris coloboma, oculosympathetic palsy, retinal varicosities, choroidal angiomas, Marcus Gunn pupil, strabismus, orbital varices, disc anomalies, glaucoma, and buphthalmos.[102] Ocular findings may occur in the absence of a facial hemangioma.

The glaucoma may occur with or without buphthalmos.[67,99,108,145] In most of these cases patients have also had a facial nevus. In the one patient with a pure form of the Klippel-Trenaunay-Weber syndrome (i.e., not combined with the Sturge-Weber syndrome), elevated intraocular pressures, and unilateral vein occlusion,[67] the association may have been circumstantial.

ANGIOMATOSIS RETINAE (VON HIPPEL–LINDAU SYNDROME)

A retinal hemangioma was illustrated for the first time in 1879 by Panas and Remy.[103] Von Hippel[143] described the progression of retinal involvement (1904) and later identified the lesion as a hemangioblastoma. Lindau[84] (1926) discovered angiomatous cysts of the cerebellum in many cases of von Hippel's disease. Subsequently, the com-

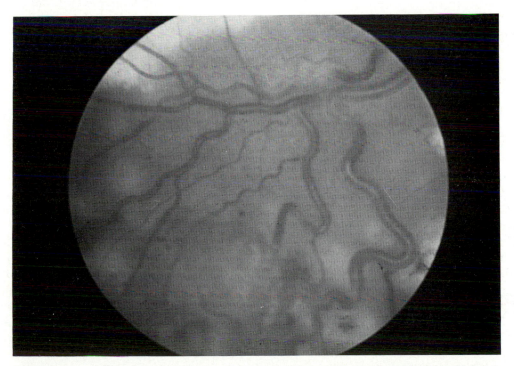

Fig. 52-21 Retinal angioma in von Hippel–Lindau syndrome. Artery and vein feeding and draining angiomas are markedly enlarged.

bination of angiomas of the retina and central nervous system was referred to as von Hippel–Lindau disease (retinocerebellar angiomatosis). Ballantyne[10] (1930) first reported the occurrence of secondary glaucoma. Nicholson et al.[100] (1976) classified the lesion as a capillary hemangioma on the basis of ultrastructural findings.

The inheritance pattern is autosomal dominant with incomplete penetrance, and the disease usually present in the second and third decades of life. In addition to the retinal and cerebellar hemangiomas, other viscera may be involved. Symptoms are usually related to the retinal and cerebellar lesions and include headache, vertigo, and cerebellar dysfunction.

Approximately 13% of patients have retinal angiomas.[121] These are reddish, globular tumors approximately 1 to 2 disc diameters in size. They are usually located in the periphery and contain arteriovenous capillary shunts (Fig. 52-21). The artery and vein leading to and from the hemangioma are characteristically dilated and tortuous. Some 50% of cases occur bilaterally, and approximately one third of patients have more than one angioma per eye. Occasionally the angioma may occur adjacent to or involve the disc. The presence of a retinal angioma should alert the examiner to search carefully for others that might be at a much earlier stage of development. Fluorescein angiography is often helpful.

The retinal involvement, when untreated, progresses from vascular dilation to transudation into the retina and subretinal space, and to exudation and hemorrhage. Exudation may occur at sites distant from the angioma, and macular exudates with star figures may be the presenting symptom. At this stage the patient may appear to have Coats' disease. Eventually, massive exudation, retinal detachment, and neovascular glaucoma may develop.

The usual course in untreated eyes consists of relentless progression. The hemangiomas should be treated as soon as they are discovered by either cryotherapy, or photocoagulation, or a combination of the two.[2,53,148,159] Eye wall resection has been reported for large angiomas resistant to cryotherapy or photocoagulation.[106]

TUBEROUS SCLEROSIS (BOURNEVILLE'S DISEASE)

Tuberous sclerosis was described by Bourneville[20] in 1881. It is inherited through an autosomal dominant gene with low penetrance and variable expressivity. Signs of the disease may be manifest at birth, but the clinical diagnosis is usually made in the first or second decade of life.

The most frequent clinical manifestations consist of a triad of epilepsy, adenoma sebaceum, and mental deficiency. The "ash leaf" sign, a hypopigmented skin spot seen under ultraviolet light, is believed to be pathognomonic. Intracranial calcified hamartomas seen radiologically are diagnostic. A wide range of other lesions occurs, including subungual fibromas, cardiac rhabdomyomas, and hamartomas of the kidney, liver, thyroid, and gastrointestinal tract.

The classic ocular lesion is the peripapillary astrocytic hamartoma, or "mulberry lesion," which may be single or multiple. These may undergo cystic degeneration and rarely mimic necrotizing retinochoroiditis.[27] Loss of vision is unusual. Sebaceous adenomas of the upper lid and glands of Zeis are less common. Hypopigmented iris and fundus lesions, retinal angiomas and poliosis have been reported.[7,65,125]

One case of glaucoma without associated cause has been reported.[112] Secondary glaucoma is also extremely rare and results from vitreous hemorrhage,[114] rubeosis iridis, and retinal detachment.[164]

OCULODERMAL MELANOCYTOSIS

Oculodermal melanocytosis, or nevus of Ota, is characterized by deep dermal pigmentation, usually unilateral, in the distribution of the first and second divisions of the trigeminal nerve (Fig. 52-22). It is commonly found in Orientals, usually women. Hereditary occurrence is extremely rare.[76,137] Most patients have concomitant hyperpigmentation of the globe, which may involve the sclera (Fig. 52-23), conjunctiva, cornea, iris (Fig. 52-24), and fundus. The iridocorneal angle may be extremely hyperpigmented without elevation of intraocular pressure. There is an increased incidence of uveal and orbital melanoma.* Angioid streaks have been reported.[8]

What appear to be primary angle-closure[47] and open-angle[47,50] glaucomas have been reported. Shaffer and Weiss[127] reported elevated intraocular pressure in a patient with nevus of Ota and melanocytic infiltration of the anterior chamber angle. Weiss and Krohn[154] postulated that the melanocytes increased outflow resistance, resulting in "benign melanocytic glaucoma." Secondary glaucomas have been associated with increased numbers of iris processes,[34] malignant melanoma of the iris,[49]

*References 18, 41, 61, 85, 140, 155, 166.

Fig. 52-22 Oculodermal melanocytosis involving first and second divisions of trigeminal nerve.

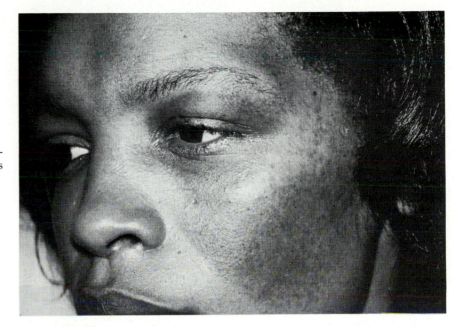

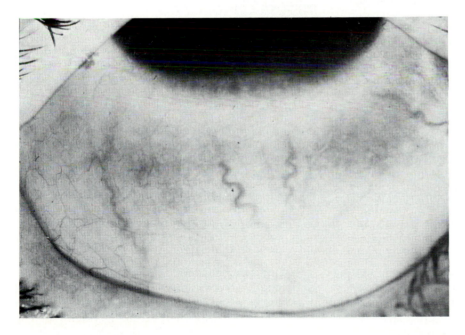

Fig. 52-23 Involvement of sclera in oculodermal melanocytosis.

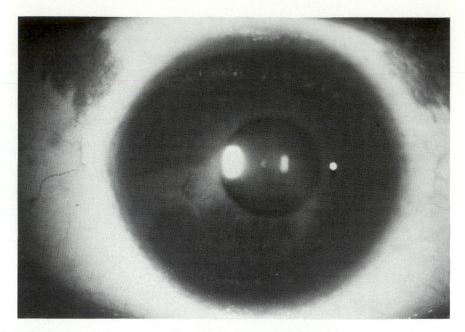

Fig. 52-24   Extensively involved iris in patient with oculodermal melanocytosis. Sclera is involved superiorly.

and nevus flammeus with retinal angiomatosis.[110] However, a study of 33 cases of ocular and oculodermal melanocytosis found no correlation between melanocytic involvement of the trabecular meshwork and elevation of intraocular pressure.[62]

BASAL CELL NEVUS SYNDROME

The basal cell nevus syndrome is a rare disease transmitted by a highly penetrant autosomal dominant gene. It is characterized by multiple skin tumors that are histologically indistinguishable from basal cell carcinomas. Dental cysts, frontal bossing, and skeletal, neurologic, genital, and skin anomalies are seen. Defective renal tubular phosphate reabsorption is common. Hermans et al.[68] classified the disease as a phakomatosis on the basis of the characteristic ocular findings.

The skin tumors may be present at birth, but usually become noticeable in adolescence. They are found most often on the eyelids, nose, cheeks, and trunk.[88] Clinically they may resemble nevi, neurofibromas, or skin tags, and their true nature may not be appreciated until pathologic diagnosis. Most lesions are benign but may become invasive. Unlike basal cell carcinoma, the nevus appears in younger individuals and in areas not exposed to sunlight.

Reported ocular findings have included orbital involvement by tumor, hypertelorism, congenital cataract, strabismus, coloboma of the choroid and optic nerve, corneal leukoma, and glaucoma.[63,73] The mechanisms involved and incidence of glaucoma have not been described.

DIFFUSE CONGENITAL HEMANGIOMATOSIS

Diffuse congenital hemangiomatosis is a rare disease in which multiple small cutaneous hemangiomas are associated with visceral hemangiomas. Death usually occurs within the first few months of life, usually as a result of cardiac failure associated with a large hepatic hemangioma.

The incidence of ocular findings in 16 reported cases was 50% and includes hemangiomas of the iris, conjunctiva, and lid, abnormal chorioretinal vasculature, and microphthalmos. Neuro-ophthalmic involvement includes cortical blindness as well as third and sixth nerve palsies secondary to CNS hemangiomas. Glaucoma was found in 12.5% of cases.[66]

One case has been associated with infantile glaucoma.[156] Neovascularization of the iris was present and extended into the angles, which were open. The pressures were normalized with a combination of cyclocryotherapy in both eyes and goniotomy in the left eye after the abnormal vessels had cleared. In a second case, a cavernous hemangioma of the iris compressed the ciliary body and occluded the angle adjacent to it, but glaucoma was not present.[98]

REFERENCES

1. Alberti, W, et al: Radiotherapy of the hemangioma of the choroid, Strahlentherapie 159:160, 1983
2. Amalric, P: Capillary microangiography and laser photocoagulation in Hippel Lindau disease, Bull Mem Soc Fr Ophthalmol 93:76, 1981
3. Alexander, GL: The Sturge-Weber syndrome. In Vinken, PJ, and Bruyn, GW, editors: Handbook of clinical neurology: the phakomatoses, vol 14, Amsterdam, 1972, North Holland Publishing Co
4. Alexander, GL, and Norman, RM: The Sturge-Weber syndrome, Bristol, England, 1960, John Wright & Sons, Ltd
5. Anderson, JR: Hydrophthalmia or congenital glaucoma, London, 1939, Cambridge University Press
6. Asano, Y, and Kimura, R: Glaucoma associated with Sturge-Weber syndrome: a case report, Glaucoma 5:186, 1983
7. Awan, KJ: Leaf-shaped lesions of ocular fundus and white eyelashes in tuberous sclerosis, South Med J 75:227, 1982
8. Awan, KJ: Ocular melanocytosis and angioid streaks, J Pediat Ophthalmol Strabismus 17:300, 1980
9. Babel, J, and Younessian, S: Buphthalmie ohne Hypertension: ein Fall von familiärer Neurofibromatose, Ber Dtsch Ophthalmol Ges 69:221, 1968
10. Ballantyne, A: Buphthalmos with facial nevus and allied conditions, Br J Ophthalmol 14:481, 1930
11. Bär, C: Ein bemerkenswerter Fall von Feuermal und Glaukom, Z Augenheilkd 57:628, 1925
12. Barkan, O: Goniotomy for glaucoma associated with nevus flammeus, Am J Ophthalmol 43:545, 1957
13. Barker, D, et al: Gene for von Recklinghausen enurofibromatosis is in the pericentromeric region of chromosome 17, Science 236:1100, 1987
14. Beck, RW, and Hanno, R: The phakomatoses, Int Ophthalmol Clin 25:97, 1985
15. Bellows, AR, Chylack, LT Jr, Epstein, DL, and Hutchinson, BT: Choroidal effusion during glaucoma surgery in patients with prominent episcleral vessels, Arch Ophthalmol 97:493, 1979
16. Beltman, J: Ueber angeborene Telangiektasien des Auges als Ursache von Glaucoma simplex, v Graefe's Arch Klin Exp Ophthalmol 59:502, 1904
17. Berkow, TW: Retinitis pigmentosa associated with Sturge-Weber syndrome, Arch Ophthalmol 75:72, 1966
18. Blodi, FC: Ocular melanocytosis and melanoma, Am J Ophthalmol 80:389, 1975
19. Board, RJ and Shields, MB: Combined trabeculotomy-trabeculectomy for the management of glaucoma associated with Sturge-Weber syndrome, Ophthalmic Surg 12:817, 1981
20. Bourneville, DM: Sclérose tubéreuse des circonvolutions cérébrales: idiotie et épilepsie hémiplégique, Arch Neurol (Paris) 1:390, 1881
21. Cabannes, C.: La buphthalmie congénitale dans ses rapports avec l'hémihypertrophie de la face, Arch d'Ophthalmol 29:368, 1909
22. Callender, GR, and Thigpen, CA: Two neurofibromas in one eye, Am J Ophthalmol 13:121, 1930
23. Christensen, RG, and Records, RE: Glaucoma and expulsive hemorrhage mechanisms in the Sturge-Weber syndrome, Ophthalmology 86:1360, 1979
24. Cibis, GW, Tripathi, RC and Tripathi, BJ: Glaucoma in Sturge-Weber syndrome, Ophthalmol 91:1061, 1984
25. Clausen, W: Discussion on Voegel's paper, Klin Monatsbl Augenheilkd 81:393, 1928
26. Collins, T, and Batten, RD: Neurofibroma of the eyeball and its appendages, Trans Ophthalmol Soc UK 25:248, 1905
27. Coppeto, JR, Lubin JR, and Albert, DM: Astrocytic hamartoma in tuberous sclerosis mimicking necrotizing retinochoroiditis, J Pediatr Ophthalmol Strabismus 19:306, 1982
28. Crowe, FW, Schull, WJ, and Neel, JV: A clinical, pathological and genetic study of multiple neurofibromatosis, Springfield, Ill, 1956, Charles C Thomas Publisher
29. Cushing, H: Cases of spontaneous intracranial hemorrhage associated with trigeminal naevi, JAMA 47:178, 1906
30. Danis, P: Aspects ophthalmologiques des angiomatoses du systeme nerveux, Acta Neurol Psychiatr Belg 50:615, 1950
31. Davis, FA: Plexiform neurofibromatosis of orbit and globe with associated glioma of the optic nerve and brain: report of a case, Arch Ophthalmol 22:761, 1939
32. de Haas, HL: Glaukom beim Naevus flammeus, Ned Tijdschr Geneeskd 2:4326, 1928
33. Dejean, C, Hervouet, F, and Leplat, G: L'embryologie de l'oeil et sa tératologie, Paris, 1958, Masson Editeur
34. Dev, S, Jain, IS, and Nayo, K: Naevus of Ota associated with glaucoma, Orient Arch Ophthalmol 7:251, 1969
35. Dimitri, V: Tumeur cérébrale congénitale (angiome caverneux), Rev Assoc Med Argent 6:63, 1923
36. Djacos, C, and Joannidés, T: La Maladie de Sturge-Weber-Krabbe, Ann Ocul 184:994, 1951
37. Duhamel, E, and Goetz, G: A propos de l'angiomatose encéphalotrigeminée, Bull Soc Ophthalmol Fr 6:541, 1954
38. Duke-Elder, S: System of ophthalmology: diseases of the uveal tract, vol 9, St Louis, 1966, The CV Mosby Co
39. Duke-Elder, S: System of ophthalmology: diseases of the lens and vitreous; glaucoma, and hypotony, vol 11, St. Louis, 1969, The CV Mosby Co
40. Dunphy, EB: Glaucoma accompanying nevus flammeus, Am J Ophthalmol 18:709, 1935
41. Dutton, JJ, et al: Orbital malignant melanoma and oculodermal melanocytosis: report of two cases and

review of the literature, Ophthalmol 91:497, 1984

42. Ehrlich, LM: Bilateral glaucoma associated with unilateral neus flammeus, Arch Ophthalmol 25:1002, 1941

43. Elschnig, A: Naevus vasculosis mit gleichseitigem Hydrophthalmus, Z Augenheilkd 39:189, 1918

44. Fabricant, RN, Todaro, GJ, and Eldridge, R: Increased levels of a nerve-growth-factor cross-reacting protein in "central" neurofibromatosis, Lancet 1:4, 1979

45. Faivre, G, Pernot, C, Gilgenkrantz, JM, and Cherrier, F: Les shunts arterioveneux des émembres: à propos d'une observation, Soc Med Nancy, May 11, 1960

46. Falk, W: Beitrag zur Aetiologie and Klinik der Sturge Weberschen Krankheit, Osten Z Kinderheilkd 5:175, 1950

47. Fishman, FRA, and Anderson, R: Nevus of Ota, Am J Ophthalmol 54:453, 1962

48. Font, RL, and Ferry, AP: The phakomatoses, Int Ophthalmol Clin 12:1, 1972

49. Font, RL, Reynolds, AN, and Zimmerman, LE: Diffuse malignant melanoma of the iris in the nevus of Ota, Arch Ophthalmol 77:513, 1967

50. Foulks, GN, and Shields, MB: Glaucoma in oculodermal melanocytosis, Ann Ophthalmol 9:1299, 1977

51. François, J: Ocular aspects of the phakomatoses. In Vinken, PJ, and Bruyn, GW, editors: Handbook of clinical neurology: the phakomatoses, vol 14, Amsterdam, 1972, North Holland Publishing Co

52. François, J, and Katz, C: Association homolatérale d'hydrophalmie de névrome plexiforme de la paupiére supérieure et d'hemihypertrophie faciale dans la maladie de Recklinghausen, Ophthalmologica 142:549, 1961

53. François, P, Madelain F, and Fallas, MC: Difficulties in the treatment of Von Hippel's retinal lesions, Bull Soc Ophthalmol Fr 80:1115, 1980

54. Freeman, D: Neurofibromata of the choroid, Arch Ophthalmol 11:641, 1934

55. Freese, L: Hydrophthalmus bein Erwachsenen, Verchardl Berl Augenarztl Ges Nov 25, 1910

56. Freidenwald, JS: Ophthalmic pathology atlas and textbook, Philadelphia, 1952, WB Saunders Co

57. Friedman, MW, and Ritchey, CL: Unilateral congenital glaucoma, neurofibromatosis and pseudoarthrosis, Arch Ophthalmol 70:294, 1963

58. Gartner, S: Malignant melanoma of the choroid in von Recklinghausen's disease, Am J Ophthalmol 23:73, 1940

59. Gass, JDM: The phakomatoses. In Smith, JL, editor: Neuroophthalmology, vol 2, St Louis, 1965, The CV Mosby Co

60. Ginzburg, J: Glaukom und Feuermal mit Akromegalie, Klin Monatsbl Augenheilkd 76:393, 1926

61. Gonder, JR, Shields, JA, and Albert DM: Malignant melanoma of the choroid associated with oculodermal melanocytosis, Ophthalmology 88:372, 1981

62. Gonder, JR, Nichol, J, Augsburger, JJ, and Shields, JA: Ocular and oculodermal melanocytosis, Can J Ophthalmol 20:176, 1985

63. Gorlin, RJ, Vickers, RA, Kellen, E, and Williamson, JJ: The multiple basal-cell nevi syndrome, Cancer 18:89, 1965

64. Grant, WM, and Walton, DS: Distinctive gonioscopic findings in glaucoma due to neurofibromatosis, Arch Ophthalmol 79:127, 1968

65. Gutman, I, et al: Hypopigmented iris spot: an early sign of tuberous sclerosis, Ophthalmology 89:1155, 1982

66. Haik, BG, Clancy, P, Ellsworth, RM, Perina, A, and Zimmerman, K: Ocular manifestations in diffuse neonatal hemangiomatosis, J Ped Ophthalmol Strabismus 20:101, 1983

67. Heinhold, P, and Nover, A: Augenveränderungen beim Klippel-Trenaunay-Weber Syndrom, Fortschr Med 89:91, 1971

68. Hermans, EH, Grosfeld, JCM, and Valk, LEM: Naevus epitheliomatides multiplex, een vijfde Facomatose, Ned Tijdschr Geneeskd 103:1795, 1959

69. Hogan, M, and Zimmerman, L: Ophthalmic pathology, an atlas and textbook, Philadelphia, 1962, WB Saunders Co

70. Hoyt, CM, and Billson, F: Buphthalmos in neurofibromatosis: is it an expression of regional giantism? J Pediatr Ophthalmol 14:228, 1977

71. Hudelo, A: Glaucome et naevus facial, Ann Ocul 166:889, 1929

72. Joy, HH: Nevus flammeus associated with glaucoma, Trans Am Ophthalmol Soc 47:93, 1949

73. Kahn, LB, and Gordon, W: Basal cell naevus syndrome, S Afr Med J 41:832, 1967

74. Kalischer, S: Demonstration des Gehirns eines Kindes mit Telangiectasie der linksseitigen Gesichtskopfhaut und Hirnoberflache, Berl Klin Wochenschr 34:1059, 1897

75. Kandarkis, A, et al: The effect of nitrates on intraocular pressure in Sturge-Weber syndrome, Glaucoma 7:120, 1985

76. Kiewe, P, and Maneff, I: Congenital bilateral melanosis occurring in the eye and face: a contribution to the problem of consanguinity, Ann d'Ocul 172:723, 1934

77. King, G, and Schwartz, GA: Sturge-Weber syndrome, Arch Int Med 94:743, 1954

78. Kissel, P, and Dureux, JB: Limites nosoligiques et conception générale des phakomatoses. In Michaux, L, and Feld, M, editors: Les phakomatoses cérébrales, Paris, 1963, SPEI

79. Klippel, M, and Trenaunay, P: Du naevus variqueux ostéohypertrophique, Arch Gén Méd 77:641, 1900

80. Knight, MS: A critical survey of neoplasms of the choroid, Am J Ophthalmol 8:791, 1925

81. Kwitko, ML: Glaucoma in infants and children, New York, 1973, Appleton-Century-Crofts

82. Lawford, JB: Naevus of left side of face: naevus of choroid, subretinal hemorrhage and detached retina in left eye, Trans Ophthalmol Soc UK 5:136, 1885

83. Lieb, WA, Wirth, WA, and Geeraets, WJ: Hydrophthalmos and neurofibromatosis, Confin Neurol 19:230, 1958

84. Lindau, A: Studien uber Kleinhirncysten, Acta Pathol Microbiol Scand 1(suppl):1, 1926

85. Makley, TA, and King, CM: Malignant melanoma in melanosis oculi, Trans Am Acad Ophthalmol Otolaryngol 71:38, 1967

86. Mann, I: Developmental abnormalities of the eye, London, 1957, British Medical Association

87. Mansheim, BJ: Aqueous outflow measurements by continuous tonometry in some unusual forms of glaucoma, Arch Ophthalmol 50:580, 1953

88. Markovits, AS, and Quickert, MH: Basal cell nevus, Arch Ophthalmol 88:397, 1972

89. Martyn, I, and Knox, DL: Glial hamartoma of the retina in generalized neurofibromatosis, Br J Ophthalmol 56: 487, 1972

90. Meeker, LH: Two tumors of the eye, Arch Ophthalmol 16:152, 1936

91. Mehney, GH: Naevus flammeus associated with glaucoma, Arch Ophthalmol 17:1018, 1937

92. Miani, P, and Brusini, P: Krupin-Denver filtering valve implant for glaucoma in Sturge-Weber syndrome, Glaucoma, 6:194, 1984

93. Michelson-Rabinowitsch, C: Beitrag zur Kenntnis des Hydrophthalmus congenitus, Arch Augenheilkd 55:245, 1906

94. Miller, RM, and Sparkes, RS: Segmental neurofibromatosis, Arch Dermatol 113:837, 1977

95. Miller, SJH: Symposium: the Sturge-Weber syndrome, Proc R Soc Med 56:419, 1963

96. Moore, RF: Diffuse neurofibromatosis with proptosis, Br J Ophthalmol 15: 272, 1931

97. Murakami, S: Zur pathologischen Anatomie und Pathogenes des Buphthalmus bei Neurofibromatosis, Klin Monatsbl Augenheilkd 51:514, 1913

98. Naidoff, MA, Kenyon, KR, and Green, WR: Iris hemangioma and abnormal retinal vasculature in a case of diffuse congenital hemangiomatosis, Am J Ophthalmol 72:633, 1971

99. Nakamura, B: Angeborener halbseitiger Naevus flammeus mit Hydrophthalmus und Knochenverdickung derselben Seite, Klin Monatsbl Augenheilkd 69:312, 1922

100. Nicholson, DH, Green, WR, and Kenyon, KR: Light and electron microscopic study of early lesions in angiomatosis retinae, Am J Ophthalmol 82:193, 1976

101. Nicolai, C: Un névrome plexiforme, Arch Ophthalmol (Paris) 29:59, 1909

102. O'Connor, PS, and Smith, JD: Optic nerve variant in the Klippel-Trenaunay-Weber syndrome, Ann Ophthalmol 10:131, 1978

103. Panas, F, and Remy, DA: Anatomie pathologique de l'oiel, Paris, 1879, Delahaye & Cie

104. Paton, L, and Collins, ET: Angioma of the choroid, Trans Ophthalmol Soc UK 39:157, 1919

105. Perry, HD, and Font, RL: Iris nodules in Von Recklinghausen's neurofibromatosis—electron microscopic confirmation of their melanocytic origin, Arch Ophthalmol 100:1635, 1982

106. Peyman, GA, Redman, KR, Mottow-Lippa, L, and Flood, T: Treatment of large von Hippel tumors by eye wall resection, Ophthalmology 90:840, 1983

107. Phelps, CD: The pathogenesis of glaucoma in Sturge-Weber syndrome, Ophthalmology 85:276, 1978

108. Pietruschka, G: Zur Symptomatic der Syndrome nach Sturge-Weber und Klippel-Trenaunay, Klin Monatsbl Augenheilkd 137:545, 1960

109. Politi, F, Sachs, R, and Barishak, R: Neurofibromatosis and congenital glaucoma, Ophthalmologica 176:155, 1978

110. Reinke, RT, Haber, K, and Josselson, A: Ota nevus, multiple hemangioma and Takayasu arteritis, Arch Dermatol 110:447, 1974

111. Renard, G: Aspects pathologiques du fond d'oeil dans les affections de la retine, Paris, 1946, Masson, Editeur

112. Riccardi, FM: Von Recklinghausen neurofibromatosis, N Engl J Med 305:1617, 1981

113. Ritch, R, Forbes, M, Hetherington, J Jr, Harrison, R, and Podos, SM: Congenital ectropion uveae with glaucoma, Ophthalmol 91:326, 1984

114. Robertson, DM: Ophthalmic findings. In Gomez, M, editor: Tuberous sclerosis, New York, 1979, Raven Press

115. Robin, AL, and Pollack, IP: Argon laser trabeculoplasty in the secondary glaucomas. In Henkind P, Shimuzu K, Blodi FC, Polack FM, and Veronneau-Troutman S, editors: ACTA: XXIV, International Congress of Ophthalmology, vol 1, Philadelphia, 1983, JB Lippincott Co

116. Ross, AH, et al: The nerve gowth factor receptor in normal and transformed neural crest cells. In Rubenstein, AE, Burge, RP, and Housman, DE, editors: Neurofibromatosis, vol 486, New York, 1986, Ann New York Acad Sci

117. Rotth, A: Muttermal und Glaukom (abstract), Zentralbl Gesamte Ophthalmol 20:588, 1929

118. Rubenstein, AE: Neurofibromatosis: a review of the clinical problem. In Rubenstein, AE, Bunge, RP, and Housman, DE, editors: Neurofibromatosis, Ann NY Acad Sci 486:1, 1986

119. Sachsalber, A: Uber das Rankenneurom der Orbita mit sekundaren Buphthalmus, Beitr Z Prakt Augenheilkd 27:1, 1978

120. Safar, K: Histologischer Beitrag zur Frage des ursächlichen Zusammenhangenzwischen Hydrophthalmos congenitus und Naevus Flammeus, Z Augenheilkd 51:301, 1897

121. Salazar, F, and Lamiell, JM: Early identification of retinal angiomas in a large kindred of von Hippel Lindau disease, Am J Ophthalmol 89:540, 1980

122. Salus, R: Glaukom und Feuermal, Klin Monatsbl Augenheilkd 71:305, 1923

123. Schiess-Gemuseus: Vier Fälle angeborener Anomalie des Auges, v Graefe's Arch Klin Exp Ophthalmol 30:191, 1884

124. Schirmer, R: Ein Fall von Teleangiektasie, v Graefe's Arch Klin Exp Ophthalmol 7:119, 1860

125. Schwartz, PL, Beards, JA, and Maris, PJ: Tuberous sclerosis associated with a retinal angioma, Am J Ophthalmol 90:485, 1980

126. Sedlacek, J, and Vrabec, F: Angioma of the choroid and Sturge-Weber-Krabbe's syndrome, Cesk Oftal 17:232, 1961

127. Shaffer, RN, and Weiss, DI: Congenital and pediatric glaucomas, St Louis, 1970, The CV Mosby Co

128. Shihab, ZM, and Kristan, RW: Recurrent intraoperative choroidal effusion in Sturge-Weber syndrome, J Pediatr Ophthalmol Strabismus 20:250, 1983

129. Siggers, DC, Boyer, SH, and Eldridge, R: Nerve growth factor in disseminated neurofibromatosis, N Engl J Med 292:1134, 1978

130. Snell, S, and Collins, ET: Plexiform neuroma of temporal region, orbit, eyelid and eyeball, Trans Ophthalmol Soc UK 23:157, 1903

131. Stoermer, J: Krankheitsbild und Ätiologie der Sturge-Weberschen Erkrankung, Medizinische 6:221, 1956

132. Stoll, KL: Nevus flammeus and glaucoma, Trans Am Acad Ophthalmol Otolaryngol 41:534, 1936

133. Sturge, WA: A case of partial epilepsy due to a lesion of one of the vasomotor centers of the brain, Trans Clin Soc London 12:162, 1879

134. Susac, JO, Smith, JL, and Scelfo, RJ: The "tomato-catsup" fundus in Sturge-Weber syndrome, Arch Ophthalmol 92:69, 1974

135. Sutherland, GA, and Mayou, MS: Neurofibromatosis of the fifth nerve with buphthalmus, Trans Ophthalmol Soc UK 27:79, 1907

136. Theodossiadis, G, Damanakis, A, and Koutsandrea, C: Aderhauteffusion Während einer antiglaukomatosen Operation bei einem Kind mit Sturge-Weber Syndrom, Klin Mbl Augenheilkd 186:300, 1985

137. Treese, MT, Pettit, TH, Foos, RY, Hofbauer, J: Familial nevus of Ota, Ann Ophthalmol 7:855, 1981

138. Tyson, HH: Nevus flammeus of the face and the globe, Arch Ophthalmol 8:365, 1932

139. Vannas, M: Naevus flammeus pa hogra armen och handen och glaucoma pa hogra ogat, Finska Lak-Sallsk Handl 76:399, 1934

140. Velazques, N, and Jones, IS: Ocular and oculodermal melanocytosis associated with uveal melanomas, Ophthalmol 90:1472, 1983

141. Verhoeff, FH: Discussion of paper by Snell and Collins, Trans Ophthalmol Soc UK 23:176, 1903

142. Von Baerensprung: Naevus unius lateris, Ann Charite-Krankenh Berlin 11:91, 1863

143. von Hippel, E: Über eine sehr seltene Erkrankung der Netzhaut, v Graefe's Arch Klin Exp Ophthalmol 59:83, 1904

144. von Recklinghausen, F: Über die multiplen Fibrome der Haut und ihre Beziehung zu den multiplen Neuromen, Berlin, 1882, Hirschwald

145. Waardenburg, PJ, Franceschetti, A, and Klein, D: Genetics and ophthalmology, vol 2, Springfield, Ill, 1973, Charles C Thomas, Publishers

146. Walsh, FB, and Hoyt, WF: Clinical neuroophthalmology, vol 3, ed 3, Baltimore, 1969, The Williams & Wilkins Co

147. Walton, DS: Hemangioma of the lid with glaucoma. In Chandler, PA, and Grant, WM, editors: Glaucoma, Philadelphia, 1979, Lea & Febiger

148. Watzke, RC, Weingeist, TA, and Constantine, JB: Diagnosis and management of von Hippel-Lindau disease. In Peyman, GA, Apple, DJ, and Sanders, DR, editors: Intraocular tumors, New York 1977, Appleton-Century-Crofts

149. Weber, FP: Angioma-formation in connection with hypertrophy of limbs and hemihypertrophy, Br J Dermatol 190:231, 1907

150. Weber, FP: On the association of extensive hemangiomatosis nevus of the skin with cerebral (meningeal) hemangioma, Proc R Soc Med 22:431, 1928

151. Weekers, R, et al.: Le diagnostic précoce du glaucome débutant, Bull Soc Belge Ophthalmol 121:1, 1959

152. Weinstein, A: Ein Fall von Buphthalmus mit kongenitaler Hypertrophie des Oberlides, Klin Monatsbl Augenheilkd 47:577, 1909

153. Weiss, DI: Dual origin of glaucoma in encephalotrigeminal angiomatosis, Trans Ophthalmol Soc UK 93:477, 1973

154. Weiss, DI, and Krohn, DL: Benign melanocytic glaucoma complicating oculodermal menlanocytosis, Ann Ophthalmol 3:958, 1971

155. Weiss, JS, and Albert, DM: Ocular melanoma. In DeVita, JE, Hellman, S, and Rosenberg, SA, editors: Cancer: principles and practice of oncology, ed 2, vol 2, Philadelphia, 1985, JB Lippincott Co

156. Weiss, MJ, and Ernest, JT: Diffuse congenital hemangiomatosis with infantile glaucoma, Am J Ophthalmol 81:216, 1976

157. Wheeler, JM: Plexiform neurofibromatosis involving the choroid, ciliary body and other structures, Am J Ophthalmol 20:368, 1937

158. Wiener, A: A case of neurofibromatosis with buphthalmus, Arch Ophthalmol 54:481, 1925

159. Witmer, R: Die retinalen Angiomatosen, Klin Mbl Augenheilkd 187:434, 1985

160. Wiznia, RA, Freedman, JK, Mancini, AD, Shields, JA: Malignant melanoma of the choroid in neurofibromatosis, Am J Ophthalmol 86:684, 1978

161. Wolter, JR: Nerve fibrils in ovoid bodies, Arch Ophthalmol 73:696, 1965

162. Wolter, JR, and Butler, R: Pigment spots of the iris and ectropion uveae with glaucoma in neurofibromatosis, Am J Ophthalmol 56:964, 1963

163. Wolter, JR, Gonzales-Sirit, R, and Mankin, WJ: Neurofibromatosis of the choroid, Am J Ophthalmol 54:217, 1962

164. Wolter, JR, and Mertus, JM: Exophytic retinal astrocytoma in tuberous sclerosis, J Pediatr Ophthalmol 6:186, 1969

165. Yamanaka, R: Naevus Flammeus mit gleichseitigem Glaukom, Klin Monatsbl Augenheilkd 78:372, 1927

166. Yanoff, M, and Zimmerman, L: Histogenesis of malignant melanoma of the uvea, Arch Ophthalmol 77:331, 1967

167. Yumita, A, Shirato, S, Yamamato, T, and Kitazawa, Y: Goniotomy with Q-switched Nd:YAG laser in juvenile developmental glaucoma: a preliminary report, Jpn J Ophthalmol 2:349, 1984

168. Zaun, W: Ueber die Beziehungen zwischen Naevus flammeus and angeborenem Glaukom, Klin Mbl Augenheilkd 72:57, 1924.

169. Zelkowitz, M: Neurofibromatosis fibroblasts: abnormal growth and binding to epidermal growth factor. In Riccardi, VM, and Mulvihill, JJ, editors: neurofibromatosis (von Recklinghausen disease) vol 29, New York, 1981, Raven Press

170. Zelkowitz, M, and Stambouly, J: Diminished epidermal growth factor binding by neurofibromatosis fibroblasts, Ann Neurol 8:296, 1980

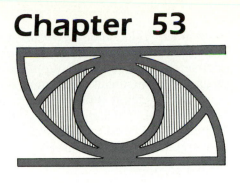

Chapter 53

Glaucoma Associated with Congenital Disorders

Louis B. Cantor

Nearly half of all known syndromes, malformations, or anatomic variants that either have a mendelian mode of transmission, or are caused by teratogenic agents, spontaneous mutation, or chromosomal anomaly may affect the eye, ocular adnexa, or orbit. In some of these syndromes, the ocular abnormalities are distinctive and the ophthalmologist may play an important role in diagnosis.

A chromosomal disorder is present in one of every 200 newborn infants. These disorders result from either duplication or absence of entire chromosomes or chromosomal segments, resulting in multiple defects. Although many of the congenital disorders to be discussed have known chromosomal abnormalities, most are of unknown etiology. The recent developments in recombinant DNA technology and chromosome banding techniques should define chromosomal abnormalities for many congenital disorders of unknown etiology.

The disorders discussed in this chapter include glaucoma as one of their many features. The glaucoma may resemble primary congenital glaucoma, juvenile or adult onset open-angle glaucoma, primary angle-closure glaucoma, or it may be secondary to other ocular anomalies with either an open or closed angle. Understanding the underlying cause of the glaucoma is important in any treatment considerations.

GLAUCOMA ASSOCIATED WITH SYSTEMIC CONGENITAL SYNDROMES, WITH KNOWN CHROMOSOMAL ABNORMALITIES

Trisomy 13 Syndrome

Trisomy 13 syndrome, also known as trisomy D syndrome, Patau's syndrome, and 13-15 trisomy syndrome, is a rare congenital disorder that results when an extra chromosome is present in the D group (chromosomes 13-15). Multiple systemic and ocular abnormalities are associated with this disorder. Though trisomy 13 syndrome is usually fatal in the first few months of life, milder forms have been reported. Systemic findings include apneic spells, developmental deficiency of the nervous system, seizures, deafness, cleft lip and palate, malformed ears, sloping forehead, capillary hemangiomata, cryptorchidism, hyperconvex fingernails, horizontal palmar creases, holoprosencephaly, truncus arteriosus, polydactyly, rocker bottom feet, renal abnormalities, pancreatic abnormalities, and intestinal malformations.*

Ocular abnormalities vary from severe involvement in the majority of cases to relatively minor anomalies. The most common are microphthalmia; retinal dysplasia; colobomata of the iris, ciliary body, and choroid; and cataracts. Other ocular findings may include anophthalmia, optic nerve

---

*References 7, 11, 106, 194, 210, 211, 229, 257, 274, 282-284, 303, 304, 307, 310, 328, 332, 341.

colobomas, iridogoniodysgenesis, persistent hyperplasia primary vitreous, optic atrophy, hypotelorism, epicanthal folds, cyclopia, and intraocular cartilage.* Congenital glaucoma resulting from poor differentiation of the angle structures has also been reported.[153,188] Standard surgical treatment for congenital glaucoma may be undertaken if the patient's general condition allows.

Ullrich's Syndrome

Ullrich's syndrome, also called Ullrich-Feichtiger syndrome or dyscraniopylophalangy, belongs to the 13-15 trisomy group, but is considered separately by some authors. Systemic findings include a hypoplastic mandible, ear malformations, congenital heart disease, spina bifida, polydactyly, genital anomalies, and a broad nose. Ocular findings may include microphthalmos, hypertelorism, narrow lid fissures, uveal colobomata, strabismus, aniridia, cloudy corneas, corneal ulcers, and glaucoma.[95,318,334] The ocular findings have not been well described histopathologically; however, the glaucoma may result from abnormal differentiation of the angle structures as noted in trisomy 13-15, or may be related to microphthalmos.[153]

Partial Deletion Syndromes of Chromosome 18

Short arm deletion (Wolf's syndrome)

A deletion of the short arm of chromosome 18 (18p−) may result in mild to moderate mental retardation, short stature, a long nasal root, ear abnormalities, and webbing of the neck, similar to that seen in Turner's and Noonan's syndromes. Ocular abnormalities include iris and/or retinal colobomas, hypertelorism, epicanthus, strabismus, ptosis, and microphthalmos. Rarely, keratoconus, corneal opacities, and cataracts have been reported. Glaucoma has not been reported as a finding in this syndrome.†

Long arm deletion (deGrouchy's syndrome)

Deletion of the long arm of chromosome 18 (18q−) presents a much more distinctive picture than deletion of the short arm. The facial characteristics consist of deep set eyes, midfacial hypoplasia, down-turned corners of the mouth, and abnormal ear canals. Microcephaly, mental retardation, and short stature are also commonly present.[178,179,184,217] Common ocular abnormalities are microcornea, nystagmus, colobomata, optic

atrophy, and congenital glaucoma. The glaucoma is associated with immaturity of the anterior chamber angle.[184,347]

Ring chromosome 18 syndrome

The ocular and systemic manifestations of Ring chromosome 18 resemble those seen in the 18q− syndrome.[60,217,347]

Trisomy 18 Syndrome (Trisomy E-syndrome, Edward's Syndrome)

Trisomy 18 syndrome includes Trisomy E-syndrome and Edward's syndrome and is secondary only to trisomy 21 as the most frequent chromosomal trisomy. It is associated with advanced maternal age, and the majority of affected patients die within the first few months of life.[34,121] This syndrome appears mostly in females. Systemic findings may include low-set ears, high-arched hard palate, ventricular septal defects, cryptorchidism, micrognathia, microstomia, hypertonia, short sternum, rocker-bottom feet, a small pelvis, and various abnormalities of the central nervous system.*

Ocular anomalies may include ptosis, narrow palpebral fissures, blepharophimosis, hypertelorism, hypotelorism, corneal opacities, lenticular opacities, uveal colobomas, blue sclerae, microphthalmos, myopia, abnormal retinal pigmentation, shallow orbits, abnormalities of the eyelashes and eyebrows, nystagmus, and strabismus.† Congenital glaucoma related to immaturity of the anterior chamber angle with anomalies of the iris and ciliary body or related to sclerocornea with anterior chamber dysgenesis has also been described.[36,100,132,162,312]

Trisomy 21

Trisomy 21 is also known as Down's syndrome, trisomy G syndrome, mongolism, and mongoloid idiocy. First described by John Down in 1866,[71] Down's syndrome is the most frequent of the autosomal trisomy syndromes, with an incidence of approximately 1 in 800 births.[308] As with most trisomies, the incidence increases with advanced maternal age, with an incidence of approximately 1 in 30 births when maternal age is over 45 years. The majority of trisomy 21 patients demonstrate a nondisjunction of chromosome 21, with translocation accounting for the majority of other cases.

Multiple systemic manifestations have been re-

---

*References 48, 99, 125, 132, 153, 208, 212, 246, 304, 328, 346.
†References 60-63, 177, 180, 181, 184, 217, 342.

*References 75, 82, 96, 105, 112, 129, 163, 187, 204, 226, 228, 254, 255, 283, 285, 292, 311, 317, 322, 323, 336, 351.
†References 34, 96, 100, 121, 129, 134, 208, 216, 255, 285, 292, 336.

ported, which are detailed in numerous references. Most common among these are mental deficiency, short stature, cardiac anomalies, hypotonia, and characteristic facial features.[30,54,332]

External ocular abnormalities are common and include mongoloid slant, epicanthus, strabismus, nystagmus, myopia, decreased interpupillary distance, ectropion, and blepharoconjunctivitis. Common intraocular abnormalities include iris hypoplasia, Brushfield spots, iris colobomas, adherent leukoma, and heterochromia iridis.* As the individual ages, keratoconus and cataracts become common. Acute hydrops resulting from keratoconus is common[56,57,242] (Fig. 53-1). Congenital glaucoma is rarely associated with trisomy 21 but has been reported. One reported patient had a strong family history of Rieger's anomaly, and it was felt that the ocular abnormalities may have been related to this rather than to trisomy 21. Whether or not glaucoma is truly associated with trisomy 21 remains uncertain, and the nature of any possibly associated glaucoma is unknown.[59,132]

Turner's Syndrome

Approximately 1 in 5,000 to 10,000 phenotypically normal females possess only one X chromosome rather than two.[86] Other X chromosome abnormalities, such as mosaicism (XO/XX), or ring X chromosome have been identified. Such abnormalities generally present with a clinical picture very similar to that described by Turner in 1938.[269,315] Turner's syndrome primarily affects females but may occasionally occur in males. Systemic findings in females include ovarian dysgenesis, webbed neck, pterygium coli, short stature, mandibulofacial disproportion, underdeveloped breasts, infantile genitalia, late appearance of pubic and axillary hair, primary amenorrhea, cubitus valgus, congenital deafness, mental retardation, coarctation of the aorta, multiple pigmented nevi, and congenital lymphedema. Diabetes and hypothyroidism have also been frequently associated with Turner's syndrome.[106,315]

Multiple ocular abnormalities have been reported in conjunction with Turner's syndrome. The most common ocular findings are ptosis and strabismus. Other ocular abnormalities may include hyperopia, myopia, cataract, epicanthus, hypertelorism, blue sclera, antimongoloid slant, red/green color blindness, exophthalmos, choroidal colobomas, persistent pupillary membrane, microcornea, microphthalmos, nystagmus, absence of

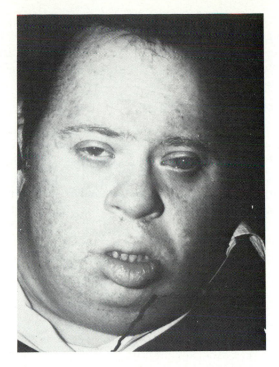

Fig. 53-1 Clinical photograph of patient with trisomy 21 and keratoconus with corneal hydrops.

the caruncle, decreased retinal pigmentation, lid hemangiomata, abducens palsy, retinitis pigmentosa, hypoplasia of the lacrimal gland, oval cornea, Duane's syndrome, retinal detachment, Coats' disease, and primary open-angle glaucoma.* Whether primary open-angle glaucoma is associated with Turner's syndrome or merely a coincidental disorder is unknown.[183] Congenital glaucoma has also been reported in association with Turner's syndrome.[172] Angle-closure glaucoma may occur secondary to other ocular abnormalities associated with Turner's syndrome.[31,156]

Ring Chromosome 6 Syndrome

Ring chromosome 6 is a rare disorder associated with multiple neural crest disorders of the anterior segment of the eye and central nervous system. The phenotypic expression of this syndrome is highly variable.[214,220,230] Reported systemic findings have included short stature, psychomotor retardation, microcephaly, malformed ears and nose, and micrognathia.[40,91,348] The most frequent reported eye abnormality is microphthalmia. Other ocular abnormalities may include strabismus, epicanthal folds, hypertelorism, nystagmus, iris co-

---

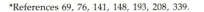

*References 69, 76, 141, 148, 193, 208, 339.

*References 4, 38, 45, 106, 183, 208, 276.

lobomas, aniridia, congenital ectropion uveae, Reiger's anomaly, cataract, megalocornea, and congenital glaucoma.[40,185,212,262,309,348] Other anomalies, such as translocations of chromosome 6, are also associated with congenital glaucoma.[309]

Prader-Willi Syndrome

The Prader-Willi syndrome is characterized by muscular hypotonia, mental retardation, obesity, and hypogonadism. Systemic features also include short stature, small hands and feet, diminished pain sensitivity, and dental anomalies.[142] An interstitial deletion of the proximal long arm of chromosome 15, 15[del(15q) (q11-q13)], has been identified in approximately 50% of patients with this syndrome, with other anomalies of chromosome 15 also being reported.[123,164,173,174]

Common ocular findings are strabismus and oculocutaneous albinoidism. Congenital ectropion uveae, which eventually results in open-angle glaucoma, is also found in this syndrome[249] (see Plate IV, Fig. 4). It is important, therefore, that any patient with congenital ectropion uveae in Prader-Willi syndrome be followed for the development of glaucoma. An abnormality of the iridocorneal angle with variable amounts of iris stromal hypoplasia are frequently seen. Angle abnormalities usually consist of large iris processes, irregular iris insertion into the ciliary body, abnormal pigmented tissue covering the meshwork, or broad peripheral anterior synechiae.

GLAUCOMA ASSOCIATED WITH SYSTEMIC CONGENITAL DISORDERS OF UNKNOWN ETIOLOGY

Atopic Dermatitis

Atopic dermatitis, also known as atopic eczema and Besnier's prurigo, is an eczematous skin disorder that often occurs in childhood but that may also be seen in adolescence and adulthood. There is an inherited abnormal skin reactivity that lowers the cutaneous threshhold to pruritis. Systemically, the cutaneous manifestations of atopic dermatitis are usually symmetrically distributed and are most commonly located in the anticubital and popliteal areas, the sides and back of the neck, shoulders, axilla, thorax, head, and face.[92]

The most commonly described ocular findings are keratoconjunctivitis, cataracts, keratoconus, and atopic dermatitis of the eyelids. The association of a secondary glaucoma with atopic dermatitis is somewhat suspect. It is likely that glaucoma seen in these individuals is secondary in most cases to topical and systemic corticosteroids, which are used to treat the ocular symptoms of the disease.[6,92,126]

Other ocular and periocular manifestations of atopic dermatitis include conjunctival chemosis, filamentary keratitis, giant papillary hypertrophy, hyperemia of the conjunctiva, linear or stellate scarring of the conjunctiva, Trantas' dots, corneal punctate staining with corneal vascularization, cataracts, and retinal detachments.[6,126]

Corticosteroids should not be used liberally for the ocular and skin manifestations, as cataracts, glaucoma, and secondary infections may develop in atopic patients treated excessively with corticosteroids. Cataract surgery in patients with atopic dermatitis has been associated with many complications including hemorrhage, retinal detachment, iridocyclitis, and corneal edema.

Cystinosis

Cystinosis is a rare autosomal recessive congenital disorder of amino acid metabolism. It is characterized by widespread intracellular deposition of cystine crystals in various organs including the kidneys, liver, spleen, lymph nodes, bone marrow, and the eyes. This disorder is characterized by three phenotypic forms: childhood, adolescent, and adult. Childhood (nephropathic) cystinosis is the most common form and is characterized by renal rickets, growth retardation, progressive renal failure, and a short life expectancy. Adult (benign) cystinosis is characterized by mild ocular symptoms from corneal crystals without renal disease. In the adult form, there is no hereditary pattern, and life expectancy is normal. Intermediate between these two forms is an adolescent form of cystinosis, which often has a mild nephropathy with diminished life expectancy. Inheritance of the adolescent cystinosis is thought to be autosomal recessive.[28,49,103,176]

Ocular findings are most notable in patients with childhood cystinosis. Corneal crystals were first described by Burki in 1941, and conjunctival crystals may be demonstrated on microscopy.[33,68] Cystine crystals have been identified in the iris, ciliary body, choroid, retinal pigment epithelium, and in the optic nerve. In addition, a retinal pigmentary disturbance in the peripheral fundus is noted in patients with childhood cystinosis, but not in the adult form.[47,49,88,344,345]

Pupillary block glaucoma has been reported to be associated with childhood cystinosis.[327] Angle closure was felt to be secondary to thickening and stiffening of the iris from cystine crystal deposition within the iris resulting in pupillary block.

Dental-Ocular-Cutaneous Syndrome

This is a rare congenital syndrome, which has been reported in a large kindred. Systemic abnormalities include defects of the upper lip, syndactyly, cutaneous hyperpigmentation overlying the interphalangeal joints, and abnormal teeth and eyelids. Juvenile onset glaucoma was present in the proband and in two other siblings in the pedigree. Description of the angle appearance was not provided.[3]

Familial Histiocytic Dermatoarthritis

Familial histiocytic dermatoarthritis is a rare autosomal dominant disorder that becomes manifest in childhood and adolescence. It is characterized by a papulonodular eruption, destructive arthritis, and ocular abnormalities.[263,350] There are multiple histiocytic cutaneous nodules, thickened skin, and a severe arthritis, mainly of the hands and wrists, but which may also be seen in other joints.

These patients suffer from cataracts, bilateral uveitis, and glaucoma. Angle abnormalities have been mentioned, but it is unclear whether the glaucoma is primary or secondary to the uveitis.

The familial incidence, nature of the arthritis, type of cutaneous lesions, and the ocular lesions serve to differentiate this syndrome from multicentric reticulohistiocytosis.

Fetal Alcohol Syndrome

It is well recognized that heavy alcohol consumption by pregnant women may have many severe and adverse toxic effects on their offspring. Facial abnormalities, mental retardation, abnormalities of the cardiovascular and skeletal systems, and small weight and height are commonly reported clinical findings. Ophthalmic manifestations are also reported, but less commonly. The more common ophthalmic findings are small palpebral fissures, epicanthus, ptosis, strabismus, microphthalmia, and myopia. Eight patients have been reported with anterior segment anomalies resembling those of the Axenfeld-Rieger syndrome and Peters' anomaly. In this series, two of the patients with Peters' anomaly had glaucoma, and the patient with Axenfeld anomaly also had glaucoma in one eye. Little information was given on the angle appearance of these eyes, and the exact mechanism of the glaucoma is not clear.[213]

Hallermann-Streiff Syndrome

Hallermann-Streiff syndrome is also known as dyscephalic mandibulooculofacial syndrome and François' dyscephalic syndrome and involves mainly the face, eyes, and skin. Abnormal development of the first and second branchial arches is responsible for the characteristic "birdlike" facies resulting from marked hypoplasia of the mandible and a narrow nose. Brachycephaly is also common. Teeth may be erupted at birth, and there may be diminished hair growth, hyperextensibility of joints, atrophic appearing skin, and dwarfism.*

Ocular manifestations are a significant part of this syndrome, with microphthalmos being especially common. Other common eye abnormalities include congenital cataracts, proptosis, nystagmus, strabismus, optic atrophy, and colobomas. Also, microcornea, iris atrophy, persistent pupillary membrane, and uveitis may be present. Microkeratoglobus has also been described.[137,256]

Cataracts are common, and a high incidence of complications as a result of (or during) cataract extraction has been reported. Secondary glaucoma, which may be very difficult to treat, may result from the cataract surgery.

There is histologic evidence to suggest that diffuse connective tissue and/or elastin disorders occur in patients with this syndrome, which may be due to a primary abnormality of glycosaminoglycan metabolism. Multiple mechanisms may account for glaucoma in a patient with Hallermann-Streiff syndrome. Abnormal accumulation of glycosaminoglycans in the trabecular meshwork may contribute to glaucoma in some patients. Abnormalities of the anterior chamber angle are also present in many cases and are apparently common, suggesting dysgenesis. Inflammatory glaucoma has been reported in several cases, possibly related to lens anomalies and a hypersensitivity to cataractous lens material. Aniridia with glaucoma has also been described.[264] Treatment must be individualized based on clinical findings with special attention given to the lens, anterior chamber angle, and any evidence of inflammation.[8,131]

Hereditary Angioedema

Hereditary angioedema is the most common congenital disorder of the complement system. It is characterized by recurrent episodes of nonpitting, nonerythematous, nonpainful, and nonpruritic edema of subcutaneous or submucosal tissues and must be differentiated from urticaria. The face and extremities are most frequently involved, but other areas of the body may also be affected, especially the gastrointestinal tract. Involvement of the gastrointestinal tract frequently leads to nausea

---

*References 80, 87, 89, 90, 118, 239, 291, 297.

and vomiting. Occasionally, the upper airway may be compromised. This disorder is inherited as an autosomal dominant trait and is characterized by a deficiency of C_1-esterase inhibitor.[12,22,24,306,316]

The relationship of hereditary angioedema and glaucoma is tenuous. Fourteen patients reviewed by Theil for drug side effects from treatment of this disorder had normal intraocular pressure. Acute glaucoma may occur in isolated cases of hereditary angioedema, but little ocular information was given for these cases and the exact nature of the ocular condition is not known.[324]

Krause's Syndrome

Krause's syndrome or congenital encephalo-ophthalmic dysplasia probably results from a chromosomal anomaly, though the exact defect is not known. There is congenital cerebral dysplasia, mental retardation, and occasionally hydrocephalus or microcephaly.

Multiple ocular defects have been described including microphthalmos, enophthalmos, ptosis, strabismus, iris atrophy, anterior and posterior synechiae, and scleral atrophy. In addition, hyaloid artery remnants may be seen, as well as intraocular hemorrhages and exudates. Cyclitic membranes, retinal detachment, cataracts, retinal hypoplasia, and retinal hyperplasia have been described pathologically. Glaucoma may result from a number of causes, including a shallow or flat anterior chamber, peripheral anterior synechiae, neovascularization, posterior synechiae, and immaturity of the anterior chamber angle. Treatment of the glaucoma, therefore, must be individualized depending on the etiology of the glaucoma and the general status of the patient.[11,114,165]

Lowe's Syndrome

The oculocerebral-renal syndrome of Lowe is characterized by renal, ocular, and musculoskeletal abnormalities and mental, psychomotor, and growth retardation.[1,83,120,147,191] This disorder occurs predominantly in male infants, though there have been isolated reports in females.[195,300] A sex-linked recessive mode of inheritance has been suggested, and progressive lenticular opacities have been noted in female carriers.[46,208,314] It has been postulated that this syndrome results from an essential enzyme abnormality, which results in the multiple ocular and systemic manifestations, though the specific enzyme defect remains unknown. Recent chromosomal studies have indicated that Lowe's syndrome can be localized to the distal long arm of the X chromosome at Xq24-q26. If this localiza-

tion is confirmed, carrier detection and prenatal diagnosis would be greatly enhanced.[279]

Renal abnormalities usually become apparent during the first year of life and consist primarily of aminoaciduria, albuminuria, glycosuria, oligoammoniuria, and renal tubular acidosis. Musculoskeletal abnormalities commonly include rickets, osteomalacia, hyporeflexia, and decreased muscle tone. Mental, psychomotor, and growth retardation are also common. Bilateral cryptorchidism is also reported.

Ophthalmic findings are often the earliest, most prominent, and consistent clinical features of this syndrome.[340] The most common ocular disorders are cataracts and congenital glaucoma. The congenital cataracts are typically dense nuclear or posterior cortical cataracts and are present in nearly all patients, with glaucoma being noted in at least two thirds of all cases. A consistent finding is the configuration of the lens, which is small in both the equatorial and anterior/posterior dimensions.

Histopathologically, there is an absence of demarcation between the nucleus and cortex, suggesting an early defect in lens embryogenesis. The nuclear bow is also small, and maturation of the lens cells appears retarded. These factors are felt to be responsible for the small size of the lens in these patients. Excrescences are also seen on the anterior and equatorial lens capsule. Clinically, the existence of congenital cataracts in patients affected with Lowe's syndrome before systemic, metabolic, and biochemical abnormalities; and the presence of lens abnormalities in female carriers supports a primary genetic defect in the lens cells (Fig. 53-2).

Congenital glaucoma may be secondary to the microphakia, or it may be secondary to angle abnormalities.[58,147,325] Lowe attributed glaucoma in some of his cases to anomalies of the canal of Schlemm or to posterior synechiae between the iris and lens. Though the precise mechanism for the glaucoma is unknown, it has been postulated that the small lens exerts anterior traction on the structures in the anterior segment by excessive zonular tension. The ciliary processes are drawn anteriorly, and the retina is also drawn anteriorly over the ciliary body. This primary lens abnormality may then prevent the normal differentiation of the anterior chamber angle.[15,147] Treatment of the congenital glaucoma has been generally unrewarding. Because of the poor life expectancy and severe mental retardation, decisions on treatment must be made on an individual basis. Where treatment appears to be indicated, standard goniotomy or filtration surgery may be attempted.

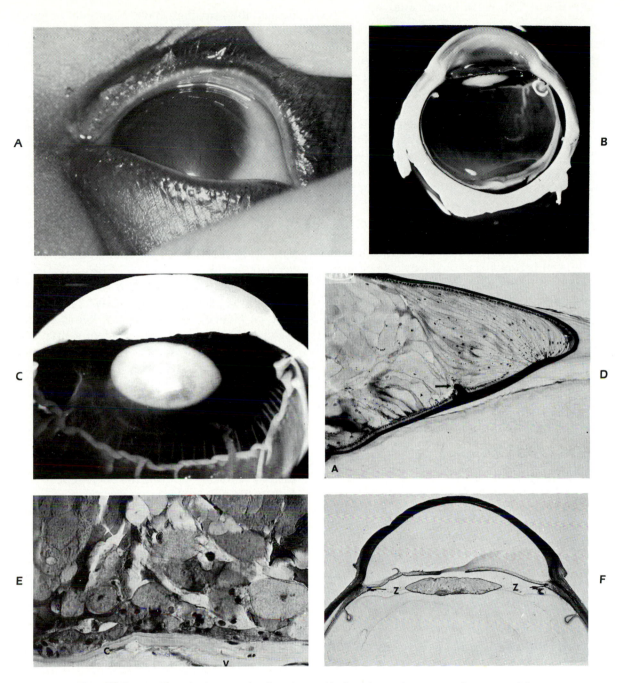

Fig. 53-2 **A,** Clinical photograph of patient with Lowe's syndrome revealing corneal haze.
B, Gross photograph of autopsy specimen taken from 8-month-old boy with Lowe's syndrome.
Cataractous lens is quite small and disc shaped. There is a densely opaque subcapsular lesion with
prominent convexity projecting from posterior pole *(arrows).* Cornea and anterior chamber are larger
than normal because of congenital glaucoma. **C,** Oblique view of posterior surface of same lens.
D, Photomicrograph showing irregular thickening of lens capsule. Wartlike excrescences *(arrow),*
posterior migration of lens epithelium, and disorganization of cortical architecture are evident. **E,**
In region of posterior polar opacity, lens capsule *(c)* is deficient, and proliferated lenticular cells are
observed among fibrils of anterior vitreous *(V).* **F,** Anterior chamber angle is incompletely formed.
Iris is incompletely separated from trabecular meshwork. Ciliary processes appear to be drawn in
toward small lens by taut zonular ligaments *(Z)* and are farther forward than normal. Ora serrata
is also farther forward than normal. (**B** to **F** from Zimmerman, LE, and Font, RL: JAMA 196:684,
1966. Copyright 1966, American Medical Association)

Multiple Basal Cell Nevi Syndrome

Multiple basal cell nevi syndrome or Gorlin-Goltz syndrome is a rare autosomal dominant syndrome involving many organs, but principally affecting the skin, endocrine, skeletal, and nervous systems. The onset of the skin lesions is usually in early childhood or around puberty. Clinically, multiple basal cell nevi are noted, which involve the nose, eyelids, face, neck, trunk, and arms. Multiple jaw cysts and rib abnormalities are frequent. In addition, kyphoscoliosis may be seen. Atypical facies with a mild degree of frontal tempoparietal bossing is usually present.

Multiple eye findings have been described but are not present in all cases. Most commonly, there may be hypertelorism with dystopia canthorum. Strabismus and corneal leukoma may also be seen. Congenital blindness has been reported secondary to a congenital cataract associated with a coloboma of the optic nerve and choroid and glaucoma. The nature of the glaucoma was not clear.[106,108,110,111,281]

Nieden's Syndrome

Nieden's syndrome, or telangiectasia-cataracta syndrome, is a familial syndrome of unknown etiology characterized by multiple small telangiectasia on the face and upper extremities. The skin may become thickened with pigmented changes noted around the neck area. Congenital heart defects have also been noted.[219]

Ocular findings may consist of cataracts, glaucoma, iris abnormalities, and sparse eyebrows. Gonioscopic appearance of the angle has not been described and the type of glaucoma remains unknown. Peterson describes "slightly increased tension" in the eyes of one of his patients. Another patient had glaucoma with tensions as high as 50 mm Hg, which responded poorly to medical treatment at that time.[232]

Oculodentodigital Dysplasia

Oculodentodigital dysplasia, known also as Meyer-Schwickerath and Weyers' syndrome and microphthalmos syndrome, is a rare congenital syndrome, which is probably inherited in an autosomal dominant fashion.[247] Meyer-Schwickerath suggested the term oculodentodigital dysplasia in 1957, though the syndrome was first recognized by Lohmann in 1920.[189,209] This syndrome consists of a characteristic facies with a thin nose and hypoplastic alae, with narrow nostrils, syndactyly and camptodactyly of the fourth and fifth fingers, hypoplastic dental enamel, microphthalmos, and iris abnormalities. The most consistently described ocular abnormalities have been microphthalmos and microcornea.*

Glaucoma has been reported rather prominently in cases of oculodentodigital dysplasia, with varying etiologies. Angle-closure glaucoma has been reported.[150,298] Additionally, angle abnormalities have been described with "patchy mesodermal tissue" and multiple iris processes to Schwalbe's line, suggesting a tendency for congenital or juvenile onset glaucoma.[66,149] Adult onset open-angle glaucoma has also been reported.[72]

Osteogenesis Imperfecta

Though many aspects of osteogenesis imperfecta had previously been described, it was not until 1918 that Van der Hoeve and de Kleyn described the clinical syndrome. The classic triad that characterizes this syndrome consists of brittle bones, blue sclerae, and deafness.[67] Also known as Van der Hoeve's syndrome, Lobstein's syndrome, brittle bone disease, and osteopsathyrosis idiopathica, osteogenesis imperfecta has an incidence of approximately 1 in 50,000 births, with no race or sex predilection. It is usually inherited as an autosomal dominant, although autosomal recessive and sporadic cases have also been reported.[17] The etiology remains undetermined, but there appears to be a diffuse collagen disorder.

Osteogenesis imperfecta is divided into two distinct clinical syndromes, osteogenesis imperfecta congenita, and osteogenesis imperfecta tarda. The congenita form manifests early in life, has more severe symptoms, and often results in early death.[35] The tarda form manifests during childhood and may run a variable course that is usually benign and prolonged. Systemic manifestations may include deafness due to otosclerosis, brittle bones, soft skull, caput medusae, short stature, dental defects, hypotonia, hyperflexibility, and a small facies.[106] Death often occurs as a result of intracranial hemorrhage resulting from the soft calvarium.

Ocular abnormalities are varied. Blue sclerae resulting from decreased thickness and increased translucency of the sclerae allowing uveal coloration to be visible are the most characteristic ocular abnormalities. Shallow orbits (pseudoproptosis), hypertelorism, megalocornea, keratoconus, cataracts, and optic atrophy are also seen. In addition, open-angle glaucoma may occur, usually manifesting in the first or second decade.[35,260] Surgical management of glaucoma, if necessary, should be undertaken with great care because of the abnor-

---

*References 23, 98, 109, 150, 234, 243, 247, 299, 338.

mal sclerae. In addition to the difficulties in performing the actual filtering procedure, the low scleral rigidity may predispose to postoperative scleral collapse, flat chamber, or suprachoroidal hemorrhage.[151]

Pierre Robin Syndrome

Pierre Robin syndrome, known also as Robin's syndrome and micrognathia-glossoptosis syndrome, is characterized by micrognathia, cleft palate, and glossoptosis. Also noted is a particular "birdlike" facies, with or without cleft palate. At birth, these infants frequently have difficulty breathing and nursing.[250,251,270] Common ocular conditions include microphthalmos, proptosis, ptosis, high myopia, and congenital glaucoma. Strabismus, retinal abnormalities, and cataracts may also be seen.[287]

Stickler's syndrome, or hereditary progressive arthroophthalmopathy may be seen in association with Pierre Robin syndrome.[267] In many cases, reports of Pierre Robin syndrome have also included descriptions of ocular findings consistent with Stickler's syndrome.[231] Stickler's syndrome is a rare autosomal dominant connective tissue disorder characterized by ocular, orofacial, and generalized skeletal abnormalities.[19] Associated ocular manifestations are high myopia, cataracts, vitreoretinal degeneration, retinal detachment, and glaucoma.[294]

The mechanism of congenital glaucoma in Pierre Robin syndrome is poorly defined. A translucent membrane over the angle and an anterior iris insertion have been described. Neovascular glaucoma, related to chronic retinal detachment, or open-angle glaucoma may be associated with Stickler's syndrome.[286,349] With improved treatment, and prolonged life expectancy, the early diagnosis of glaucoma or retinal detachment may have profound effects on the life of these children.

Rubinstein-Taybi Syndrome

This disorder is characterized by broad thumbs and toes, highly arched palate, mental and motor retardation, and cardiac abnormalities. An abnormal facies is also present, which is similar to that seen in cri-du-chat syndrome.[259]

Ocular manifestations include antimongoloid slant of the lid fissures, epicanthus, high arched brows, long eyelashes, refractive errors, and strabismus. Cataracts, nystagmus, ptosis, optic atrophy, colobomas of the iris and retina, blepharoptosis, and nasolacrimal duct obstruction are less commonly seen.[258] Juvenile glaucoma associated

with a developmental anomaly of the anterior chamber angle may be associated with this syndrome.[277,335] The iris has been described as inserting high into the trabeculum. Goniotomy and trabeculectomy have both been reported as successful in controlling the glaucoma in these patients.[20,186,203,275] Anesthetic difficulties related to the cardiac anomalies have been reported; therefore, caution is advised when using neuromuscular blocking agents on these patients to minimize the risks of arrhythmia.[295,296]

Senior-Loken Syndrome

Senior-Loken syndrome is also known as familial renal-retinal dystrophy, and is characterized by familial juvenile nephronophthisis and progressive tapetoretinal degeneration. There is impaired urinary concentrating ability with progressive renal failure resulting in polyuria, polydipsia, anemia, and a relatively normal, though dilute urine. It may be distinguished from familial juvenile nephronophthisis in that it is inherited as an autosomal recessive trait, rather than autosomal dominant, and is associated with tapetoretinal degeneration. Consanguinity is often reported.*

Infrequently, the tapetoretinal degeneration may be complicated by an exudative retinopathy, which may lead to neovascular glaucoma, similar to what has been described in other types of tapetoretinal degeneration.[85,170,268] It may be useful to obtain an ERG in homozygotes because this test may be abnormal before the appearance of clinical signs of tapetoretinal degeneration at a time when renal function may also be relatively unremarkable.[64,127]

Weber-Christian Syndrome

Weber-Christian syndrome or Pfeifer-Weber-Christian syndrome occurs primarily in relatively young white females and is characterized by recurrent, nodular, inflammatory panniculitis. The involvement is predominantly located on the trunk, arms, and legs. Clinical features may include arthralgias, myalgias, abdominal pain, anorexia, and hepatosplenomegaly.[44,227,240,333]

Ocular findings are apparently unusual but may include anterior uveitis with secondary glaucoma and also acute exudative retinochoroiditis. Treatment of the inflammatory glaucoma should probably parallel treatment of the cystic disease, including aqueous suppressants for the increased intraocular pressure and corticosteroids. Systemi-

*References 13, 81, 190, 207, 223, 236, 266, 272, 273, 320.

cally, antimalarials and corticosteroids have appeared to be most effective with immunosuppressive therapy used in only those patients who are resistent to both of these medications.

Zellweger Syndrome

The cerebrohepatorenal syndrome of Zellweger is a rare congenital autosomal recessive syndrome characterized by an abnormal facies, cerebral dysgenesis, hepatic dysfunction, and polycystic kidneys. The etiology of this syndrome is unknown; however, a variety of oxidative defects have been identified, associated with abnormalities of mitochondria and peroxisomes. Other clinical findings may include craniofacial anomalies (macrocephaly, large anterior fontanel, hypertelorism, shallow supraorbital ridges, high arched palate, posterior cleft palate, abnormal ear helices), central nervous system anomalies (hypotonia, severe mental retardation, nystagmus, seizures), cardiac defects, and hepatomegaly.[115,154,281]

Ocular findings may include cataracts with a prominent Y suture, corneal clouding, Brushfield's spots, microphthalmia, optic nerve dysplasia and hypoplasia, pigmentary retinopathy, and blindness with an extinguished ERG. Glaucoma may also occur but the pathogenesis is not clear. Iridocorneal adhesions with angle closure were reported histopathologically in one case.[116,289]

GLAUCOMA ASSOCIATED WITH OCULAR CONGENITAL DISORDERS

Congenital Ectropion Uveae

Congenital ectropion uveae is a rare nonprogressive entity in which iris pigment epithelium is present on the anterior surface of the iris stroma. The extent is variable, but normally it does not extend into the angle. The majority of patients with this disorder present with glaucoma in the affected eye. The onset of glaucoma is usually as a late congenital glaucoma or juvenile glaucoma. There are usually associated angle abnormalities with angle dysgenesis and anterior insertion of the iris root.[70,241,249]

Congenital ectropion uveae is frequently associated with neurofibromatosis, though it has also been associated with other abnormalities, including Rieger's syndrome, primary facial hemihypertrophy, the Prader-Willi syndrome, and chromosome 15 abnormalities.[249,343]

Because glaucoma develops in most, if not all of these patients, it is imperative that they be followed closely for the development of elevated intraocular pressure and also to screen for manifestations of neural crest disorders, particularly neurofibromatosis. Treatment of the glaucoma is often difficult. Attempts at medical control are initiated first, but surgery frequently becomes necessary. Because of the relatively young age at which the glaucoma often develops, the prognosis for standard glaucoma surgery is guarded.

Congenital Corneal Staphyloma

Congenital corneal staphyloma is a rare developmental anomaly characterized by an opacified, ectatic cornea. The condition is usually unilateral and the anterior segment of the involved eye is usually markedly abnormal. The ectatic cornea usually protrudes through the palpebral fissure and may be vascularized. Associated ocular abnormalities may include microphthalmos, keratoglobus, cornea plana, and congenital leukoma. A severe glaucoma is frequently reported and is due to an obliterated anterior chamber with iris adherent to the posterior aspect of the cornea. The posterior segment of the eye is usually unremarkable.[175,224,265]

Congenital corneal staphyloma is presumed to be secondary to a failure of normal migration of neural crest cells, possibly placing this disorder in a continuum with Peters' anomaly.[330,337] In selected cases, the corneal staphyloma may be treated by penetrating keratoplasty with salvage of some vision.

Cornea Plana

Cornea plana is a rare congenital disorder, which may be seen in association with sclerocornea or microcornea. Diffuse corneal stromal opacities are common and the anterior chamber may appear shallow because of the flat cornea. The limbus is often poorly defined and the corneal refractive power is diminished, though the refractive error of the eye may vary from hyperopia to myopia, depending on the axial length of the globe. Other associated ocular anomalies may include iris colobomata, congenital cataract, ectopia lentis, retinal and macular aplasia, microphthalmos, amblyopia, sclerocornea, and glaucoma. Both autosomal recessive and autosomal dominant modes of inheritance have been described. It is felt that this disorder results from a developmental arrest of the corneal tissue in the fourth month of gestation when the corneal curvature changes relative to that of the sclera.*

Glaucoma is present in approximately 20% of

---

*References 14, 77, 78, 84, 133, 171, 278, 301.

cases and usually results from progressive angle closure related to the shallow anterior chamber. Mechanical crowding of the angle, and not pupillary block, is probably the predominant mechanism. An iridectomy may be helpful, especially if it is a broad based surgical iridectomy. However, filtration surgery is usually necessary for long-term pressure control.

Iridoschisis

This unusual progressive ocular disorder has its onset in approximately the sixth to seventh decade of life. There is bilateral iris cleavage with shedding of the anterior iris leaf. Anterior synechiae develop which may be in the periphery, or even more centrally where the iris contacts the corneal endothelial surface. Full-thickness holes do not develop, as the disorder is limited to the iris stroma. There is no discernible inheritance pattern and no other noted ocular or systemic abnormalities.[55]

Glaucoma occurs in approximately 50% of cases. The precise etiology is unknown but is probably related to peripheral anterior synechia. Standard medical therapy for glaucoma may be instituted, but the glaucoma may become progressively worse necessitating filtration surgery.

Megalocornea

Megalocornea is a developmental, nonprogressive anomaly of the cornea and anterior segment in which there are no clinical signs of congenital glaucoma.[271,319] In the newborn, the average horizontal corneal diameter is 10 mm, and the average adult horizontal corneal diameter of approximately 11.6 mm is obtained by 2 years of age. According to most authors, a corneal diameter of at least 12 mm in the newborn is necessary to diagnose megalocornea. Megalocornea is most commonly inherited as an X-linked recessive trait, though autosomal dominant and autosomal recessive inheritance patterns have also been reported.[208,253]

Congenital glaucoma and megalocornea have been reported together in many pedigrees.[93] Megalocornea and congenital glaucoma also have many clinical features in common, leading some authors to consider that megalocornea may be an incomplete form of congenital glaucoma.[146] In these pedigrees, magalocornea is usually defined as a horizontal corneal diameter exceeding 12 mm, a deep anterior chamber, abnormal tissue in the angle, and a normal intraocular pressure. The noting of an angle abnormality with enlarged corneas and

no clinical sign of glaucoma is not well understood, and the relationship between congenital glaucoma and megalocornea has not been resolved.[200]

Two types of megalocornea have been described. In incomplete megalocornea, the cornea and anterior segment appear normal, and multiple iris processes may be present with pigmentation of the trabecular meshwork. In complicated, or anterior megalophthalmos, there is megalocornea, posterior embryotoxon, Krukenberg spindles, pigmentation of the trabecular meshwork, iris tissue bridging the angle, lax zonular fibers, iridodonesis, and a cataract or dislocated lens. Congenital glaucoma, keratoglobus, and high myopia must be considered in the differential diagnosis of megalocornea. In keratoglobus, the cornea is globular shaped with thinning of the stroma, most pronounced at the periphery.

Microcoria

Congenital microcoria, in which the pupil size is less than 2 mm, is a rare familial, autosomal dominant disorder. The primary anomaly is maldevelopment of the iris dilator muscle.[9,73,130,238,302] A late onset congenital glaucoma, as well as iris abnormalities, have frequently been associated with this disorder. Typically, the angle reveals goniodysgenesis with multiple iris processes bridging the angle with an anterior iris insertion. Histopathologic studies reveal immaturity of the angle structures, identical to what has been described in congenital glaucoma. Treatment is similar to that of congenital glaucoma in the younger patient, or to late onset congenital or juvenile glaucoma in older patients. Angle-closure glaucoma with pupillary block may also occur and should be treated by an iridectomy.[135,321]

Microcornea

This rare ocular congenital disorder is defined by a corneal diameter less than 10 mm. The eye may be otherwise normal, or there may be other associated ocular anomalies including anterior chamber dysgenesis with an anterior iris insertion and glaucoma. Often, microcornea is found in association with anterior microphthalmos, with crowding of the anterior segment that may result in angle-closure glaucoma.[193] Occasionally, microcornea is associated with other systemic syndromes, such as Ehlers-Danlos.[74] Other ocular conditions associated with microcornea are glaucoma, congenital cataracts, and Peters' anomaly.[113] A syndrome involving congenital cataracts, abnormal iris, nystagmus, and congenital glaucoma has also

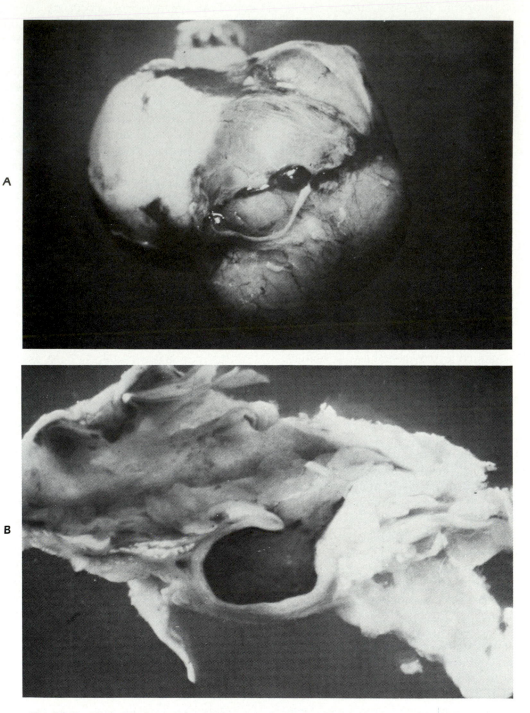

Fig. 53-3   Microphthalmos with orbital cyst. **A,** Gross photograph of globe at left with large orbital cyst attached to globe. **B,** Cut section reveals globe at right with communication to cyst above and at left.

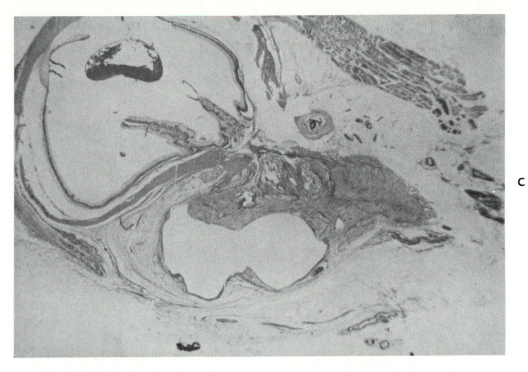

Fig. 53-3 cont'd   C, Photomicrograph of globe above and cyst below. Retina is dysplastic.

been described.[41] Microcornea has also been associated with uveal coloboma, high myopia, posterior staphyloma, and microphthalmia.[16]

Microphthalmos

Three general forms of microphthalmos are described: "pure" microphthalmos (nanophthalmos), microphthalmos with cyst, and microphthalmos associated with other systemic anomalies. Inheritance may be sporadic, autosomal dominant, autosomal recessive, or rarely X-linked.[102,222] Glaucoma associated with microphthalmos is usually due to chronic angle closure.

Nanophthalmos is a familial clinical syndrome characterized by hypermetropia, short axial length, small corneal diameters, thickened sclera, narrow anterior chamber angles, and glaucoma. Glaucoma related to chronic angle closure generally has its onset between the third to the fifth decade. Every attempt is made to treat the glaucoma resulting from nanophthalmos medically or with laser, as surgical intervention may be complicated by choroidal effusions and other difficulties.[26,37,157,261,280]

Microphthalmos with an orbital cyst is caused by failure of the choroidal fissure to close during embryologic development when the eye is between the 7 to 14 mm stage.[169] The retinal tissue proliferates through the fissure into the orbital space and is covered by connective tissue, producing a cyst. The globe is generally quite small and malformed, whereas the cyst may be extremely large and may produce pseudoproptosis (Fig. 53-3). This disorder is generally unilateral, though bilateral cases occur. The treatment *generally* consists of surgical excision of both the orbital cyst and the malformed globe.* Microphthalmos may also be seen in a wide variety of congenital systemic disorders, congenital infectious syndromes, and congenital ocular disorders† on p. 944.

As the mechanism for the glaucoma is generally angle closure, treatment is directed at initially attempting to relieve any pupillary block by iridectomy and then to treat medically. If this is not sufficient, then filtration surgery may be indicated, depending on the status of the eye. Intraocular surgery may be prone to hazards in these eyes, however, and the visual prognosis is generally guarded.

Morning Glory Syndrome

The term morning glory syndrome was first used by Kindler in 1970 to describe 10 cases of an unusual ocular anomaly, which was characterized

---

*References 10, 51, 143, 161, 169, 199, 331.
†References 89, 102, 136, 138, 182, 209, 218, 347.

DISORDERS ASSOCIATED WITH MICROPHTHALMOS

CONGENITAL SYSTEMIC DISORDERS

Trisomy 13
Ring chromosome 13
Chromosome 18 deletion syndrome
Hallermann-Streiff syndrome
Oculodentodigital dysplasia
Pierre Robin syndrome
Treacher Collins' syndrome
Oculovertebral dysplasia
Oculoauriculovertebral syndrome
Ullrich's syndrome
Focal dermal hypoplasia (Goltz's syndrome)
Meckel's syndrome
Myotonic dystrophy
François dyscephalic syndrome
Conradi's syndrome

CONGENITAL INFECTIOUS DISORDERS

Congenital rubella
Congenital toxoplasmosis
Cytomegalic inclusion disease

CONGENITAL OCULAR DISORDERS

Sclerocornea
Congenital cataracts
Iris and uveal colobomata
Cornea plana
Microcornea

---

by a large staphylomatous optic disc, covered with glial tissue. In each of these cases, the peripapillary area was also surrounded by a region of chorioretinal pigment abnormality, and the retinal vessels radiated from the disc in an anomalous fashion. Krause also emphasized the typical features of morning glory syndrome as an excavated optic disc with an elevated circumpapillary ring of chorioretinal pigmentary abnormality.[144,158,166]

Several systemic abnormalities have been reported in conjunction with morning glory syndrome including midline facial anomalies, basal encephaloceles, and agenesis of the corpus callosum.[160] It has been advised that patients with the morning glory syndrome have evaluation of the nasopharynx and radiographic examination of the skull to rule out these or other associated disorders.[39,140,160,235]

Associated ocular anomalies include strabismus, myopia, anisometropia, nonrhegmatogenous retinal detachments, hyaloid artery remnants, congenital cataracts, lid hemangioma, and peripheral retinal pigmentary changes.[5,65,101,293] Brini et al.[25] had also suggested that there are changes in the anterior segment consistent with anterior segment dysgenesis as well. Open-angle glaucoma in a pa-

tient with morning glory syndrome has also been described, and it was theorized that this may have been the result of a congenital malformation of the anterior chamber angle, though there was no histopathologic evidence to support this, and the gonioscopic appearance of the angle was unremarkable.[248]

Persistent Hyperplastic Primary Vitreous

Persistent hyperplastic primary vitreous (PHPV) is usually unilateral and is recognizable at birth in full-term infants. Microphthalmos is usually evident with leukocoria resulting from a retrolental fibrovascular mass (Fig. 53-4). The lens is usually clear, though there may be variable degrees of posterior lens opacification. If left untreated, most eyes with PHPV develop spontaneous intraocular hemorrhage, corneal opacification, secondary glaucoma, retinal detachment, or phthisis. In the past, many of these eyes have come to enucleation, most due to intractable glaucoma or phthisis bulbi.[117,202,244,245]

The fundamental abnormality is a persistence and overgrowth of the primary vitreous and its associated blood vessels, the hyaloid artery, vasa hyaloidea propria, and branches contributed by the ciliary vessels. The ciliary processes are incorporated into the periphery of the membrane and are drawn centrally as the eye grows, resulting in a dense fibrovascular retrolental mass. The posterior lens capsule may rupture as the lens and the remainder of the eye grow at a rate that exceeds that of the vascular retrolental membrane. This often results in a cataract, which may be slow or rapid in onset, and which will often become intumescent. Spontaneous hemorrhage may occur into the membrane, vitreous, or lens. Fibrous tissues and blood vessels may extend to the defect in the posterior lens capsule. Elements of the peripheral retina are continuous with the mass and as traction develops a retinal detachment may result. Other associated findings may include rupture of the anterior lens capsule; unusual vascularity of the iris; ectopia lentis; and coloboma of the iris, choroid, or optic nerve. The anterior chamber is often shallow, either due to forward displacement of the lens-iris diaphragm from the fibrovascular membrane or due to enlargement of the lens with cataract formation.

Glaucoma associated with PHPV is caused by angle closure either secondary to an intumescent cataract, forward movement of the lens-iris diaphragm associated with contracture of the retrolental membrane, or hemorrhage from persistent vessels within the fibrovascular membrane.

Early surgical intervention with removal of the

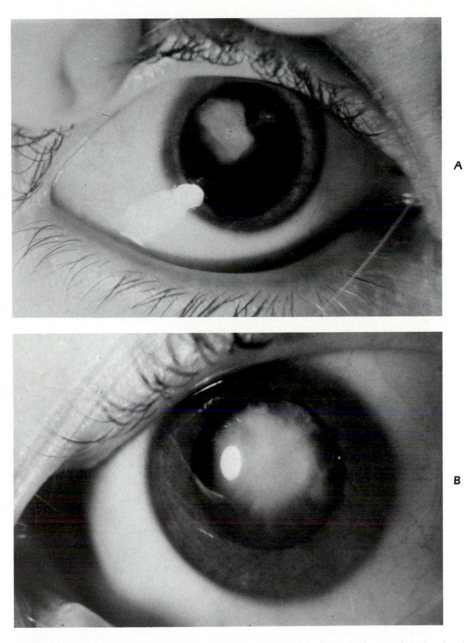

Fig. 53-4 Persistent hyperplastic primary vitreous. **A,** Clinical photograph revealing localized white retrolental opacity. **B,** More advanced example. Eye is microphthalmic as well.

Continued.

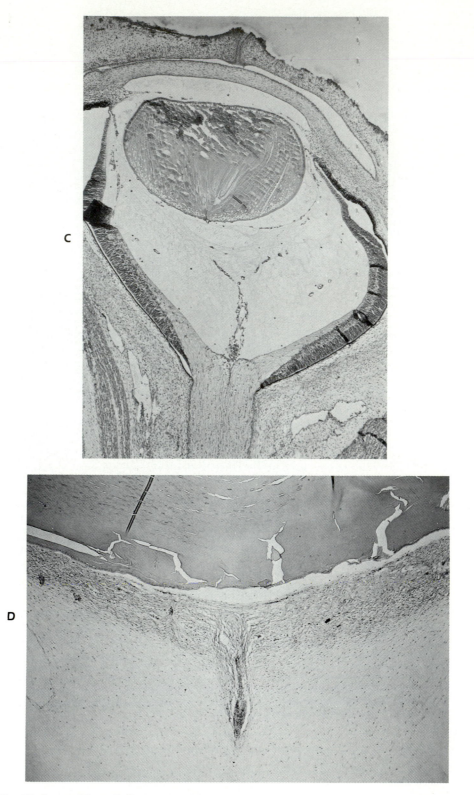

Fig. 53-4, cont'd   **C,** Fully developed hyaloid system in 16 mm embryonic eye. Note that lids have not separated. **D,** PHPV with retrolental fibrovascular mass.

lens, fibrovascular postlenticular membrane, vitrectomy, and cauterization or removal of the hyaloid stalk has shown promise in preventing the usually progressive pathologic sequence of events that may result in secondary glaucoma and phthisis.* In addition to avoiding severe complications, early surgery seems to allow for a better potential visual prognosis and for better growth of the eye for cosmetic purposes. In those cases that have not undergone early surgery and have developed secondary angle-closure glaucoma, treatment is aimed at removing the lens and performing a peripheral iridectomy, often associated with a vitrectomy as well. Because of the small size of these eyes, care must be taken when incisions are placed into the eye to avoid intraoperative complications.

Retinal Degeneration with Nanophthalmos, Cystic Macular Degeneration, and Angle-closure Glaucoma

This syndrome was recently reported in a pedigree of seven related patients with an autosomal recessive mode of inheritance.[197] All had progressive tapetoretinal degeneration, cystic macular degeneration, high hyperopia, nanophthalmos, and angle-closure glaucoma. Another pedigree with autosomal dominant nanophthalmos, angle-closure glaucoma, and tapetoretinal degeneration has been described. In this pedigree, all affected members had myopia, and there was no cystic macular degeneration.[122] Another case report described a patient with nanophthalmos, angle-closure glaucoma, retinal degeneration, and cystic macular degeneration. No pedigree was given, and the inheritance was unknown.[97]

The management of nanophthalmos with angle-closure glaucoma may prove difficult.[26,37,157,221,280] The eyes are generally hyperopic with a short axial length, and angle-closure glaucoma frequently occurs in the fourth to the sixth decades of life. Surgery is frequently complicated by uveal effusions. Medical therapy may be effective; however, miotics may paradoxically increase the pupillary block and precipitate further angle closure. Laser iridotomy or peripheral iridoplasty have apparently the highest rate of success. If surgery becomes necessary, uveal effusions may be a problem, and in some cases, vortex vein decompression has been suggested,[27] or simultaneous drainage of the suprachoroidal space with a sclerotomy may be helpful.

*References 2, 79, 94, 233, 288, 290.

Retinopathy of Prematurity

Because of the improved treatment and survival of premature infants, retinopathy of prematurity, or retrolental fibroplasia, remains a significant cause of childhood blindness. Ophthalmologists are increasingly involved in the early care of these infants and must be able to document the stages of disease, recognize complications, and treat or refer these patients for management of complications.

Effort directed to developing a standardized classification system has resulted in the International Classification of Retinopathy of Prematurity (ICROP). In addition to the more detailed descriptions concerning the posterior segment and retina, information concerning the anterior segment has also been stressed in the ICROP, because it may have important consequences for the structure and integrity of the eye, and in particular, for the development of glaucoma.[18,53,139]

Secondary angle-closure glaucoma has been recognized as a complication of the later stages of retinopathy of prematurity for many years (Fig. 53-5). Most commonly, this glaucoma occurs in the first years of life, though it may occur in the third decade.[124, 237,326] Signs of the development of angle-closure glaucoma in small infants or young children may be difficult. If the intraocular pressures are extremely high, the child will appear ill and will usually stop eating or drinking. It has been estimated that this complication may occur in as many as 30% of eyes with advanced retinopathy of prematurity.[168] Progressive myopia related to changes within the configuration of the lens rather than to corneal myopia or increasing changes in axial length is often associated with the shallowing of the anterior chamber.[107] Microphthalmos has also been reported in association with advanced retinopathy of prematurity, which may also predispose to chronic angle-closure glaucoma.[155]

Walton et al.[326] recommended an iridectomy in cases of angle-closure glaucoma due to retinopathy of prematurity but found that this procedure was not always helpful.[326] They observed that the iris in some cases will fall posteriorly, and the angle will open only if significant peripheral anterior synechia has not formed. Prophylactic iridectomy was recommended when signs of increasing cicatrization and shallowing of the anterior chamber were seen and were progressing even without glaucoma. It has been observed, however, that the peripheral iridectomies may frequently reclose as the anterior chamber shallows and the coloboma in the iris comes into contact with the peripheral cornea

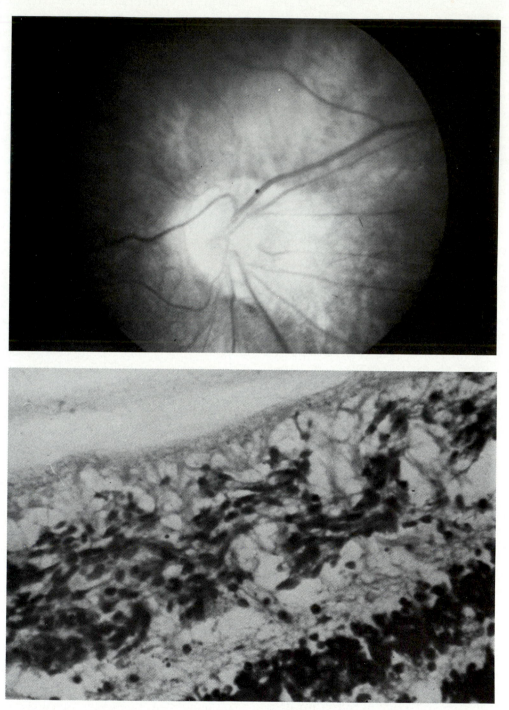

Fig. 53-5 Retinopathy of prematurity. **A,** Fundus photograph of young child with arrested retinopathy of prematurity with traction of retinal vessels. Note how vessels are all pulled to right side, which is temporally in left eye. **B,** Photomicrograph revealing glomeruloid tufts of proliferated endothelial cells in peripheral temporal retina of child.

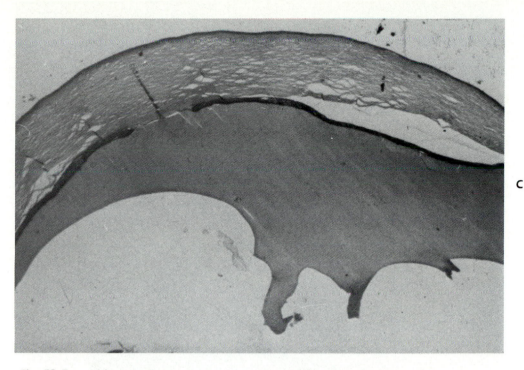

Fig. 53-5 cont'd   C, End-stage retinopathy of prematurity with totally obliterated anterior chamber. Lens has fallen out during tissue processing.

and angle. Because of this complication, a sector iridectomy was recommended. However, Walton demonstrated that iridectomies were not uniformly beneficial in altering the course of the chronic angle-closure glaucoma, which was occurring in retinopathy of prematurity, suggesting that pupillary block was not the primary mechanism.[326] It was suggested that forward displacement of the lens-iris diaphragm was the cause of the chronic angle closure and lens extraction was recommended.[21,52,124] Lens extraction alone or combined with vitrectomy has since proven helpful in many patients.[152,206,237] Kushner[167] reported that cycloplegics were initially helpful in some cases of angle closure related to ciliary block, but for an eventual cure vitrectomy and lensectomy were required.

Although successful treatment of the glaucoma with preservation of the eye using pars plana lensectomy and anterior vitrectomy can be obtained, visual results continue to be poor due to the cicatricial changes and retinal detachment. Some recent attempts to reattach the retina after lensectomy and vitrectomy have resulted in improved vision in some cases.[196,313] If only one eye develops severe cicatricial changes with secondary angle-closure glaucoma, with useful vision in the fellow eye, alternatives to intraocular surgery have been suggested because of the rare possibility of sympathetic ophthalmia. These alternatives would

include enucleation, retrobulbar alcohol, or cyclocryotherapy to alleviate the symptoms of the more severely involved eye.

Another mechanism for glaucoma in late stages of retinopathy of prematurity is rubeosis with development of neovascular glaucoma where a chronic retinal detachment has been present.[43] Treatment for these cases is very difficult. When the eye becomes uncomfortable, cyclocryotherapy or enucleation may be considered.

Sclerocornea

Sclerocornea is a rare congenital anomaly affecting the cornea either peripherally or diffusely. With only peripheral involvement, the vision may be normal and the diagnosis made only as an incidental finding. With diffuse involvement, there is severe limitation of vision. Sclerocornea is usually bilateral, though unilateral cases occur. This disorder may occur as an isolated disorder, or in conjunction with many other ocular and systemic defects.[104,133,201] A chromosomal translocation defect has been reported in one case of sclerocornea, and another case was associated with trisomy 18.[162,252] Systemic defects reported in association with sclerocornea include cerebellar dysfunction, deafness, cryptorchidism, brachycephaly, mental retardation, skin anomalies, facial anomalies, and the Smith-Lemli-Opitz syndrome.[119]

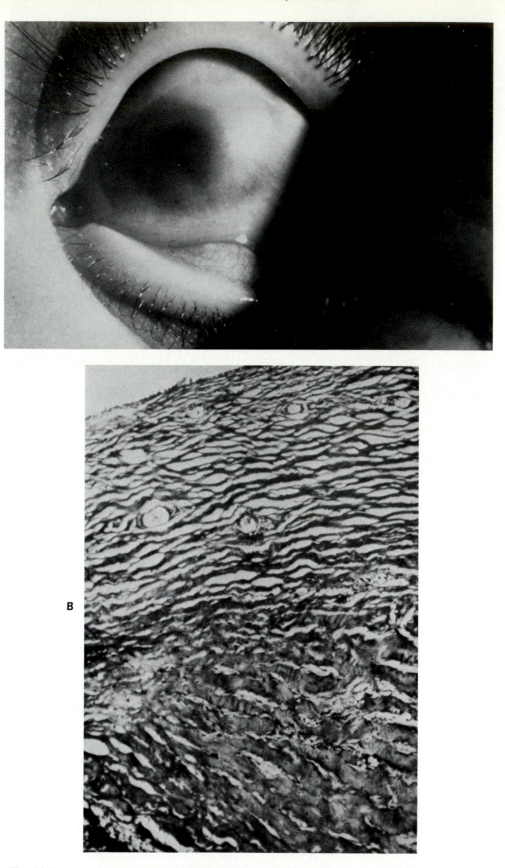

Fig. 53-6   Sclerocornea. **A,** Clinical photograph of left eye of 8-month-old child with sclerocornea. Condition was present bilaterally. Central cornea is translucent. Peripheral cornea is hazy and vascularized. There is no corneoscleral sulcus. Scleral curvature is continuous with corneal curvature. **B,** Photomicrograph of cornea revealing marked vascularization at all levels. Note markedly thickened corneal lamellae inferiorly.

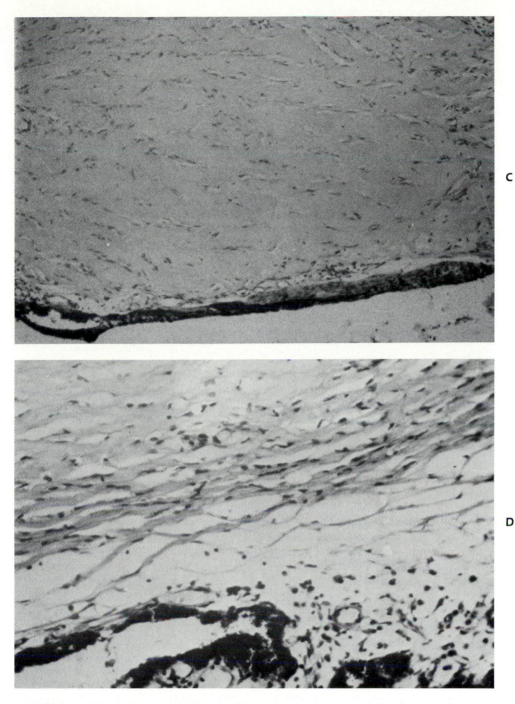

Fig. 53-6 cont'd   C, Photograph showing obliteration of anterior chamber with total iridocorneal adhesion. Corneal lamellae are markedly thickened. Iris possesses no stroma. There is no Decemet's membrane or corneal epithelium. **D,** There are no angle structures. There is total iridocorneal adhesion but no ciliary musculature, scleral spur, or trabecular meshwork.

Associated ocular anomalies are many and may include enophthalmos, blepharoptosis, microphthalmos, macrophthalmos, nystagmus, strabismus, cornea plana,[14,171,301] shallow anterior chamber, anterior synechiae, posterior embryotoxon, iris anomalies, cataracts, uveal colobomas, and glaucoma. The etiology of the glaucoma may vary. A congenital angle anomaly has been described by Goldstein suggesting a type of developmental glaucoma. Cases have also been described where glaucoma was associated with a narrow angle and pupillary block was suspected (Fig. 53-6).[104]

REFERENCES

1. Abassi, V, Lowe, CU, and Calcagno, PL: Oculo-cerebro-renal syndrome; a review, Am J Dis Child 115:145, 1968
2. Acers, TE, and Coston, TO: Persistent hyperplastic primary vitreous, Am J Ophthalmol 64:734, 1967
3. Ackerman, JL, Ackerman, AL, and Ackerman, AB: A new dental, ocular and cutaneous syndrome, Int J Dermatol, 12:285, 1973
4. Adhikary, HP: Ocular manifestations of Turner's syndrome, Trans Opthalmol Soc UK 101:395, 1981
5. Akiyama, K, et al: Retinal detachment in morning glory syndrome, Ophthalmic Surg 15:841, 1984
6. Amemiya, T, Matsuda, H, Uehara, M: Ocular findings in atopic dermatitis with special reference to the clinical features of atopic cataract, Ophthalmologica 180:129, 1980
7. Angelman, H: Syndrome of coloboma with multiple congenital abnormalities in infancy, Br Med J 1:1212, 1961
8. Aracena, T, and Sangueza, P: Hallermann-Streiff-François syndrome, J Pediatr Ophthalmol 14:373, 1977
9. Ardouin, M, Urvoy, M, and Lefranc, J: Microcorie congénitale, Bull Mem Soc Fr Ophtalmol 77:356, 1964
10. Arstikaitis, M: A case report of bilateral microphthalmos with cysts, Arch Ophthalmol 82:480, 1969
11. Atkins, L, and Rosenthal, MK: Multiple congenital abnormalities associated with chromosomal trisomy, N Engl J Med 265:314, 1962
12. Atkinson, JP: Diagnosis and management of hereditary angioedema (HAE), Ann Allergy 42:348, 1979
13. Avasthi, PS, Erikson, DG, and Gardner, KD: Hereditary renal-retinal dysplasia and the medullary cystic disease-nephronophthisis complex, Ann Intern Med 84:157, 1976
14. Barkan, H, and Borley, WE: Familial cornea plana, complicated by cataracta nigra and glaucoma, Am J Ophthalmol 19:307, 1936
15. Bartsocas, CS: Manifestations in Lowe's syndrome, Ann Ophthalmol, 2:369, 1970
16. Bateman, JB, and Maumenee, IH: Colobomatous macrophthalmia with microcornea, Ophthalmic Paediatr Genet 4:59, 1984
17. Beighton, P, Winship, I, and Behari, D: The ocular form of osteogenesis imperfecta: a new autosomal recessive syndrome, Clin Genet 28:69, 1985
18. Biglan, AW, Brown, DR, and Macpherson, TA: Update on retinopathy of prematurity, Semin Perinatol 10:187, 1986
19. Blair, NP, et al: Hereditary progressive arthro-ophthalmopathy of Stickler, Am J Ophthalmol 88:876, 1979
20. Blanck, MF, Braun-Vallon, S, and Guillaumat, ML: Deux cas de nanisme constitutionnel (syndrome de Rubinstein et Taybi) avec glaucome, Bull Soc Opthalmol Fr 68:173, 1968
21. Blodi, F: Symposium: retrolental fibroplasia (retinopathy of prematurity) management, Trans Am Acad Ophthalmol Otolaryngol 59:35, 1955
22. Bork, K, Kreuz, W, and Witzke, G: Hereditares angioneurotisches Ödem, Dtsch Med Wochenschr 109:1331, 1984
23. Brailey, WA: Double microphthalmos with defective development of iris, teeth, and anus. Glaucoma at an early age, Trans Opthalmol Soc UK 10:139, 1890
24. Brickman, CM, and Hosea, SW: Hereditary angioedema, Int J Dermatol 22:141, 1983
25. Brini, A, Charton, MN, and Baumgartner, M: Staphylome scléral péripapillaire avec ectopie postérieure de la papille (Morning glory syndrome), J Fr Ophthalmol 3:323, 1980
26. Brockhurst, RJ: Nanophthalmos with uveal effusion, Arch Ophthalmol 92:1289, 1975
27. Brockhurst, RJ: Vortex vein decompression for nanophthalmic uveal effusion, Arch Ophthalmol 98:1987, 1980
28. Brubaker, RF, et al: Benign cystinosis, the clinical, biochemical and morphologic findings in a family with two affected siblings, Am J Med 49:546, 1970
29. Deleted in proofs
30. Brushfield, T: Mongolism, Br J Dis Child 21:16, 1924
31. Buckley, CA, and Cheng, H: Intraocular melanoma, diabetes, and Turner's syndrome: presentation with proptosis, Br J Ophthalmol 65:460, 1981
32. Deleted in proofs
33. Burki, E: Ueber die Cystinkrankheit in Kleinkindersalter unter besonderer Berucksichtigung des Augendes, Ophthalmologica 101:257, 1941
34. Butler, LJ, et al: E(16-18) trisomy syndrome: analysis of 13 cases, Arch Dis Child 40:600, 1965
35. Buyse, M, and Bull, MJ: A syndrome of osteogenesis imperfecta, microcephaly, and cataracts, Birth Defects 14:95, 1978
36. Calderone, JP, et al: Intraocular pathology of trisomy 18 (Edward's syndrome): report of a case and review of the literature, Br J Ophthalmol 67:162, 1983
37. Calhoun, FP: The management of glaucoma in nanophthalmos, Trans Am Ophthalmol Soc 73:97, 1975
38. Cameron, JD, Yanoff, M, and Frayer, WC: Coats' disease and Turner's syndrome, Am J Ophthalmol 78:852, 1974
39. Caprioli, J, and Lesser, RL: Basal encephalocele and morning glory syndrome, Br J Ophthalmol, 67:349, 1983
40. Carnevale, A, et al: Ring chromosome 6 in a child with minimal abnormalities, Am J Med Genet 4:271, 1979
41. Cebon, L, and West, RH: A syndrome involving congenital cataracts of unusual morphology, microcornea, abnormal irides, nystagmus and congenital glaucoma, inherited as an autosomal dominant trait, Aust J Ophthalmol 10:237, 1982
42. Cennamo, G, Sammartino, A, and Fioretti, F: Morning glory syndrome with contractile peripapillary staphyloma, Br J Ophthalmol 67:346, 1983

43. Chong, LP, Machemer, R, and de Juan, E: Vitrectomy for advanced stages of retinopathy of prematurity Am J Ophthalmol, 102:710, 1986

44. Christian, HA: Relapsing febrile nodular nonsupprative panniculitis, Arch Intern Med 42:338, 1928

45. Chrousos, GA, et al: Ocular findings in Turner's syndrome: a prospective study, Ophthalmology 91:926, 1984

46. Cibis, GW, et al: Lenticular opacities in carriers of Lowe's syndrome, Ophthalmology 93:1041, 1986

47. Cogan, DG, and Kuwabara, T: Ocular pathology of cystinosis, Arch Ophthalmol 13:75, 1960

48. Cogan, DG, and Kuwabara, T: Ocular pathology of the 13-15 trisomy syndrome, Arch Ophthalmol 72:246, 1964

49. Cogan, DG, et al: Ocular manifestations of systemic cystinosis, Arch Ophthalmol 55:36, 1956

50. Deleted in proofs

51. Collins, ET: Congenital abnormalities, Trans Opthalmol Soc UK 17:254, 1897

52. Collyer, R, Arstikaitis, M, and Pashby, T: Glaucoma in children, Trans Can Ophthalmol Soc 21:92, 1959

53. Committee for the Classification of Retinopathy of Prematurity: The international classification of retinopathy of prematurity, Arch Ophthalmol 102:1130, 1984

54. Crawford, Md'A: Multiple congenital anomalies associated with an extra autosome, Lancet 2:22, 1961

55. Cross, HE, and Maumenee, AE: Progressive spontaneous dissolution of the iris, Surv Ophthalmol 18:186, 1973

56. Cullen, JF: Blindness in mongolism (Down's syndrome), Br J Ophthalmol 47:331, 1963

57. Cullen, JF, and Butler, HG: Mongolism (Down's syndrome) and keratoconus, Br J Ophthalmol 47:321, 1963

58. Curtin, VT, Joyce, EE, and Ballin, N: Ocular pathology in the oculo-cerebro-renal syndrome of Lowe, Am J Ophthalmol 64:533, 1967

59. Dark, AJ, and Kirkham, TH: Congenital corneal opacities in a patient with Rieger's anomaly and Down's syndrome, Br J Ophthalmol 52:631, 1968

60. deGrouchy, J: Chromosome 18: a topologic approach, J Pediatr 66:414, 1965

61. deGrouchy, J, et al: Chromosome 17-18 en anneau et malformations congénitales chez un fille, Ann Genet (Paris) 27:189, 1963

62. deGrouchy, J, et al: Délétion partielle des bras longs du chromosome 18, Pathol Biol (Paris) 12:579, 1964

63. deGrouchy, J, and Turleau, C: Clinical atlas of human chromosomes, ed 2, New York, 1984, John Wiley & Sons

64. Delleman, JW, and van Balen, AT: Carrier detection in tapetoretinal degeneration in association with medullary cystic disease, Am J Ophthalmol 95:487, 1983

65. Dempster, AG, Lee, WR, and Forrester, JV: The 'morning glory syndrome'—a mesodermal defect? Ophthalmologica 187:222, 1983

66. d'Épinay, SL, and Reme, C: Klinische und mophologische Untersuchungen eines kongenitalen Glaukoms bei Okulo-digito-dentalem Syndrom, Klin Monatsbl Augenheilkd 168:113, 1976

67. Dessoff, J: Blue sclerotics, fragile bones and deafness, Arch Ophthalmol 12:60, 1934

68. Dodd, MJ, Pusin, SM, and Green, WR: Adult cystinosis, Arch Ophthalmol 96:1054, 1978

69. Donaldson, DD: The significance of spotting of the iris in mongoloids, Arch Ophthalmol 65:50, 1961

70. Dowling, JL, et al: Primary glaucoma associated with iridotrabecular dysgenesis and ectropion uveae, Ophthalmology 92:912, 1985

71. Down, JHL: Observations on ethnic classification of idiots, Clin Lect and Rep, London Hosp 111:259, 1866

72. Dudgeon, J, and Chisholm, IA: Oculo-dento-digital dysplasia, Trans Opthalmol Soc UK 94:203, 1974

73. Duke-Elder, S, editor: System of Ophthalmology III, part 2, Congenital deformities, St. Louis, 1963, The CV Mosby Co

74. Durham, DG: Cutis hyperelastica (Ehlers-Danlos syndrome) with blue scleraes, microcornea, and glaucoma, Arch Ophthalmol 49:220:1953

75. Edwards, JH, et al: A new trisomic syndrome, Lancet 1:787, 1960

76. Eissler, R, and Longnecker, LP: The common eye findings in mongolism, Am J Ophthalmol 54:398, 1962

77. Elliott, JH, et al: Hereditary sclerocornea, Arch Ophthalmol 103:676, 1985

78. Eriksson, AW, Lehman, W, and Forsius, H: Congenital cornea plana in Finland, Clin Genet 4:301, 1973

79. Federman, JL, et al: The surgical and nonsurgical management of persistent hyperplastic primary vitreous, Ophthalmology 89:20, 1982

80. Feingold, M, and Gellis, S: Ocular abnormalities associated with first and second arch syndromes, Surv Ophthalmol 14:30, 1969

81. Fillastre, JP, et al: Néphropathie interstitielle chronique et dystrophie rétinenne familiales (syndrome de Senior-Loken), Nouv Presse Med 9:309, 1974

82. Finley, WH, Finley, SC, and Carte, ET: 17-18 trisomy syndrome, Am J Dis Child 106:591, 1963

83. Fisher, NF, Hallett, J, and Carpenter, G: Oculocerebrorenal syndrome of Lowe, Arch Ophthalmol 77:642, 1967

84. Fishman, AJ, et al: Cornea plana: a case report, Ann Ophthalmol 14:47, 1982

85. Fogle, JA, Welch, RB, and Green, WR: Retinitis pigmentosa and exudative vasculopathy, Arch Ophthalmol 96:969, 1978

86. Ford, CE, et al: A sex chromosome anomaly in a case of gonadal dysgenesis (Turner's syndrome), Lancet, 1:711, 1959

87. François, J: A new syndrome, dyscephalia with bird face and dental anomalies, nanism, hypotrichosis, cutaneous atrophy, microphthalmia, and congenital cataract, Arch Ophthalmol 60:842, 1958

88. François, J, et al: Cystinosis, Am J Ophthalmol 73:643, 1972

89. François, J, and Pierard, J: The François dyscephalic syndrome and skin manifestations, Am J Ophthalmol 71:1241, 1971

90. François, J, and Victoria-Troncoso, V: François' dyscephalic syndrome and skin manifestations, Ophthalmologica 183:63, 1981

91. Fried, K, et al: Mental retardation and congenital malformations associated with a ring chromosome 6, Clin Genet 7:192, 1975

92. Friedlaender, MH: Atopic dermatitis. In Fraunfelder, F, Roy, H, editors: Current ocular therapy, Philadelphia, 1985, WB Saunders

93. Friedmann, AI, and Etzine, S: Familial co-existence of congenital glaucoma and megalo-cornea, Ophthalmologica, 142:629, 1961

94. Gass, JDM: Surgical excision of persistent hyperplastic primary vitreous, Arch Ophthalmol 83:163, 1970

95. Geeraets, WJ: Ocular syndromes, Philadelphia, 1976, Lea & Febiger

96. German, JL, III, et al: Autosomal trisomy of a group 16-18 chromosome, J Pediatr, 60:503, 1962

97. Ghose, S, Sachdev, MS, and Kumar, H: Bilateral nanophthalmos, pigmentary retinal dystrophy, and angle closure glaucoma-a new syndrome? Br J Ophthalmol 69:624, 1985

98. Gillespie, FD: A hereditary syndrome: "dysplasia oculodentodigitalis," Arch Ophthalmol, 71:95, 1964

99. Ginsberg, J, and Bove, KE: Ocular pathology of trisomy 13, Ann Ophthalmol 6:113, 1974

100. Ginsberg, J, Perrin, EV, and Sueoka, WT: Ocular manifestations of trisomy 18, Am J Ophthalmol 66:59, 1968

101. Giuffre, G: Morning glory syndrome: clinical and electrofunctional study of three cases, Br J Ophthalmol 70:229, 1986

102. Goldberg, MF, and McKusick, VA: X-linked colobomatous microphthalmos and other congenital anomalies, Am J Ophthalmol 71:1128, 1971

103. Goldman, H, et al: Adolescent cystinosis, comparisons with infantile and adult forms, Pediatrics 47:979, 1971

104. Goldstein, JE, and Cogan, DG: Sclerocornea and associated congenital anomalies, Arch Ophthalmol 67:99, 1962

105. Goldstone, RM, and Motsay, DS: Trisomy 18 syndrome: case report with chromosomal analysis, Guthrie Clin Bull 30:108, 1964

106. Goodman, M, and Gorlin, RJ: The face in genetic disorders, St. Louis, 1970, The CV Mosby Co

107. Gordon, RA, and Donzis, PB: Myopia associated with retinopathy of prematurity, Ophthalmology 93:1593, 1986

108. Gorlin, RJ, and Goltz, RW: Multiple basal-cell epithelioma, jaw cysts and bifid rib, N Engl J Med 262:908, 1960

109. Gorlin, RJ, Meskin, LH, and Geme, JW: Oculodentodigital dysplasia, J Pediatr 63:69, 1963

110. Gorlin, RJ, Vickers, RA, Kelln, E, and Williamson, JJ: The multiple basal-cell nevi syndrome, Cancer 18:89, 1965

111. Gorlin, RJ, Yunis, JJ, and Tuna, N: Multiple nevoid basal cell carcinoma, odontogenic keratocysts and skeletal anomalies, Acta Derm Venereol (Stockh) 43:39, 1963

112. Gottlieb, MI, et al: Trisomy-17 syndrome, report of three cases and review of the literature, Am J Med 33:763, 1962

113. Green, JS, and Johnson, GJ: Congenital cataract with microcornea and Peters' anomaly as expressions of one autosomal dominant gene, Ophthalmic Paediatr Genet 7:187, 1986

114. Grutzner, P: Augensymptome bei kongenitaler Encephalo-Ophthalmo-Dysplasie (persistierende Pupillarmembran, peripherer Netzhautwulst und Meningocele bei zwei Geschwistern mit generalisierten Anfallen), Bericht; Dtsch Ophthalmol Ges, 67:258, 1966

115. Gustafsson, J, et al: Zellweger's cerebro-hepato-renal syndrome—variations in expressivity and in defects of bile acid synthesis, Clin Genet 24:313, 1983

116. Haddad, R, Font, RL, and Friendly, DS: Cerebro-hepato-renal syndrome of Zellweger, Arch Ophthalmol 94:1927, 1976

117. Haddad, R, Font, RL, and Reeser, F: Persistent hyperplastic primary vitreous. A clinicopathologic study of 62 cases and review of the literature, Surv Ophthalmol 23:123, 1978

118. Hallermann, W: Vogelgesicht und Cataracta congenita, Klin Monatsbl Augenheilkd 113:315, 1948

119. Harbin, RL, et al: Sclerocornea associated with the Smith-Lemli-Opitz syndrome, Am J Ophthalmol 84:72, 1977

120. Harris, LS, et al: Oculo-cerebro-renal syndrome: report of a case in a baby girl, Br J Ophthalmol 54:278, 1970

121. Hecht, F, et al: The no. 17-18 (E) trisomy syndrome, J Pediatr 63:605, 1963

122. Hermann, P: Le syndrome microphthalmie-retinite pigmentaire-glaucome, Arch Ophtalmol (Paris), 18:17, 1958

123. Hittner, HM, et al: Oculocutaneous albinoidism as a manifestation of reduced neural crest derivatives in the Prader-Willi syndrome, Am J Ophthalmol 94:328, 1982

124. Hittner, HM, Rhodes, LM, and McPherson, AR: Anterior segment abnormalities in cicatricial retinopathy of prematurity, Ophthalmology 86:803, 1979

125. Hoepner, J, and Yanoff, M: Ocular anomalies in trisomy 13-15, Am J Ophthalmol 74:729, 1972

126. Hogan, MJ: Atopic keratoconjunctivitis, Am J Ophthalmol 36:937, 1953

127. Hogewind, BL, et al: Electro-retinal abnormalities in heterozygotes of renal-retinal dysplasia, Acta Med Scand 202:323, 1977

128. Deleted in proofs

129. Holman, GH, et al: The 18-trisomy syndrome–two new clinical variants, N Engl J Med 268:982, 1963

130. Holth, S, and Berner, O: Congenital miosis or pinhole pupils owing to developmental faults of the dilator muscle, Br J Ophthalmol 7:401, 1923

131. Hopkins, DJ, and Horan, EC: Glaucoma in the Hallermann-Streiff syndrome, Br J Ophthalmol 54:416, 1970

132. Howard, RO: Classification of chromosomal eye syndromes, Int Ophthalmol 4:77, 1981

133. Howard, RO, and Abrahams, IW: Sclerocornea, Am J Ophthalmol 71:1254, 1971

134. Huggert, A: The trisomy 18 syndrome: a report of three cases in the same family, Acta Ophthalmol (Copenh), 44:186, 1966

135. Hyams, SW, and Neumann, E: Congenital microcoria and combined mechanism glaucoma, Am J Ophthalmol 68:326, 1969

136. Ide, CH, Miller, GW, and Wollschlaeger, PB: Familial facial dysplasia, Arch Ophthalmol 84:427, 1970

137. Ide, CH, and Webb, RW: Hallermann-Streiff syndrome, Am J Ophthalmol 67:151, 1969

138. Ide, CH, Wollschlaeger, PB, Wollschlaeger, G: Oculovertebral syndrome associated with cardiovascular abnormalities, Ann Ophthalmol, 4:836, 1972

139. International Committee for the Classification of the Late Stages of Retinopathy of Prematurity: an international classification of retinopathy of prematurity: II. The classification of retinal detachment, Arch Ophthalmol 105:906, 1987

140. Jackson, WE, and Freed, S: Ocular and systemic abnormalities associated with morning glory syndrome, Ophthalmic Paediatr Genet 5:111, 1985

141. Jaeger, EA: Ocular findings in Down's syndrome, Trans Am Ophthalmol Soc 78:808, 1980

142. Jeffcoate, WJ, et al: Endocrine function in the Prader-Willi syndrome, Clin Endocrinol (Oxf) 12:81, 1980

143. Jensen, OA: Microphthalmia with associated pseudogliomatosis of the retina and pseudogliomatous orbital cyst, Acta Ophthalmol (Copenh), 43:240, 1965

144. Jensen, P, and Kalina, RE: Congenital anomalies of the optic disk, Am J Ophthalmol 82:27, 1976

145. Deleted in proofs

146. Jerndal, T: Goniodysgenesis and hereditary juvenile glaucoma, Acta Ophthalmol (Copenh) [Suppl] 107:5, 1970

147. Johnson, BL, and Hiles, DA: Ocular pathology of Lowe's syndrome in a female infant, J Pediatr Ophthalmol 13:204, 1976

148. Journel, H, et al: Eye manifestations of trisomy 21: study of 53 cases and review of the literature, Ann Pediatr (Paris) 33:387, 1986

149. Judisch, GF, et al: Oculodentodigital dysplasia, four new reports and a literature review, Arch Ophthalmol 97:878, 1979

150. Kadrnka-Lovrenčić, M, et al: Die oculo-dento-digitale Dysplasie (das Meyer-Schwickerath-syndrom), Monatsschr Kinderheilkd 121:42, 1973

151. Kaiser-Kupfer, MI, et al: Low ocular rigidity in patients with osteogenesis imperfecta, Invest Ophthalmol Vis Sci 20:807, 1981

152. Kalina, RE: Treatment of retrolental fibroplasia, Surv Ophthalmol 24:229, 1980

153. Keith, CG: The ocular manifestations of trisomy 13-15, Trans Ophthalmol Soc UK 86;435, 1966

154. Kelley, RI: Review: the cerebrohepatorenal syndrome of Zellweger, morphologic and metabolic aspects, Am J Med Genet 16:503, 1983

155. Kelley, SP, and Fielder, AR: Microcornea associated with retinopathy of prematurity, Br J Ophthalmol 71:201, 1987

156. Khodadoust, A, and Paton, D: Turner's syndrome in a male: report of a case with myopia, retinal detachment, cataract, and glaucoma, Arch Ophthalmol 77:630, 1967

157. Kimbrough, RL, et al: Angle-closure glaucoma in nanophthalmos, Am J Ophthalmol 88:572, 1979

158. Kindler, P: Morning glory syndrome: unusual congenital optic disk anomaly, Am J Ophthalmol 69:376, 1970

159. Deleted in proofs

160. Koenig, SB, Naidich, TP, and Lissner, G: The morning glory syndrome associated with sphenoidal encephalocele, Ophthalmology 89:1368, 1982

161. Kok-van Alphen, CC, et al: Microphthalmus and orbital cyst, Ophthalmologica 167:389, 1973

162. Kolbert, GS, and Seelenfreund, M: Sclerocornea, anterior cleavage syndrome, and trisomy 18, Ann Ophthalmol 2:26, 1970

163. Koulischer, L, Pelc, S, and Perier, O: A case of trisomy-18 mosaicism, Lancet 2:945, 1963

164. Kouseff, BG: The cytogenetic controversy in the Prader-Labhart-Willi syndrome, Am J Med Genet 13:431, 1982

165. Krause, AC: Congenital encephalo-ophthalmic dysplasia, Arch Ophthalmol 36:387, 1946

166. Krause, U: Three cases of the morning glory syndrome, Acta Ophthalmol (Copenh), 50:188, 1972

167. Kushner, BJ: Ciliary block glaucoma in retinopathy of prematurity, Arch Ophthalmol 100:1078, 1982

168. Kwitko, M: Secondary glaucoma in infancy and childhood. In Kwitko, M, editor: Glaucoma in infants and children, New York, 1973, Appleton-Century-Crofts

169. Ladenheim, J, and Metrick, S: Congenital microphthalmos with cyst formation, Am J Ophthalmol 41:1059, 1956

170. Lanier, JD, McCrary, JA, and Justice, J: Autosomal recessive retinitis pigmentosa and Coats' disease. A presumed familial incidence, Arch Ophthalmol 94:1737, 1976

171. Larsen, V, and Eriksen, A: Cornea plana, Acta Ophthalmol (Copenh), 27:275, 1949

172. Laurent, C, Royer, J, and Noel, G: Syndrome de Turner et glaucome congénitale, Bull Soc Ophtalmol Fr 5:367, 1961

173. Ledbetter, DH, et al: Chromosome 15 abnormalities and the Prader-Willi syndrome: a follow-up report of 40 cases, Am J Hum Genet 34:278, 1982

174. Ledbetter, DH, et al: Deletions of chromosome 15 as a cause of the Prader-Willi syndrome, N Engl J Med 304:325, 1981

175. Leff, SR, et al: Congenital corneal staphyloma: clinical, radiological, and pathological correlation, Br J Ophthalmol 70:427, 1986

176. Lietman, PS, et al: Adult cystinosis-a benign disorder, Am J Med 40:511, 1966

177. Lejeune, J, and Berger, R: Sur deux observations familiales de translocations complexes, Ann Genet (Paris) 8:21, 1965

178. Lejeune, J, et al: La délétion partielle du bras long du chromosome 18. Individualisation d'un novel état morbide, Ann Genet 9:32, 1966

179. Lejeune, J, et al: Partial deletion of long arm of chromosome 18—A new autosomal syndrome, Presented at the Third International Congress on Human Genetics, Chicago, Sept, 1966,

180. Lejeune, J, et al: Monosomie partielle pour un petit acrocentrique, CR Acad Sci (Paris), 259:4187, 1964

181. Lejeune, J, et al: Sur un cas de délétion partielle du bras court du chromosome 18, resultant d'une translocation familiale 18-17, Ann Genet 9:27, 1966

182. Lessell, S, Coppeto, J, and Samet, S: Ophthlamoplegia in myotonic dystrophy, Am J Ophthalmol 71:1231, 1971

183. Lessell, S, and Forbes, AP: Eye signs in Turner's syndrome, Arch Ophthalmol 76:211, 1966

184. Levenson, JE, Crandall, BF, and Sparkes, RS: Partial deletion syndromes of chromosome 18, Ann Ophthalmol 3:756, 1971

185. Levin, H, et al: Aniridia, congenital glaucoma and hydrocephalus in a male infant with ring chromosome 6, Am J Med Genet 25:281, 1986

186. Levy, NS: Juvenile glaucoma in the Rubinstein-Taybi syndrome, J Pediatr Ophthalmol 13:141, 1976

187. Lewis, AJ: The pathology of 18 trisomy, J Pediatr 65:92, 1964

188. Lichter, PR, and Schmickel, RD: Posterior vortex vein and congenital glaucoma in a patient with trisomy 13 syndrome, Am J Ophthalmol 80:939, 1975

189. Lohmann, W: Beitrag zur Kenntnis des reinen Mikrophthalmus, Arch Augenheilkd 86:136, 1920

190. Loken, AC, et al: Hereditary renal dysplasia and blindness, Acta Pediatr Scand 50:177, 1961

191. Lowe, CU, Terrey, M, and MacLachlan, EA: Organic-aciduria, decreased renal ammonia production hydrophthalmos, mental retardation, Am J Dis Child 83:164, 1952

192. Deleted in proofs

193. Lowe, RF: The eyes in mongolism, Br J Ophthalmol 33:131, 1949

194. Lubs, HA, Koenig, EU, and Brandt, IK: Trisomy 13-15: a clinical syndrome, Lancet 1:1001, 1961

195. Lythgoe, C, and Ramsey, MS: Possible case of oculo-cerebro-renal (Lowe's) syndrome in a female infant, Can J Ophthalmol 8:591, 1973

196. Machemer, R: Closed vitrectomy for severe retrolental fibroplasia in the infant, Ophthalmology 90:436, 1983

197. MacKay, CJ, et al: Retinal degeneration with nanophthalmos, cystic macular degeneration, and angle-closure glaucoma. A new recessive syndrome, Arch Ophthalmol 105:366, 1987

198. Deleted in proofs

199. Makley, TA, and Battles, M: Microphthalmos with cyst, report of two cases in the same family, Surv Ophthalmol 13:200, 1969

200. Malbran, E, and Dodds, R: Megalocornea and its relation to congenital glaucoma, Am J Ophthalmol 49:908, 1960

201. Malik, SR, et al: Sclero-cornea, Br J Ophthalmol 49:602, 1965

202. Manschot, WA: Persistent hyperplastic primary vitreous, Arch Ophthalmol 59:188, 1958

203. Manzitti, E, and Lavin, JR: Le glaucome congénitale dans le syndrome de Rubinstein-Taybi, Ann Ocul (Paris) 205:1005, 1972

204. Matsuda, H, and Tanaka, H: A case of 16-18 trisomy syndrome, Tokushima J Exp Med 10:231, 1964

205. Deleted in proofs

206. McCormick, AQ, and Pratt-Johnson, JA: Angle closure glaucoma in infancy, Ophthalmic Surg 2:91, 1971

207. Meier, DA, and Hess, JW: Familial nephropathy with retinitis pigmentosa, A new oculorenal syndrome in adults, Am J Med 39:58, 1965

208. Mets, MB, and Maumenee, IH: The eye and the chromosome, Surv Ophthalmol 28:20, 1983

209. Meyer-Schwickerath, G, Grüterich, E, and Weyers, H: Mikrophthalmussyndrome, Klin Monatsbl Augenheilkd 131:18, 1957

210. Miller, JQ, et al: A specific congenital defect of brain associated with 13-15 trisomy, Am J Dis Child 104:532, 1962

211. Miller, JQ, et al: A specific congenital brain defect (arhinencephaly) in 13-15 trisomy, N Engl J Med 268:120, 1963

212. Miller, M, et al: A chromosomal anomaly with multiple ocular defects, Am J Ophthalmol 55:901, 1963

213. Miller, MT, et al: Anterior segment anomalies associated with the fetal alcohol syndrome, J Pediatr Ophthalmol Strabismus 21:8, 1984

214. Moore, CM, Heller, RH, and Thomas, GH: Developmental abnormalities associated with a ring chromosome 6, J Med Genet 10:299, 1973

215. Deleted in proofs

216. Mullaney, J: Ocular pathology in trisomy 18 (Edwards' syndrome), Am J Ophthalmol 76:246, 1973

217. Neu, RL, and Takashi, K: Partial deletion of long arm of chromosome 18 and deletion of short arm of chromosome 18. In Gardener, LI, editor: Endocrine and genetic diseases of childhood, Philadelphia, 1969

218. Niebuhr, E: Partial trisomies and deletions of chromosome 13. In Yunis, JJ, editor: New chromosomal syndromes, New York, 1977, Academic Press

219. Nieden, A: Cataractbildung bei Teleangiectatischer Ausdehnung der Capillaren der Ganzen Gesichtshaut, Zentralb Parkt Augenheilkd 113:53, 1887

220. Nishi, Y, et al: Ring chromosome 6: case report and review, Am J Med Genet 12:109, 1982

221. O'Grady, RB: Nanophthalmos, Am J Ophthalmol 71:1251, 1971

222. Ogunye, OO, Murray, RF, and Osgood, T: Linkage studies in Lenz microphthalmia, Hum Hered 25:493, 1975

223. Olmer, M, Salvadori, JM, and Pherron, H: Syndrome de Senior-Loken, Nouv Presse Med 3:1032, 1974

224. Olson, JA: Congenital anterior staphyloma. Report of two cases, J Pediatr Ophthalmol 8:177, 1971

225. Deleted in proofs

226. Ozonoff, MB, Steinbach, HL, and Mamunes, P: The trisomy 18 syndrome, Am J Roentgenol 91:618, 1964

227. Panush, RS, et al: Weber-Christian disease, analysis of 15 cases and review of the literature, Medicine 64:181, 1985

228. Passarge, E, et al: Malformations of the central nervous system in trisomy 18 syndrome, J Pediatr 69:771, 1966

229. Patau, K, et al: Multiple congenital anomaly caused by an extra autosome, Lancet 1:790, 1960

230. Peeden, JN, et al: Ring chromosome 6: variability in phenotypic expression, Am J Med Genet 16:563, 1983

231. Perkins, T: Pierre-Robin syndrome, Trans Opthalmol Soc UK 90:179, 1970

232. Peterson, HP: Telangiectasis and cataract, Acta Ophthalmol (Copenh) 32:565, 1954

233. Peyman, GA, Sanders, DR, and Nagpal, KC: Management of persistent hyperplastic primary vitreous, Br J Ophthalmol 60:756, 1976

234. Pfeiffer, RA, Erpenstein, H, and Jünemann, G: Oculo-dento-digitale dysplasie, Klin Monatsbl Augenheilkd 152:247, 1968

235. Pišteljić, DT, et al: Poland syndrome associated with 'morning glory' syndrome (coloboma of the optic disc), J Med Genet 23:364, 1986

236. Polak, BCP, Hogewind, BL, and Van Lith, FHM: Tapetoretinal degeneration associated with recessively inherited medullary cystic disease, Am J Ophthalmol 84:645, 1977

237. Pollard, ZF: Secondary angle-closure glaucoma in cicatricial retrolental fibroplasia, Am J Ophthalmol 89:651, 1980

238. Polomeno, RC, and Milot, J: Congenital miosis, Can J Ophthalmol 14:43, 1979

239. Ponte, F: Further contributions to the study of the syndrome of Hallermann and Streiff (congenital cataract with bird's face), Ophthalmologica 143:399, 1962

240. Popoff, N, and Wheelock, MC: Relapsing febrile nodular nonsupprative panniculitis, Arch Intern Med 97:39, 1956

241. Quigley, HA, and Stanish, FS: Unilateral congenital iris pigment epithelial hyperplasia associated with late-onset glaucoma, Am J Ophthalmol 86:182, 1978

242. Rados, A: Conical cornea and mongolism, Arch Ophthalmol 40:454, 1948

243. Rajic, DS, and Veber, LL: Hereditary oculodentoosseous dysplasia, Ann Radiol (Paris) 9:224, 1966

244. Reese, AB: Persistence and hyperplasia of primary vitreous; retrolental fibroplasia-two entities, Arch Ophthalmol 41:527, 1949

245. Reese, AB: Persistent hyperplastic primary vitreous, Trans Am Acad Ophthalmol Otolaryngol 59:271, 1955

246. Reese, AB, and Straatsma, BR: Retinal dysplasia, Am J Ophthalmol 45:199, 1958

247. Reisner, SH, et al: Oculodentodigital dysplasia, Am J Dis Child 118:600, 1969

248. Rinaldi, E, et al: Morning glory syndrome with chronic simple glaucoma, Ophthalmic Paediatr Genet 7:69, 1986

249. Ritch, R, et al: Congenital ectropion uveae with glaucoma, Ophthalmology 91:326, 1984

250. Robin, MP: La chute de la base de la langue considérée comme une nouvelle cause de géne dans la respiration nasopharyngienne, Bull Acad Natl Med (Paris) 89:37, 1923

251. Robin, P: Glossoptosis due to atresia and hypotrophy of the mandible, Am J Dis Child 48:542, 1934

252. Rodrigues, MM, Calhoun, J, and Weinreb, S: Sclerocornea with an unbalanced translocation (17p,10q), Am J Ophthalmol 78:49, 1974

253. Rogers, GL, and Polomeno, RC: Autosomal-dominant inheritance of megalocornea associated with Down's syndrome, Am J Ophthalmol 78:526, 1974

254. Rogers, TR, Hagstrom, JWC, and Engle, MA: Origin of both great vessels from the right ventricle associated with the trisomy-18 syndrome, Circ Res 32:802, 1965

255. Rohde, RA, Hodgman, JE, and Cleland, RS: Multiple congenital anomalies in the E-trisomy (Group 16-18) syndrome, Pediatrics 33:258, 1964

256. Ronen, S, et al: The early management of a baby with Hallermann-Streiff-François syndrome, J Pediatr 16:119, 1979

257. Rosenfield, RL, et al: Trisomy of chromosomes 13-15 and 17-18: its association with infantile arteriorsclerosis, Am J Med Sci 135:763, 1962

258. Roy, FH, Summitt, RL, Hiatt, RL, and Hughes, JG: Ocular manifestations of the Rubinstein-Taybi syndrome, Arch Ophthalmol, 79:272, 1968

259. Rubinstein, JH, and Taybi, H: Broad thumbs and toes and facial abnormalities, a possible mental retardation syndrome, Am J Dis Child, 105:88, 1963

260. Ruedemann, AD: Osteogenesis imperfecta congenita and blue sclerotics, a clinicopathologic study, Arch Ophthalmol 49:6, 1953

261. Ryan, EA, Zwann, J, and Chylack, LT: Nanophthalmos with uveal effusion. Clinical and embryologic considerations, Ophthalmology 89:1013, 1982

262. Salamanca-Gomez, F, Nava, S, and Armendares, S: Ring chromosome 6 in a malformed boy, Clin Genet 8:370, 1975

263. Saudan, Y: Diagnostic differential clinique des arthrites peripheriques, Radiol Clin Biol 43:283, 1974

264. Schanzlin, DJ, Goldberg, DB, and Brown, SI: Hallermann-Streiff syndrome associated with sclerocornea, aniridia, and a chromosomal abnormality, Am J Ophthalmol 90:411, 1980

265. Schanzlin, DJ, et al: Histopathologic and ultrastructural analysis of congenital corneal staphyloma, Am J Ophthalmol 95:506, 1983

266. Schimke, RN: Hereditary renal-retinal dysplasia, Ann Intern Med 70:735, 1969

267. Schreiner, RL, et al: Stickler syndrome in a pedigree of Pierre Robin syndrome, Am J Dis Child 126:86, 1973

268. Schuman, JS, et al: Senior-Loken syndrome (familial renal-retinal dystrophy) and Coats' disease, Am J Ophthalmol 100:822, 1985

269. Schwartz, DE: Noonan's syndrome associated with ocular abnormalities, Am J Ophthalmol 73:955, 1972

270. Schwartz, L: Ateliosis of the mandibular arch, Arch Otolaryngol 31:491, 1940

271. Schweitzer, NMJ: Megalocornea, Ophthalmologica 144;304, 1962

272. Senior, B: Familial renal-retinal dystrophy, Am J Dis Child 125:442, 1973

273. Senior, B, Friedmann, FR, and Braudo, MR: Juvenile familial nephropathy with tapetoretinal degeneration, Am J Ophthalmol 52:625, 1961

274. Sergovich, F, et al: The D trisomy syndrome: a case report with a description of ocular pathology, Can Med Assoc J 89:151, 1963

275. Shaffer, RN, and Weiss, DJ, editors: Congenital and pediatric glaucomas, St. Louis, 1970, The CV Mosby Co

276. Shapiro, MB, and France, TD: The ocular features of Down's syndrome, Am J Ophthalmol 99:659, 1985

277. Shihab, ZM: Pediatric glaucoma in Rubinstein-Taybi syndrome, Glaucoma 12:288, 1984

278. Shorb, SR: Bilateral ametropic amblyopia resulting from bilateral cornea plana, Am J Ophthalmol 73:663, 1972

279. Silver, DN, Lewis, AL, and Nussbaum, RL: Mapping the Lowe oculocerebrorenal syndrome to Xq24-q26 by use of restriction fragment length polymorphisms, J Clin Invest 79:282, 1987

280. Singh, OS, et al: Nanopthalmos, a perspective on identification and therapy, Ophthalmology 89:1006, 1982

281. Smith, DW: Recognizable patterns of human malformation, Philadelphia, 1970, WB Saunders

282. Smith, DW, Patau, K, and Therman, E: Autosomal trisomy syndromes, Lancet 1:211, 1961

283. Smith, DW, et al: A new autosomal trisomy syndrome: multiple congenital anomalies caused by an extra chromosome, J Pediatr 57:338, 1960

284. Smith, DW, et al: The D₁ trisomy syndrome, J Pediatr 62:326, 1963

285. Smith, DW, et al: The no. 18 trisomy syndrome, J Pediatr 60:513, 1962

286. Smith, JL, Cavanaugh, JA, and Stowe, FC: Ocular manifestations of the Pierre Robin syndrome, Arch Ophthalmol 63:110, 1960

287. Smith, JL, and Stowe, FR: The Pierre Robin syndrome (glossoptosis, micrognathia, cleft palate), a review of 39 cases with emphasis on associated ocular lesions, Pediatrics 27:128, 1961

288. Smith, RE, and Maumenee, AE: Persistent hyperplastic primary vitreous, results of surgery, Trans Am Acad Ophthalmol 78:911, 1974

289. Stanescu, B, and Dralands, L: Cerebro-hepato-renal (Zellweger's) syndrome, Arch Ophthalmol 87:590, 1972

290. Stark, WJ, et al: Persistent hyperplastic primary vitreous, surgical treatment, Ophthalmology 90:452, 1983

291. Steele, RW, and Bass, JW: Hallermann-Streiff syndrome, clinical and prognostic considerations, Am J Dis Child 120:462, 1970

292. Steinberg, JB, and Jackson, JF: The 16-18 trisomy syndrome, Am J Dis Child 105:213, 1963

293. Steinkuller, PG: The morning glory disk anomaly: case report and literature review, J Pediatr Ophthalmol Strabismus, 17:81, 1980

294. Stickler, GB, et al: Hereditary progressive arthro-ophthalmopathy, Mayo Clin Proc 40:433, 1965

295. Stirt, JA: Anesthetic problems in Rubinstein-Taybi syndrome, Anesth Analg 60:534, 1981

296. Stirt, JA: Succinylcholine in Rubinstein-Taybi syndrome, Anesthesiology 57:429, 1982

297. Streiff, EB: Dysmorphie mandibulo-faciale (tête d'-oiseau) et altérations oculaires, Ophthalmologica 120:79, 1950

298. Sugar, HS: Oculodentodigital dysplasia syndrome with angle closure glaucoma, Am J Ophthalmol 86:36, 1978

299. Sugar, HS, Thompson, JP, and Davis, JD: The Oculo-dento-digital dysplasia syndrome, Am J Ophthalmol 61:1448, 1966

300. Svorc, J, et al: Oculo-cerebro-renal syndrome in a female child, Am J Dis Child 114:124, 1970

301. Swett, WE: Congenital cornea plana, Am J Ophthalmol 7:437, 1924

302. Tawara, A, and Inomata, H: Familial cases of congenital microcoria associated with late onset con-

genital glaucoma and goniodysgenesis, Jpn J Opthalmol 27:63, 1983

303. Taylor, AI: Patau's, Edwards' and Cri du Chat syndromes: a tabulated summary of current findings,
Dev Med Child Neurol 9:78, 1967

304. Taylor, AI: Autosomy trisomy syndromes: a detailed study of 27 cases of Edwards' syndrome and
27 cases of Patau's syndrome, J Med Genet 5:227,
1968

305. Taylor, DSI: The genetic implications of optic disc
anomalies, Trans Ophthalmol Soc UK 104:853, 1985

306. Theil, PL: Ophthalmological examination of patients in long-term treatment with tranexamic acid,
Acta Ophthalmol (Copenh) 59:237, 1981

307. Therman, E, et al: The D trisomy syndrome and
XO gonadal dysgenesis: dysgenesis in two sisters,
Am J Hum Genet 13:193, 1961

308. Thompson, and Thompson, editors: Genetics in
medicine, Philadelphia, 1980, WB Saunders

309. Tinning, S, Jacobsen, P, and Mikkelsen, M: A (1;6)
translocation associated with congenital glaucoma
and cleft lip and palate, Hum Hered 25:453, 1975

310. Townes, PL, et al: Trisomy 13-15 in a male infant,
J Pediatr 60:528, 1962

311. Townes, PL, et al: Observations on the pathology
of the trisomy 17-18 syndrome, J Pediatr, 62:703,
1963

312. Townes, PL, Manning, JA, and Dehart, GK, Jr: Trisomy 18(16-18) associated with congenital glaucoma and optic atrophy, J Pediatr 61:755, 1962

313. Trese, MT: Surgical results of stage V retrolental
fibroplasia and timing of surgical repair, Ophthalmology 91:461, 1984

314. Tripathi, RC, Cibis, GW, and Tripathi, BJ: Pathogenesis of cataracts in patients with Lowe's syndrome, Ophthalmology, 93:1046, 1986

315. Turner, HH: A syndrome of infantilism, congenital
webbed neck, and cubitus valgus, Endocrinology
23:566, 1938

316. Twarog, FJ: Urticaria in childhood: pathogenesis
and management, Pediatr Clin North Am 30:887,
1983

317. Uchida, IA, Bowman, JM, and Wang, HC: The 18-
trisomy syndrome, New Engl J Med 266:1198, 1962

318. Ullrich, O: Der status Bonnevie-Ullrich im Rahmen
anderer dyscranio-dysphalangien, Ergeb Inn Med
Kinderheilkd 2:412, 1951

319. Vail, DT: Adult hereditary anterior megalophthalmos sine glaucoma: a definite disease entity, Arch
Ophthalmol 6:39, 1931

320. van Balen, ATM, and van Collenburg, JJM: Tapetoretinal degeneration and familial juvenile nephronophthisis (FJN), J Pediatr Ophthalmol 13:329, 1976

321. Veirs, ER, and Brown, W: Congenital miosis, Arch
Ophthalmol 65:83, 1961

322. Voorhess, ML, Aspillaga, MJ, and Gardner, LI: Trisomy 18 syndrome with absent radius, varus deformity of hand, and rudimentary thumb, J Pediatr
65:130, 1964

323. Voorhess, ML, Vaharu, T, and Gardner, LI: Trisomy
16-18 syndrome, Lancet, 1:992, 1962

324. Walsh, FB, and Hoyt, WF: Clinical neuro-ophthalmology II, ed 3, Baltimore, 1969, Williams & Wilkins

325. Walton, DS: Congenital glaucoma associated with
congenital cataract, J Pediatr Ophthalmol 15:221,
1972

326. Walton, DS: Retrolental fibroplasia with glaucoma.
In Chandler, DA, and Grant, WM, editors: Glaucoma, ed 2, Philadelphia, 1979, Lea & Fibiger

327. Wan, WL, Minckler, DS, Rao, NA: Pupillary-block
glaucoma associated with childhood cystinosis, Am
J Ophthalmol 101:700, 1986

328. Warburg, M, and Mikkelsen, M: A case of 13-15
trisomy or Bartholin-Patau's syndrome, Acta Ophthalmol (Copenh), 41:321, 1963

329. Deleted in proofs

330. Waring, GO, Rodrigues, MM, and Laibson, PR: Anterior chamber cleavage syndrome. A stepladder
classification, Surv Ophthalmol 20:3, 1975

331. Waring, GO, Roth, AM, and Rodrigues, MM: Clinicopathologic correlation of microphthalmos with
cyst, Am J Ophthalmol 82:714, 1976

332. Warkany, J, Passarge, E, and Smith, LB: Congenital
malformations in autosomal trisomy syndromes,
Am J Dis Child 112:502, 1966

333. Weber, FP: A case of relapsing non-suppurative
nodular panniculitis, showing phagocytosis of subcutaneous fat-cells by macrophages, Br J Dermatol
37:301, 1925

334. Weber, JW, and Schwarz, H: Der Typus Rostockien-
sis Ullrich-Feichtiger Dyskranio-pyo-phalangie,
Helv Paediatr Acta 15:163, 1960

335. Weber, U, and Bernsmeier, H: Rubinstein-Taybi-
Syndrom und Juveniles Glaukom, Klin Monatsbl
Augenheilkd 183:47, 1983

336. Weber, WW, et al: Trisomy 17-18(E): studies in long-
term survival with report of two autopsied cases,
Pediatrics 34:533, 1964

337. Weizenblatt, S: Congenital malformations of cornea
associated with embryonic arrest of ectodermal and
mesodermal structures, Arch Ophthalmol 52:415,
1954

338. Weintraub, DM, Baum, JL, and Pashayan, HM: A
family with oculodentodigital dysplasia, Cleft Palate J 12:323, 1975

339. Williams, RDB: Brushfield spots and Wofflin nodules in the iris: an appraisal in handicapped children, Dev Med Child Neurol 23:646, 1981

340. Wilson, WA, Richards, W, and Donnell, GN: Oculocerebral-renal syndrome of Lowe, Arch Ophthalmol 70:5, 1963

341. Wilson, WG, et al: Trisomy 18/Trisomy 13, mosaicism in an adult with profound mental retardation
and multiple malformations, Am J Med Genet
16:131, 1983

342. Wolf, U, et al: Deletion on short arms of a B-chro-
mosome without "Cri du Chat" syndrome, Lancet,
1:769, 1965

343. Wolter, JR, and Butler, RG: Pigment spots of the iris and ectropion uveae, with glaucoma in neurofibromatosis, Am J Ophthalmol 56:964, 1963

344. Wong, VG: The eye and cystinosis. In Schulman, JD, editor: Cystinosis, Washington, D.C., 1972, U.S. Dept Health, Education, and Welfare

345. Wong, VG, Lietman, PS, and Seegmiller, JE: Alterations of pigment epithelium in cystinosis, Arch Ophthalmol 77:361, 1967

346. Yanoff, M, Frayer, WC, and Scheie, HG: Ocular findings in a patient with 13-15 trisomy, Arch Ophthalmol 70:372, 1963

347. Yanoff, M, Roarke, LB, and Niederer, BS: Ocular and cerebral abnormalities in chromosome 18 deletion defect, Am J Ophthalmol 70:391, 1970

348. Young, RS, et al: Deletions of the long arm of chromosome 6: two new cases and review of the literature, Am J Med Genet 20:21, 1985

349. Young, NJA, et al: Stickler's syndrome and neovascular glaucoma, Br J Ophthalmol 63:826, 1979

350. Zayid, I, and Farraj, S: Familial histiocytic dermatoarthritis, a new syndrome, Am J Med 54: 793, 1973

351. Zellweger, H, Beck, K, and Hawtrey, CE: Trisomy 18 report of a case and discussion of the syndrome, Arch Intern Med 113:598, 1964

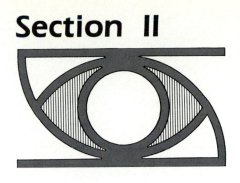
Glaucomas Associated with Ocular Disease

Chapter 54

Glaucomas Associated with Primary Disorders of the Corneal Endothelium

M. Bruce Shields
John E. Bourgeois

The common denominator of the glaucomas discussed in this chapter is a primary abnormality of the corneal endothelium. Two of these conditions, the iridocorneal endothelial syndrome and posterior polymorphous dystrophy, represent spectra of clinical and histopathologic abnormalities in which there is strong evidence that the corneal endothelial disorder leads to, or is directly associated with, the changes responsible for the glaucoma. In a third disorder, Fuchs' endothelial dystrophy, the relationship between the corneal disorder and associated glaucoma is not as well understood.

IRIDOCORNEAL ENDOTHELIAL SYNDROME

History and Terminology

In 1903, Harms[31] described a form of secondary glaucoma associated with extreme atrophy of the iris and hole formation. The condition has been called *essential iris atrophy*, or *progressive essential iris atrophy*. Chandler,[17] in 1956, reported cases that were similar to essential iris atrophy but different in that changes in the iris were limited to slight corectopia and mild stromal atrophy. In addition, corneal edema, which may also be seen in essential iris atrophy, appeared to be a more consistent feature, often occurring at intraocular pressures that were normal or only slightly elevated. In all cases, Chandler noted an abnormality of the corneal endothelium, which he described as having the ap-

pearance of fine, hammered silver. The condition became known as *Chandler's syndrome*. In both essential iris atrophy and Chandler's syndrome, the glaucoma is associated with progressive closure of the anterior chamber angle.

In 1969, Cogan and Reese[21] described two patients with pigmented nodules of the iris, associated with some features similar to essential iris atrophy and Chandler's syndrome. Enucleation for suspected melanoma was performed in both cases, but the nodules were found to be benign, composed of tissue resembling that of the iris stroma. Subsequent studies[66,68] revealed that these nodules may occur on the surface of the iris in association with the complete spectrum of changes seen with essential iris atrophy and Chandler's syndrome,[61,68] and such a condition has become known as the *Cogan-Reese syndrome*. Scheie and Yanoff[61] also described similar cases with diffuse nevi, rather than nodules, on the surface of iris. This condition has been called the *iris nevus syndrome*.

Continued study of these conditions has led to the theory that each one represents a clinical variation within a single spectrum of disease.[16,67,69] The common denominator is a characteristic abnormality of the corneal endothelium that leads, in some cases, to variable degrees of corneal edema, progressive closure of the anterior chamber angle with secondary glaucoma, and the spectrum of iris changes described above. Yanoff[82] suggested the

Table 54-1 *Iridocorneal endothelial (ICE) syndrome*

Major clinical variations	Characteristic features
Progressive iris atrophy	Iris features predominate with marked corectopia, atrophy, and hole formation
Chandler's syndrome	Changes in the iris are mild to absent, whereas corneal edema, often at normal intraocular pressures, is typical
Cogan-Reese syndrome	Nodular, pigmented lesions of the iris are the hallmark and may be seen with the entire spectrum of corneal and other iris defects

name *iridocorneal endothelial (ICE) syndrome* for this spectrum of clinical and histopathologic abnormalities, and this has become the most commonly used term. It has been common practice, however, to retain the identity and terminology of the major clinical variations (Table 54-1). Since atrophy of the iris is not an essential or fundamental aspect of these disorders, the term *progressive iris atrophy* may be preferable for the variation previously known as essential iris atrophy. Chandler's syndrome is distinguished from progressive iris atrophy by milder or absent iris changes and possibly more common corneal edema. There are also intermediate variations between progressive iris atrophy and Chandler's syndrome, in which changes in the iris are more extensive than in Chandler's syndrome, but lack the hole formation of progressive iris atrophy. The Cogan-Reese syndrome is characterized by iris nodules, which have a histologic appearance resembling that of iris stroma, associated with any degree of corneal edema or iris atrophy. The iris nevus syndrome differs from the Cogan-Reese syndrome by the presence of more diffuse, flat iris lesions with the histologic structure of nevi. There has been a tendency to lump the Cogan-Reese and iris nevus syndromes together as a single entity, but further study is needed to determine whether the iris nevus syndrome is truly a variation of the ICE syndrome or a separate entity.[72]

General Features

The ICE syndrome is almost always clinically unilateral, although subclinical abnormalities in the corneal endothelium of the fellow eye are common. The condition is usually recognized in early to middle adulthood, with a predilection for women. Familial cases are rare, and there is no consistent association with systemic diseases.[66,67]

The most common manifestations of the ICE syndrome are abnormalities of the iris, reduced visual acuity, and pain. The patients may first notice an abnormal shape or position of their pupil, or they may describe a localized or diffuse dark spot on the iris, which usually represents an area of stromal atrophy or full-thickness hole formation. The reduced vision and pain are typically the result of the corneal edema but may result from the secondary glaucoma later in the course of the disease. Patients commonly note a mild blur in the morning hours when the cornea is slightly swollen as the result of lid closure during sleep. With exposure to air, however, the cornea may begin to dehydrate during the day, resulting in gradual improvement in vision. As the severity of the disease progresses, the corneal edema may persist throughout the day, with marked visual loss and pain. This may occur with or without elevated intraocular pressure. However, as secondary glaucoma develops, the ocular tension can aggravate the corneal edema and associated symptoms. In addition, advanced stages of glaucoma may lead to visual reduction from optic atrophy and occasional pain from the high intraocular pressure.

Clinicopathologic Features

Corneal alterations

A common feature throughout the ICE syndrome is a corneal endothelial abnormality, which can be seen by slit-lamp biomicroscopy as a fine, hammered silver appearance of the posterior cornea, similar to that of Fuchs' dystrophy (Fig. 54-1). This defect may occur by itself without symptoms or may cause corneal edema with variable degrees of reduced vision and pain, as noted above. In some cases, islands of the endothelial abnormality may be seen in the fellow eye, which is otherwise unaffected by the disease process.

Specular microscopy of the corneal endothelial cells reveals a characteristic, diffuse abnormality with variable degrees of pleomorphism in size and shape, dark areas within the cells, and loss of the clear hexagonal margins (Fig. 54-2).[34,46,65,75,77] These morphologic changes have been seen in patients with progressive iris atrophy, Chandler's syndrome, and the Cogan-Reese syndrome, although we are not aware of any such reports in patients with the iris nevus syndrome. Some studies have revealed focal areas of normal and abnormal cells separated by a distinct border,[10,46] with gradual disappearance of the normal areas over time.[10] Decreased endothelial cell counts and cellular pleo-

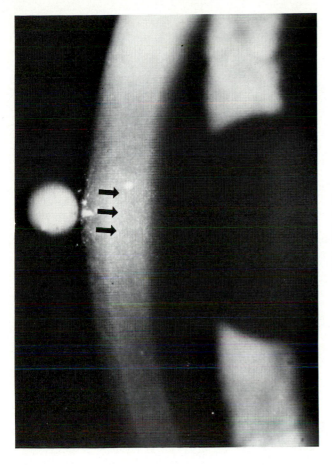

Fig. 54-1 Slit-lamp view showing fine beaten silver appearance of corneal endothelial abnormality *(arrows)* in ICE syndrome (Reprinted with permission from Shields, MB, Campbell, DG, and Simmons, R Jr: Am J Ophthalmol 85:749, 1978. Published with permission from The American Journal of Ophthalmology. Copyright by The Ophthalmic Publishing Company)

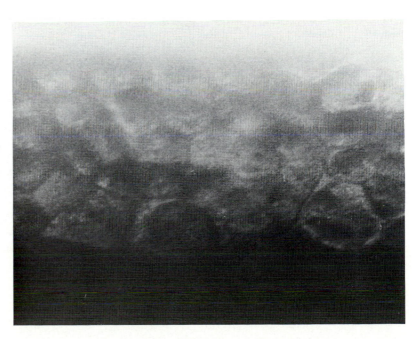

Fig. 54-2 Specular microscopic appearance of corneal endothelial cells in ICE syndrome showing pleomorphism in size, shape, dark areas within cells, and loss of clear hexagonal margins. (Courtesy LW Hirst, MD)

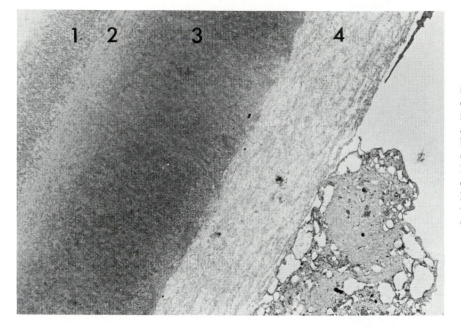

Fig. 54-3 Transmission electron microscopic view of inner corneal surface in ICE syndrome showing part of abnormal cell on four-layered membrane, composed of anterior nonbanded *(1)* and posterior banded *(2)* portions of Descemet's membrane with abnormal compact collagenous *(3)* and loose collagenous *(4)* layers (×6,875). (Reprinted with permission from Shields, MB, et al: Ophthalmology 86:1533, 1979)

Fig. 54-4 Gonioscopic view of patient with ICE syndrome showing peripheral anterior synechiae *(PAS)* extending beyond trabecular meshwork *(TM)* to Schwalbe's line *(SL)*. (Reprinted with permission from Shields, MB, et al: Ophthalmol 85:749, 1978. Published with permission from The American Journal of Ophthalmology. Copyright by The Ophthalmic Publishing Company)

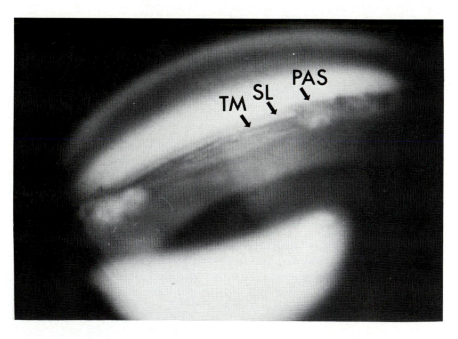

morphism have also been observed in fellow, asymptomatic eyes of patients with the ICE syndrome.[42] Endothelial permeability, studied by fluorophotometry, was markedly decreased in the eye with the clinically apparent disorder, but normal in the fellow eye.[11]

Electron microscopic study of the posterior cornea in advanced cases has revealed grossly abnormal cells lining multilayered collagenous tissue posterior to Descemet's membrane* (Fig. 54-3). There is considerable variation, however, in the reported appearance of this cellular layer. In some cases, the cells are markedly attenuated or absent, exposing areas of the underlying collagenous layer,[69] whereas other specimens reveal multiple cellular layers, suggesting loss of contact inhibition.[1] Some cells have filopodial cytoplasmic projections, indicative of cellular migration.[1,59] Some cells show evidence of metabolic activity, while others appear disrupted and necrotic.[1] There are conflicting reports regarding the basic nature of the cells, with some describing evidence of epithelial cells.[33,50] Most studies, however, suggest that the cells are endothelial in structure, and immunohistochemical studies have revealed no evidence of epithelial characteristics.[59] Occasional lymphocytes have been seen on or within this cellular layer.[1,59] The underlying collagenous layer consists of a thin, normally appearing Descemet's membrane bounded posteriorly by thickened layers with banded and fibrillar tissue. The latter observations suggest that the abnormal collagen was deposited by the abnormal endothelial cells in postnatal life, years before clinical recognition of the disease.[2] Histologic study of the fellow eye of a 75-year-old woman with the ICE syndrome revealed severe corneal endothelial dystrophy with marked corneal guttata.[27]

Anterior chamber angle alterations

Peripheral anterior synechiae, usually extending to or beyond Schwalbe's line, are common to all variations of the ICE syndrome (Fig. 54-4). Histologic studies reveal a cellular membrane consisting of a single layer of endothelial cells and a Descemet-like membrane extending down from the peripheral cornea. The membrane may cover an open anterior chamber angle in some areas or may be associated with synechial closure of the angle elsewhere in the same eye.[16,25,49,57,58]

The synechial closure of the anterior chamber

angle is typically progressive, eventually leading to intraocular pressure elevation in a large percentage of cases. However, the secondary glaucoma does not correlate precisely with the degree of synechial closure,[67] and it has been reported to occur when the entire angle was open, but apparently covered by the cellular membrane.[5,80] Presumably, obstruction to aqueous outflow may result from either the membrane covering the trabecular meshwork or synechial closure of the anterior chamber angle.

Alterations of the iris

The abnormalities of the iris constitute the primary basis for distinguishing clinical variations within the ICE syndrome.

Progressive iris atrophy. Progressive iris atrophy is characterized by marked atrophy of the iris, associated with variable degrees of corectopia and ectropion uveae. The latter two features are usually directed toward the quadrant with the most prominent area of peripheral anterior synechiae.[16,67] The hallmark of progressive iris atrophy is hole formation of the iris, which occurs in two forms: stretch holes, and melting holes.[67] With stretch holes, the iris is markedly thinned in the quadrant away from the direction of pupillary distortion, and the holes develop within the area that is being stretched (Fig. 54-5). In other eyes, melting holes develop without associated corectopia or thinning of the iris (Fig. 54-6). Fluorescein angiographic studies suggest that thinning of the iris is associated with iris ischemia (Fig. 54-7).[68]

Histopathologic findings of the iris in this and all variations of the ICE syndrome include a cellular membrane on portions of the anterior surface of the iris (Fig. 54-8), which is similar to and continuous with that seen over the anterior chamber angle.[16,25,49] The membrane is most often found in the quadrant toward which the pupil is distorted, with marked iris atrophy and hole formation in the opposite quadrant.[16]

Chandler's syndrome. In Chandler's syndrome, there is typically minimal corectopia and mild atrophy of the iris stroma (Fig. 54-9).[17] In some cases there may be no detectable change in the iris. Intermediate variations may also be seen, in which the degree of corectopia and stromal iris atrophy is more extensive than that typically seen in Chandler's syndrome, but the characteristic hole formation of progressive iris atrophy is lacking. The histopathologic findings are the same as those

---

*References 1, 2, 25, 33, 49-51, 53, 59, 69, 78.

Text continued on p. 972.

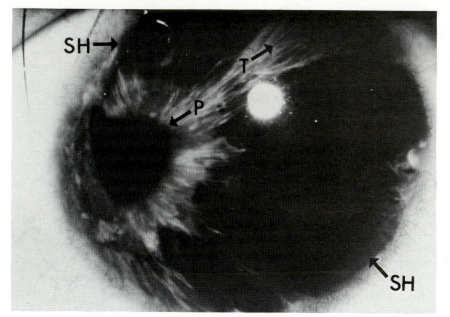

Fig. 54-5 Progressive iris atrophy, a variation of ICE syndrome, with pupillary distortion *(P)*, thinning of iris *(T)*, and stretch holes *(SH)*. (Reprinted with permission from Shields, MB: Surv Ophthalmol 24:3, 1979; Courtesy RJ Simmons, MD)

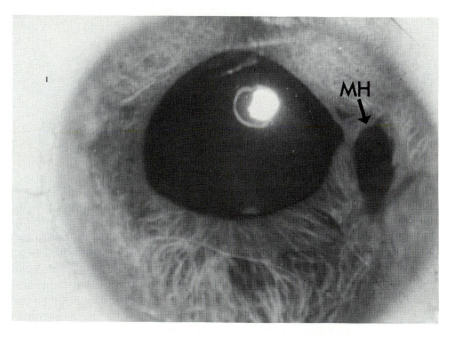

Fig. 54-6 Progressive iris atrophy, a variation of ICE syndrome, with melting hole *(MH)*. (Reprinted with permission from Shields, MB, et al: Am J Ophthalmol 85:749, 1978. Published with permission from The American Journal of Ophthalmology. Copyright by The Ophthalmic Publishing Company)

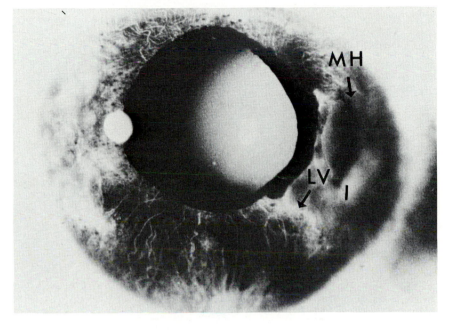

Fig. 54-7 Fluorescein angiographic view of eye in Fig. 54-6, showing ischemia *(I)* and leakage *(arrows)* around melting hole. (Reprinted with permission from Shields, MB, et al: Am J Ophthalmol 85:749, 1978. Published with permission from The American Journal of Ophthalmology. Copyright by The Ophthalmic Publishing Company)

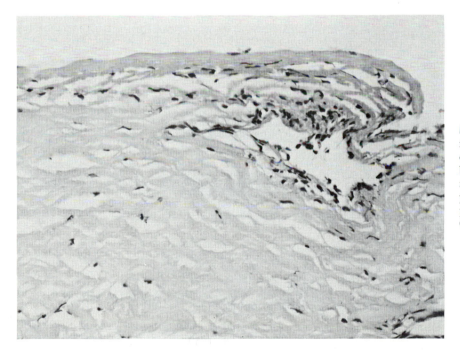

Fig. 54-8 Light microscopic view of iris specimen from eye with ICE syndrome showing Descemet-like membrane and scant monolayer of cells *(arrow)* extending across stroma (Hematoxylin-eosin, × 250). (Reprinted with permission from Shields, MB, et al: Ophthalmology 86:1533, 1979)

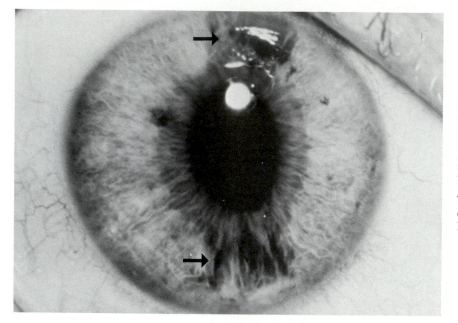

Fig. 54-9 Chandler's syndrome, a variation of ICE syndrome, with slight pupillary distortion and thinning of iris stroma at vertical poles *(arrows)*. (Reprinted with permission from Shields, MB, et al: Am J Ophthalmol 85:749, 1978. Published with permission from The American Journal of Ophthalmology. Copyright by The Ophthalmic Publishing Company)

Fig. 54-10 Cogan-Reese syndrome, a variation of ICE syndrome, showing ectropion uveae *(white arrow)*, numerous dark nodules *(black arrows)* on area of flattened iris stroma. (Reprinted with permission from Shields, MB, et al.: Arch Ophthalmol 94:406, 1976. Copyright 1976, American Medical Association)

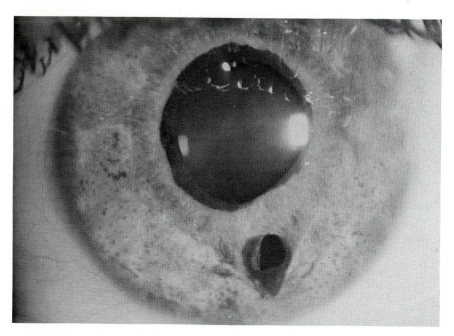

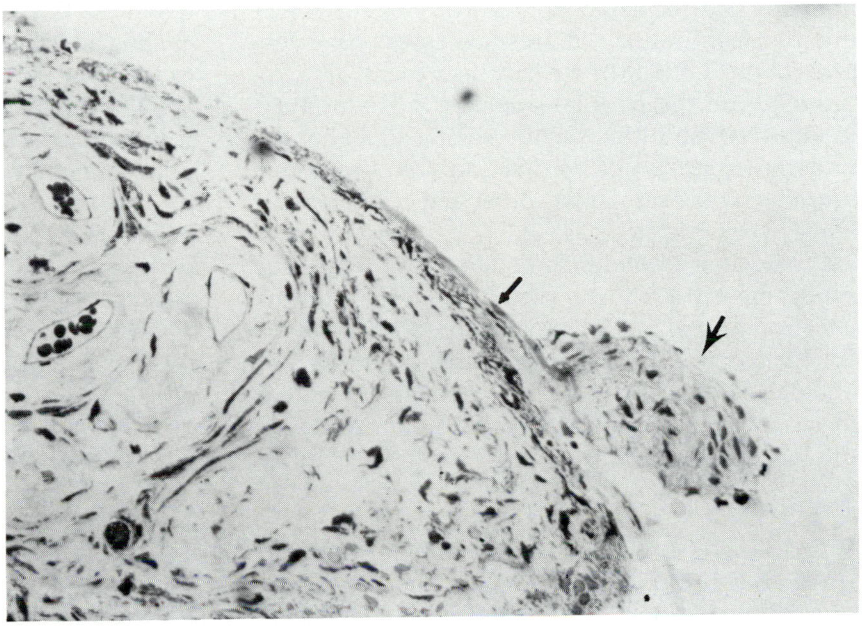

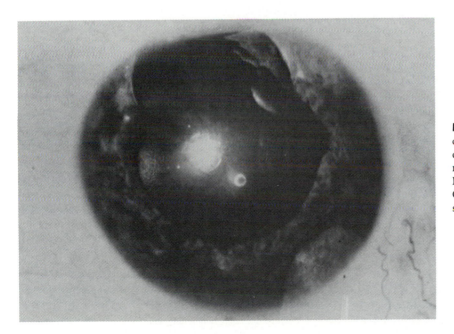

Fig. 54-11 Light microscopic view of iridectomy specimen from eye with Cogan-Reese syndrome showing nodule composed of cells resembling iris stroma *(large arrow)*, portion of monolayer of spindle-shaped cells *(small arrow)*. (Toluidine blue and basic fuchsin, ×200). (Reprinted with permission from Shields, MB, et al: Arch Ophthalmol 94:406, 1976)

Fig. 54-12 Example of iris nevus syndrome with diffuse, pigmented lesion on surface of iris. (Reprinted with permission from Scheie, HG, and Yanoff, M: Arch Ophthalmol 93:963, 1976. Copyright 1976, American Medical Association)

seen in progressive iris atrophy, with the exception of the extensive iris atrophy and hole formation.

Cogan-Reese syndrome.   The eyes with Cogan-Reese syndrome may have any degree of iris atrophy but are distinguished by the presence of pigmented, pedunculated nodules on the surface of the iris (Fig. 54-10).[21,61,68] In some cases, other features of the ICE syndrome may be present for many years before the nodules appear.[22,68] The nodular lesions have an ultrastructure similar to that of the underlying stroma of the iris and are always surrounded by the previously described cellular membrane* (Fig. 54-11).

Iris nevus syndrome.   The hallmark of iris nevus syndrome is the diffuse, pigmented lesions on the iris stroma (Fig. 54-12), which are reported to have the histologic appearance of nevi.[61] As previously noted, however, it has yet to be confirmed whether these cases have the other features that characterize the ICE syndrome.

Theories of Mechanism

The precise etiologic factors of the ICE syndrome are unknown. The infrequency of familial cases and the histologic evidence that corneal alterations begin in postnatal life argue against an inherited or congenital disorder. The observation of lymphocytes on or in the corneal endothelial layer[1,2,59] suggests the presence of chronic inflammation and has led to the theory of a viral cause.[1,2] However, occasional lymphocytes have also been seen within the corneal endothelium of an eye with posterior polymorphous dystrophy, an inherited corneal disease, suggesting that these may be normal *passenger* cells migrating in the endothelial layer.[59] Therefore, the underlying cause of the corneal endothelial abnormality in the ICE syndrome is not known, although there is strong evidence that it is this fundamental abnormality that leads to the other clinicopathologic features in this spectrum of disease.

The membrane theory of Campbell et al.[16] maintains that the abnormality of the corneal endothelium in the ICE syndrome causes the corneal edema and also leads to the proliferation of the cellular membrane across the anterior chamber angle and onto the surface of the iris (Fig. 54-13). Contracture of the cellular portion of this membrane causes the formation of peripheral anterior synechiae, the corectopia, and the ectropion uveae.

Stretching of the iris in the direction away from the corectopia is believed to contribute to the atrophy and hole formation, although additional factors, such as ischemia, may also be involved.[66] The cellular membrane is also thought to be responsible for the development of the nodular lesions of the iris in the Cogan-Reese syndrome, possibly by encircling and pinching off portions of the iris stroma to form the nodules.[15,26]

The mechanism of secondary glaucoma in the ICE syndrome is also believed to be related to the cellular membrane. In some cases, the membrane may cover the trabecular meshwork, which is still visible gonioscopically, thereby obstructing aqueous outflow. In most cases, however, the intraocular pressure does not begin to rise until contracture of the membrane has led to some degree of synechial closure of the anterior chamber angle.

Differential Diagnosis

There are several other disorders of the cornea and iris, many of which have associated glaucoma, that could be confused with the various forms of the ICE syndrome. It is helpful to think of these in the following three categories[66,67]: corneal endothelial disorders, dissolution of the iris, and nodular lesions of the iris.

Corneal endothelial disorders

Posterior polymorphous dystrophy may have associated glaucoma, as well as changes of the anterior chamber angle and iris that resemble the ICE syndrome. However, the difference in appearance of the posterior corneal abnormalities, as well as the familial tendency and bilateral nature of posterior polymorphous dystrophy, help distinguish these two spectra of disease. Fuchs' endothelial dystrophy has corneal changes that are clinically similar to those of the ICE syndrome, but none of the chamber angle or iris features of the latter condition. Both of these conditions are discussed in more detail later in this chapter.

Dissolution of the iris

The Axenfeld-Rieger syndrome (see Chapter 50) has striking clinical and histopathologic similarities to the ICE syndrome, but the congenital nature and bilaterality, as well as the systemic features of this developmental disorder, help separate the two conditions. Some advanced cases of progressive iris atrophy might resemble aniridia, but the bilaterality of aniridia is again a helpful differential feature. Iridoschisis is characterized by separation of superficial layers of iris stroma and may

---

*References 15, 16, 22, 25, 26, 52.

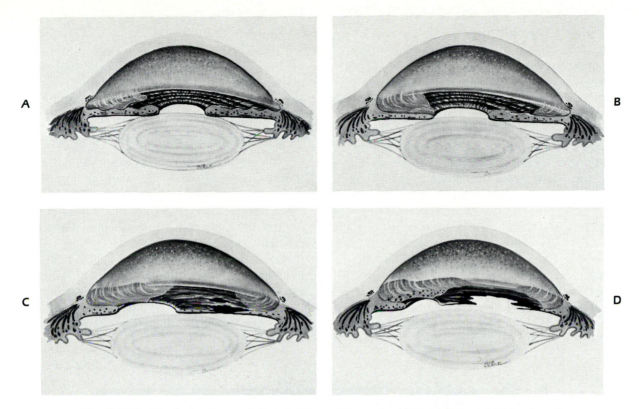

Fig. 54-13   Membrane theory of Campbell for pathogenesis of ICE syndrome: **A,** Extension of membrane from corneal endothelium over anterior chamber angle, onto iris. **B,** Contraction of membrane, creating peripheral anterior synechiae, corectopia. **C,** Thinning, atrophy of iris in quadrants away from corectopia. **D,** Hole formation in area of atrophy (in progressive iris atrophy), ectropion uveae in direction of corectopia, and nodules in area of membrane (in Cogan-Reese syndrome). (Reprinted with permission from Shields, BM Surv Ophthalmol 24:3, 1979)

be associated with glaucoma. However, it is typically a disease of the elderly.

Nodular lesions of the iris

Patients with the Cogan-Reese syndrome have had enucleation for presumed melanomas of the iris. Melanosis of the iris may also be confused with the Cogan-Reese syndrome by characteristic verrucous-like elevations in the former. This is usually unilateral, although a bilateral case has been described.[73] In addition, differentiation must be made from the nodular lesions of neurofibromatosis, as well as nodular inflammatory disorders, such as sarcoidosis.

Management

Patients with the ICE syndrome may require treatment for corneal edema, secondary glaucoma, or both. The glaucoma can often be controlled medically in the early stages, especially with drugs that reduce aqueous production, such as beta-blockers and carbonic anhydrase inhibitors. Lowering the intraocular pressure may also control the corneal edema, although the additional use of hypertonic saline solutions and soft contact lenses are often required.

When the intraocular pressure can no longer be controlled medically, surgical intervention is indicated. Laser trabeculoplasty is usually not effective in these cases. Filtering surgery is reasonably successful,[67] although late failures occur, which in some cases may be caused by endothelialization of the filtering bleb.[22] In some cases, surgical reduction of the intraocular pressure may relieve the corneal edema. However, even an extremely low intraocular pressure will usually not reverse advanced corneal edema. Furthermore, corneal edema may develop as a postoperative complication of glaucoma filtering surgery in patients with the ICE syndrome. Therefore, filtering surgery is not recommended as a specific treatment for the corneal edema. Penetrating keratoplasty is usually required for these cases after the glaucoma has been controlled.[13,49,69]

POSTERIOR POLYMORPHOUS DYSTROPHY

History and Terminology

The spectrum of disease that is now commonly referred to as *posterior polymorphous dystrophy* (PPD) represents a wide range of clinical and histopathologic variations. It is not surprising therefore that the related history and terminology are confusing. The earliest descriptions may have been those of Koeppe[38] (1916), who called it "keratitis bullosa interna," and Schnyder[62] (1924), who referred to it as "herpes of the posterior cornea." In 1958, Snell and Irwin[70] noted the involvement of the posterior corneal stroma and coined the term *hereditary deep dystrophy of the cornea.* The asociation with glaucoma was first described by Rubenstein and Silberman[60] (1968), who referred to the disorder as "hereditary mesodermal dystrophy." It was primarily the work of Grayson[30] and Cibis, et al.[18,19] in the 1970's, however, that led to our present understanding of the varied manifestations of PPD.

Clinical Features

General features

PPD is considered to be congenital, often progressive, and usually bilateral. Although autosomal dominant in its inheritance pattern, its expression is highly variable among family members both in age of clinical manifestation and in severity.

Ocular findings

On slit-lamp examination, vesicular, geographic, or bandlike opacities are seen on the posterior corneal surface (Fig. 54-14). Visual acuity is often normal, although in patients with extensive involvement, stromal and epithelial edema can occur with significant reduction in vision. Whereas the changes are progressive, the corneal abnormalities can at any age be segmental and limited, or diffuse with involvement of the entire cornea. Although PPD is usually bilateral, asymmetry of ocular involvement can be significant to the extent

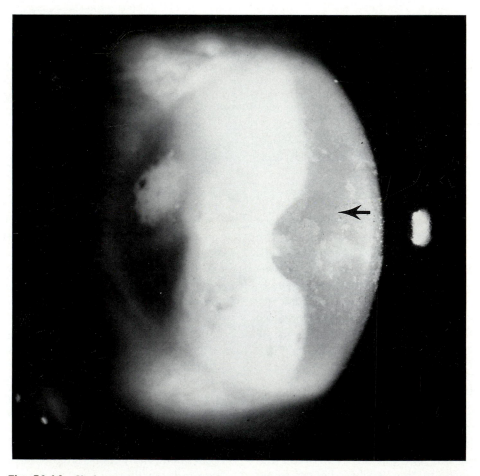

Fig. 54-14 Slit-lamp view of patient with posterior polymorphous dystrophy showing typical, irregular lesions *(arrow)* of posterior corneal surface. (Reprinted with permission from Bourgeois, J, Shields, MB, and Thresher, R: Ophthalmology 91:420, 1984)

that, clinically, only unilateral abnormalities are apparent.

Associated glaucoma

Secondary glaucoma occurs in approximately 13% of patients with PPD.[57] Three clinical forms of glaucoma have been described: adult open-angle, adult closed-angle, and juvenile.[18,19] Patients with the open-angle or juvenile forms have gonioscopically normal anterior chamber angles except for a high insertion of the iris. The angle-closure form of glaucoma is characterized by iridocorneal adhesions that range in severity from fine, or broad-based adhesions that are seen only on gonioscopy to large adhesions that are seen easily by slit-lamp examination.[40] The angle-closure cases may have associated iris atrophy and corectopia, and patients with the broad-based adhesions will nearly always have elevated intraocular pressure.[40]

Histopathologic Features of the Cornea

Electron microscopic studies of the posterior cornea in patients with PPD have demonstrated abnormalities of the endothelium and underlying Descemet's membrane. Most reports have described endothelial cells with epithelial-like characteristics, including microvilli, few mitochondria, the presence of cytoplasmic keratin filaments, and multilayering with desmosomal junctions.[8,30,32,63] Descemet's membrane is typically thickened and multilayered with a normal-banded anterior layer, but an abnormal posterior collagenous layer, which contains nonbanded fibrils, basement membrane-like material, and a wide-banded material.[30,74,78] Clinically, the severity of the corneal opacification and edema depend on the extent to which the normal mosaic of endothelial cells are replaced by abnormal epithelial-like cells. Specular microscopy[35] and cell culture techniques[56] have demonstrated the presence of both endothelial and epithelial-like cells in patients with PPD.

The structure of Descemet's membrane can serve as a historical record of the fetal and postnatal function of the endothelium.[4,79,81] The endothelial deposition of Descemet's membrane in the human eye changes at or around the time of birth. Anterior Descemet's collagen is synthesized in the fetal period and is banded, whereas collagen in the posterior Descemet's layer is deposited postnatally and is nonbanded. The normal-banded anterior layer with the abnormal posterior layer in PPD suggest that the disorder may result from abnormalities associated with perinatal endothelial cell reorganization and final differentiation.[4]

Histopathologic studies of corneal buttons from infants (2 and 3 months of age) have been reported.[23,54] The posterior cellular layers were predominantly epithelial in nature, although endothelial cells were also seen. Focal alterations were noted in Descemet's membrane with thinner or absent membrane under the epithelial-like cells. The findings suggested an onset of the disease in the early period of intrauterine life corresponding to the beginning of Descemet's membrane production.

Mechanisms of Glaucoma

Patients with angle-closure glaucoma have extensive iridocorneal adhesions and occasional corectopia.[18,19,30,40] Histologic examination has revealed a membrane extending down from the cornea, across the chamber angle, and onto the surface of the iris (Fig. 54-15).[57] Presumably, contraction of

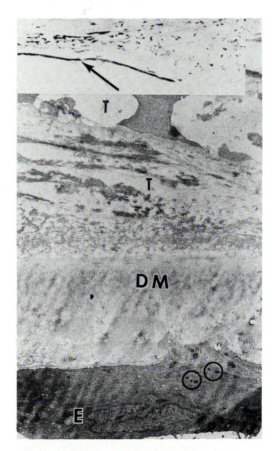

Fig. 54-15 Transmission electron microscopic view of trabeculectomy specimen from eye with posterior polymorphous dystrophy showing trabecular beams *(T)* covered by Descemet-like membrane *(DM)* and transformed endothelial cells *(E)* with numerous microvillous projections and desmosomal attachments *(circles)* (×8,200). *Inset:* light microscopic appearance of membrane on trabecular meshwork *(arrow)* (Toluidine blue, ×130). (Reprinted with permission from Rodrigues, MM, Phelps, CD, Krachmer, JH, et al: Arch Ophthalmol 98:688, 1980. Copyright 1980, American Medical Association)

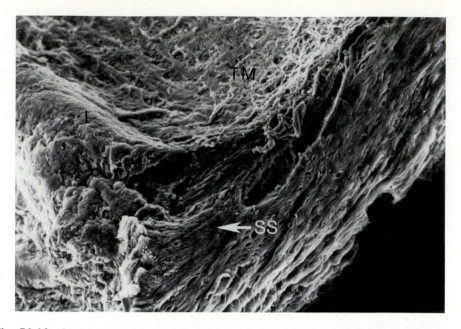

Fig. 54-16 Scanning electron microscopic view of trabeculectomy specimen from eye with posterior polymorphous dystrophy showing high insertion of iris *(I)* into posterior aspect of trabecular meshwork *(TM)* well anterior to scleral spur (SS) (×230). (Reprinted with permission from Bourgeois, J, Shields, MB, and Thresher, R: Ophthalmology 91:420, 1984)

this membrane results in iridocorneal adhesions, angle closure, and corectopia[19] (similar to the membrane theory of mechanism in the ICE syndrome). The cellular nature of the membrane is consistent with endothelial cells having microvilli and other epithelial-like characteristics.[57]

The mechanism of glaucoma in the patients with the open-angle form of glaucoma has not been fully elucidated, although one adult patient with PPD and open-angle glaucoma was found by histologic examination to have a high insertion of the iris into the posterior portion of the trabecular meshwork with collapse of the intertrabecular spaces (Fig. 54-16).[9] Presumably, abnormal tension exerted by the high insertion of the iris results in collapse of the trabecular meshwork and increased resistance to outflow. Similar anterior chamber anomalies have been described in patients with primary congenital glaucoma.[3] Although not proven by histologic studies, it may be postulated that some juveniles with PPD and glaucoma have similar anterior chamber angle anomalies.

Differential Diagnosis

Conditions that may be confused with PPD include other forms of posterior corneal dystrophy, such as Fuchs' endothelial dystrophy, congenital hereditary corneal dystrophy, and posterior amorphous corneal dystrophy. The latter is characterized by diffuse gray-white, sheetlike opacities of the posterior stroma, with occasional fine iris processes extending to Schwalbe's line for 360 degrees, and various abnormalities of the iris; but no glaucoma.[24] When iridocorneal adhesions are present, the Axenfeld-Rieger syndrome and the ICE syndrome should also be considered. The bandlike thickenings of posterior polymorphous dystrophy may be confused with the Haab's striae of congenital glaucoma, although the latter can usually be recognized by the thinned areas with thickened edges.[20]

Management

Treatment of the corneal abnormalities associated with PPD must be tailored to the extent of corneal decompensation. If the endothelial changes are limited and segmental without significant stromal edema, no treatment may be required. When necessary, limited stromal edema can be improved with topical sodium chloride 5% drops or ointment. Once the disease progresses to visually limiting stromal and epithelial edema, penetrating keratoplasty may be required.

Krachmer[40] has described the difficulties in performing penetrating keratoplasty in patients with PPD and associated glaucoma secondary to iridocorneal adhesions. In a series of 22 transplants, 9 grafts (41%) failed, and 6 of these 9 had glaucoma. All eyes with iridocorneal adhesions had both preoperative and postoperative glaucoma. He concluded that this factor most prominently influences keratoplasty for PPD, and that patients with these findings should not undergo keratoplasty until absolutely necessary.

Management of the glaucoma in PPD is similar to that for patients with the ICE syndrome. Miotics should be reserved for patients with open angles, and even these may not be effective. Beta-blockers and carbonic anhydrase inhibitors may be beneficial in both open- or closed-angle situations. Epinephrine compounds may also be efficacious in both forms of the glaucoma.

Laser trabeculoplasty is rarely effective and should be used with caution, since it could accelerate angle closure in patients with membrane growth across the angle. Filtering surgery is usually required in patients who are not controlled with maximum tolerable medical therapy. It has a success rate that is comparable to that for other forms of chronic glaucoma.

FUCHS' ENDOTHELIAL DYSTROPHY
Terminology and Clinicopathologic Features
Cornea guttata

Cornea guttata is a common condition, the incidence of which increases significantly with age.[29,44] Slit-lamp biomicroscopy reveals a beaten silver appearance of the central posterior cornea, similar to that seen in the ICE syndrome. However, by specular microscopic study a more characteristic pattern is seen, consisting of enlarged endothelial cells with dark areas that overlap the cell borders.[6,43] The primary pathologic finding is an alteration in the corneal endothelium that leads to a deposition of collagen on the posterior surface of Descemet's membrane. Histologically, this may appear as warts or excrescences in the pure form of cornea guttata. In other cases, focal accumulations may be covered by additional basement membrane or there may be a uniform thickening of the posterior collagen layers.[45]

Fuchs' endothelial dystrophy

The vast majority of individuals with cornea guttata have otherwise normal corneas with no visual impairment. A small number of patients with the same posterior corneal changes as described above, however, will develop edema of the corneal stroma and endothelium. The clinical entity was described by Fuchs[28] in 1910, and the association with a dystrophy of the corneal endothelium was subsequently recognized. The disorder is bilateral with a predilection for women and an onset usually between the ages of 40 and 70 years. There is a strong familial tendency, and an autosomal dominant inheritance has been described.[45] The condition may lead to severe visual reduction often requiring penetrating keratoplasty.

Association with Glaucoma
Influence of intraocular pressure on corneal endothelium

Reports are conflicting regarding the association of glaucoma with cornea guttata and Fuchs' endothelial dystrophy. This may be the result, at least in part, of the fact that elevated intraocular pressure often induces secondary changes in the corneal endothelium. Reduced cell densities have been reported in association with open-angle glaucoma,[36] angle-closure glaucoma,[7,48,52] and some secondary glaucomas.[63,64,75] However, the degree of endothelial alteration does not always correlate with the height of intraocular pressure elevation, suggesting that other factors may also influence the association between glaucoma and corneal endothelial changes.[36] It has been shown, for example, that the structure of corneal endothelium is altered by anterior uveitis, including glaucomatocyclitic crises,[47,63,64] as well as increasing age.[37] These observations must be taken into consideration with any reported association between glaucoma and an alteration of the corneal endothelium.

Cornea guttata and aqueous outflow

It was reported that patients with cornea guttata have a high incidence of abnormal tonographic facilities of outflow.[14] However, in a subsequent study using wide-field specular microscopy, the mean value for facility of outflow in patients with cornea guttata was not statistically different from the normal population, and there was no correlation between the extent of guttata and facility of outflow.[55] Another study of patients with cornea guttata showed a lower mean intraocular pressure in this group compared with a matched population without guttata.[12]

Fuchs' endothelial dystrophy and glaucoma

Two forms of glaucoma have been reported in association with Fuchs' endothelial dystrophy: open-angle glaucoma and angle-closure glaucoma.

Open-angle glaucoma. It was once estimated that 10% to 15% of patients with Fuchs' endothelial dystrophy have open-angle glaucoma.[39] However, a study of 64 families with Fuchs' endothelial dystrophy revealed only 1 case of open-angle glaucoma.[41] In another study, no genetic overlap between Fuchs' endothelial dystrophy and primary open-angle glaucoma was found on the basis of in vitro lymphocyte responsiveness to corticosteroids.[76]

Angle-closure glaucoma. Although the association between open-angle glaucoma and Fuchs' endothelial dystrophy remain uncertain, it has been well documented that patients with shallow anterior chambers and Fuchs' dystrophy may develop angle-closure glaucoma, apparently as a result of a gradual thickening of the cornea with eventual closure of the anterior chamber angle.[71]

Management

Although glaucoma is usually not present in eyes with Fuchs' endothelial dystrophy, medical efforts to further reduce the normal intraocular pressure may sometimes help to minimize the corneal edema. When glaucoma is present, the open-angle form is managed in the same manner as primary open-angle glaucoma, whereas the angle-closure form requires an iridectomy or filtering procedure. Prophylactic miotic therapy has not been effective in cases with impending angle-closure.[71]

REFERENCES

1. Alvarado, JA, Murphy, CG, Maglio, M, and Hetherington, J: Pathogenesis of Chandler's syndrome, essential iris atrophy and the Cogan-Reese syndrome. I. Alterations of the corneal endothelium, Invest Ophthalmol Vis Sci 27:853, 1986
2. Alvarado, JA, Murphy, CG, Juster, RP, and Hetherington, J: Pathogenesis of Chandler's syndrome, essential iris atrophy and the Cogan-Reese syndrome. II. Estimated age of disease onset, Invest Ophthalmol Vis Sci 27:873, 1986
3. Anderson, DR: The development of the trabecular meshwork and its abnormality in primary infantile glaucoma, Trans Am Ophthalmol Soc 79:458, 1981
4. Bahn CR, et al: Classification of corneal endothelial disorders based on neural crest origin, Ophthalmology 91:558, 1984
5. Benedikt, O, and Roll, P: Open-angle glaucoma endothelialization of the anterior chamber angle, Glaucoma 2:368, 1980
6. Bigar, F, Hurzeler, R, and Rejman, P: Cornea guttata, Klin Monatsbl Augenheilkd 176:644, 1980
7. Bigar, F, and Witmer, R: Corneal endothelial changes in primary acute angle-closure glaucoma, Ophthalmology 89:596, 1982
8. Boruchoff, SA, and Kuwabara, T: Electron microscopy of posterior polymorphous degeneration, Am J Ophthalmol 72:879, 1971
9. Bourgeois, J, Shields, MB, and Thresher, R: Open angle glaucoma associated with posterior polymorphous dystrophy: a clinicopathologic study, Ophthalmology 91:420, 1984
10. Bourne, WM: Partial corneal involvement in the iridocorneal endothelial syndrome, Am J Ophthalmol 94:774, 1982.
11. Bourne, WM, and Brubaker, RF: Decreased endothelial permeability in the iridocorneal endothelial syndrome, Ophthalmology 89:591, 1982
12. Burns, RR, Bourne, WM, and Brubaker, RF: Endothelial function in patients with cornea guttata, Invest Ophthalmol Vis Sci 20:77, 1981
13. Buxton, JN, and Lash, RS: Results of penetrating keratoplasty in the iridocorneal endothelial syndrome, Am J Ophthalmol 98:297, 1984
14. Buxton, JN, Preston, RW, Riechers, R, and Guilbault, N: Tonography in cornea guttata: a preliminary report, Arch Ophthalmol 77:602, 1967
15. Campbell, DG: Formation of iris nodules in primary proliferative endothelial degeneration. Paper presented at Association for Research in Vision and Ophthalmology, Sarasota, Fla, April 30-May 4, 1979
16. Campbell, DG, Shields, MB, and Smith, TR: The corneal endothelium and the spectrum of essential iris atrophy, Am J Ophthalmol 86:317, 1978
17. Chandler, PA: Atrophy of the stroma of the iris: endothelial dystrophy, corneal edema, and glaucoma, Am J Ophthalmol 41:607, 1956
18. Cibis, GW, Krachmer, JH, Phelps, CD, and Weingeist, TA: Iridocorneal adhesions in posterior polymorphous corneal dystrophy, Trans Am Acad Ophthalmol Otolaryngol 81:770, 1976
19. Cibis, GW, Krachmer, JH, Phelps, CD, and Weingeist, TA: The clinical spectrum of posterior polymorphous dystrophy, Arch Ophthalmol 95:1529, 1977
20. Cibis, GW, and Tripathi, RC: The differential diagnosis of Descemet's tears (Haab's striae) and posterior polymorphous dystrophy bands: a clinicopathologic study, Ophthalmology 89:614, 1982
21. Cogan, DG, and Reese, AB: A syndrome of iris nodules, ectopic Descemet's membrane, and unilateral glaucoma, Doc Ophthalmol 26:424, 1969
22. Daicker, B, Sturrock, G, and Guggenheim, R: Clinicopathological correlation in Cogan-Reese syndrome, Klin Monatsbl Augenheilkd 180:531, 1982
23. de Felice, GP, et al: Posterior polymorphous dystrophy of the cornea: an ultrastructural study, v Graefe's Arch Klin Exp Ophthalmol 223:265, 1985
24. Dunn, SP, Krachmer, JH, and Ching, SST: New findings in posterior amorphous corneal dystrophy, Arch Ophthalmol 102:236, 1984
25. Eagle, RC, Jr, Font, RL, Yanoff, M, and Fine, BS: Proliferative endotheliopathy with iris abnormalities: the iridocorneal endothelial syndrome, Arch Ophthalmol 97:2104, 1979

26. Eagle, RC, Jr, Font, RL, Yanoff, M, and Fine, BS: The iris naevus (Cogan-Reese) syndrome: light and electron microscopic observations, Br J Ophthalmol 64:446, 1980

27. Eagle, RC, Jr, and Shields, JA: Iridocorneal endothelial syndrome with contralateral guttate endothelial dystrophy: a light and electron microscopic study, Ophthalmology 94:862, 1987

28. Fuchs, E: Dystrophia epithelialis cornealis, Arch Ophthalmol 76:478, 1910

29. Goar, E: Dystrophy of the cornea endothelium, Am J Ophthalmol 17:215, 1934

30. Grayson, M: The nature of hereditary deep polymorphous dystrophy of the cornea: its association with iris and anterior chamber dysgenesis, Trans Am Ophthalmol Soc 72:516, 1974

31. Harms, C: Einseitige spontane Luckenbildung der Iris durch Atrophie ohne mechanische Zerrung, Klin Monatsbl Augenheilkd 41:522, 1903

32. Henriquez, AS, et al: Morphologic characteristics of posterior polymorphous dystrophy: a study of nine corneas and review of the literature, Surv Ophthalmol 29:139, 1984

33. Hirst, LW, et al: Epithelial characteristics of the endothelium in Chandler's syndrome, Invest Ophthalmol Vis Sci 24:603, 1983

34. Hirst, LW, Quigley, HA, Stark, WJ, and Shields, MB: Specular microscopy of iridocorneal endothelial syndrome, Am J Ophthalmol 89;11, 1980

35. Hirst, LW, and Waring GO, III: Clinical specular microscopy of posterior polymorphous endothelial dystrophy, Am J Ophthalmol 95:143, 1983

36. Hong, C, Kandori, T, Kitazawa, Y, and Tanishima, T: Corneal endothelial cells in ocular hypertension, Jpn J Ophthalmol 26:183, 1982

37. Kaufman, HE, Capella, JA, and Robbins, JE: The human corneal endothelium, Am J Ophthalmol 61:835, 1966

38. Koeppe, L: Klinische Beobachtungen mit der Lampe und dem Hornhautmikroskop, v Graefe's Arch Klin Exp Ophthalmol 91:363, 1916

39. Kolker, AE, and Hetherington, J, Jr: Becker-Shaffer's diagnosis and therapy of the glaucomas, ed. 4, St Louis, 1976, The CV Mosby Co

40. Krachmer, JH: Posterior polymorphous corneal dystrophy: a disease characterized by epithelial-like endothelial cells which influence management and prognosis, Trans Am Ophthalmol Soc 83: 413, 1985

41. Krachmer, JH, Purcell, JJ, Jr, Yound, CW, and Bucher, KD: Corneal endothelial dystrophy: a study of 64 families, Arch Ophthalmol 96:2036, 1978

42. Kupfer, C, Kaiser-Kupfer, MI, Datiles, M, and McCain, L: The contralateral eye in the iridocorneal endothelial (ICE) syndrome, Ophthalmology 90: 1343, 1983

43. Laing, RA, et al: Endothelial mosaic in Fuchs' dystrophy: a qualitative evaluation with the specular microscope, Arch Ophthalmol 99:80, 1981

44. Lorenzetti, DWC, Uotila, MH, Parikh, N, and Kaufman, HE: Central cornea guttata: incidence in the general population, Am J Ophthalmol 64:1155, 1967

45. Magovern, M, et al: Inheritance of Fuchs' combined dystrophy, Ophthalmology 86:1897, 1979

46. Neubauer, L, Lund, OE, and Leibowitz, HM: Specular microscopic appearance of the corneal endothelium in iridocorneal endothelial syndrome, Arch Ophthalmol 101:916, 1983

47. Olsen, T: Changes in the corneal endothelium after acute anterior uveitis as seen with the specular microscope, Acta Ophthalmol 58:250, 1980

48. Olsen, T: The endothelial cell damage in acute glaucoma: on the corneal thickness response to intraocular pressure, Acta Ophthalmol 58:257, 1980

49. Patel, A, et al: Clinicopathologic features of Chandler's syndrome, Surv Ophthalmol 27:327, 1983

50. Portis, JM, Stamper, RL, Spencer, WH, and Webster, RG, Jr.: The corneal endothelium and Descemet's membrane in the iridocorneal endothelial syndrome, Trans Am Ophthalmol Soc 83:316, 1985

51. Quigley, HA, and Forster, RF: Histopathology of cornea and iris in Chandler's syndrome, Arch Ophthalmol 96:1878, 1978

52. Radius, RL, and Herschler, J: Histopathology in the iris-nevus (Cogan-Reese) syndrome, Am J Ophthalmol 89:780, 1980

53. Richardson, RM: Corneal decompensation in Chandler's syndrome: a scanning and transmission electron microscopic study, Arch Ophthalmol 97:2112, 1979

54. Richardson, WP, and Hettinger, ME: Endothelial and epithelial-like cell formations in a case of posterior polymorphous dystrophy, Arch Ophthalmol 103:1520, 1985

55. Roberts, CW, Steinert, RF, Thomas, JV, and Boruchoff, SA: Endothelial guttata and facility of aqueous outflow, Cornea 3:5, 1984

56. Rodrigues, MM, Newsome, DA, Krachmer, JH, and Sun, TT: Posterior polymorphous dystrophy of the cornea: cell culture studies, Exp Eye Res 33:535, 1981

57. Rodrigues MM, et al: Glaucoma due to endothelialization of the anterior chamber angle: a comparison of posterior polymorphous dystrophy of the cornea and Chandler's syndrome, Arch Ophthalmol 98:688, 1980

58. Rodrigues, MM, Streeten, BW, and Spaeth, GL: Chandler's syndrome as a variant of essential iris atrophy: a clinicopathologic study, Arch Ophthalmol 96:643, 1978

59. Rodrigues, MM, Stulting, RD, and Waring GO, III: Clinical, electron microscopic, and immunohistochemical study of the corneal endothelium and Descemet's membrane in the iridocorneal endothelial syndrome, Am J Ophthalmol 101:16, 1986

60. Rubenstein, RA, and Silberman, JJ: Hereditary deep dystrophy of the cornea associated with glaucoma and ruptures in Descemet's membrane, Arch Ophthalmol 79:123, 1968

61. Scheie, HG, and Yanoff, M: Iris nevus (Cogan-Reese) syndrome: a cause of unilateral glaucoma, Arch Ophthalmol 93:963, 1975

62. Schnyder, WF: Herpetiforme Erkrankung der Hornhautruck Flache, Klin Monatsbl Augenheilkd 73:385, 1924

63. Setala, K: Response of human corneal endothelial cells to increased intraocular pressure: a specular microscopic study, Acta Ophthalmol Suppl 144:547, 1980

64. Setala, K, and Vannas, A: Endothelial cells in the glaucomato-cyclitic crisis, Adv Ophthalmol 36:218, 1978

65. Setala, K, and Vannas, A: Corneal endothelial cells in essential iris atrophy: a specular microscopic study, Acta Ophthalmol 57:1020, 1979

66. Shields, MB: Progressive essential iris atrophy, Chandler's syndrome, and the iris nevus (Cogan-Reese) syndrome: a spectrum of disease, Surv Ophthalmol 24:3, 1979

67. Shields, MB, Campbell, DG, and Simmons, RJ: The essential iris atrophies, Am J Ophthalmol 85:749, 1978

68. Shields, MB, Campbell, DG, Simmons, RJ, and Hutchinson, BT: Iris nodules in essential iris atrophy, Arch Ophthalmol 94:406, 1976

69. Shields, MB, McCracken, JS, Klintworth, GK, and Campbell, DG: Corneal edema in essential iris atrophy, Ophthalmology 86:1533, 1979

70. Snell, AC, and Irwin, ES: Hereditary deep dystrophy of the cornea, Am J Ophthalmol 45:636, 1958

71. Stocker, FW: The endothelium of the cornea and its clinical implications, ed 2, Springfield, 1971, Charles C Thomas, Publisher

72. Sugar, HS: The iris nevus and Cogan-Reese syndromes: separate entities? Ann Ophthalmol 13:405, 1981

73. Traboulsi, EI, and Maumenee, IH: Bilateral melanosis of the iris, Am J Ophthalmol 103:115, 1987

74. Tripathi, RC, Casey, TA, and Wise, G: Hereditary posterior polymorphous dystrophy: an ultrastructural and clinical report, Trans Ophthalmol Soc UK 94:211, 1974

75. Vannas, A, Setala, K, and Ruusuvaara, P: Endothelial cells in capsular glaucoma, Acta Ophthalmol 55:951, 1977

76. Waltman, SR, Palmberg, PF, and Becker, B: In vitro corticosteroid sensitivity in patients with Fuchs' dystrophy, Doc Ophthalmol Proc Series 18:321, 1979

77. Wang, Y: Specular microscopic studies of the corneal endothelium in iridocorneal endothelial (ICE) syndrome, Eye Science 1:53, 1985

78. Waring, GO, III: Posterior collagenous layer of the cornea: ultrastructural classification of abnormal collagenous tissue posterior to Descemet's membrane in 30 cases, Arch Ophthalmol 100:122, 1982

79. Waring, GO, Laibson, PR, and Rodrigues, M: Clinical and pathological alterations of Descemet's membrane, with emphasis on endothelial metaplasia, Surv Ophthalmol 18:325, 1974

80. Weber, PA, and Gibb, G: Iridocorneal endothelial syndrome: glaucoma without peripheral anterior synechias, Glaucoma 6:128, 1984

81. Wulle, KG: Electron microscopy of the fetal development of the corneal endothelium and Descemet's membrane of the human eye, Invest Ophthalmol 11:897, 1972

82. Yanoff, M: In discussion of Shields, MB, McCracken, JS, Klintworth, GK, and Campbell, DG: Corneal edema in essential iris atrophy, Ophthalmology 86:1549, 1979

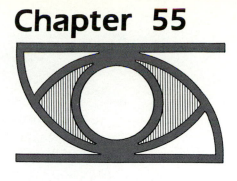

Chapter 55

Pigmentary Glaucoma

Thomas M. Richardson

HISTORICAL BACKGROUND

More than three fourths of a century ago, von Hippel[64] suggested that glaucoma could be caused by obstruction of the aqueous outflow system by pigment. Levinsohn[34] detected pigment in the anterior chamber angle of certain patients with glaucoma and believed that these particles originated from the pigmented layer of the iris. A cause-and-effect relationship between pigment and glaucoma was therefore supported by some investigators (for example, Koeppe[31] and Jess[28]) but was opposed by others (for example, Vogt,[63] Birch-Hirschfeld,[7] and Evans et al.[18]).

In 1940, Sugar[58] described a 29-year-old man with a form of glaucoma accompanied by degeneration of the pigment epithelium of the iris and ciliary body and deposition of pigment on surfaces within the anterior chamber. By 1949 Sugar and Barbour[61] had applied the term *pigmentary glaucoma* to this entity and had delineated the clinical features that are now well recognized as the hallmarks of an unusual type of glaucoma. The pigment particles observed in this condition arise from the pigmented neuroepithelium of the iris and perhaps the ciliary body.[5,50,59]

Many cases of pigmentary glaucoma were subsequently reported, and in 1966, Sugar[59] reviewed 147 cases in which additional features of this disease were highlighted. His findings were confirmed in a large series by Scheie and Cameron.[49]

CLINICAL FEATURES

Pigmentary glaucoma is a bilateral disorder commonly associated with a moderate degree of myopia. It occurs with a greater incidence in men than in women and at a relatively young age of onset in comparison with that of primary open-angle glaucoma. It is characterized by loss of pigment from the pigmented epithelium of the iris, particularly in the midperipheral region (Fig. 55-1). This loss of pigment produces radial trans-illumination defects in the iris and dispersion of melanin pigment into the aqueous humor. The pigment is deposited on various surfaces in the anterior segment, including the lens, zonules, iris, cornea, and trabecular meshwork (Fig. 55-2). The

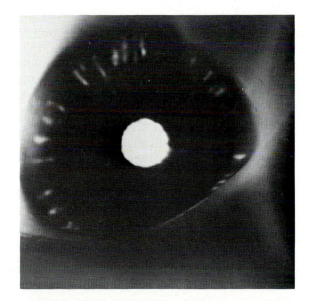

Fig. 55-1 Iris transillumination in patient with pigmentary glaucoma showing spokelike, midperipheral, radial defects resulting from loss of pigment from pigment epithelium. See Plate III, Fig. 5.

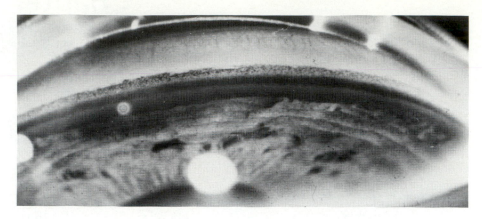

Fig. 55-2   Goniophotograph of anterior chamber angle from patient with pigmentary glaucoma showing dense band of pigment on trabecular meshwork. See Plate III, Fig. 6.

accumulation of pigment in the aqueous outflow system is believed to be the cause of the associated glaucoma.

Pigment deposited on the corneal endothelium generally assumes the configuration of a central, vertical, brown band (Krukenberg's spindle). The spindle varies in length from 1 to 6 mm and is up to 3 mm wide. Its vertical form is probably attributable to the vertical meeting of aqueous convection currents. Occasionally, pigment deposition takes the form of more diffusely distributed punctate deposits. Endothelial pigment has no known deleterious effect on endothelial function and patients with pigmentary dispersion syndrome have no significant difference in central endothelial cell density and corneal thickness when compared with age-, sex-, and refractive error-matched control eyes.[53]

In the iris, regions of pigment loss appear as radial, slitlike, midperipheral transillumination defects detected by careful retroillumination (see Plate III, Fig. 5). The defects can best be observed by a dark-adapted examiner using a fiberoptic transilluminator as a light source. The probe of the illuminator is positioned over the sclera to achieve a bright red reflex through the pupil. The radial pattern of iris defects common to pigmentary glaucoma should be present if the diagnosis is to be made reliably. Pigment deposition may also be noted on the anterior iris surface.

The anterior chamber is characteristically deep, and the iris assumes a concave configuration most marked in the midperiphery. Gonioscopic examination reveals open angles, a characteristic homogeneous and dense band of hyperpigmentation on the trabecular meshwork, and a ring of pigment along Schwalbe's line (Sampaolesi line) (see Plate III, Fig. 6).

Pigment deposition has also been noted on the zonular fibers and on the lens surface, where it is usually found on the posterior capsule at the insertion of the posterior zonular fibers.

The observation by Gillies[20] that pigmentary dispersion syndrome is accompanied by vascular hypoperfusion of the iris, which may precede changes in the iris pigment epithelium, suggests that fluorescein angiography could also be beneficial in early diagnosis of this condition.

Individuals with pigmentary glaucoma appear clinically like those with the pigmentary dispersion syndrome except for the elevated pressures and signs of glaucomatous damage.

NATURAL HISTORY

Heredity

Families with multiple members having pigmentary dispersion syndrome were reported only sporadically until recently. Krukenberg's spindles had been reported in mother and daughter in three families,[51,57,62] and in twin brothers in another.[40] Stankovic[56] described a family in which pigmentary glaucoma was observed through four generations, but he considered these cases to show autosomal recessive inheritance. Kaiser-Kupfer et al.[29] reported pigmentary dispersion syndrome in two brothers, their father, and a paternal uncle.

More recently, however, Mandelkorn et al.[38] reported 4 families in whom 6 of 19 relatives of probands had pigmentary dispersion syndrome and suggested an autosomal dominant mode of inheritance. McDermott et al.[41] detected pigmentary dispersion syndrome in 25% of 48 immediate relatives of 21 probands and 47% of immediate adult relatives, suggesting an autosomal dominant inheritance with phenotypic expression usually appearing after the second decade.

Age of Onset

Little is known about the age of onset of pigmentary dispersion syndrome. The youngest patient in the series of Scheie and Cameron[49] was 14 years of age. The age at diagnosis is about 35 to 45 years for men and 40 to 50 years for women. The mean age at the time of diagnosis of patients with pigmentary dispersion syndrome with normal intraocular pressures is younger than those with glaucoma, as would be expected.

Risk Factors

In most pigmentary glaucoma series, males outnumber females. The ratio of males to females with pigmentary dispersion syndrome and normal intraocular pressure is equal or even shows a greater proportion of females, suggesting that males may be more prone to the development of glaucoma. The majority of patients with pigmentary dispersion syndrome with and without glaucoma are myopic. Berger et al.,[4] in correlating age, refraction, and intraocular pressure status, found that the higher the myopia, the younger the age at which glaucomatous damage tended to develop.

Davidson et al.[13] found a deeper anterior chamber in patients with pigmentary dispersion syndrome than in controls. Kaiser-Kupfer et al.[29] found three of four related patients with pigmentary dispersion syndrome with markedly asymmetric pigment dispersion and normal intraocular pressures in both eyes to have an anterior chamber depth 0.2 mm greater in the affected eye.

Most patients with pigmentary dispersion syndrome are white. The disease is rare in blacks and Orientals. Five patients in one family in the series of Scheie and Cameron[49] were described as mulatto. Pigmentary glaucoma has been reported in a black albino.[65] Duncan[14] reported the development of Krukenberg's spindles during pregnancy in four black women, only one of whom was slightly myopic. It is uncertain whether this represented true pigmentary dispersion syndrome.

Progression

Eyes with pigmentary dispersion syndrome often have a normal intraocular pressure. The true prevalence of pigmentary dispersion syndrome in the population is unknown, and it is difficult to estimate the frequency with which glaucoma develops. The time between diagnosis of pigment dispersion and the onset of glaucoma varies considerably and may take up to 12 to 20 years.[42,59,60] Some patients with diffuse pigment dispersion have not developed abnormal pressures even after 20 years of follow up.[16] A recent long-term retrospective

analysis involving 65 patients revealed glaucoma in 36% of male and 33% of female patients with pigmentary dispersion syndrome after a mean follow up of 17 years.[42] Although the ratio of male to female patients with pigmentary dispersion syndrome was 1.6:1, once a given patient was identified as having the syndrome, both sexes appeared to have an equal chance of developing glaucoma.

In a recent prospective study, Richter et al.[44] reported that the disease is usually progressive. Of 110 eyes of 55 patients with pigmentary dispersion syndrome or pigmentary glaucoma followed for a mean of 27 months (6 to 43 months), 62% remained stable, 34% had worsening of their glaucoma, and 5% improved. During the course of the study, 45 eyes (41%) had clinically detectable active dispersion of pigment. There was a significant association between progression of glaucoma and active pigment dispersion, which was more commonly associated with an elevated intraocular pressure than with increased optic nerve cupping or visual field loss at stable intraocular pressures. Interestingly, when patients aged less than 44 years, 45 to 64 years, and greater than 65 years were compared, there were no differences in the frequency of active pigment dispersion and worsening of glaucoma. The results of this study suggest that in patients with pigmentary glaucoma or pigmentary dispersion syndrome, increasing iris transillumination defects, increasing corneal pigmentation, and the presence of pigment granules on the anterior lens capsule in the undilated pupillary zone may be risk factors for increasing intraocular pressure.

Whereas pigmentary glaucoma is usually a progressive disease requiring medical or surgical management to prevent damage to the optic disc and glaucomatous visual field loss, it sometimes has a mild course or occasionally becomes less severe, particularly with increasing age. Lichter and Shaffer[36] observed a definite decrease in the amount of pigment in the trabecular meshwork in 10% of 102 patients and concluded that the pigment could pass out of the meshwork as the patient aged. On occasion, transilluminating areas of the iris have been observed to disappear,[11,16] suggesting that these areas can be resurfaced by pigment epithelium or pigment-containing cells. In a few patients, the intraocular pressure has been noted to return toward normal after several years of treatment.[16,22,55] In such patients it has been possible to reduce or discontinue treatment for glaucoma.

Ritch[45] reported on four patients with glaucomatous damage and pigmentary dispersion syndrome in whom the intraocular pressures were normal. These patients showed no progression of their glaucomatous cupping or visual field damage. These patients were all much older than the average patient with pigmentary glaucoma and none of them had had a diagnosis of glaucoma made at the time at which the damage developed. A presumptive diagnosis was made of pigmentary glaucoma that had remitted spontaneously.

PATHOPHYSIOLOGY AND MECHANISMS
Development of Glaucoma

Although the clinical features of pigmentary glaucoma have been described in detail, knowledge of its pathophysiology remains obscure, because of both the limited availability of histopathologic specimens and because of the lack of a readily available animal model in which to test various hypotheses relative to the pathophysiology of the disease. The pathogenetic mechanism that adequately explains the cause-and-effect relationship between pigment in the anterior segment and the elevation of intraocular pressure has long been a topic of debate.

One hypothesis suggests that patients who develop pigmentary glaucoma have a mesodermal angle anomaly,[10,35,36] and that the presence of pigment in the trabecular meshwork is secondary to a developmental defect in the anterior chamber angle structures. However, these anomalies (abnormal iris processes) seem to occur with equal frequency in similarly myopic eyes that have open angles and no excessive pigment in the meshwork.[16] Other iris abnormalities, namely hyperplasia of the iris dilator muscle and degeneration of iris nerve fibers, have been observed in the pigmentary dispersion syndrome,[19,33] but their relevance to the development of glaucoma is unknown.

Recently, fluorescein angiographic studies of 10 patients with pigmentary dispersion syndrome or pigmentary glaucoma showed evidence of vascular hypoperfusion of the iris, decreased radial vessels, and leakage of dye from the pupillary margin and peripupillary area.[20] In cases in which the fellow eye was virtually unaffected by the pigment dispersion, vascular changes were present but less marked, suggesting that they precede the changes in the pigment epithelium. These findings are consistent with the hypothesis that a deficiency of the mesodermal support tissues of the iris contributes to the cause of pigmentary glaucoma.

Others have suggested that pigmentary glaucoma is simply a variant of primary open-angle glaucoma. This view is supported by a study indicating that patients with the pigmentary dispersion syndrome who develop an elevated intraocular pressure after the administration of topical corticosteroids belong to a class of individuals genetically predisposed to open-angle glaucoma.[1] Another study of pressure responses to corticosteroids suggested that pigmentary glaucoma is not simply a variant of primary open-angle glaucoma, but is in fact a separate and distinct entity.[2] Results from neither study, however, have been confirmed.

A view that has gained increasing support is that the intraocular pressure elevation is caused, at least initially, by accumulation of melanin pigment in the trabecular meshwork (Fig. 55-3), and that this blocks the flow of aqueous humor through the outflow channels.[58] Pigment particles obtained from the iris pigment epithelium and perfused into enucleated human and primate eyes increase the resistance to fluid flow through the aqueous outflow system.[3,21] This is confirmed clinically by tonography when patients with pigmentary disper-

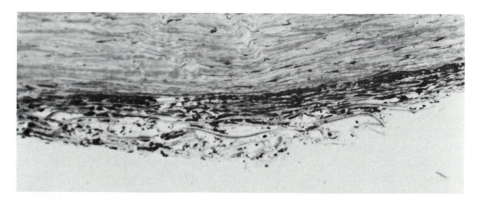

Fig. 55-3 Light microscopic appearance of trabecular meshwork in pigmentary glaucoma. Heavy deposits of melanin pigment extend through entire depth of meshwork.

sion syndrome who develop a shower of pigment, either spontaneously or after vigorous exercise, have an acute rise in intraocular pressure and a concomitant decrease in the facility of outflow.[17]

Occasionally, complaints of diminished vision and halos may be elicited. These are thought to correlate with pigment dispersion and resultant significant pressure elevations. Transient rises in intraocular pressure have also been observed after release of pigment into the anterior chamber following pupillary dilation.[32] Topically administered mydriatics, especially sympathomimetics such as phenylephrine, often result in the liberation of pigment into the aqueous humor.[24,39] However, in normal individuals or those with primary open-angle glaucoma, phenylephrine either reduces or has no effect on intraocular pressure.[24] Patients with either pigmentary or exfoliative glaucoma may develop an acute rise in intraocular pressure associated with pigment release, suggesting that these eyes are more susceptible to temporary obstruction of the aqueous outflow system by pigment particles.[32] A similar conclusion can be reached from Mapstone's study.[39]

To determine the prognostic value of intraocular pressure responses to phenylephrine in identifying those patients predisposed to pressure elevation as a result of pigment release, Epstein et al.[17] performed provocative testing on a selected group of patients who had bilateral pigmentary dispersion syndrome with or without glaucoma. Phenylephrine 10% was administered topically to one eye while the second eye served as the control. Only 2.5% of the patients developed 4+ pigment reaction in the anterior chamber, and less than 15% developed a rise in intraocular pressure greater than 2 mm Hg. As in Kristensen's study,[32] the majority of patients who developed a rise in intraocular pressure already had either pigmentary glaucoma or exfoliative glaucoma. Few, if any, with only the pigmentary dispersion syndrome developed increased pressure.

It is interesting that pigment liberation tended to be greatest in the older patient with pigment dispersion who already had glaucoma and who also had been treated with topical antiglaucoma medication. It seems paradoxical that pigment liberation should be increased with increasing age, when it is well known that the incidence of pigmentary glaucoma actually decreases with advancing years. Although there seems to be no correlation between the extent of iris transillumination and the grade of phenylephrine-induced pigment liberation, Kristensen[32] showed that repeated mydriasis resulted in smaller and smaller showers of pigment into the anterior chamber. However, mydriasis induced after about 2 weeks' recovery from mydriatics produced pigment liberation approxi-

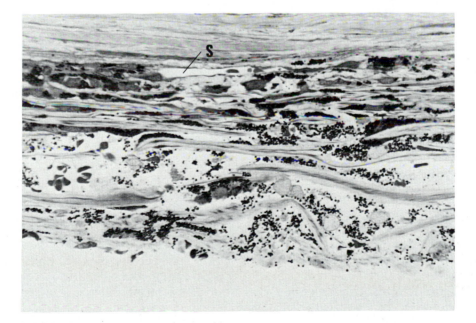

Fig. 55-4 Light micrograph of trabecular meshwork and portion of Schlemm's canal (S) from patient with pigmentary glaucoma. Free pigment granules are located mainly in uveal meshwork and beginning of the corneoscleral meshwork. Deeper deposits of pigment are mainly intracellular. Free pigment is not found within the lumen of Schlemm's canal.

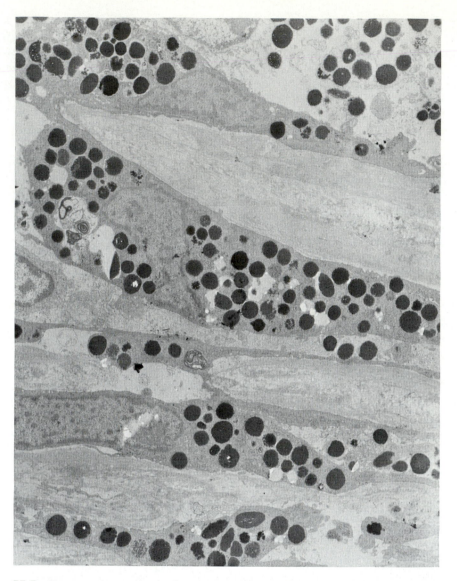

Fig. 55-5 Electron micrograph of trabecular meshwork in which cells lining trabecular sheets are heavily laden with pigment granules. Some granules are fragmented and could be undergoing digestion. Except for heavy pigment deposits, trabecular cells appear relatively healthy. A few free pigment granules are located in intertrabecular spaces.

mately the same as in the initial response. This suggests that pigment or pigment-containing cells expand to cover the sites of previously liberated pigment.[11] A correlation between pigment liberation and worsening of glaucoma has been observed by Richter et al.[44] in a study of the natural evolution of pigmentary dispersion syndrome and pigmentary glaucoma. Thus active dispersion of pigment is clinically detectable, is correlated with elevation of intraocular pressure, and continues to occur in older patients.

Although the above studies demonstrate that pigment particles can temporarily obstruct aqueous outflow, dense pigmentation of the trabecular meshwork can occur without pressure elevation.[19] Some individuals with pigment dispersion may not develop an elevated pressure or abnormal outflow facility after up to 20 years of observation.[16] The mere presence of pigment particles in the meshwork is not sufficient to account for glaucoma.

What factors determine the fate of pigment particles in the aqueous outflow system, and how are these factors translated into elevation of intraocular pressure? It is common to find on gonioscopy a dense band of pigment in the trabecular meshwork of persons with the pigmentary dispersion syn-

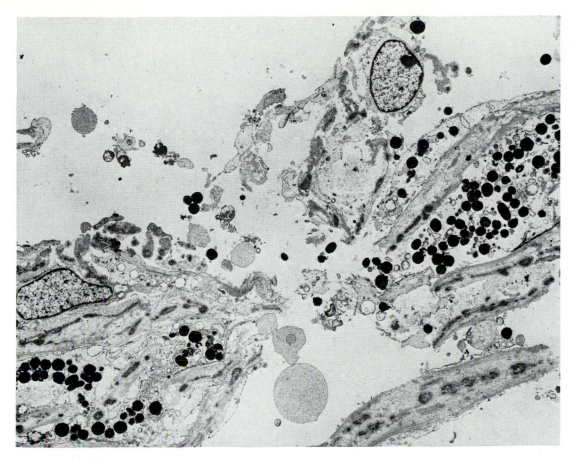

Fig. 55-6   Electron micrograph of trabecular meshwork in which trabecular cells have undergone degeneration, leaving trabecular beams partially denuded of cells. Connective tissue of some beams is disorganized. Pigment particles and cell debris fill intertrabecular spaces.

drome (see Fig. 55-2). The pigment particles are located both within and outside the cells that line the trabeculae[19,25,27,44,46] (Figs. 55-4 and 55-5). Occasionally, a pigment-containing cell, ostensibly derived from the iris stroma, is seen in the intertrabecular spaces. Commonly, from examination of histopathologic specimens, the amount of pigment within and outside the cells of the trabecular meshwork appears to severely restrict the intertrabecular spaces. Such restriction alone is probably sufficient to impede the flow of aqueous humor and cause elevation of intraocular pressure.

There seems, however, to be another stage in the obstructive process in the patient who is unresponsive to medical therapy. Electron microscopic studies of such patients have revealed degeneration of endothelial cells of the trabecular meshwork, trapping of cell debris or breakdown products of pigment-containing cells (Fig. 55-6), and sclerosis of the trabecular beams[43] (Figs. 55-7

and 55-8). There is evidence that the endothelial cells that line the trabeculae behave as local purveyors of materials passing through the corneoscleral meshwork.[6,11] These cells appear to have a selective capacity to phagocytize various types of particles and cells that can potentially obstruct the outflow channels.[47,52] Excessive phagocytosis often appears to lead to migration of the endothelial cells away from the trabeculae[46,51] (Fig. 55-9), or to autolysis of the cells in situ[43] (see Fig. 55-6), which contributes to the cell debris. In either case the trabeculae are left denuded and unprotected from the aqueous humor and its contents. A similar process occurs in pigmentary glaucoma, where denudation of the trabeculae leads to breakdown and collapse of the intertrabecular spaces with degeneration and sclerosis of the trabeculae (see Figs. 55-7 and 55-8).

These observations have led us to postulate that obstruction of the aqueous outflow system and

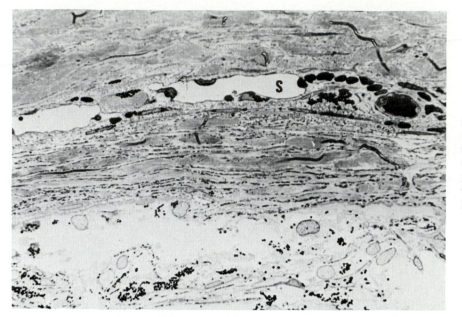

Fig. 55-7 Light micrograph of severely damaged trabecular meshwork in pigmentary glaucoma. Corneoscleral meshwork is collapsed and appears relatively acellular. Schlemm's canal *(S)* is patent and free of pigment particles.

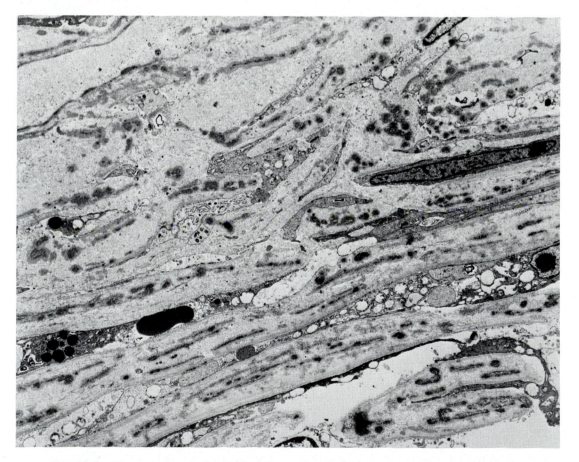

Fig. 55-8 Electron micrograph of trabecular meshwork demonstrated in Fig. 55-7. Trabecular sheets have collapsed and fused, leading to obliteration of aqueous pathway. Cell debris, scattered pigment-containing cells, and an occasional normal-appearing cell are located throughout sclerotic tissue.

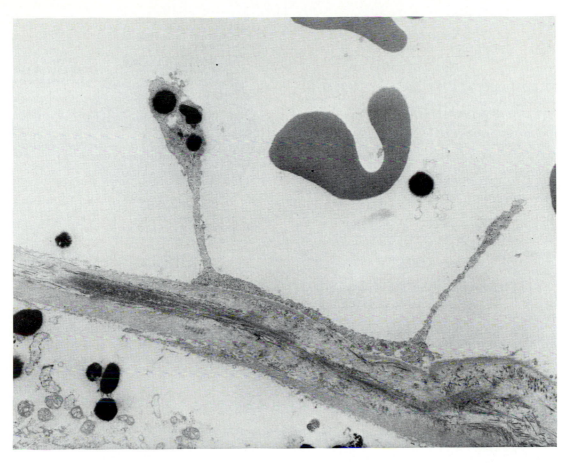

Fig. 55-9   Portion of trabecular endothelial cell in contact with trabecular beam. Trabecular cell contains ingested pigment particles. Portions of cell have lost contact with beam, leaving underlying connective tissue exposed.

the development of glaucoma probably occur in two stages, as diagrammed in Fig. 55-10. In the first stage, pigment liberated mainly from the iris neuroepithelium accumulates in the cells and spaces of the otherwise normal-appearing trabecular meshwork. Accumulation of pigment in moderate amounts over a short period may acutely obstruct the intertrabecular space and result in transient elevation of intraocular pressure. Excessive phagocytosis of pigment leads to migration of the trabecular cells away from the beams. These cells may undergo autolysis, resulting in further accumulation of cell debris and pigment in the meshwork. The remaining attached cells spread over the denuded portions of the trabeculae in an apparent attempt to keep them covered (Fig. 55-11).

During the first stage, the pigment dispersion cycle probably remains static, with only an occasional or low-grade elevation of intraocular pressure. This stage is probably clinically reversible, provided that the trabecular meshwork maintains

the capacity to undergo self-repair. When it loses this capacity, the trabecular beams degenerate and the second stage is entered. The second stage is probably irreversible and is the result of irreparable damage to the trabeculae (see Fig. 55-8).

Such a scheme could explain the great variability in individual behavior in this disease. The transient rises in pressure observed after a pigment shower following mydriasis and the acute obstruction of outflow after injection of iris pigment into the anterior chamber of human or animal eyes fit well with the first stage, which can be transient with only a temporary rise in intraocular pressure.[36] The key to reversibility appears to reside in the capacity of trabecular endothelial cells to migrate away from the beams and be replaced by new or healthier cells (see Fig. 55-11) that repair mildly damaged trabecular sheets before they undergo degeneration and collapse. Inability of the trabecular meshwork to achieve the latter may represent a primary defect in the endothelial cells. This would

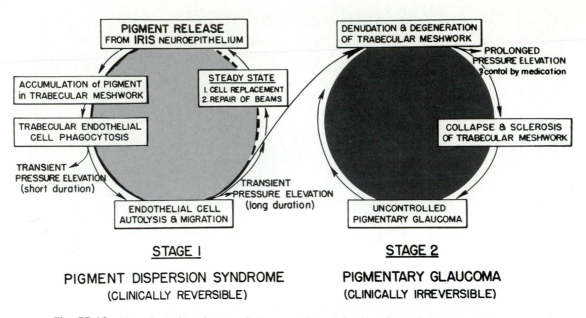

STAGE 1

PIGMENT DISPERSION SYNDROME
(CLINICALLY REVERSIBLE)

STAGE 2

PIGMENTARY GLAUCOMA
(CLINICALLY IRREVERSIBLE)

Fig. 55-10 Hypothetical mechanism that may explain pathophysiology of pigmentary glaucoma. First stage of disease is clinically reversible and gives rise to transient rises in intraocular pressure. Second stage, characterized by irreparable damage to trabecular tissues, is irreversible and is accompanied by uncontrolled glaucoma.

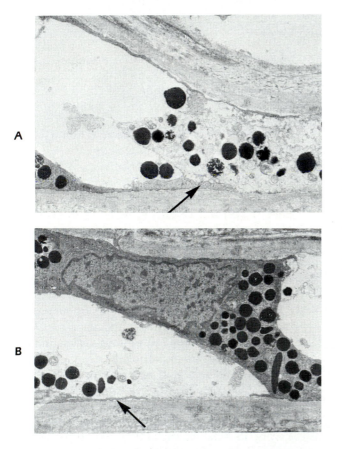

Fig. 55-11 Trabecular meshwork in which single trabecular cells support opposing beams. Thin processes of healthy trabecular cells spread to cover denuded beams or replace damaged or degenerating cells. **A,** A pale, disintegrating trabecular cell has partially lifted from beam and is being undermined by a process from healthier trabecular cell *(arrow).* Bottom surface of upper beam has been covered by a thin cell process, whereas upper surface of beam is still denuded of cells. **B,** A small cell process from a large trabecular cell has extended to cover a portion of denuded lower beam. A second healthy trabecular cell has extended under and is replacing damaged trabecular cell *(arrow).*

explain why certain individuals with pigmentary dispersion syndrome develop severe glaucoma, whereas others with an identical clinical picture have a normal intraocular pressure. Those who have mild to moderate pressure elevation and who apparently recover from the disease can be thought of as having a less severe endothelial incapacitation.

Loss of Pigment from the Iris

The loss of pigment from the iris has been considered to be the result of congenital atrophy or degeneration of the iris neuroepithelium.[9,46] Campbell[11] has documented a pathogenetic mechanism that appears to account for this pigment release (Fig. 55-12). Alternate back-and-forth rubbing of the posterior peripheral iris surface against packets of zonules inserted anteriorly on the lens surface appears to mechanically dislodge pigment granules from the pigmented epithelium of the iris. The loss of pigment and cells that overlie the zonules correspond well with the midperipheral radial pattern of iris transillumination defects (Fig. 55-13). Loss of pigment, however, can progress to involve the entire neuroepithelial layer. Kampik et al.,[30] using scanning electron microscopy, confirmed that the iris defects consistently follow the course of the zonular fibers.

This theory also provides explanations for two questions regarding pathophysiology. First, why pigmentary glaucoma predominantly affects younger white men with mild to moderate myopia; and second, why the severity and incidence of the disease decrease with increasing age. Campbell[11] believes that in eyes of patients predisposed to pigmentary glaucoma, the peripheral iris assumes a concave configuration, allowing it to rub against the zonules during normal physiologic movement, causing pigment liberation. The young myopic eye may continue to enlarge into the patient's 20s or early 30s, and this increase in diameter of the globe may be associated with an enlargement of the ciliary body ring in relation to the lens. This enlargement causes the peripheral iris to sag and establish contact with the zonules. Male predominance may occur because the greater size of the eye in men may increase the chance of the peripheral iris configuration being sufficiently concave to permit iridozonular rubbing. Except in the young myope, the eye generally ceases to enlarge when maturity is reached. The lens, however, continues to grow slowly until late in life. Since the average size of the pupil decreases with increasing age, the combination of increasing lens diameter and decreasing pupil size creates a relative pupillary block, which causes an anterior shift in the peripheral iris away from the zonules.[11] This may explain the decrease in incidence and severity of pigmentary glaucoma in elderly patients.

Another puzzling feature of pigmentary glaucoma is its relative rarity in blacks and Orientals, even though their uveae are heavily pigmented and

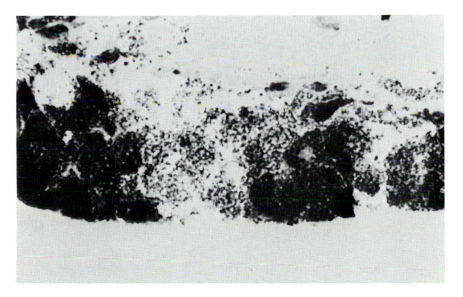

Fig. 55-12 Light micrograph of a region of pigmented epithelium of iris where pigment has been liberated. Sharply delineated regions of pigment loss may represent paths of zonular fibers.

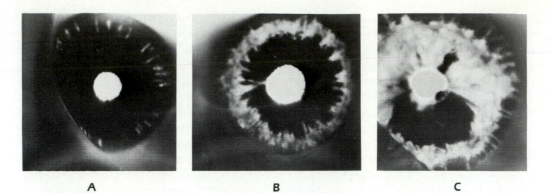

Fig. 55-13   Photographs of transilluminated irides depicting three stages of pigment loss in pigmentary glaucoma. Characteristic early midperipheral pattern of transillumination defects shown in **A** may become confluent in some patients and extend toward the pupillary margin as shown in **B**. Rarely, pigment loss may progress to involve most of iris, as shown in **C**.

pigment in the angle is not an uncommon finding. In a comparative study of aqueous humor dynamics in normotensive eyes of black and white patients, Boles-Carenini et al.[8] were unable to demonstrate a difference in intraocular pressure, facility of outflow, or rate of aqueous humor production between the two groups. The higher incidence in whites might be related more specifically to the degree of iris pigmentation and stromal compactness.

The iris in darkly pigmented individuals is heavily laden with pigment, and its anterior surface commonly appears velvety smooth and homogeneously compact. By contrast, in more lightly pigmented persons the iris is not only lighter in color, but also appears to have a more lacy texture, deep crypts, and easily visible stromal blood vessels. The lightest irides also appear thinner, often to a point where the slit-beam can be focused through the stroma to the level of the pigmented layer. Although attempts to demonstrate histologically that the darker iris is thicker have not been successful, it does appear to be more compact with a larger number of melanocytes in the stroma.[67] The velvety appearance of the iris under slit-lamp observation is borne out histologically by evidence of a semiconfluent anterior surface.

Evidence of a more compact stroma in darkly pigmented irides is suggested by the fact that the darker iris does not respond initially as well as the lighter colored iris to miotics or mydriatics. Chen and Poth[12] in 1929 found that pupils of whites were most responsive to several different mydriatics, blacks were least responsive, and Orientals had an intermediate response.

A possible explanation for the slower response

of blacks to miotics and mydriatics was provided by Emiru.[15] Comparing African blacks with European whites, he administered homatropine 4% to one eye and phenylephrine 4% to the other. Both onset of mydriasis and attainment of full mydriasis took less time in the European than in the heavily pigmented African. Interestingly, the irides of albino Africans dilated more briskly than those of either group, suggesting that these differences are more related to iris color than to race. Furthermore, homatropine, a cholinergic blocking agent, had a faster onset of action than phenylephrine, an adrenergic stimulator. The site of action of homatropine is the sphincter pupillae, and the site of action of phenylephrine is the dilator pupillae, which lies deeper in the stroma. The difference in accessibility to these muscles by topically applied drugs is argued as being the reason for the different individual responses found in such studies.[15] The more heavily pigmented compact stroma of dark irides may not only impede the penetration of various drugs, but might also limit the extent to which such irides dilate. Such stromal characteristics as heavy pigmentation and compactness might prevent peripheral iris sagging, which is believed to be essential for the development of the pigmentary dispersion syndrome.[11]

DIFFERENTIAL DIAGNOSIS

Pigmentary dispersion, with or without elevated intraocular pressure, can usually be easily distinguished from most other abnormalities in which dissemination of pigment is part of the disease process. These include uveitis, pigment in the angle caused by dispersion of melanoma cells, cysts of the iris and ciliary body, postoperative conditions, and aging changes. Most of these occur unilaterally and are evident on history and examination. In addition, trabecular pigmentation is less dense and is usually unevenly distributed throughout the circumference of the trabecular meshwork in these conditions.

The disease most similar to pigmentary glaucoma is pseudoexfoliation syndrome with glaucoma. In this condition, there is loss of pigment from the iris neuroepithelium; iris transillumination, pigment dispersion in the anterior segment, including Krukenberg's spindle; trabecular pigmentation; and elevation of intraocular pressure. Careful biomicroscopic examination easily separates the two diseases.

The age of onset for pseudoexfoliative glaucoma is usually over 60 and rare under 40. There is no sexual or racial predilection for the pseudoexfoliation syndrome, although reports seem to indicate a higher prevalence of the disease in Scandinavians. The size and shape of the eye (myopia) appear to be unrelated to the incidence of the disease. The pigmentation of the trabecular meshwork is not as intense as in pigmentary glaucoma. Iris transillumination characteristically begins at the pupillary border and not the midperiphery. Unlike pigmentary dispersion, approximately 50% of patients with pseudoexfoliation syndrome are clinically affected in only one eye. Finally, the presence of white flakes of pseudoexfoliation material at the pupillary border and on the anterior lens surface is diagnostic of the syndrome.

Several reports[26,48,54,66] have appeared recently describing a secondary form of pigmentary glaucoma that can occur after the implantation of posterior chamber intraocular lenses. The pigment liberation is thought to be caused by excessive trauma of the iris at the time of lens implantation or continued contact of the intraocular lens with the iris postoperatively. This entity can be distinguished from the naturally occurring disease by its presence in the operated eye alone, a history of posterior chamber lens implantation, and mild to marked iris pigment atrophy in areas contingent with or adjacent to the lens. Intraocular pressure elevation is usually transient or easily controlled, but laser trabeculoplasty has been required in some instances.

MANAGEMENT

Medical Therapy

The rationale for the institution of medical therapy in pigmentary glaucoma may be different from that used in other forms of open-angle glaucoma. In pigmentary glaucoma, there is often a rather insidious rise in intraocular pressure, with ocular tensions commonly rising to 60 mm Hg or more. Patients with pigmentary dispersion syndrome are also subject to rather wide fluctuations in intraocular pressure.

The early age of onset and the wide fluctuations in intraocular pressure require a somewhat different approach to management from that of primary open-angle glaucoma. If the trabecular meshwork has the capacity to undergo self-repair and remain in stage I of the disease, only the occasional "crisis" of pressure elevation will require therapy, and the condition may eventually go into remission. However, if the meshwork has limited or no capacity to recover and the disease goes into stage II, the management will be determined by the effectiveness of the medication and the remaining functional capacity of the trabecular meshwork.

The approach to the medical therapy of pigmentary glaucoma is basically the same as that for primary open-angle glaucoma. Theoretically, drugs that constrict the pupil and tauten the peripheral iris might decrease iridozonular rubbing and eliminate pigment accumulation in the meshwork. However, miotics in young individuals are poorly tolerated because of the associated spasm of accommodation and blurring of vision. Miotics should be used cautiously in young myopic patients with pigmentary glaucoma, because of the reported association with retinal detachment in patients with associated chorioretinal degeneration. All patients with pigmentary glaucoma being considered for miotic therapy should have a careful peripheral retinal examination.

An alpha-adrenergic blocking agent such as thymoxamine hydrochloride, which constricts the pupil but does not affect accommodation or aqueous humor dynamics could prove beneficial.[11] Thymoxamine is not approved for this purpose, however, and is unavailable for general use. In its present formulation, the ocular irritation that the drug causes makes it unlikely that patients would tolerate it. Mechanistically, such a drug has interesting possibilities, and its usefulness should be explored.

Epinephrine compounds alone, or in combination with other agents, have proven effective.[16] Scheie and Cameron[49] felt that epinephrine alone or combined with pilocarpine appeared to be more effective in lowering intraocular pressure in pigmentary glaucoma than in primary open-angle glaucoma.

Beta-adrenergic blocking agents are also effective and have a relatively low incidence of undesirable side effects. Carbonic anhydrase inhibitors may be used on a short-term basis to lessen the severity of an acute pressure rise or on a long-term basis when indicated and tolerated by the patient.

Laser trabeculoplasty may be performed as an interim treatment in the management of advanced pigmentary glaucoma. Although the initial result from laser trabeculoplasty is good, a larger proportion of patients lose control of intraocular pressure over time when compared with primary open-angle glaucoma patients, and the loss of control can occur in less time (9 months versus 2 to 3 years). Lunde[37] found that the loss of control tended to occur in patients who were older and who had glaucoma for a longer period. Hagadus et al.,[23] using life-table analysis, found an inverse correlation between age of the patient and duration of successful control in a series of 50 eyes with pigmentary glaucoma undergoing laser trabeculoplasty. Extra caution must be exercised to watch these patients carefully since laser trabeculoplasty can result in worsening of the glaucoma.

Surgical Therapy

The surgical management of patients with pigmentary glaucoma follows the same principles and considerations used in the management of primary open-angle glaucoma. The appearance and change in the optic nerve along with visual field defects should be the principal guidelines used in deciding whether surgery is needed. Most patients respond well to standard filtration operations.

REFERENCES

1. Becker, B, and Podos, SM: Krukenberg's spindles and primary open-angle glaucoma, Arch Ophthalmol 76:635, 1966
2. Becker, B, Shin, DH, Cooper DG, and Kass, MA: The pigment dispersion syndrome, Am J Ophthalmol 83:161, 1977
3. Bellows, AR, Jocson, VL, and Sears, ML: Iris pigment granule obstruction of the aqueous outflow channels in enucleated monkey eyes, Paper presented at the Association for Research in Vision and Ophthalmology, 1974
4. Berger, A, Ritch, R, McDermott, JA, and Wang, RF: Pigmentary dispersion, refraction and glaucoma, Invest Ophthalmol Vis Sci Suppl 28:114, 1987
5. Bick, MW: Pigmentary glaucoma in females, Arch Ophthalmol 58:483, 1957
6. Bill, A: Blood circulation and fluid dynamics in the eye, Physiol Rev 55:383, 1975
7. Birch-Hirschfeld, A: Menschlichen Auges durch Rontgenstrahlen, Z Augenheilkd 45:199, 1921
8. Boles-Carenini, B, Buten, RE, Spurgeon, WM, and Ascher, KW: Comparative tonographic study of nor-

motensive eyes of white and Negro persons, Am J Ophthalmol 40:224, 1955
9. Brini, A, Porte, A, and Roth, A: Atrophie des couches epitheliales de l'iris: étude d'un cas de glaucome pigmentaire au microscope optique et au microscope electronique, Doc Ophthalmol 26:403, 1969
10. Calhoun, FP, Jr: Pigmentary glaucoma and its relation to Krukenberg's spindles, Am J Ophthalmol 36:1398, 1953
11. Campbell, DG: Pigmentary dispersion and glaucoma: a new theory, Arch Ophthalmol 97:1667, 1979
12. Chen, KK, and Poth, EJ: Racial difference as illustrated by the mydriatic action of cocaine, euphthalmine, and ephedrine, J Pharm Exp Ther 36:429, 1929
13. Davidson, JA, Brubaker, RF, and Ilstrup, DM: Dimensions of the anterior chamber in pigment dispersion syndrome, Arch Ophthalmol 101:81, 1983
14. Duncan, TE: Krukenberg spindles in pregnancy, Arch Ophthalmol 91;355, 1974
15. Emiru, VP: Response to mydriatics in the African, Br J Ophthalmol 55:538, 1971
16. Epstein, DL: Pigment dispersion and pigmentary glaucoma. In Chandler, PA, and Grant, WM, editors: Glaucoma, Philadelphia, 1979, Lea & Febiger
17. Epstein, DL, Boger, WP, III, and Grant, WM: Phenylephrine provocative testing in the pigmentary dispersion syndrome, Am J Ophthalmol 85:43, 1978
18. Evans, WH, Odom, RE, and Wenass, EJ: Krukenberg's spindle: a study of 202 collected cases, Arch Ophthalmol 26:1023, 1941
19. Fine, BS, Yanoff, M, and Scheie, HG: Pigmentary "glaucoma": a histologic study, Trans Am Acad Ophthalmol Otolaryngol 78:314, 1974
20. Gillies, WE: Pigmentary glaucoma: a clinical review of anterior segment pigment dispersal syndrome, Aust N Z J Ophthalmol 13:325, 1985
21. Grant, WM: Experimental aqueous perfusion in enucleated human eyes, Arch Ophthalmol 69:783, 1963
22. Grant WM: Personal communication, 1981
23. Hagadus, J et al: Argon laser trabeculoplasty in pigmentary glaucoma, Invest Ophthalmol Vis Sci Suppl 25:94, 1984
24. Havener, VH: Ocular pharmacology, ed 4, St Louis, 1978, The CV Mosby Co
25. Hoffmann, F, Dumitrescu, L, and Hager, H: Pigment-glaucom, Klin Monatsbl Augenheilkd 166:609, 1975
26. Huber, C: The gray iris syndrome: an iatrogenic form of pigmentary glaucoma, Arch Ophthalmol 102:397, 1984
27. Iwamoto, T, Witmer, R, and Landolt, E: Light and electron microscopy in absolute glaucoma with pigment dispersion phenomena and contusion angle deformity, Am J Ophthalmol 72:420, 1971
28. Jess, A: Zur Frage des Pigmentglaukoms, Klin Monatsbl Augenheilkd 71:175, 1923
29. Kaiser-Kupfer, MI, Kupfer, C, and McCain, L: Asymmetric pigment dispersion syndrome, Trans Am Ophthalmol Soc 81:310, 1983

30. Kampik, A, Green, WR, Quigley, HA, and Pierce LH: Scanning and transmission electron microscopic studies of two cases of pigment dispersion syndrome, Am J Ophthalmol 91:573, 1981

31. Koeppe, L: Die Rolle des Irispigment beim Glaukom, Ber Dtsch Ophthalmol Ges 40:478, 1916

32. Kristensen, P: Mydriasis-induced pigment liberation in the anterior chamber associated with acute rise in intraocular pressure in open-angle glaucoma, Acta Ophthalmol 43:714, 1965

33. Kupfer, C, Kuwabara, T, and Kaiser-Kupfer, M: The histopathology of pigmentary dispersion syndrome with glaucoma, Am J Ophthalmol 80:857, 1975

34. Levinsohn, G: Beitrag zur pathologische Anatomie und Pathologie des Glaukoms, Arch Augenheilkd 62:131, 1909

35. Lichter, PR: Pigmentary glaucoma: current concepts, Trans Am Acad Ophthalmol Otolaryngol 78:309, 1974

36. Lichter, PR, and Shaffer, RM: Diagnostic and prognostic signs in pigmentary glaucoma, Trans Am Acad Ophthalmol Otolaryngol 74:984, 1970

37. Lunde, MW: Argon laser trabeculoplasty in pigmentary dispersion syndrome with glaucoma, Am J Ophthalmol 96:721, 1983

38. Mandelkorn, RM, et al: Inheritance and the pigmentary dispersion syndrome, Ann Ophthalmol 15:577, 1983

39. Mapstone, R: Pigment release, Br J Ophthalmol 65:258, 1981

40. Mauksch H: Zerfall des retinalen Pigmentblattes der Iris bei zwei Brudern, Ztrschr f Augenheilkd 57:262, 1925

41. McDermott, JA, Ritch, R, Berger, A, and Wang, RF: Inheritance of pigmentary dispersion syndrome, Invest Ophthalmol Vis Sci Suppl 28:153, 1987

42. Migliazzo, CV, Shaffer, RN, Nykin, R, and Magee, S: Long-term analysis of pigmentary dispersion syndrome and pigmentary glaucoma, Ophthalmology 93:1528, 1986

43. Richardson, TM, Hutchinson, BT, and Grant WM: The outflow tract in pigmentary glaucoma: a light and electron microscopic study, Arch Ophthalmol 195:1015, 1977

44. Richter, CU, Richardson, TM, and Grant WM: Pigmentary dispersion syndrome and pigmentary glaucoma: a prospective study of the natural history, Arch Ophthalmol 104:211, 1986

45. Ritch, R: Nonprogressive low-tension glaucoma with pigmentary dispersion, Am J Ophthalmol 94:190, 1982

46. Rodrigues, MM, Spaeth, GL, Weinreb, S, and Sivalingam, E: Spectrum of trabecular pigmentation in open-angle glaucoma: a clinicopathologic study, Trans Am Acad Ophthalmol Otolaryngol 81:258, 1976

47. Rohen, JW, and van der Zypen, E: The phagocytic activity of the trabecular meshwork endothelium: an electron microscopic study of the vervet (cercopi-

thecus aethiops), v Graefe's Arch Klin Exp Ophthalmol 175:143, 1968

48. Samples, JE, Van Buskirk, EM, Shults, WT, and Van Dyk, HJL, Jr: Optic nerve head drusen and glaucoma, Arch Ophthalmol 103:1678, 1985

49. Scheie, HG, and Cameron JD: Pigment dispersion syndrome: a clinical study, Br J Ophthalmol 65:264, 1981

50. Scheie, HG, and Fleischauer, HW: Idiopathic atrophy of the epithelial layers of the iris and ciliary body, Arch Ophthalmol 59:216, 1958

51. Seissiger, J: Weitere Beitrage zur Kenntnis der Axenfeld-Krukenberg'schen Pigmentspindel, Klin Monatsbl Augenheilkd 77:37, 1926

52. Sherwood, M, and Richardson, TM: Evidence for in vivo phagocytosis by trabecular endothelial cells, Invest Ophthalmol Vis Sci Suppl 21:66, 1980

53. Shihab, Z, Murrell, WJ, Lamberts, DW, and Avera, B: The corneal endothelium and central corneal thickness in pigmentary dispersion syndrome, Arch Ophthalmol 104:845, 1986

54. Smith, JP: Pigmentary open-angle glaucoma secondary to posterior chamber intraocular lens implantation and erosion of the iris pigment epithelium, J Am Intraocul Implant Soc 11:174, 1985

55. Speakman, JS: Pigmentary dispersion, Br J Ophthalmol 65:249, 1981

56. Stankovic, J: Den Beitrag zur Kenntnis der Vererbung des Pigmentglaukom, Klin Monatsbl Augenheilkd 139:165, 1961

57. Strebel, J, and Steiger, O: Korrelation der Vererbung von Augenleiden (Ectopia lentium cong, Ectopia pupillae, Myopie) und sog nicht angeborenen Herzfehlern, Arch f Augenheilkd 78:208, 1915

58. Sugar, HS: Concerning the chamber angle. I. Gonioscopy, Am J Ophthalmol 23:853, 1940

59. Sugar, HS: Pigmentary glaucoma: a 25-year review, Am J Ophthalmol 62:499, 1966

60. Sugar, HS: Symposium: glaucoma-discussion of the three preceding papers, Trans Am Acad Ophthalmol Otolaryngol 78:328, 1974

61. Sugar, HS, and Barbour, FA: Pigmentary glaucoma: a rare clinical entity, Am J Ophthalmol 32:90, 1949

62. Vogt, A: Weitere Ergebnisse der Spaltlampenmikroskopie des vorderen Bulbaschnittes (Cornea, vorderer Glaskorper, Conjunctiva, Lidrander). I. Abschnitt, Hornhaut, Arch f Ophthalmol 106:63, 1921

63. Vogt, A: Atlas der Spaltlampenmikroskopie, Klin Monatsbl Augenheilkd 81:711, 1928

64. von Hippel, E: Zur pathologischen Anatomie des Glaucoma, Arch Ophthalmol 52:498, 1901

65. Weber, PA, and Dingle, JB: Pigmentary glaucoma in a black albino, Ann Ophthalmol 15:454, 1983

66. Woodhams, JT, and Lester, JC: Pigmentary dispersion glaucoma secondary to posterior chamber intraocular lenses, Ann Ophthalmol 16:852, 1984

67. Yanoff, M, and Fine, BS: Ocular pathology: a text and atlas, New York, 1975, Harper & Row, Publisher

Chapter 56

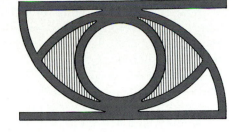

Exfoliation Syndrome

William E. Layden

HISTORICAL BACKGROUND

In 1917, Lindberg[76] first described the presence of grayish flecks on the pupillary border in 50% of his patients with chronic glaucoma. In describing this condition, the terms *senile exfoliation* and *glaucoma capsulare* were suggested by Vogt,[146] who considered exfoliation material to originate from the lens capsule and associated it with open-angle glaucoma. Others argued that it was merely deposited on the normal lens capsule.[24,80]

Emphasis on this syndrome was lost, however, until 1951, when Weekers et al.[148] coined the term *senile uveal exfoliation*. Wilson[149] suggested the term *glaucoma senilis* to indicate that exfoliation was a result of aging, and Dvorak-Theobald[38] suggested *pseudoexfoliation of the lens capsule* to differentiate it from true exfoliation in glassblowers. Other terms coined to reflect the presumed origin and nature of the material have included *iridociliary exfoliation with capsular pseudoexfoliation*,[10] *exfoliation of the pseudocapsule*,[68] *fibrillopathia epitheliocapsularis*,[21] and *complex pigmentary glaucoma*.[117]

Eagle et al.[39] suggested that the exfoliation syndrome is a basement membrane disease, terming it the *basement membrane exfoliation syndrome*. Bergmanson et al.[20] suggested the term *exfoliation of the lens capsule* to cover all the aspects of this syndrome. Garner and Alexander[44] suggested *oxytalanosis of the aqueous* based on studies of histochemical similarity of exfoliation material to zonular fibers.

Sunde[132] proposed the term *exfoliation syndrome*, which may be the most inclusive description of the clinical, biochemical, and histopathologic findings. For purposes of discussion, we will differentiate exfoliation syndrome *with* and *without* glaucoma.

EPIDEMIOLOGY

Incidence without Glaucoma

Reported prevalence rates of exfoliation vary widely in different geographic locations.[35] Reasons for such variations include the racial and ethnic composition of the population studied, patient selection, clinical criteria for diagnosis, thoroughness of examination, and definition of glaucoma. As a result, comparison of reports is difficult even when age-specific rates are available. Although originally associated with the Scandinavian countries, it is now well established that exfoliation occurs worldwide, virtually no area being spared.* It should be noted that many cases go undetected because of failure to dilate the pupil or to examine the lens by the slit-lamp after dilation, and because of a low index of suspicion.[74,112]

The prevalence of exfoliation ranges from 0% among the Eskimos to as high as 38% in Navaho Indians.[41,43] Age is an important determinant in the incidence of exfoliation in patients both with and without glaucoma, prevalence rates increasing markedly from age 50 to the late 80s.[7] In the Framingham Eye Study, age-specific prevalence rates for exfoliation in patients not identified specifically as having glaucoma rose from 0.6% for ages 52 to 64 to as high as 5% for ages 75 to 85.[63] Aasved[5] similarly found a 0.4% rate for ages 50 to 59 and a 7.9% rate at ages 80 to 89. South African Bantu have the onset of the pregranular stage at about the age of 40.[15] Taylor et al.[140] found a range of 1.3% to 16% in Australian aborigines, depending on the age.

---

*References 1, 15, 35, 41, 43, 79, 136, 139.

Incidence With Glaucoma

The reported incidence of exfoliation in patients with glaucoma varies according to author and population studied, ranging from practically zero to as high as 93%.[5,16,56,136] Luntz[79] found exfoliation in 1.4% of whites and 20% of blacks with open-angle glaucoma in South Africa. Exfoliation was reported in 8.1% of Australian aborigines with glaucoma[140] and 46% to 57% of glaucoma patients in Iceland.[134] In all reviews, the incidence of exfoliation and glaucoma increases with age. The youngest reported patient was 22 years of age.[130] Overall, however, it is a disease of the elderly.

Odland and Aasved[85] studied the occurrence of glaucoma in eyes with exfoliation followed for 2 to 9 years and found the greatest risk of glaucoma to be in the initial years. However, adequate follow-up is often difficult,[119] and this has been disputed.[70,120] Linner[77] suggested that exfoliation may remain stable for a long period of time and then suddenly increase in intensity with a concomitant rise in intraocular pressure. Patients with exfoliation who have glaucoma tend to be younger than those who do not have glaucoma.[3,53,136]

Glaucoma occurs more commonly in eyes with exfoliation syndrome than in those without it. Kozart and Yanoff found glaucomatous optic nerve or visual field damage in 7% and ocular hypertension in 15% of 100 consecutive patients with exfoliation syndrome. Henry et al.[61] found the 5- and 10-year cumulative probabilities of initially nonglaucomatous eyes with exfoliation syndrome developing glaucoma to be 5.3% ± 0.1% and 15.4% ± 2%, respectively, a significantly higher rate than would be expected in a similar group of patients without exfoliation syndrome.

Women have predominated in some studies of exfoliation syndrome without glaucoma.[1,2,5,56,136] However, in exfoliation syndrome with glaucoma, no sex predilection seems to occur.*

Recent findings showing that eyes with elevated intraocular pressure and signs of loss of pigment from the iris sphincter region may be found to have exfoliation material on conjunctival biopsy in the absence of clinically visible exfoliation on the lens suggest that exfoliation syndrome may be much more common than previously realized.[95]

Monocular versus Binocular Involvement

Monocular involvement seems to be more common in exfoliation syndrome than binocular in-

volvement; at least in the American literature.[63,70,147] Tarkkanen[136] described unchanged unilateral occurrence in 47 patients followed for 5 years. Hansen and Sellevold[57] found, however, that exfoliation developed in the second eye in 40% of men and in 31% of women over 5 years. Aasved[2] found that 43% of patients with unilateral occurrence developed binocular involvement after 6 or 7 years. Henry et al.[61] found the probability of exfoliation developing in the opposite eye was 6.8% after 5 years and 16.8% after 10 years. Most evidence points to the fact that unilateral exfoliation is often the precursor of bilateral exfoliation. Bilateral glaucoma and exfoliation syndrome occur at a slightly older age than unilateral exfoliation and glaucoma.[49,63,70,136]

Systemic Associations

No clear-cut association of exfoliation with any systemic disease has been shown. There does not seem to be any correlation with diabetes mellitus, cardiovascular disease, or hypertension. Tsukahara and Matsuo[142] described patients with both primary familial amyloidosis and exfoliation, but age was a predominant factor in both conditions, and a cause-and-effect association could not be established.

Association with cataract formation is not clear.[74,115,136] Since both entities occur in the aging population, it is difficult to ascribe a common etiologic association.[72,115,122,136] No correlation with other diseases of the vitreous or retina has been found, and no difference from normals has been found on HLA typing.[121]

Heredity

No clear pattern of inheritance has been discerned.[66,92,138] Gifford[49] reported a father and son with exfoliation. Tarkkanen[136] found no clear familial tendency but did note such an association in primary open-angle glaucoma and postulated that a gene was responsible for open-angle glaucoma, exfoliation, and pigment dispersion.[136] However, patients with exfoliation but without glaucoma respond to topical steroid testing similarly to the normal population.[50,93,137] The possibility of both exfoliation and primary open-angle glaucoma occurring in the same pedigree further confuses the issue.

CLINICAL PICTURE

Conjunctiva and Cornea

Clinically the conjunctiva is normal in exfoliation syndrome. Fluorescein angiography reveals

---

*References 1, 2, 56, 64, 70, 134, 136.

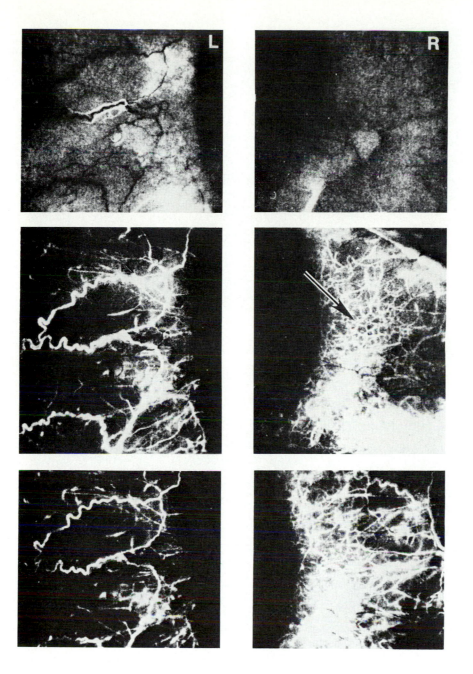

Fig. 56-1   Fluorescein angiography of limbus. **L,** Eye with open-angle glaucoma. **R,** Exfoliation glaucoma. Arrow illustrates loss of regular pattern and neovascularization. (From Laatikainen, L: Acta Ophthalmol 111(suppl):3, 1971)

loss of the regular limbal vascular pattern and areas of neovascularization in advanced cases (Fig. 56-1), as well as congestion of the anterior ciliary vessels.[73]

Small areas of flakes or clumps of exfoliation may be found on the endothelial surface of the cornea. There is usually a small amount of pigment inferiorly on the endothelium. Rarely there may be sufficient pigmentation to form a Krukenberg's spindle, but most often it is a diffuse, nonspecific form of pigmentation of the endothelium. Vannas et al.[145] noted a decrease in endothelial cell count by specular microscopy that could not be correlated with the duration of treatment or severity of the glaucoma. Spheroidal degeneration of the cornea has also been noted in eyes with exfoliation.[17]

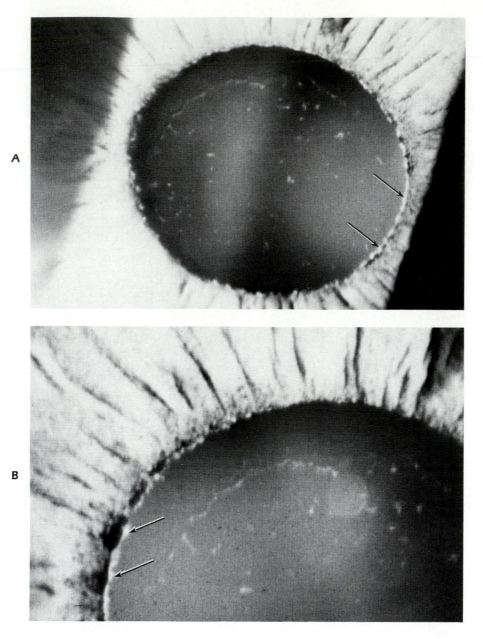

Fig. 56-2 **A,** Flecks in pupillary border *(arrows).* **B,** Close-up view of material lining pupil edge *(arrows).*

Iris and Pupil

Small flakes on the pupillary margin of the iris are a hallmark of exfoliation syndrome (Fig. 56-2). These can be best observed by moving the slit-lamp at 30 to 45 degrees using high magnification and a moderately narrow slit-beam. There may be fine pigmentation on the iris surface, especially in the folds and crypts.[94] This is more commonly seen in blue irides and may be difficult to detect in darkly pigmented ones. Prince and Ritch[94] noted particulate pigment deposition on the sphincter to be a characteristic sign of exfoliation syndrome.

Transillumination defects occur at the pupillary ruff and margin (see Plate IV, Fig. 2), in contrast to the midstromal slit-like transillumination defects found in pigmentary glaucoma.[6] However, if a sufficient amount of depigmentation has occurred,

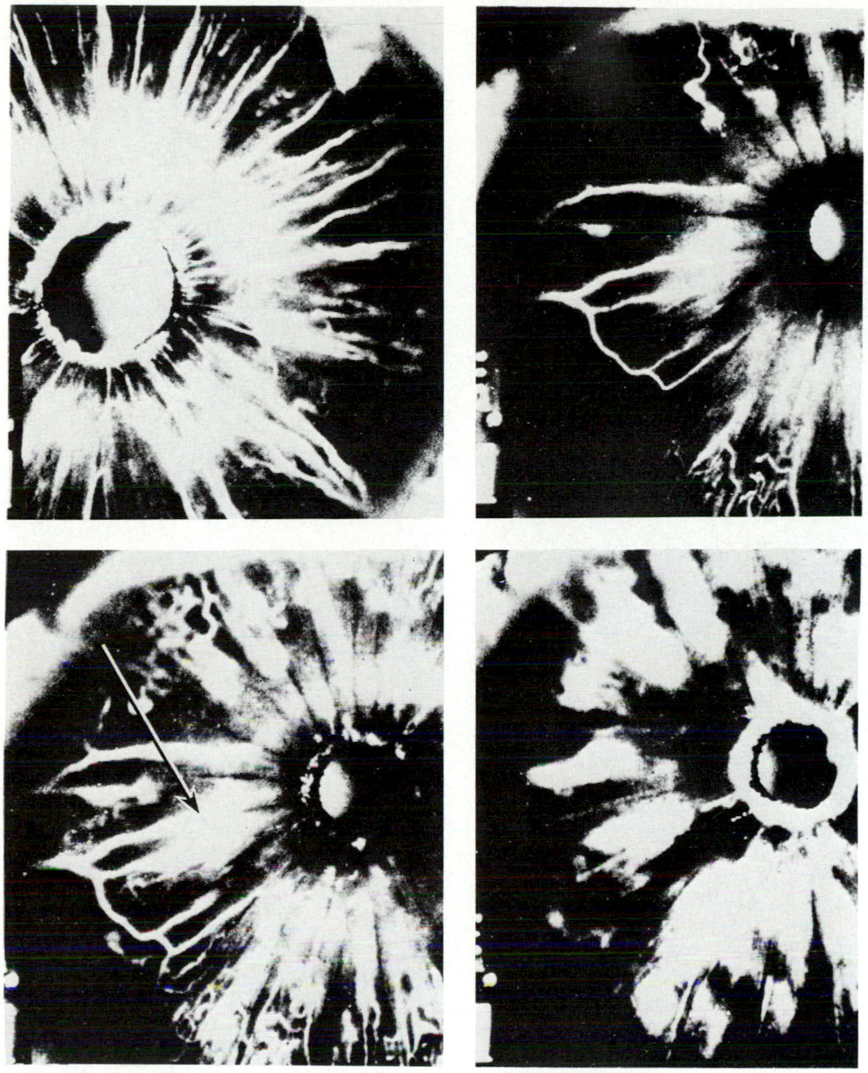

Fig. 56-3 **A,** Healthy fellow eye. **B** to **D,** Exfoliation with progressive filling showing neovascularization and profound leakage of dye *(arrow).*

defects may be noted over the entire sphincter region. Phakodonesis and iridodonesis may be present more commonly than previously thought.[55] Heavily pigmented synechiae may be present between the pupillary margin and the anterior lens capsule. Whether these are related to chronic miotic therapy or are intrinsic to the disease process is unknown. These adhesions may create difficulties in performing an adequate anterior capsulotomy during cataract extraction.

Angiographic abnormalities of the iris vessel include diminution in number, lack of normal radial pattern, neovascular clumps, and leakage of fluorescein[23,144] (Fig. 56-3).

Anterior Chamber and Angle

Rarely, small pigment floaters or small exfoliation particles can be seen floating in the aqueous in the undilated eye. After mydriasis, pigment dispersion is often seen, reminiscent of the liberation of pigment into the anterior chamber during mydriasis in the pigment dispersion syndrome.[71,81] Baba[11] observed gelatinous material liberated after dilation, which he linked to a high concentration of albuminoids in the aqueous.

Pigmentation of the trabecular meshwork is a prominent aspect of exfoliation syndrome[74,150] and may be an early diagnostic finding before the appearance of deposits on the pupillary margin or

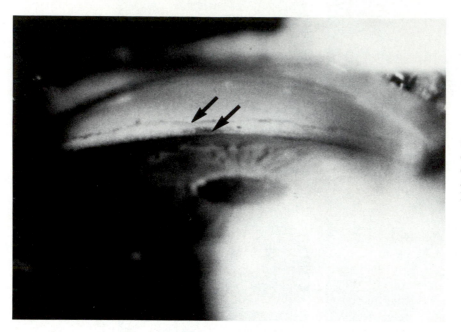

Fig. 56-4   Angle in exfoliation syndrome showing blotchy pigmentation of trabecular meshwork *(long arrow)* and pigment deposition on Schwalbe's line *(short arrow)*.

Fig. 56-5   Three zones on anterior lens capsule. Clear area is between central disc and peripheral zone with exception of bridge of material *(double arrows)*.

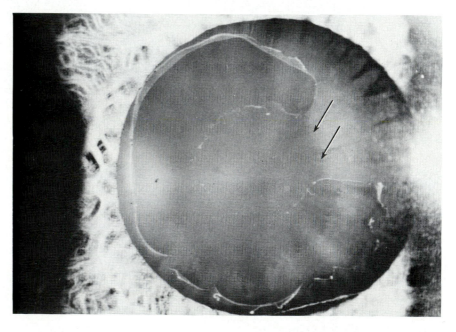

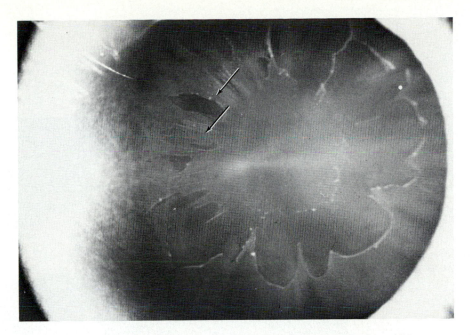

Fig. 56-6 Radial striations of material on lens capsule, perhaps a reflection of iris movement (*arrows*).

anterior lens capsule[95] (Fig. 56-4). Pigmentation in the superior portion of the meshwork should suggest the presence of exfoliation.[150] Pigmentation in unilateral cases is always more marked in the eye with exfoliation.[74,94]

The pigment is much less distinct in exfoliation syndrome than that seen in the pigment dispersion syndrome, and the pigment band is spotty and not as well defined. Pigment deposition on Schwalbe's line[113] is often present but may also be seen in other entities, such as the pigment dispersion syndrome. Less commonly, small flecks of exfoliation material can be observed in the angle.

Angle-closure glaucoma may be associated with exfoliation, but the majority of patients have open angles.[54]

Lens, Zonules, and Ciliary Body

Exfoliation material on the surface of the lens is the syndrome's most consistent and important diagnostic feature.* Three distinct zones may be present: a translucent central disc, a granular girdle around the periphery, and a clear zone separating these two areas (Fig. 56-5). The central disc is present in approximately 20% of cases, accounting for the occasional lack of pupillary flecks.[74] The intermediate clear zone is apparently caused by pupillary rubbing in eyes not on miotic therapy.[131] A curled-up edge of the central zone may be seen

*References 9, 76, 114, 132, 136.

after dilation. The peripheral zone is always present; it may be granular in the periphery and frosty white centrally, and radial striations are often seen (Fig. 56-6 and Plate IV, Fig. 3).

Deposits of exfoliation material on the zonules may explain the tendency to spontaneous subluxation or dislocation of the lens in advanced cases[13] (Fig. 56-7). Recent studies indicate the zonules are coated with exfoliation material without clear evidence of dehiscence of the zonular fibers themselves.[44] Deposits occur on the anterior hyaloid face after intracapsular cataract extraction (Fig. 56-8), suggesting that the lens is not the only source of exfoliation material.[25,51,96,129]

Cycloscopic examination of the zonules and ciliary processes has revealed accumulations of exfoliation material in all eyes in which it was present on the anterior lens surface and in over 50% of fellow eyes of unilateral cases[84] (see Plate IV, Fig. 1).

Intraocular Pressure

Mean intraocular pressures in normotensive eyes with exfoliation are usually higher than in those without exfoliation.[4] In patients with elevated intraocular pressure, the mean pressure is higher at the time of detection than it is in primary open-angle glaucoma.[4,58] Glaucomatous optic nerve head and visual field damage also tends to be greater in patients with exfoliation glaucoma than in patients with primary open-angle glau-

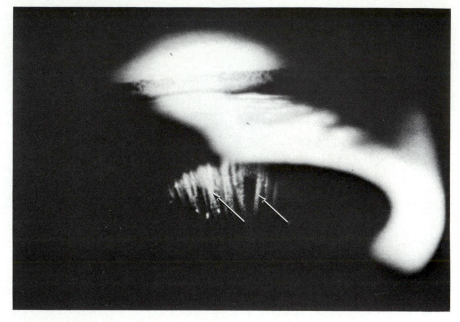

Fig. 56-7 Zonules coated with exfoliation material *(arrows)*. (Courtesy RN Shaffer, MD)

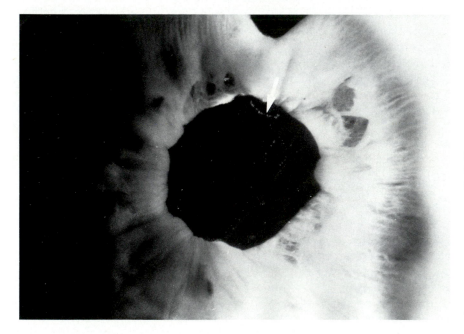

Fig. 56-8 Exfoliation material on anterior vitreous face after cataract extraction *(arrow)*.

coma.[3] This probably reflects the effects of the higher intraocular pressure on the optic nerve. Surgical treatment for glaucoma is more often necessary in eyes with exfoliation than with primary open-angle glaucoma.[3]

It has been thought that the degree of pigmentation may play a role in the high pressures encountered in some cases, but the extent of pigmentation and the severity of the glaucoma do not always correlate.[74] Only rarely is low-tension glaucoma associated with the presence of exfoliation.[131]

PATHOPHYSIOLOGY

Origin of the Exfoliation Material

Sunde[132] maintained that exfoliation originated as a degenerative condition of the lens capsule and that the characteristic deposition patterns were caused by the iris rubbing the material away from the anterior capsular surface. Bergmanson et al.[20] confirmed involvement of the lens capsule and underlying epithelium. Nonpigmented ciliary epithelium and iris pigment epithelium are also sources of exfoliation material. Electron microscopic studies indicate that not only the lens capsule, but other ocular structures such as the ciliary body, iris, and conjunctiva contain deposits of exfoliative material* (Fig. 56-9).

_____

*References 9, 18, 29, 46-48, 99, 101-103, 108.

Anterior Segment

Exfoliation material appears to be intimately involved with the adventitia of the iris vessels[47,74,99] (Fig. 56-10). Obliteration of the lumen, resulting in neovascularization and leakage of dye, correlates well with these findings.[105] Recent studies with fluorophotometry confirm these findings.[67] Deposits on the anterior surface of the iris and in the crypts and furrows are exogenous, as are those on the cornea, which does not appear to be a source of exfoliation. Extensive atrophy of pigment epithelial cells and deposits on the posterior surface have been described by both light and electron microscopy.[24,36,38]

Deposits occur on the trabecular meshwork and in the intertrabecular spaces. Ringvold and Vegge[108] found eyes with higher pressures to have greater involvement of the trabecular meshwork by exfoliation material. Exfoliation material may be present in the intertrabecular spaces, trabecular endothelium, juxtacanalicular tissue, and beneath the endothelium of Schlemm's canal, but not in the canal itself.[107] Material may be brought to the angle by the aqueous humor or produced by the basement membrane of trabecular endothelial cells. Harnisch[59] described both intercellular and intracellular pigment granules in the trabecular cells. There is an indication that the endothelial cells of the trabecular beams are not as severely involved as in the pigmentary dispersion syndrome.[98]

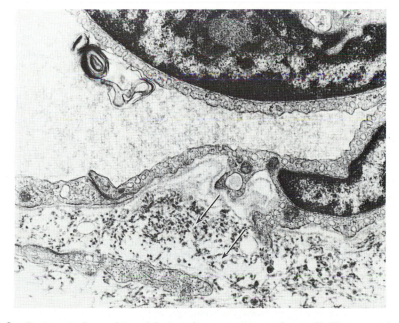

Fig. 56-9 Conjunctival vessel in exfoliation glaucoma. Arrows denote fibrillar material. (×3200.) (Courtesy RN Shaffer, MD)

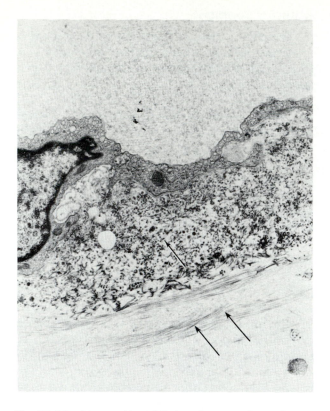

Fig. 56-10 Iris vessel in exfoliation glaucoma. Arrow denotes fibrillar material; doubles arrows denote normal collagen. (×16,000.) (From Layden, WE, and Shaffer, RN: Published with permission from the American Journal of Ophthalmology 78:835-841, 1974. Copyright by the Ophthalmic Publishing Co)

Lens and Zonules

Busacca[24] found minute vacuoles in the deep and superficial layers of the lens capsule, with exfoliation material appearing to flake off the capsular surface. Several other investigators also indicated involvement of the lens capsule[9,21,29,38,45] (Figs. 56-11, and 56-12). However, debate continues as to whether there is primary involvement of the capsule and epithelial cells of the lens, or whether it is a secondary deposit. Sugar et al.[131] suggested the lens, iris, and ciliary body epithelia as sources of exfoliation fibrils. Dickson and Ramsay[36] confirmed the presence of material on the lens capsule, but felt that it might originate from the iris pigment epithelium. Bergmanson et al.[20] found involvement of the lens capsule and underlying epithelium, especially on the peripheral third of the capsule. The capsule and epithelium at the pole of the lens were free of this material.

Dvorak-Theobald[38] supposed that zonules may be fragile and lead to lens displacement. No histologic confirmation of zonular weakness exists. Sunde[132] found flakes on the zonules but described elasticity of the zonular fibers as being normal. Deposits on the zonules may be of exogenous origin[135] (Fig. 56-13 and Plate IV, Fig. 3).

Involvement of the nonpigmented ciliary epithelium appears to be consistent[36,46,135] (Fig. 56-14). Sunde[132] found exfoliation on the pars plana in

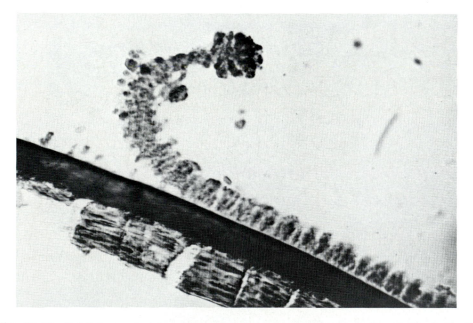

Fig. 56-11 Exfoliation material peeling off anterior lens capsule. (From Dvorak-Theobald, G: Am J Ophthalmol 37:1, 1954)

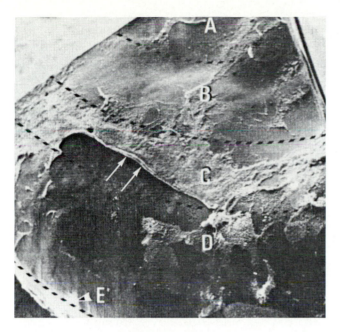

Fig. 56-12 Scanning electron micrograph of anterior lens surface with exfoliation material *(arrows)*. (×35.) *A,* Central area. *B,* Connection of peripheral-central area. *C,* Peripheral zone. *D,* Far periphery. *E,* Equator. (From Dickson, DH, and Ramsay, MS: Can J Ophthalmol 10:148, 1975)

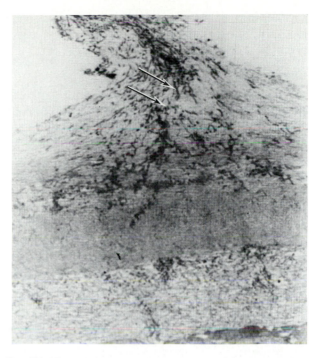

Fig. 56-13 Exfoliation material near zonular insertion. Arrows denote fibrillar material. (Courtesy JS Speakman, MD)

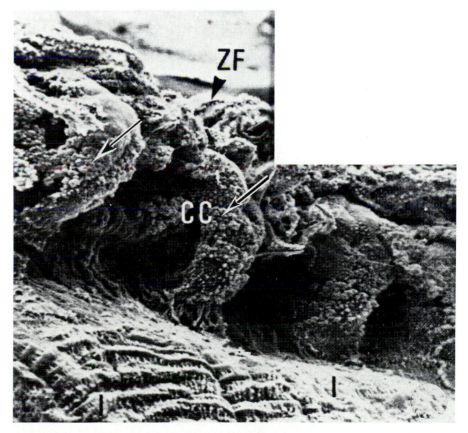

Fig. 56-14 Scanning electron micrograph of ciliary processes showing accumulation of material *(arrows)*. (×55.) *ZF,* Zonular fibers; *CC,* ciliary concretions (exfoliation material). (From Dickson, DH, and Ramsay, MS: Can J Ophthalmol 10: 148, 1975) See also Plate IV, Fig. 1.

about 50% of eyes. No exfoliation material has been found in the vessels or the stroma of the ciliary body or processes.

Other Tissues

Routine light microscopy shows no conjunctival alteration. With transmission electron microscopy, characteristic fibrillar granular material occurs near the basement membranes of the endothelial cells of the limbal conjunctival vessels.[74,99,114,123] Drainage of exfoliation materal from the aqueous does not account for its presence in the conjunctiva.[101]

Eagle et al.[39] found exfoliation material in the wall of a short posterior ciliary artery, as well as in the anterior iris stroma adjacent to a newly formed abnormal endothelial basement membrane. They suggested that exfoliation material is an abnormal basement membrane synthesized at multiple sites by aging cells. These may lead to replacement of normal basement membranes and subsequent epithelial atrophy.[39] This work has been recently confirmed by Spinelli.[124]

Although the palpebral conjunctiva may be involved, biopsies of the skin or oral mucosa do not reveal any abnormal material, suggesting an absence of systemic involvement.[103]

Nature of the Exfoliation Material

The biochemical nature of the exfoliation material remains unknown. It has been suggested that exfoliation material is amyloid-like,[29,34,104,106,127] or an amyloid.[82] The material consists of an irregular meshwork of randomly oriented cross-banded fibrils measuring about 30 nm in diameter[30,33] within a loose fibrogranular matrix containing 6 to 10 nm microfibrils.[125] "Classic" exfoliation fibers at high magnification appear to be composites of the microfibrils, aggregated laterally with added dense binding material.[28]

Davanger[31,32] concluded that the filament is a proteoglycosaminoglycan consisting of a protein core surrounded by polysaccharide side chains. Harnisch et al.[60] using the indirect immunoperoxidase method found that the fibrils contained a basement membrane proteoglycan. Anti–basement membrane proteoglycan antibodies to lens material reacted strongly with exfoliation material, implicating lens epithelium in its production. Mizuno et al.[83] found histochemical evidence of high acid phosphatase activity, suggesting that lysozymes were involved in the production of exfoliation material. Possible rupture of pigment epithelial cells may account for lysosomal involvment.[83]

Zirm[152] noted a high concentration of IgG in the aqueous in exfoliation but not in primary open-angle glaucoma. Baba[11] demonstrated alpha$_1$-lipoprotein in exfoliation material and felt that this might be the result of the high permeability of vessels in the anterior segment in exfoliation. He also found that the material was a sulfated glycosaminoglycan and suggested that abnormal glycosaminoglycan metabolism precedes the formation of the exfoliation material.[12]

Garner and Alexander[44] found exfoliation material to stain differently than zonules and suggested that the zonules were coated rather than being a source of production of the exfoliation material. They suggested that oxytalan, a microfibrillar component of elastic tissue, is a constituent of the exfoliation fibrils. Oxytalan is present in the body in areas of mechanical stress. In the eye, accommodation involves the equatorial lens capsule, the zonules, and the ciliary epithelium.

Lectin staining of exfoliation material has suggested a complex carbohydrate composition, with both O-linked sialomucin-type and N-linked oligosaccharide chains.[128]

Roh et al.[111] found mature, intermediate, and microfibrils adjacent to fibroblasts in close proximity to elastic tissue in the conjunctiva and suggested that the microfibrils may be involved in the formation of exfoliation material. Streeten et al.[126] found histochemical similarities between zonular elastic microfibrils and exfoliation material and a resemblance of the larger microfibrils of the ground substance to zonular and other oxytalan microfibrils.[125] The strong anatomic association between exfoliation fibers with elastosis in conjunctival specimens led the authors to suggest that exfoliation fibers themselves might be a form of elastosis. The close association of exfoliation fibers with fibroblasts suggested that exfoliation fibers can derive from cells that do not normally form basement membrane.[125]

MECHANISM OF GLAUCOMA

The debate as to whether exfoliation is an incidental finding in open-angle glaucoma or is actually the cause of the glaucoma continues. Glaucoma in eyes with exfoliation syndrome may be the result of blockage of the trabecular meshwork by exfoliation material or pigment liberated from the iris, dysfunction of trabecular endothelial cells, or concomitant primary open-angle glaucoma.

Exfoliation often exists in the absence of glaucoma[137] and may arise independently of glaucoma in some patients.[26] Extensive deposits of exfoliation material have been found in the trabecular meshwork of normotensive eyes.[19]

Severe pigment dispersion in exfoliation may also cause glaucoma. The concept of trabecular blockage fits well with the results of topical steroid testing and with the finding that in unilateral cases, the meshwork in the affected eye is the more pigmented one. However, a recent study by Richardson and Epstein,[98] using perfusion and ultrastructural studies, indicates that the trabecular meshwork was free of exfoliation material and that the main pathology involved destruction of Schlemm's canal and the accumulation of material in the juxtacanalicular region. However, the ultrastructural studies were done after perfusion and particulate material could have been washed from the meshwork.

In patients with unilateral exfoliation and open angles, glaucoma may also occur in the uninvolved fellow eye, suggesting an underlying defect in the aqueous dynamics.[88,136] This concept is also consistent with the finding of greater pigmentation in the affected eye. It is possible that in eyes with normal aqueous dynamics, exfoliation may exist without glaucoma, whereas in eyes with underlying impaired aqueous dynamics, glaucoma may result.

The observation that some patients with unilateral exfoliation have bilateral glaucoma counters the idea of a simple obstruction. Electron microscopic examination of the conjunctiva, however, has revealed the presence of exfoliation material in virtually all of these fellow eyes. The recent finding that exfoliation material may be found in the conjunctiva in eyes with increased pigmentation of the trabecular meshwork in the absence of clinically visible exfoliation on the lens[95] underscores the importance of further elucidation of its role in the development of glaucoma.

Angle-closure glaucoma has been described as occurring often in association with exfoliation.[54,62,78,150] Herbst[62] suggested that exfoliation may be causally related to acute angle-closure through the production of pupillary block. This is in contrast to the studies of Bartholomew[18] and Forsius et al.[42] Increased adherence of the pigment epithelium to the lens capsule could facilitate the development of pupillary block.[131] Another factor that may play a role in the development of secondary glaucoma is the possible relationship of phakodonesis as a sign of zonular weakness[14] or the complication of central anterior lens capsule adhesions to iris pigmentation.[29] Both could cause increased pupillary block.

It appears that the most current, reasonable explanation of the association between exfoliation syndrome and open-angle glaucoma is the presence of the material in an already glaucomatous eye as indicated by work where the noninvolved eye may be classified as having glaucoma in up to 24% of the cases.[112] Another possible explanation is that secondarily induced glaucoma may be present with a great deal of exfoliation material or a high association of adhesions of the pupillary area with the lens.

DIAGNOSIS

Diagnostic Techniques

Careful examination of the pupillary border is of great help in the diagnosis. If, after dilation, the diagnosis is still in question, placing the slit beam at 45 degrees to the axis of observation may help highlight the deposition on the endothelium of the cornea and slit-lamp transillumination of the pupillary edge may also be helpful.

Koeppe gonioscopy appears to be more revealing than gonioscopy with Zeiss or Goldmann lenses. When one sweeps across the iris to the angle, small deposits on the pupillary border can be highlighted (Fig. 56-15). Cycloscopy may also be helpful in making the diagnosis. However, the identification of small amounts of pigment on the endothelium of the cornea, elevated intraocular pressure, characteristic pigmentation on gonioscopy, and deposits on the anterior surface of the pupil and lens are generally sufficient.

Differential Diagnosis

The most important entity in the differential diagnosis is the pigment dispersion syndrome, which usually has a more distinct pigment band in the angle and a Krukenberg's spindle. It characteristically occurs in younger myopes and transillumination defects are peripheral and slit-like in contrast to those found in the exfoliation syndrome.

True exfoliation of the lens capsule is seen in those with exposure to high temperatures, such as glassblowers; is associated with cataract; and is rarely associated with glaucoma. The deposit from the heat-induced cataract is rolled up in a characteristic thin sheet, in contrast to the frosty appearance of exfoliation (Fig. 56-16). Iritis with pigment dispersion in the meshwork and adhesions of the pupillary margin to the anterior lens capsule can be differentiated by the lack of exfoliation material on the anterior lens capsule. Toxic exfoliation from iridocyclitis or foreign bodies such as copper or brass can usually be differentiated easily. A trau-

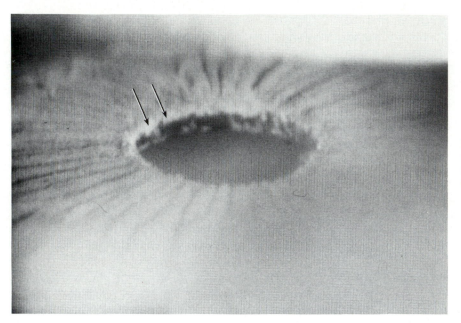

Fig. 56-15 Arrows highlight material on pupil viewed through Koeppe lens. (Courtesy RN Shaffer, MD)

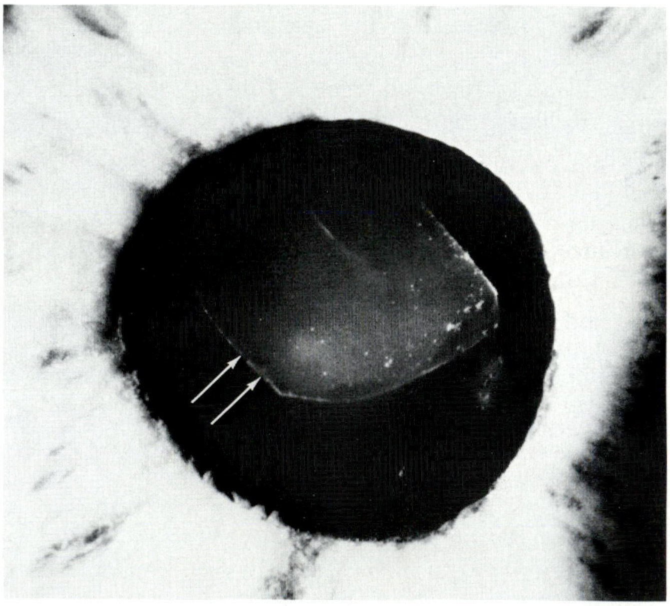

Fig. 56-16 True exfoliation *(arrows)*—splitting of capsule—seen in glassblower's cataract.

matic exfoliation or peeling of the lens capsule can occur but appears to be extremely rare.

Other conditions characterized by pigment changes, such as Fuchs' heterochromic iridocyclitis, pigmentation of the chamber angle with aging or after surgery, and pigmentation secondary to intraocular tumors can usually be readily distinguished.

MANAGEMENT

Medical Therapy

The initial approach to treatment of open-angle glaucoma associated with exfoliation is the same as that for primary open-angle glaucoma and includes beta-adrenergic antagonists, epinephrine compounds, and miotics. Glaucoma associated with exfoliation may be more resistant to medical therapy than primary open-angle glaucoma.*

The addition of epinephrine derivatives to beta-adrenergic blockers may be more effective than in primary open-angle glaucoma.[86] Miotic treatment may lead to synechiae between the pupillary margin and anterior lens capsule. Therefore miotic use should be accompanied by frequent dilation. However, dilation may also result in acute rises in intraocular pressure accompanied by diffuse pigment dispersion in the anterior chamber.[81,112] Routine dilation of patients with open-angle glaucoma treated with miotics was considered potentially hazardous by Shaw and Lewis.[116] Carbonic anhydrase inhibitors do not appear to be more or less effective than in primary open-angle glaucoma.

Laser and Surgical Therapy

Argon laser trabeculoplasty has been reported successful in open-angle glaucoma.† In exfoliation syndrome with glaucoma, it may be associated with sudden, late rises of intraocular pressure.[90,109] Patients with exfoliation may have a further upward drift of intraocular pressure in long-term studies.[109] There also are reports of a higher and greater percentage of pressure spikes immediately after argon laser trabeculoplasty in eyes with exfoliation.[143] Retreatment with lasers may help in some of the eyes.[109]

Laser iridectomy is the accepted treatment for angle-closure glaucoma associated with exfoliation. Use of the Nd:YAG laser may afford less closure of the iridectomy and more ease of penetration than the argon laser.[110]

The results of trabeculectomy are comparable to those in primary open-angle glaucoma.[39] There do not appear to be unusual complications.[65] Trabeculotomy has been advocated as an alternative surgical procedure,[52] although the effectiveness of this procedure in adult patients is subject to question.

Despite occasional reports that lens extraction in exfoliation might help pressure control, most investigators have noted that deposition of material on the hyaloid membrane continues after lens extraction.[49,51,96,129] Therefore cataract extraction should be performed only for visual reasons. Complications of extracapsular cataract surgery are more common in patients with exfoliation and include capsular rupture; lens dislocation, and zonular dialyses; and insufficient mydriasis.[55,97,118]

Prognosis

The prognosis is poorer with exfoliation syndrome and glaucoma compared with primary open-angle glaucoma. Ocular hypertensives with exfoliation are much more likely to develop glaucomatous damage on long-term follow-up than are those without exfoliation.[91] However, many patients with exfoliation never develop elevated intraocular pressures. It would be interesting to follow those patients who have had extracapsular cataract extraction and posterior chamber lens implantation to see if there is any adverse or beneficial effect on the long-term prognosis. More studies are needed not only to clarify the exact nature of the material but also to determine whether there are any true systemic associations.

REFERENCES

1. Aasved, H: The geographical distribution of fibrillopathia epitheliocapsularis, Acta Ophthalmol 47: 792, 1969
2. Aasved, H: The frequency of fibrillopathia epitheliocapsularis (so-called senile exfoliation or pseudoexfoliation) in patients with open-angle glaucoma, Acta Ophthalmol 49:194, 1971
3. Aasved, H: The frequency of optic nerve damage and surgical treatment in chronic simple glaucoma and capsular glaucoma, Acta Ophthalmol 49:589, 1971
4. Aasved, H: Intraocular pressure in eyes with and without fibrillopathia epitheliocapsularis, Acta Ophthalmol 49:601, 1971
5. Aasved, H: Mass screening for fibrillopathia epitheliocapsularis, Acta Ophthalmol 49:334, 1971
6. Aasved, H: Incidence of defects in the pigmented pupillary ruff in eyes with and without fibrillopathia epitheliocapsularis, Acta Ophthalmol 51: 710, 1973

---

*References 8, 22, 27, 37, 40, 69, 74, 87.
†References 75, 89, 90, 109, 133, 141, 143, 151.

7. Aasved, H: Prevalence of fibrillopathia epithelio-capsularis (pseudoexfoliation) and capsular glaucoma, Trans Ophthalmol Soc UK 1979, 99:293

8. Airaksinen, PJ: The long-term hypotensive effect of timolol maleate compared with the effect of pilocarpine in simple and capsular glaucoma, Acta Ophthalmol 57:425, 1979

9. Ashton, N, Sharit, M, Coelzer, R, and Black, R: Electron microscopic study of pseudoexfoliation of the lens capsule. I. Lens capsule and zonular fibers, Invest Ophthalmol 4:141, 1965

10. Audibert, J: Cited in Tarkkanen, A: Pseudoexfoliation of the lens capsule. Acta Ophthalmol Suppl 71:1, 1962

11. Baba, H: Investigation of the pathogenesis of glaucoma capsulare with special discussion of alpha-1 Lp and CP: in aqueous humor, v Graefe's Arch Klin Exp Ophthalmol 218:283, 1982

12. Baba, H: Histochemical and polarization optical investigation for glycosaminoglycans in exfoliation syndrome, v Graefe's Arch Klin Exp Ophthalmol 221:106, 1983

13. Bartholomew, RS: Lens displacement associated with pseudocapsular exfoliation, Br J Ophthalmol 54:744, 1970

14. Bartholomew, RS: Phakodonesis, Br J Ophthalmol 54:663, 1970

15. Bartholomew, RS: Pseudocapsular exfoliation in the Bantu of South Africa. I. Early or pregranular clinical stage, Br J Ophthalmol 55:693, 1971

16. Bartholomew, RS: Pseudocapsular exfoliation in the Bantu of South Africa. II. Occurrence and prevalence, Br J Ophthalmol 57:41, 1973

17. Bartholomew, RS: Spheroidal degeneration of the cornea, Doc Ophthalmol 43:325, 1977

18. Bartholomew, RS: Anterior chamber depths in eyes with pseudoexfoliation, Br J Ophthalmol 64:322, 1980

19. Benedikt, O, and Roll, P: The trabecular meshwork of a non-glaucomatous eye with the exfoliation syndrome, Virch Arch 384:347, 1979

20. Bergmanson, JPG, Jones, WL, and Chu WF: Ultrastructural observations on (pseudo-) exfoliation of the lens capsule: a re-examination of the involvement of the lens epithelium, Br J Ophthalmol 68:118, 1984

21. Bertelson, RI, Drablos, PA, and Flood, PR: The so-called senile exfoliation (pseudoexfoliation) of the anterior lens capsule, a product of the lens epithelium, Acta Ophthalmol 42:1096, 1964

22. Blika, S, and Saunte, E: Timolol maleate in the treatment of glaucoma simplex and glaucoma capsulare, Acta Ophthalmol 60:967, 1982

23. Brooks, AMV, and Gillies, WE: The development of microneovascular changes in the iris in pseudoexfoliation of the lens capsule, Ophthalmology 1987, 94:1090

24. Busacca, A: Struktur and Bedeutung der Hautchennieder-Schlaze in der vorderen and hinteren Augenkammer, v Graefe's Arch Klin Exp Ophthalmol 119:135, 1927

25. Caccamise, WC: The exfoliation syndrome in the aphakic eye, Am J Ophthalmol 1981, 91:111

26. Ceban, L, and Smith, RJH: Pseudoexfoliation of lens capsule and glaucoma, Br J Ophthalmol 60:279, 1976

27. Chandler, PA, and Grant WM: Glaucoma, ed 2, Philadelphia, 1979, Lea & Febiger

28. Dark, AJ, and Streeten, BW: Pseudoexfoliation syndrome. In: Garner, A and Klintworth, GK, editors: Pathobiology of ocular disease: a dynamic approach, Part B, New York, 1982, Marcel Dekker

29. Dark AJ, Streeten, BW, and Conward, CC: Pseudoexfoliative diseases of the lens: a study in electron microscopy and histochemistry, Br J Ophthalmol 61:462, 1977

30. Davanger, M: On the molecular composition and physico-chemical properties of the pseudoexfoliation material, Acta Ophthalmol 55:621 1977

31. Davanger, M: A note on the pseudoexfoliation fibrils, Acta Ophthalmol 56:114, 1978

32. Davanger, M: Studies on the pseudoexfoliation material, v Graefe's Arch Klin Exp Ophthalmol 208:65, 1978

33. Davanger M: Pseudo-exfoliation material: electron microscopy after the application of lanthanum as tracer particles and ionic stain, Acta Ophthalmol 58:512, 1980

34. Davanger M, and Pederson, OO: Pseudoexfoliation material on the anterior lens surface: demonstration of an interfibrillar ground substance, Acta Ophthalmol 53:3, 1975

35. Dell, WM: The epidemiology of the pseudo-exfoliation syndrome, J Am Optometric Assoc 56:113, 1985

36. Dickson, DH, and Ramsay, MS: Fibrillopathia epitheliocapsularis (pseudoexfoliation): a clinical and electron microscope study, Can J Ophthalmol 10:148, 1975

37. Duke-Elder, S: System of ophthalmology, vol 11, St Louis, 1969, The CV Mosby Co

38. Dvorak-Theobald, G: Pseudoexfoliation of the lens capsule: relation to "true" exfoliation of the lens capsule as reported in the literature and role in the production of glaucoma capsulocuticulare, Am J Ophthalmol 37:1, 1954

39. Eagle, RC, Jr, Font, RL, and Fine, BS: The basement membrane exfoliation syndrome, Arch Ophthalmol 6:273, 1971

40. Eustace, P, McAuliffe-Curtin, D, and Dwyer, P: Timolol response in the pseudoexfoliation syndrome, Res Clin Forums 3:55, 1981

40a. Eustace, P, McAuliffe-Curtain, D, and Dwyer, JP: HLA antigens in the pseudoexfoliation syndrome, Trans Ophthalmol Soc UK 100:510, 1980

41. Faulkner, HW: Pseudo-exfoliation of the lens among the Navajo Indians, Am J Ophthalmol 72:206, 1971

42. Forsius, H, Sveinsson, K, Als, E, and Luuka, H: Pseudoexfoliation of the lens capsule and depth of anterior chamber in northern Iceland, Acta Ophthalmol 52:421, 1974

43. Forsius, H: Prevalence of pseudoexfoliation of the lens in Finns, Lapps, Icelanders, Eskimos, and Russians, Trans Ophthalmol Soc UK 99:296, 1979

44. Garner, A, and Alexander, RA: Pseudoexfoliative disease: histochemical evidence of an affinity with zonular fibers, Br J Ophthalmol 68:574, 1984

45. Ghosh, M, and Speakman, JS: Anterior central opacities of the capsule in senile lens exfoliation, Can J Ophthalmol 6:273, 1971

46. Ghosh, M, and Speakman, JS: The ciliary body in senile exfoliation of the lens, Can J Ophthalmol 8:394, 1973

47. Ghosh, M, and Speakman, JS: The iris in senile exfoliation of the lens, Can J Ophthalmol 9:289, 1974

48. Ghosh, M, and Speakman, JS: The origin of senile lens exfoliation, Can J Ophthalmol 1983, 18:340

49. Gifford, H, Jr: A clinical and pathologic study of exfoliation of the lens capsule, Am J Ophthalmol 46:508, 1958

50. Gillies, WE: Corticosteroid-induced ocular hypertension in pseudoexfoliation of lens capsule, Am J Ophthalmol 70:90, 1970

51. Gilles, WE: Effect of lens extraction in pseudoexfoliation of the lens capsule, Br J Ophthalmol 54:46, 1973

52. Gillies, WE: Trabeculotomy in pseudoexfoliation of the lens capsule, Br J Ophthalmol 61:297, 1977

53. Gillies, WE: Secondary glaucoma associated with pseudoexfoliation of the lens capsule, Trans Ophthalmol Soc UK 98:96, 1978

54. Gnanadoss, AS, and Parasuraman, A: Pseudoexfoliation and narrow angle glaucoma, Orient Arch Ophthalmol 10:55, 1972

55. Guzek, JP, et al: Risk factors for intraoperative complications in 1000 extracapsular cataract cases, Ophthalmology 94:461, 1987

56. Hansen, E, and Sellevold, OJ: Pseudoexfoliation of the lens capsule. I. Clinical evaluation with special regard to the presence of glaucoma, Acta Ophthalmol 46:1095, 1968

57. Hansen, E, and Sellevold, OJ: Pseudoexfoliation of the lens capsule. II. Development of the exfoliation syndrome, Acta Ophthalmol 47:161, 1969

58. Hansen, E, and Sellevold, OJ: Pseudoexfoliation of the lens capsule. III. Ocular tension in eyes with pseudoexfoliation, Acta Ophthamol 48:446, 1970

59. Harnisch, JP: Exfoliation material in different sections of the eye, Graefes Arch Clin Exp Ophthalmol 203:181, 1977

60. Harnisch, JP, Barrach, JH, Hassell, JR, and Sinha, PK: Identification of a basement membrane proteoglycan in exfoliation material, AVG 215:273, 1981

61. Henry, JC, et al: Long-term follow-up of pseudoexfoliation and the development of elevated intraocular pressure, Ophthalmology 1987, 94:545

62. Herbst, RW: Angle closure glaucoma in a patient with pseudoexfoliation of the lens capsule, Ann Ophthalmol 8:853, 1976

63. Hiller, R, Sperduto, RD, and Krueger, DE: Pseudoexfoliation, intraocular pressure, and senile lens changes in a population based survey, Arch Ophthalmol 100:1080, 1982

64. Horven, I: Exfoliation syndrome, Arch Ophthalmol 76:505, 1966

65. Jerndal, T, and Kriisa, U: Results of trabeculectomy for pseudoexfoliative glaucoma, Br J Ophthalmol 58:927, 1974

66. Jerndal, T, and Svedbergh, B: Goniodysgenesis in exfoliation glaucoma, Adv Ophthalmol 35:45, 1978

67. Johnson, DH, and Brubaker, RF: Dynamics of aqueous humor in the syndrome of exfoliation with glaucoma, Am J Ophthalmol 93:629, 1982

68. Jones, B: Cited in Tarkkanen, A: Pseudoexfoliation of the lens capsule, Acta Ophthalmol Suppl 71:1, 1962

69. Kolker, AE, and Hetherington, J, Jr: Becker and Shaffer's diagnosis and therapy of the glaucomas, ed 5, St Louis, 1983, The CV Mosby Co

70. Kozart, DM, and Yanoff, M: Intraocular pressure status in 100 consecutive patients with exfoliation syndrome, Ophthalmology 89:214, 1982

71. Krause, U, Hine, J, and Frisius, H: Pseudoexfoliation of the lens capsule and liberation of iris pigment, Acta Ophthalmol 51:39, 1973

72. Krause, U, and Tarkkanen, A: Cataract and pseudoexfoliation, Acta Ophthalmol 56:329, 1978

73. Laatikainen, L: Fluorescein angiographic studies of the peripapillary and perilimbal regions in simple, capsular and low-tension glaucoma, Acta Ophthalmol Suppl 111:3, 1971

74. Layden, WE, and Shaffer, RN: Exfoliation syndrome, Am J Ophthalmol 78:835, 1974

75. Lieberman, MF, Hoskins, HD, Jr, and Hetherington, J, Jr: Laser trabeculoplasty and the glaucomas, Ophthalmology 90:790, 1983

76. Lindberg, JG: Kliniska undersokningar over depigmentering av pupillarranden och genomlysbarket av iris vid fall av alderstarr samit i normala ogon hos gamla personer (Clinical studies of depigmentation of the pupillary margin and transillumination of the iris in cases of senile cataract and also in normal eyes in the aged), MD thesis, Diss Helsingfors, 1917

77. Linner, E: The association of ocular hypertension with the exfoliation syndrome, the pigmentary dispersion syndrome and myopia, Surv Ophthalmol 25:143, 1980

78. Lowe, RF: Primary angle-closure with capsular exfoliation of the lens, Br J Ophthalmol 48:492, 1964

79. Luntz, MH: Prevalence of pseudoexfoliation syndrome in an urban South African clinic population, Am J Ophthalmol 74:581, 1972

80. Malling, B: Untersuchungen uber das Verhaltnis zwischen Iridocyclitis and Glaukom, Acta Ophthalmol 1:97, 1923

81. Mapstone, R: Pigment release, Br J Ophthalmol 65:258, 1981

82. Meretoja, J, and Tarkkanen, A: Occurence of amyloid in eyes with pseudo-exfoliation, Ophthalmol Res 9:80, 1977

83. Mizuno, K, Hara, S, Ishiguro, S, and Takei, Y: Acid phosphatase in eyes with pseudoexfoliation, Am J Ophthalmol 89:482, 1980

84. Mizuno, K, and Muroi, S: Cycloscopy of pseudoexfoliation, Am J Ophthalmol 87:513, 1979

85. Odland, M, and Aasved, H: Follow-up of initially nonglaucomatous patients with fibrillopathia epitheliocapsularis (so-called senile exfoliation of the anterior lens capsule), Paper presented at the twentieth meeting of Nordic Ophthalmologists, 1971

86. Ohrstrom, A, and Kattsstrom, O: Interaction of timolol and adrenaline, Br J Ophthalmol 65:53, 1981

87. Olivius, E, and Thorburn, W: Prognosis of glaucoma simplex and glaucoma capsulare, Acta Ophthalmol 56:921, 1978

88. Pohjanpelto, P: The fellow eye in unilateral hypertensive pseudoexfoliation, Am J Ophthalmol 75:216, 1973

89. Pohjanpelto, P: Argon laser treatment of the anterior chamber angle for increased intraocular pressure, Acta Ophthalmol 59:211, 1981

90. Pohjanpelto, P: Late results of laser trabeculoplasty for increased intraocular pressure, Acta Ophthalmol 1983, 61:998

91. Pohjanpelto, P: Influence of exfoliation syndrome on prognosis in ocular hypertension $> = 25$ mm: a long-term follow-up, Acta Ophthalmol 64:39, 1986

92. Pohjanpelto, P, and Hurskainen, L: Studies in relatives of patients with glaucoma simplex and patients with pseudoexfoliation of the lens capsule, Acta Ophthalmol 50:255, 1972

93. Pohjola, S, and Horsmanheimo, A: Typically applied corticosteroids in glaucoma capsulare, Arch Ophthalmol 85:150, 1971

94. Prince, AM, and Ritch, R: Clinical signs of the pseudoexfoliation syndrome, Ophthalmology, 93:803, 1986

95. Prince, AM, et al: Preclinical diagnosis of pseudoexfoliation syndrome, Arch Ophthalmol 105:1076, 1987

96. Radian, AB, and Radian, AL: Senile pseudoexfoliation in aphakic eyes, Br J Ophthalmol 59:577, 1975

97. Raitta, C, and Setala, K: Intraocular lens implantation in exfoliation syndrome and capsular glaucoma, Acta Ophthalmol 64:130, 1986

98. Richardson, M, and Epstein, DL: Exfoliation glaucoma: a quantitative perfusion and ultrastructural study, Ophthalmology 88:968, 1981

99. Ringvold, A: Electron microscopy of the walls of iris vessels in eyes with and without exfoliation syndrome, Virch Arch [Pathol Anat] 348:328, 1969

100. Ringvold, A: Ultrastructure of exfoliation material (Busacca deposits), Virch Arch 350:95, 1970

101. Ringvold, A: Electron microscopy of the limbal conjunctiva in eyes with pseudoexfoliation syndrome (p.e. syndrome), Virch Arch [Pathol Anat] 355:275, 1972

102. Ringvold, A: Light and electron microscopy of the anterior iris surface in eyes with and without pseudoexfoliation syndrome, v Graefe's Arch Klin Exp Ophthalmol 188:131, 1973

103. Ringvold, A: On the occurrence of pseudoexfoliation material in extrabulbar tissue from patients with pseudoexfoliation syndrome of the eye, Acta Ophthalmol 51:411, 1973

104. Ringvold, A: A preliminary report on the amino-acid composition of the pseudoexfoliation material, Exp Eye Res 15:37, 1973

105. Ringvold, A, and Davanger, M: Iris neovascularisation in eyes with pseudoesxfoliation syndrome, Br J Ophthalmol 65:138, 1981

106. Ringvold, A, and Husby, G: Pseudoexfoliation material—an amyloid-like substance, Exp Eye Res 17:289, 1973

107. Ringvold, A, and Davanger, M: Notes on the distribution of pseudoexfoliation material with particular reference to the uveoscleral route of aqueous humor, Acta Ophthalmol 55:807, 1977

108. Ringvold, A, and Vegge, T: Electron microscopy of the trabecular meshwork in eyes with exfoliation syndrome (pseudoexfoliation of the lens capsule), Virch Arch [Pathol Anat] 353:110,1971

109. Ritch, R, and Podos, SM: Laser trabeculoplasty in the exfoliation syndrome, Bull NY Acad Med 59:339, 1983

110. Robin, AL, and Pollack, IP: A comparison of neodymium: YAG and argon laser iridotomies, Ophthalmology 91:1011, 1984

111. Roh, YB, Ishibashi, T, Ito, N, and Inomata H: Alteration of microfibrils in the conjunctiva of patients with exfoliation syndrome, Arch Ophthalmol 105:978, 1987

112. Roth, M, and Epstein, DL: Exfoliation syndrome, Am J Ophthalmol 89:477, 1980

113. Sampaolesi, R: Neue Untersuchungen uber das Pseudo-kapselhautchen-Glaukom (Glaucoma Capsulare), Ber Deutsch Ophthal Ges 62:177, 1959

114. Seland, JH: The ultrastructure of the deep layer of the lens capsule in fibrillopathia epitheliocapsularis (FEC), so-called senile exfoliation or pseudoexfoliation, Acta Ophthalmol 56:335, 1978

115. Seland, JH, and Chylack, LT, Jr: Cataracts in the exfoliation syndrome (fibrillopathia epitheliocapsularis), Trans Ophthalmol Soc UK 102:375, 1982

116. Shaw, BR, and Lewis, RA: Intraocular pressure elevation after pupillary dilation in open angle glaucoma, Arch Ophthalmol 104:1185 1986

117. Simon Tor, JM: Glaucoma pigmentario complexus, Arch Soc Ophthalmol Hisp Am 21:121, 1961

118. Skuta, GL, et al: Zonular dialysis during extracapsular cataract extraction in pseudoexfoliation syndrome, Arch Ophthalmol 105:632 1987

119. Slagsvold, JE: The follow-up in patients with pseudoexfoliation of the lens capsule with and without glaucoma. I. Factors influencing the patients attendance in eye clinics, Acta Ophthalmol 62:177, 1984

120. Slagsvold, JE: The follow-up in patients with pseudoexfoliation of the lens capsule with and without glaucoma. II. The development of glaucoma in persons with pseudoexfoliation, Acta Ophthalmol 64:241 1986

121. Slagsvold, JE, and Nordhagen, R: The HLA system in primary open angle glaucoma and in patients with pseudoexfoliation of the lens capsule (exfoliation or fibrillopathia epitheliocapsularis). Acta Ophthalmol 58:188, 1980

122. Sood, GC, Sofat, BK, Mehrotra, SK, and Chandel, RD: Capsular exfoliation syndrome, Br J Ophthalmol 57:120, 1973

123. Speakman, JS, and Ghosh, M: The conjunctiva in senile lens exfoliation, Arch Opthalmol 94:1757, 1976

124. Spinelli, D, DeFelice, GP, Vigasio, F, and Coggi, G: The iris vessels in the exfoliation syndrome: ultrastructural changes, Exp Eye Res 41:449, 1985

125. Streeten, BW, et al: Pseudoexfoliative fibrillopathy in the conjunctiva: a relation to elastic fibers and elastosis, Ophthalmology 94:1439, 1987

126. Streeten, BW, Dark, AJ, and Barnes, CW: Pseudoexfoliative material and oxytalan fibers, Exp Eye Res 38:523, 1984

127. Streeten, BW, Gibson, SA, and Dark, AJ: Pseudoexfoliative material contains an elastic microfibrillar-associated glycoprotein, Trans Am Ophthalmol Soc 84:304, 1986

128. Streeten, BW, Gibson, SA, and Li, ZY: Lectin binding to pseudoexfoliative material and the ocular zonules, Invest Ophthalmol Vis Sci 27:1516, 1986

129. Sugar, HS: Das Exfoliations Syndrom: Ursache fibrillaren Materials auf der Linsenkapsel (English abstract), Klin Monatsbl Augenheilkd 169:1, 1976

130. Sugar, HS: Pigmentary glaucoma and the glaucoma associated with the exfoliation-pseudoexfoliation syndrome, Ophthalmology 1984, 91:307

131. Sugar, HS, Harding, C, and Barsky, D: The exfoliation syndrome, Ann Ophthalmol 10:1165, 1976

132. Sunde, OA: Senile exfoliation of the anterior lens capsule, Acta Ophthalmol Suppl 45:1, 1956

133. Svedbergh, B, and Sherwood, M: Argon laser trabeculoplasty in exfoliation glaucoma: a retrospective analysis, Dev Ophthalmol 11:116, 1985

134. Sveinsson, D: The frequency of senile exfoliation in Iceland Acta Ophthalmol 52:596, 1974

135. Takei, Y, and Mizumo, K: Electron-microscopic study of pseudoexfoliation of the lens capsule, v Graefe's Arch Klin Exp Ophthalmol 205:213, 1978

136. Tarkkanen, A: Pseudoexfoliation of the lens capsule, Acta Ophthalmol Suppl 71:1, 1962

137. Tarkkanen, A, and Horsmanheimo, A: Topical corticosteroids and non-glaucomatous pseudoexfoliation, Acta Ophthalmol 44:323, 1966

138. Tarkkanen, A, Voipio, G, and Krivusalo, P: Family study of pseudoexfoliation and glaucoma, Acta Ophthalmol 43:697, 1965

139. Taylor, HR: Pseudoexfoliation, an environmental disease? Trans Ophthalmol Soc UK 99:302, 1979

140. Taylor, HR, Hollows, FC, and Mann, D: Pseudoexfoliation of the lens in Australian aborigines, Br J Ophthalmol 61:473, 1977

141. Thomas, JV, Simmons, RJ, and Belcher, CD, III: Argon laser trabeculoplasty in the presurgical glaucoma patient, Ophthalmology 89:187, 1982

142. Tsukahara, S, and Matsuo, T: Secondary glaucoma accompanied with primary familial amyloidosis, Ophthalmologica 175:250, 1977

143. Tuulonen, A, Airaksinen, PJ: Laser trabeculoplasty in simple and capsular glaucoma, Acta Ophthalmol 61:1009, 1983

144. Vannas, A: Fluorescein angiography of the vessels of the iris in pseudoexfoliation of the lens capsule, capsular glaucoma and other forms of glaucoma, Acta Ophthalmol Suppl 105:37, 1969

145. Vannas, A, Setala, K, and Rurisuraara, P: Endothelial cells in capsular glaucoma, Acta Ophthalmol 55:951, 1977

146. Vogt, A: Ein neues Spaltlampenbild des Pupillargebietes: hellblauer Pupilearsaumfilz mit Hautchenbildunz aus der Linsenvorderkapsel, Klin Monatsabl Augenheilkd 75:1, 1925

147. Wandel, T: Disease of the internal eye: exfoliation syndrome, Clin Signs Ophthalmol 7:2, 1986

148. Weekers, L, Weekers, R, and Dednjaid, J: Pathogenie du glaucome "capsulaire," Doc Ophthalmol 5/6:555, 1951

149. Wilson, RP: Capsular exfoliation and glaucoma capsulare, Trans Ophthalmol Soc NZ 7:8, 1953

150. Wishart, PK, Spaeth, GL, and Poryzees, EM. Anterior chamber angle in the exfoliation syndrome, Br J Ophthalmol 69:103, 1985

151. Zborowski, L, Ritch, R, Podos, SM, and Boas, R: Prognostic features in laser trabeculoplasty, Acta Ophthalmol 62:142, 1984

152. Zirm, M: Proteins in aqueous humor, Adv Ophthalmol 40:100, 1980

Chapter 57

Lens-induced Open-angle Glaucoma

Claudia Richter
David L. Epstein

Lens-induced open-angle glaucoma may develop in several different clinical situations:

1. Hypermature or mature (rarely immature) cataracts may leak lens proteins into the aqueous humor and obstruct the aqueous outflow channels. This form of lens-induced secondary open-angle glaucoma is classically termed phacolytic glaucoma, although more recent studies suggest that *lens protein glaucoma* may be a more appropriate term.

2. Following extracapsular cataract surgery, lens injury, or Nd:YAG laser posterior capsulotomy, liberated lens particles and debris may obstruct the outflow pathways and cause a secondary open-angle glaucoma. This is sometimes mislabeled phacotoxic or phacoanaphylactic glaucoma because the cellular response to the liberated lens material is incorrectly assumed to be responsible for obstructing aqueous outflow. A more appropriate term is *lens particle glaucoma*.

3. When lens material is sequestered in the eye, after extracapsular cataract surgery or trauma, true phacoanaphylaxis rarely may result in glaucoma. Phacoanaphylaxis may also develop when a cataract leaks or a lens ruptures in one eye and sensitization to lens protein antigens has occurred in the fellow eye (e.g., after extracapsular surgery).

The different lens-induced reactions are complex and have multiple pathophysiologic mechanisms. Classic phacolytic glaucoma (lens protein glaucoma) is the easiest to classify and the most readily understood entity, whereas glaucoma resulting from retained lens cortex (lens particle glaucoma) and phacoanaphylaxis becomes progressively more complicated in both classification and pathogenesis. Nevertheless, it is important to differentiate these entities in light of our present knowledge.

PHACOLYTIC GLAUCOMA (LENS PROTEIN GLAUCOMA)

Background

Glaucoma associated with a macrophagic response to lens material leaking from a hypermature cataract was described by Zeeman[48] in 1943. Irvine and Irvine[17] amplified this description and suggested that blockage of the trabecular meshwork by macrophages was the principal mechanism of the glaucoma. Flocks et al.[12] proposed the term phacolytic glaucoma for the open-angle glaucoma associated with a leaking hypermature cataract. They believed that the glaucoma was caused by obstruction of the intertrabecular spaces by a combination of macrophages and escaped morgagnian fluid. Obstruction of the trabecular meshwork by macrophages distended with engulfed lens material has been emphasized in the pathogenesis of this glaucoma.[4,15,19,46] However, laboratory investigations have demonstrated that the soluble lens proteins leaking from hypermature lenses cause a severe obstruction of aqueous outflow.[8-11]

Clinical Picture

The term *phacolytic glaucoma* should be reserved for the sudden onset of open-angle glaucoma caused by a leaking mature or hypermature (rarely immature) cataract. Lens-induced glaucoma following extracapsular cataract surgery or penetrating lens trauma should not be classified as phacolytic (see Glaucoma Caused by Retained Lens Cortex later in this chapter).

Patients with phacolytic glaucoma typically have acutely elevated intraocular pressure. This pressure, often elevated to very high levels, produces ocular redness and pain as severe as that associated with acute angle-closure glaucoma. The disease process is usually monocular. Since phacolytic glaucoma occurs in eyes harboring mature or hypermature cataracts, there is usually a history of gradually diminishing vision over months or years. During an acute episode of glaucoma, vision may deteriorate further to inaccurate light projection, but this does not contraindicate cataract extraction.

On slit-lamp examination, diffuse corneal edema is usually present. An intense flare in the anterior chamber, which has been attributed to soluble lens proteins,[15,17,46] commonly is observed. The visible cells are macrophages. These are larger and more translucent than typical leukocytes, and usually only a moderate number are present. Hypopyon is uncommon and usually occurs only with a large defect in the lens capsule. Commonly, there are chunks of white material circulating in the aqueous humor that may represent small particles of lens material, cellular aggregates, or insoluble lens protein aggregates.[19] Calcium oxalate crystals also have been observed in the aqueous humor.[3]

The cataract is usually mature (totally opacified) or hypermature (with a liquid cortex and a free-floating nucleus). An immature cataract rarely may leak lens protein, usually through the posterior capsule. Soft white patches, probably representing macrophages phagocytosing lens protein at leaks in the capsule, typically are present on the lens capsule (Fig. 57-1).

On gonioscopy, the anterior chamber angle is open without obvious abnormalities. However, concomitant angle recession has been reported in 25% of patients with phacolytic glaucoma.[39]

Most often the onset of phacolytic glaucoma heralds a progressive elevation of intraocular pressure, despite antiglaucoma medical therapy. Rare cases have been observed in which a hypermature cataract leaked only intermittently, causing recurrent acute episodes of glaucoma.

If the cataract is dislocated into the vitreous, the signs of phacolysis are often subtle, making a correct diagnosis more difficult to achieve. The eye may be only slightly injected, with moderate intraocular pressure elevation and anterior chamber reaction. Observable white patches on the lens cap-

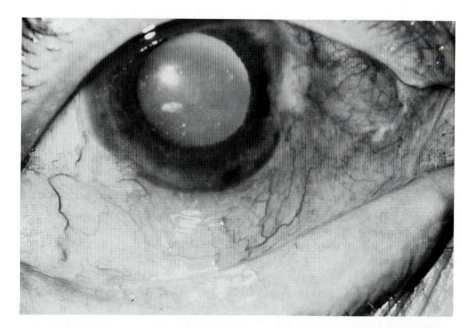

Fig. 57-1 Hypermature cataract with white patches on anterior lens capsule in phacolytic glaucoma.

sule provide an important clue to the diagnosis.

Phacolytic glaucoma has not been reported in children. In one series of 20 cases of phacolytic glaucoma, the youngest patient was 35 years old.[44]

Pathophysiology and Mechanism of Glaucoma

The amount of high-molecular-weight lens protein (molecular weight greater than 150 million g/mol) increases with age and cataract formation,[20,21,40] and is nearly absent in the lenses of infant and juvenile patients.[21,22,40,41] High-molecular-weight protein is commonly found in the nucleus, rather than in the cortex, of the lens. In phacolytic lenses, however, high concentrations of this protein are found in the liquid cortex,[10] possibly indicating either a nuclear disintegration process, or further cortical protein aggregation. By virtue of their size, high-molecular-weight soluble lens proteins may be expected to obstruct the trabecular outflow pathways, if liberated in sufficient quantities.

The lens proteins are ordinarily sequestered within the capsule and isolated from the remainder of the eye. During phacolysis, microscopic defects occur in the anterior or posterior lens capsule, through which soluble lens proteins enter the aqueous humor. These microscopic leaks probably reflect an end stage in the process of cataract formation. There is some evidence that immature senile cataracts may intermittently leak very small quantities of lens proteins into the aqueous humor.[33]

In patients with phacolytic glaucoma, the aqueous humor concentration of high-molecular-weight protein is similar to the concentrations found to produce obstruction of aqueous outflow in experimental perfusion studies.[10] The magnitude of outflow obstruction increases with the length of the lens protein perfusion time.[11]

Morphologically, eosinophilic proteinlike material and macrophages have been observed in the trabecular meshwork of eyes with phacolytic glaucoma.[16] The presence of macrophages is a natural response to the presence of lens material in the anterior chamber, and their presence does not necessarily cause glaucoma. Although fewer in number than in phacolytic glaucoma, identical engorged macrophages not associated with glaucoma have been found in the aqueous humor of children after cataracts were needled and aspirated.[47] The macrophages, probably representing the normal scavenger response to free lens material in the eye, remove liberated lens proteins from the trabecular meshwork and from the sites of lens capsule leakage. Whether lens protein–laden macrophages further impair fluid outflow through the trabecular meshwork is not clear. Dueker[7] placed large numbers of swollen rabbit macrophages, which had engulfed oil in the peritoneum, into the anterior chambers of rabbits and failed to observe any significant intraocular pressure elevation.

The available evidence suggests that phacolytic glaucoma is caused by direct lens protein obstruction of the outflow pathways.[8,10,11] It is remarkable that in excised eyes this protein obstruction cannot be relieved by vigorous irrigation of the anterior chamber or by prolonged perfusion with mock aqueous humor.[11] Yet clinically the glaucoma is rapidly reversible following the removal of the lens. This may indicate that normal cellular processes within the trabecular meshwork can alleviate the obstructed flow when the lens protein leak stops. Postoperative glaucoma rarely follows intracapsular cataract extraction with alpha-chymotrypsin. Although this suggests that alpha-chymotrypsin may reduce fluid obstruction by producing smaller fragments of accumulated lens proteins in the outflow pathways, this could not be documented experimentally.[11]

Diagnosis

Special diagnostic techniques

Diagnostic paracentesis usually reveals the typical engorged macrophages on microscopic examination (Fig. 57-2). Phase-contrast microscopy and the Millipore filter technique[14] may help identify the macrophages. Often only a few characteristic macrophages are observed, and their number does not correlate with the severity of the glaucoma. At times macrophages may not be present in the aspirated fluid, especially if topical corticosteroids were administered.

Differential diagnosis

The acute intraocular pressure elevation associated with phacolytic glaucoma must be differentiated from that of primary angle-closure glaucoma, angle-closure resulting from cataract and pupillary block, neovascular glaucoma, glaucoma associated with uveitis, and glaucoma resulting from trauma (including acute angle-recession glaucoma and ghost cell glaucoma). A prior history of known cataract-induced decreased vision is helpful in diagnosing the phacolytic glaucoma patient's condition.

If the cornea is edematous, topical glycerin should be used to facilitate slit-lamp and gonio-

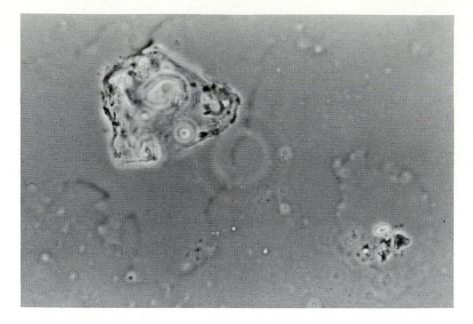

Fig. 57-2 Typical swollen macrophage with engulfed lens material seen by phase-contrast microscopy. (Courtesy Thomas M. Richardson, M.D.)

scopic examinations. On slit-lamp examination, the anterior chamber cellular reaction in phacolytic glaucoma consists of larger, translucent macrophages. This cellular reaction contrasts with the small leukocytes present in most inflammatory glaucomas and with the smaller, off-white, more numerous cells in ghost cell glaucoma. Iris blood vessels may be dilated in phacolytic glaucoma, but new vessels are not seen. On gonioscopy, the angle is usually open with no obvious abnormality.

Following trauma, a severe secondary open-angle glaucoma with variable concentrations of inflammatory cells in the anterior chamber may result from insult to the trabecular meshwork associated with the angle recession. The patient's history and the physical findings should differentiate this from a phacolytic process.

When phacolytic glaucoma occurs with a lens that is dislocated into the vitreous, the differential diagnosis includes primary open-angle glaucoma, angle-recession glaucoma, and an idiopathic type of open-angle glaucoma associated with lens dislocation without angle recession. The latter is not rare, yet the cause is unknown. Examination of the dislocated lens capsule, with a contact lens if necessary, will reveal the white patches typically present in phacolytic glaucoma.

Management

Medical therapy

Patients with suspected phacolytic glaucoma should be hospitalized because this glaucoma, po-

tentially, may worsen rapidly. Semi-emergent cataract extraction should be planned. As part of the immediate care plan, intraocular pressure should be lowered with hyperosmotic agents, carbonic anhydrase inhibitors (both intravenously and orally), and topical beta-adrenergic antagonists.[9] Although not fully evaluated, miotics do not seem effective.

Topical steroid therapy is useful to quiet the eye preoperatively. Occasionally, steroid therapy may lower the pressure temporarily, indicating an inflammatory component to the glaucoma. Despite steroid and antiglaucoma therapies, intraocular pressure often returns to high levels necessitating prompt cataract surgery. A trial of diagnostic steroid therapy may differentiate the rare case of phacolytic glaucoma in the presence of an immature cataract from uveitic glaucoma.

Surgical therapy

Because of the magnitude of pressure elevation and its refractoriness to medical therapy, it often becomes necessary to remove the cataract soon after the condition has been diagnosed.

Retrobulbar anesthetic, with epinephrine to decrease orbital vascular congestion, is preferable to general anesthetic. Intraocular pressure should be measured before surgically entering the eye. If the pressure is high, either paracentesis or a deliberate, gradual entry into the anterior chamber at the time of cataract section should be employed to avoid rapid decompression of the globe. Intracapsular cataract extraction with alpha-chymotrypsin

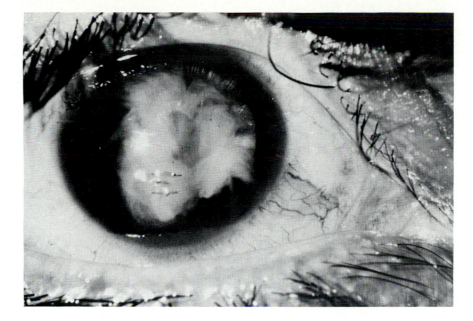

Fig. 57-3 "Fluffed up" cortical lens material in anterior chamber after penetrating trauma. (Courtesy C. Davis Belcher III, M.D.)

and a sector iridectomy is our preferred method for lens delivery. Modern extracapsular surgery, with careful aspiration of all cortical material, may be difficult when the cornea is edematous. In addition, opening the lens capsule may release large amounts of liquefied lens proteins into the aqueous humor possibly causing persistent inflammation and glaucoma. For this reason, intracapsular extraction should be performed with great care, to avoid rupturing the lens capsule. If the capsule does rupture, the nucleus should be removed and an irrigation-aspiration device should be used to remove all residual cortical material.

Following cataract surgery, the glaucoma is usually alleviated and the patient generally does quite well. The patient's postoperative vision often proves surprisingly good. Therefore remember that the usual poor preoperative vision of inaccurate light projection need not deter definitive cataract surgery.

GLAUCOMA CAUSED BY RETAINED LENS CORTEX (LENS PARTICLE GLAUCOMA)
Clinical Picture

Following planned or unplanned extracapsular cataract extraction, a penetrating lens injury, or Nd:YAG laser posterior capsulotomy, cortical and capsular lens material may be liberated and eventually obstruct trabecular outflow (Fig. 57-3). The severity of the glaucoma typically correlates with the amount of free cortical lens material present in the anterior chamber. Often a delay of days to

weeks occurs between the extracapsular surgery, or injury, and the onset of the glaucoma. During this time, progressively more cortical material enters the anterior chamber. After Nd:YAG laser posterior capsulotomy, the intraocular pressure may begin rising immediately. The magnitude of this laser-induced pressure elevation does not correlate with the amount of lens debris or inflammatory cells present in the anterior chamber.

Fragments of white cortical lens material may be seen circulating in the aqueous humor, and lens debris may deposit on the corneal endothelium. If the intraocular pressure is highly elevated, corneal edema may be present. Significant inflammation may accompany this condition with heavy flare and cellular reaction in the anterior chamber. The circulating white cells may include smaller leukocytes and larger, more translucent macrophages. If there are large amounts of free lens material, a hypopyon may be observed. On gonioscopy, the angle is open and often cortical lens material is present in the angle. Peripheral anterior synechiae may result from significant inflammation.

Sometimes a similar form of glaucoma may occur many years after extracapsular cataract surgery when lens material is freed into the anterior chamber. Circulating chunks of whitish lens material then are seen in the aqueous humor. The cellular reaction is more macrophagic than in the immediate postoperative condition previously described.

A mature or hypermature cataract may spontaneously rupture in the eye, liberating lens fragments into the aqueous humor. To what degree any resulting glaucoma is caused by lens particle obstruction or by a phacolytic process (i.e., lens protein obstruction) remains unclear.

Intraocular pressure elevation is the most common complication of Nd:YAG laser posterior capsulotomy.[5,23,31,42] Intraocular pressure elevations of 10 mm Hg above baseline pressure have been reported in 59% to 67% of patients.[5,31] The pressure elevation can be significant. Intraocular pressure elevation greater than 40 mm Hg occurred in 38% of patients,[32] and one patient with no light perception vision[43] required an anterior chamber paracentesis to relieve a pressure greater than 80 mm Hg.

The intraocular pressure elevation following Nd:YAG laser posterior capsulotomy begins immediately after capsulotomy, peaks between 3 and 4 hours after the procedure, remains elevated for 24 hours, and usually returns to baseline within 1 week. The risk of a pronounced intraocular pressure elevation after pulsed laser capsulotomy is greater in patients without an intraocular lens, patients with glaucoma, or patients receiving more than 200 millijoules total laser energy during the capsulotomy.

Pathophysiology and Mechanism of Glaucoma

Free particulate lens material readily obstructs the trabecular meshwork.[11] For this reason, the glaucoma has been called lens particle glaucoma.[8] However, the glaucoma may also be caused by the inflammatory cells usually present and by the viscoelastic agents used in cataract surgery.

Free lens material probably leaves the eye via the trabecular outflow pathways. Perfusion studies in enucleated human eyes demonstrate that very small amounts of particulate lens material cause significant obstruction of outflow.[11] The occurrence of lens particle glaucoma in only a small number of patients with free cortical material indicates that dynamic cellular processes within the meshwork, perhaps involving the macrophages seen pathologically in their eyes, alleviate rather than aggravate this mechanical, particulate obstruction.

The low occurrence of lens particle glaucoma after extracapsular surgery or penetrating lens injury probably also relates to the amount of free lens material in the aqueous humor, inflammation induced hyposecretion, and the inherent facility of the trabecular outflow pathways. In one study of intraocular pressure and extracapsular cataract extraction, patients with preexisting controlled glaucoma had more frequent intraocular pressure elevations greater than or equal to 15 mm Hg above baseline during the first postoperative 8-week period than nonglaucomatous patients.[34] The more frequent intraocular pressure elevations present in glaucomatous patients suggest that eyes with previously decreased outflow facility are more susceptible to increased intraocular pressure with any further insult to the trabecular meshwork.

It is possible that absorption of lens cortical material through the trabecular meshwork might result in trabecular dysfunction and open-angle glaucoma many years later.[8,27] Several studies have reported the development of open-angle glaucoma 6 months to 45 years after extracapsular cataract surgery in children.[6,18,28] Consequently, more adults with delayed lens particle glaucoma following extracapsular cataract extraction may be found in the future.

The intraocular pressure elevation following Nd:YAG laser posterior capsulotomy significantly correlates with reduced facility of aqueous outflow.[13,31,37] The pathophysiology of outflow obstruction has not been fully defined. Pressure elevation could not be associated with visible particulate debris or inflammatory cells,[31] although it is possible that either small lens fragments, not visible on slit-lamp examination, or soluble, nonparticulate proteins liberated by laser capsulotomy could obstruct the meshwork. Shock wave damage to the endothelial cells does not appear to be the sole cause of pressure elevation. In an animal study, optical breakdown produced by the Nd:YAG laser in the anterior chamber was not associated with intraocular pressure elevation when the crystalline lens was not damaged.[24] Finally, vitreous molecules that reach the trabecular meshwork through the opened posterior capsule may contribute to elevated intraocular pressure.[36]

Diagnosis

In the typical postoperative or postpenetrating injury patient, lens particle glaucoma usually is diagnosed when the clinical findings indicate significant quantities of free cortical lens material in the aqueous humor and elevated intraocular pressure. If small amounts of lens material are present, or in atypical clinical settings, an anterior chamber tap and microscopic examination of the fluid may aid in the diagnosis by identifying macrophages and fragments of suspected lens material. High-molecular-weight protein need not be present in the aqueous humor in lens particle glaucoma, since the glaucoma directly results from lens cortical fragments and not from their soluble lens protein content. Macrophages may simply be the normal scavenger response to free lens material in the eye. Therefore finding macrophages does not necessarily identify a glaucoma as lens-related.

Lens particle open-angle glaucoma can occur many years after extracapsular cataract surgery in children or adults. The differential diagnosis includes primary as well as secondary open-angle glaucoma, in particular the various uveitic glaucomas. It is not currently possible to distinguish this delayed-onset lens particle glaucoma, so its diagnosis depends on a high degree of suspicion.

All patients receiving Nd:YAG laser posterior capsulotomy must be considered at risk for developing postoperative elevated intraocular pressure. All patients should have a prelaser and, at least, a 1-hour postlaser intraocular pressure measurement, because a 5 mm Hg or greater elevation at 1 hour is highly predictive of a 10 mm Hg or greater maximum elevation above baseline.[31] Prophylactic treatment with timolol or pilocarpine[30] decreases the incidence of large pressure elevations, but does not completely prevent them. When prophylactic antiglaucoma medications are used, intraocular pressure still should be measured at 1 hour. In glaucomatous patients, pressure should be measured again at 3 to 4 hours, since small pressure elevations may cause additional damage to the optic nerve and permanent visual loss.

Management

Medical therapy

Medical therapy of lens particle glaucoma consists of a combination of carbonic anhydrase inhibitors, topical beta-adrenergic antagonists, and, perhaps, temporary osmotics.[9] Miotics should be avoided because these patients tend to form synechiae. Cycloplegics should be used to dilate the pupil. Topical corticosteroids are used to treat the commonly present inflammation. Corticosteroid administration may delay absorption of the lens material. Therefore, their administration should be titrated to reduce inflammation and prevent synechiae formation, while allowing the retained lens material to resolve.

Intraocular pressure elevation following Nd:YAG laser posterior capsulotomy may be treated with carbonic anhydrase inhibitors, beta-adrenergic antagonists (timolol, levobunolol, betaxolol), and hyperosmotic agents. Careful follow-up in the early postlaser period is indicated.

Surgical therapy

If glaucoma from retained lens cortex does not respond quickly and adequately to the previously mentioned medical maneuvers, the lens material should be surgically removed without delay. In the early stages of the disorder, this lens material is loose and is easily aspirated from the anterior chamber resulting in a dramatic cure of the glaucoma. If surgery is delayed, lens material may be trapped within the capsule or inflammatory membranes. Microvitrectomy instruments are valuable in removing trapped lens material through a closed incision.

Intraocular pressure elevation following Nd:YAG laser posterior capsulotomy usually responds to medical therapy. Only rarely is filtration surgery required.

PHACOANAPHYLAXIS

Clinical Picture

Phacoanaphylaxis is an uncommon granulomatous inflammation in response to liberated lens material. It rarely causes glaucoma and, in fact, usually is associated with hypotony. Phacoanaphylaxis occurs in the following clinical situations that allow sensitization to previously isolated lens proteins: (1) following extracapsular cataract extraction with or without vitreous loss; (2) following extracapsular cataract extraction in one eye, with subsequent extracapsular surgery or a leaking mature or hypermature cataract in the other involved eye; and (3) after spontaneous or traumatic rupture of the lens capsule.

The clinical presentation of phacoanaphylaxis is variable and the diagnosis often is not made until an enucleated eye is pathologically examined. The inflammatory reaction may occur within hours[38] or days,[29,35] or may be delayed for months[32] following lens injury or surgery. The uveitis may be mild or virulent. A patient initially may experience only decreased vision or an acutely inflamed eye. On examination, keratic precipitates are present on the cornea and any intraocular lens. Many inflammatory cells are present in the anterior chamber, and a hypopyon is common. Peripheral anteroposterior synechiae commonly form as a result of the inflammation, and patients may have pupillary block glaucoma. Residual lens material is always present. The uveitis usually also involves the vitreous, and inflammatory membranes may form. The duration of the latent period and the severity of the uveitis are not associated with the quantity of free lens material. Typically, the uveitis does not respond to topical, subconjunctival, or systemic corticosteroids.[45] Occasionally, the uveitis may transiently abate, following steroid therapy, only to increase again, causing a "parade of hypopyons". Removing an intraocular lens has no effect on the uveitis.[1] The process is nearly always uniocular, although there have been reports of a "sympathizing" reaction in the fellow eye.[18]

Pathophysiology and Mechanism of Glaucoma

Normally lens proteins are immunologically isolated within the lens capsule. Violation of the lens capsule, however, may allow sensitization and development of the typical, zonal, granulomatous inflammatory reaction.[26,49] Initially the damaged lens is surrounded by an extensive polymorphonuclear leukocyte infiltrate. Then a zone of granulomatous inflammation, composed of mononuclear cells, epithelioid cells, and giant cells, surrounds the damaged area. The uvea is infiltrated with lymphocytes and plasma cells. Circulating lens proteins or particles notably are lacking in the aqueous humor.

When glaucoma occurs in phacoanaphylaxis, it may result from multiple pathologic mechanisms. Residual lens material can obstruct the trabecular meshwork causing lens particle glaucoma. The inflammatory reaction may involve the trabecular meshwork, causing or aggravating the glaucoma. Topical steroids used to treat the inflammation may cause steroid-induced glaucoma. Finally, inflammation can cause peripheral anterior synechiae and secondary angle-closure glaucoma.

Diagnosis

Unfortunately, the correct diagnosis often is made after enucleation.[26] If phacoanaphylaxis is left untreated, an unremitting downhill course of chronic inflammation leading to phthisis bulbi can ensue. The preceding clinical signs should serve as a guide, but when in doubt and faced with relentless uveitis, one should surgically remove and microscopically examine the residual lens material. Diagnostic paracentesis may reveal foamy macrophages[2] identical to those seen in phacolytic glaucoma, although the clinical appearance of the eye remains distinctly different.

Differential diagnosis includes uveitis caused by an intraocular lens in pseudophakic eyes, sym-

pathetic ophthalmia, anaerobic bacterial endophthalmitis, and other causes of granulomatous uveitis.

Management

Surgical removal of the residual lens material is required to cure the condition. In traumatic cases, where the lens material is mixed with vitreous, closed vitrectomy-lensectomy is the procedure of choice. All residual lens material must be removed to stop the phacoanaphylactic inflammation.

In cases of phacoanaphylaxis following extracapsular cataract surgery, the capsule can be removed manually with forceps in a hand-over-hand technique[25] after first injecting alpha-chymotrypsin beneath the iris. Any intraocular lens should be removed before removing the lens capsule. It is possible to remove the posterior capsule, anterior capsular flaps, and residual cortex in one piece. The removed lens material should be submitted for pathologic examination to verify the diagnosis.

If a cataract develops in the opposite eye, intracapsular cataract extraction is indicated to prevent residual lens protein from remaining in that eye. This is necessary since the lens protein antibodies previously formed in response to phacoanaphylaxis in the first eye could cause, secondarily, an accelerated immunologic response in the second eye.

REFERENCES

1. Apple, DJ, et al: Complications of intraocular lenses: a historical and pathological review, Surv Ophthalmol 29:1, 1984
2. Apple, DJ, et al: Phacoanaphylactic endophthalmitis associated with extracapsular cataract extraction and posterior chamber intraocular lens, Arch Ophthalmol 102:1528, 1984
3. Bartholomew, RS, and Rebello, PF: Calcium oxalate crystals in the aqueous, Am J Ophthalmol 88:1026, 1979
4. Bellows, JG: Cataract and abnormalities of the lens, New York, 1975, Grune & Stratton, Inc
5. Channell, MM, and Beckman, H: Intraocular pressure changes after neodymium-YAG laser posterior capsulotomy, Arch Ophthalmol 102:1024, 1984
6. Chrousos, GA, Parks, MM, and O'Neill, JF: Incidence of chronic glaucoma, retinal detachment and secondary membrane surgery in pediatric aphakic patients, Ophthalmology 91:1238, 1984
7. Dueker, DK: Personal communication, 1977
8. Epstein, DL: Lens-induced glaucoma. In Chandler, PA, and Grant, WM, editors: Glaucoma, Philadelphia, 1979, Lea & Febiger

9. Epstein, DL: Phacolytic glaucoma. In Fraunfelder, FT, and Roy, FH, editors: Current ocular therapy, Philadelphia, 1980, WB Saunders Co

10. Epstein, DL, Jedziniak, JA, and Grant, WM: Identification of heavy molecular weight soluble protein in aqueous humor in human phacolytic glaucoma, Invest Ophthalmol Vis Sci 17:398, 1978

11. Epstein, DL, Jedziniak, JA, and Grant, WM: Obstruction of aqueous outflow by lens particles and by heavy molecular weight soluble lens proteins, Invest Ophthalmol Vis Sci 17:272, 1978

12. Flocks, M, Littwin, CS, and Zimmerman, LE: Phacolytic glaucoma: a clinicopathological study of one hundred thirty-eight cases of glaucoma associated with hypermature cataract, Arch Ophthalmol 54:37, 1955

13. Gaasterland, DE, Cummins, CE, III, and Weiblinger, RP: Ocular hypertensive response to pulsed Nd/YAG discission, Invest Ophthalmol Vis Sci 25 (Suppl):45, 1984

14. Goldberg, MF: Cytological diagnosis of phacolytic glaucoma utilizing millipore filtration of the aqueous, Br J Ophthalmol 51:847, 1967

15. Greer, CH: Ocular pathology, Oxford, 1972, Blackwell Scientific Publications, Ltd

16. Hogan, MJ, and Zimmerman, LE: Ophthalmic pathology: an atlas and textbook, Philadelphia, 1962, WB Saunders Co

17. Irvine, SR, and Irvine, AR: Lens induced uveitis and glaucoma. III. Phacogenetic glaucoma: lens-induced glaucoma, mature or hypermature cataract; open iridocorneal angle, Am J Ophthalmol 35:489, 1952

18. Ishikawa, Y, Sawata, K, and Ishikawa, Y: Three cases of endophthalmitis phacoanaphylactica in the fellow eye after extracapsular lens extraction, Folia Ophthalmol Jpn 28:1260, 1977

19. Jaffe, NS: Cataract surgery and its complications, ed 4, St. Louis, 1984, The CV Mosby Co

20. Jedziniak, JA, et al: On the presence and mechanism of formation of heavy molecular weight aggregates in human normal and cataractous lenses, Exp Eye Res 15:185, 1973

21. Jedziniak, JA, Kinoshita, JH, Yates, EM, and Benedek, GB: The concentration and localization of heavy molecular weight aggregates in aging normal and cataractous human lenses, Exp Eye Res 20:367, 1975

22. Jedziniak, JA, Nicoli, DG, Baram, H, and Benedek, GB: Quantitative verification of the existence of high molecular weight protein aggregates in the intact normal human lens by light-scattering spectroscopy, Invest Ophthalmol Vis Sci 17:51, 1978

23. Keates, RH, Steinert, RF, Puliafito, CA, and Maxwell, SK: Long-term follow-up of Nd:YAG posterior capsulotomy, Am Intra-Ocul Implant Soc J 10:164, 1984

24. Khodadoust, AA, Arkfeld, DF, Caprioli, J, and Sears, ML: Ocular effect of neodymium-YAG laser, Am J Ophthalmol 98:144, 1984

25. Little, JN: Outline of phacoemulsification for the ophthalmic surgeon, Oklahoma City, 1974, Semco Color Press

26. Perlman, EM, and Albert, DM: Clinically unsuspected phacoanaphylaxis after ocular trauma, Arch Ophthalmol 95:244, 1977

27. Phelps, CD, and Arafat, NI: Open-angle glaucoma following surgery for congenital cataracts, Arch Ophthalmol 95:1985, 1977

28. Pressman, SH, and Crouch, ER: Pediatric aphakic glaucoma, Ann Ophthalmol 15:568, 1983

29. Rahi, AHS, and Garner, A: Immunopathology of the eye, Oxford, 1976, Blackwell Scientific Publications, Ltd

30. Richter, CU, et al: Prevention of intraocular pressure elevation following neodymium-YAG laser posterior capsulotomy, Arch Ophthalmol 103:912, 1985

31. Richter, CU, et al: Intraocular pressure elevation following Nd:YAG laser posterior capsulotomy, Ophthalmology 92:636, 1985

32. Riise, P.: Endophthalmitis phacoanaphylactica, Am J Ophthalmol 60:911, 1965

33. Sandberg, HO: The alpha-crystallin content of aqueous humor in cortical, nuclear, and complicated cataracts, Exp Eye Res 22:75, 1976

34. Savage, JA, Thomas, JV, Belcher, CD, and Simmons, RJ: Extracapsular cataract extraction and posterior chamber intraocular lens implantation in glaucomatous eyes, Ophthalmology 92:1506, 1985

35. Schlaegel, TF: Uveitis following cataract surgery. In Bellows, JG, editor: Cataract and abnormalities of the lens, New York, 1975, Grune and Stratton, Inc

36. Schubert, HD, Morris, WJ, Trokel, SL, and Balazs, EA: The role of the vitreous in the intraocular pressure rise after neodymium-YAG laser capsulotomy, Arch Ophthalmol 103:1538, 1985

37. Smith, CB: Effect of neodymium:YAG laser posterior capsulotomy on outflow facility, Glaucoma 6:171, 1984

38. Smith, RE, and Weiner, P: Unusual presentation of phacoanaphylaxis following phacoemulsification, Ophthalmic Surg 7:65, 1976

39. Smith, ME, and Zimmerman, LE: Contusive angle recession in phacolytic glaucoma, Arch Ophthalmol 74:799, 1965

40. Spector, A, Li, S, and Sigelman, J: Age-dependent changes in the molecular size of human lens proteins and their relationship to light scatter, Invest Ophthalmol 13:795, 1974

41. Spector, A, Stauffer, J, and Sigelman, J: The human lens in relation to cataract. In Ciba Foundation Symposium, vol 19, Amsterdam, 1973, Elsevier

42. Terry, AC, Stark, WJ, Maumenee, AE, and Fagadau, W: Neodymium-YAG laser for posterior capsulotomy, Am J Ophthalmol 96:716, 1983

43. Vine, AK: Ocular hypertension following Nd:YAG laser capsulotomy: a potentially blinding complication, Ophthalmic Surg 15:283, 1984

44. Volcker, HE, and Naumann, G: Zur Klinik des phakolytischen Glaukoms, Klin Monatsbl Augenheilkd 166:613, 1975

45. Wohl, LG, Lucier, AC, Kline, OR, and Galman, BD: Pseudophakic phacoanaphylactic endophthalmitis, Ophthalmic Surg 17:234, 1986

46. Yanoff, M, and Fine, BS: Ocular pathology: a text and atlas, New York, 1975, Harper & Row, Publishers

47. Yanoff, M, and Scheie, HG: Cytology of human lens aspirate: its relationship to phacolytic glaucoma and phacoanaphylactic endophthalmitis, Arch Ophthalmol 80:166, 1968

48. Zeeman, WPC: Zwei Falle von Glaucoma phacogeneticum mit anatomischem Befund, Ophthalmologica 106:136, 1943

49. Zimmerman, LE: Lens induced inflammation in human eyes. In Maumenee, AE, and Silverstein, AM, editors: Immunopathology of uveitis, Baltimore, 1964, The Williams & Wilkins Co

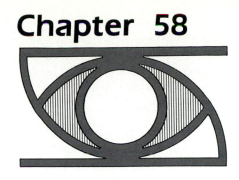

Chapter 58

Glaucoma Secondary to Lens Intumescence and Dislocation

Jeffrey M. Liebmann
Robert Ritch

Disorders of the lens may be responsible for secondarily inciting both open-angle and angle-closure glaucomas. An intact lens can produce angle-closure either by in situ enlargement or by anterior subluxation or dislocation.

LENS INTUMESCENCE

Mechanism

Although not generally considered a secondary glaucoma, primary angle-closure glaucoma itself occurs as a result of changes in the lens. The typical eye with angle-closure has a hyperopic refractive error, a larger-than-average lens thickness, and a smaller-than-average anterior chamber depth (see Chapter 42). The iridocorneal angle is widely open in youth, and angle-closure glaucoma usually does not occur until the fifth to seventh decade of life. Progressive enlargement of the lens throughout life results in gradual shallowing of the anterior chamber and alterations in the anatomic relationships of the structures of the anterior segment. The enlarging lens crowds the iris into a smaller space and, in pushing the iris forward, narrows the iridocorneal angle. Increasing iridolenticular apposition increases the resistance to aqueous flow through the pupillary aperture, leading to a relative pupillary block and an increase in aqueous pressure in the posterior chamber. This in turn distends the peripheral iris (iris bombé), further narrowing the iridocorneal angle. Various factors that cause the pupil to become mid-dilated, such as dim light, emotional stress, or drugs, induce a combination of lens-sphincter contact and angle crowding. Under these conditions the peripheral iris may balloon against the trabecular meshwork, precipitating an attack of angle-closure glaucoma. Iridectomy eliminates pupillary block by creating an alternative pathway of aqueous flow between the posterior and anterior chambers.

The lens itself may also push the iris forward, mechanically narrowing the space between the iris periphery and the trabecular meshwork. The underlying mechanism in such cases may be pressure originating posterior to the lens or lens enlargement (see Chapter 49). A gradation exists in the relative proportions of the contributions of peripheral bombé and direct pressure by the lens in inducing the narrowing of the angle. If the lens is large, a correspondingly smaller amount of bombé becomes necessary for the angle to close. Two conditions that predispose the eye to this situation are a rapidly developing intumescent senile cataract and a traumatic cataract caused by a perforating injury.[35]

Although angle-closure caused by an intumescent lens may occur in an otherwise normal eye with the opposite eye having a deep anterior chamber, it is more common in smaller eyes with preexisting narrow angles. Forward lens movement may also be a participatory factor in some cases, on the basis of zonular weakening by trauma, exfoliation syndrome, or age.

Diagnostic Clues

It is often difficult to determine the relative proportions of lens enlargement or forward displacement and pupillary block (iris bombé) preoperatively in a patient with angle-closure glaucoma. There are certain clues that one can use to distinguish these two mechanisms. Most important is a disparity in the depths of the anterior chambers or in the angle configurations between the two eyes. To determine whether a disparity exists and to rule out artifactitious alteration of the angle by bombé, these parameters should be examined when both eyes are being treated with the same topical medications. Despite the fact that they may simultaneously reduce peripheral angle crowding, miotics may exacerbate pupillary block and increase iris bombé by constricting the pupil and further increasing iridolenticular contact. Miotics also increase anteroposterior lens thickness and cause shallowing of the anterior chamber and may exacerbate angle-closure attacks when the lens is primarily responsible and pupillary block minimal.

Unequal cataract formation or progression between the two eyes should alert the examiner to the possibility of a significant contribution to angle-closure by the lens even in the absence of chamber depth or angle disparity. In the case of a mature unilateral cataract, this is easy, but in other cases the difference may be evident by only slight inequality of acuity or of anteroposterior lens thickness.

For practical purposes, the advent of laser iridectomy has reduced the need to differentiate these mechanisms preoperatively. If the cataract significantly affects visual acuity, lens extraction solves both problems. If not, laser iridectomy should be performed as the procedure of choice, since in the great majority of cases there is some element of pupillary block. If the patient has a medically unresponsive attack of angle-closure, peripheral iridoplasty is nearly always successful at opening the angle, allowing time for the eye to quiet and for laser iridectomy to be performed, and obviating the need to perform intraocular surgery on an inflamed eye with a markedly elevated intraocular pressure.[98,99]

Gonioscopy after iridectomy offers a retrospective view to assess the contribution by the lens to the angle-closure. An angle that shows marked widening implies a major contribution by bombé, whereas an angle that does not suggests a major contribution by the lens. Patients in whom the angle is narrow postoperatively should be watched for further narrowing as the lens continues to enlarge. It should not be assumed that once the patient has undergone iridectomy, angle-closure cannot recur. Eyes that have had even a large surgical iridectomy or trabeculectomy may develop angle-closure at a later date because of an intumescent lens (Fig. 58-1).

ECTOPIA LENTIS

In 1749 Berryat, who described a young patient with both lenses in the anterior chamber, was the first to report lens dislocation.[18] In 1846 Sichel[107] differentiated between traumatic and spontaneous dislocation, and Arlt suggested in 1849 that a congenital factor produced dislocations in children.[18] In 1856 Stellwag introduced the term *ectopia lentis*,[18] and Ringelhan and Elschnig[97] in 1931 classified dislocations as traumatic, secondary, or congenital. The earlier literature was extensively reviewed by Clarke.[23]

Ectopia lentis refers to displacement of the lens from its normal central position within the posterior chamber. *Subluxation* implies loosening or breakage of some of the zonules, so that the lens is no longer centered in the optical axis but still remains partially or entirely within the pupillary space and entirely behind the iris (see Plate IV, Fig. 6). In the case of *dislocation*, there are no remaining zonular attachments and, although the lens may remain behind the iris and partially or entirely within the pupillary aperture, it may also migrate into the anterior chamber or the vitreous.

Numerous entities have been reported to be either causes of or associated with ectopia lentis, as shown in the box on p. 1030. In some of these, the dislocation is clearly hereditary, whereas in others, it is secondary to trauma or ocular disease. Some disorders, such as Marfan's syndrome, homocystinuria, and Weill-Marchesani syndrome, are classically associated with lens subluxation or dislocation. Others either may be rarely associated, or the association may occur coincidentally. Further knowledge of these disorders at the molecular level and of the biochemistry of the zonular apparatus will help elucidate the causative relationships.

Clinical Findings

Symptoms

Patients with uncomplicated ectopia lentis have symptoms primarily related to disturbances of visual acuity. Minimal subluxation may be asymptomatic. Relaxation of the zonular apparatus

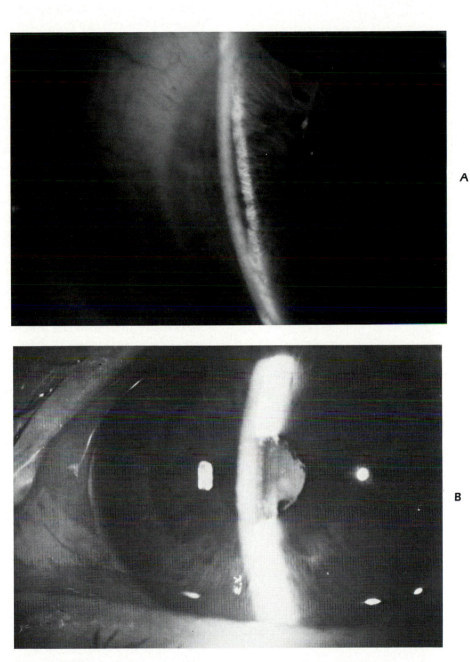

Fig. 58-1   A, This patient had undergone bilateral surgical iridectomies at age 45 after angle-closure attack in left eye. Twelve years later, he again had acute angle-closure in the same eye. Attack was broken with peripheral iridoplasty, and patient has been maintained succesfully for 2 years without surgical intervention. **B,** Slit view of the anterior chamber in patient with angle-closure caused by lens intumescence 1 year after successful trabeculectomy.

CONDITIONS ASSOCIATED WITH ECTOPIA LENTIS

I. Heritable disorders
  A. Lens dislocation common
    1. Isolated ectopia lentis[38,56,80,116]
    2. Spontaneous late subluxation of lens[48,77]
    3. Ectopia lentis et pupillae
    4. Isolated microspherophakia
    5. Weill-Marchesani syndrome
    6. Marfan's syndrome
    7. Homocystinuria
    8. Sulfite oxidase deficiency[53]
  B. Lens dislocation reported
    1. Alport's syndrome[110]
    2. Aniridia[31]
    3. Cornea plana[27]
    4. Cotlier-Reinglass syndrome[25]
    5. Craniofacial dysostosis[87]
    6. Cross-Khodadoust syndrome[26]
    7. Ehlers-Danlos syndrome[113]
    8. Familial pseudomarfanism[32]
    9. Focal dermal hypoplasia syndrome[45]
    10. Hyperlysinemia[110]
    11. Klinefelter's syndrome[6]
    12. Klippel-Feil syndrome[57]
    13. Mandibulofacial dysostosis[61,70]
    14. Megalocornea[20]
    15. Persistent hyperplastic primary vitreous[27]
    16. Oxycephaly[34]
    17. Pfändler's syndrome[89]
    18. Polydactyly[24]
    19. Primordial dwarfism[79]
    20. Retinitis pigmentosa[27,47]
    21. Rieger's syndrome[66]
    22. Sprengel's deformity[34]
    23. Sturge-Weber syndrome[57]
II. Secondary lens dislocations
  A. Extraocular causes
    1. Trauma
    2. Surgical complications
  B. Secondary to ocular disease
    1. Buphthalmos
    2. Exfoliation syndrome[4]
    3. High myopia
    4. Intraocular tumor
    5. Mature or hypermature cataract
    6. Syphilis*[55]
    7. Uveitis

*Rather than a direct relationship between syphilis and lens dislocation, it may be that patients with syphilis are more prone to trauma.

permits the lens to assume its natural spherical form, particularly in younger patients, in whom the lens is more pliable because of the absence of nuclear sclerosis. Decreasing the equatorial diameter of the lens and increasing its anteroposterior length lead to lenticular myopia, as does anterior displacement of the lens, with or without spherophakia. Tilting, rotation, or decentration of the lens around any of its axes may result in lenticular astigmatism, which cannot be corrected with lenses. A disparity between the degree of astigmatism found on refraction and that measured by keratometry, as well as a variable amount of astigmatism from one examination to another, should direct the ophthalmologist to rule out an early subluxation. The loss of zonular support also leads to defective accommodation and difficulty with near vision.

If the lens margin is within the pupillary aperture, monocular diplopia results, whereas quadriplopia can occur if the condition is bilateral. If the lens is completely away from the pupil, an aphakic refraction can be given.[75,84] A mobile lens results in constantly changing refractive states. Uncorrectable poor visual acuity may lead to amblyopia in children and may be the most common cause of diminished visual acuity in patients with ectopia lentis.[83]

Signs

Lens displacement may range in severity from a minimal, scarcely noticeable shift in axis to complete dislocation into the anterior chamber or vitreous. In early stages of subluxation, wide dilation of the pupil may be necessary to determine asymmetry of the lens position. When the zonules are loosened, the lens can move within the posterior chamber, and iridodonesis occurs. When slight, iridodonesis is best detected midway between the pupil and the periphery and appears as a faint rippling of the iris stroma. Phakodonesis may also be apparent in more advanced cases. One may observe movement of the lens and iris in infants by gently swaying them from side to side or in older patients by having them rapidly change fixation or by firmly jolting the slit-lamp stand while the patient's chin is secure in the chin rest.[57]

Examination of the anterior chamber may help detect early subluxation or differentiate angle-closure caused by subluxation from primary angle-closure. Forward movement of the lens results in shallowing of the anterior chamber in the involved eye and a disparity in the depths of the anterior chambers between the two eyes if the condition is unilateral or asymmetric. A difference between the anterior chamber depths of the two eyes should always raise the suspicion of lens subluxation. A mobile lens may also result in variable refractive errors and/or anterior chamber depths between one examination and the next.

When the lens is dislocated posteriorly, the anterior chamber is deep and the angle widely open

A

B

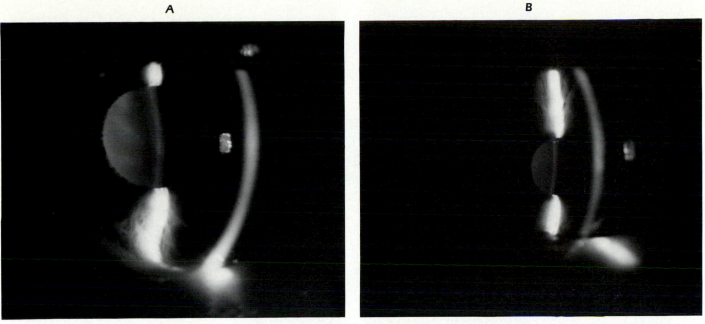

Fig. 58-2   Right, **A,** and left, **B,** eyes of patient with exfoliation syndrome OU and posteriorly subluxed lens OD. Lens subluxation in presence of exfoliation syndrome is much more common than previously realized.

(Fig. 58-2). A tilted lens may result in unequal depths between quadrants in the same chamber, the angle appearing shallow or even closed where the lens is tilted forward, and the diametrically opposite quadrants deep.

When the lens is subluxed or dislocated anteriorly, gonioscopy reveals a characteristic appearance (Fig. 58-3). When the lens is small, the peripheral iris is freed from posterior contact with the lens equator and zonules and allows it to fall backward, deepening the angle. The bulk of the lens is in contact primarily with the middle third of the iris, stretching it and creating a bulge that appears to fit the contour of the lens. The sphincter, anterior to this bulge, is angled forward because of the stretching of the middle region of the iris by the lens and appears conical, similar to the crater of a volcano, the lens surface corresponding to the base of the crater. This appearance may sometimes be differentiated from that caused by an intumescent, nondislocated lens, in which the entire iris appears to wrap around the lens. Iridodonesis may be present in the former situation but not in the latter. If pupillary block is present, the resultant iris bombé counteracts the tendency for the peripheral iris to fall backward, and the appearance of the angle is then one of angle-closure. Because of this, the characteristic gonioscopic appearance is best seen after iridectomy.

On slit-lamp examination, the zonular fibers may appear intact but stretched or thickened. Ruptured zonular fibers may be seen attached to the lens capsule (Fig. 58-4), but more often they are absent, presumably having retracted to the ciliary processes. Vitreous may be present in the pupillary space and protrude into the anterior chamber, where it may contribute to pupillary block.

Ophthalmoscopically, the edge of the lens appears as a dark crescent because of internal reflection of the light. Two images of the optic disc may be seen, one through the lens and one through the aphakic region of the pupil. Retinoscopy is also of value in delineating the edges of the lens.

When complications such as uveitis, cataract, glaucoma, or retinal detachment are present, additional symptoms and signs corresponding to these complications are also present.

Glaucoma Associated with Ectopia Lentis

Several mechanisms can contribute to glaucoma in the presence of a subluxed or dislocated lens, as shown in the box on p. 58-7. Some of these are coincidental and are not discussed in this chapter. Of those directly related to the lens, the most important are the glaucomas associated with forward movement of the lens. Syndromes whose primary manifestations are lens related are discussed below. Phakolytic glaucoma is discussed in Chapter 57, glaucoma secondary to uveitis in Chapter 67, and angle-recession glaucoma in Chapter 68.

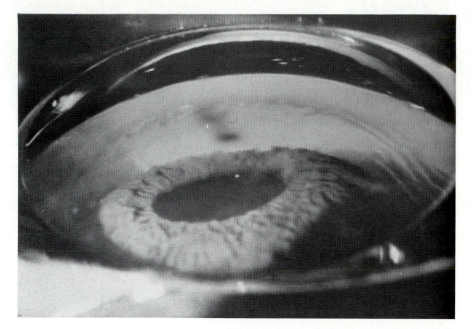

Fig. 58-3 Goniophotograph of angle-closure in a 28-year-old woman with anterior subluxation of lens. Note conical shape to iris, particularly in region of sphincter, giving structure appearance of "volcano crater."

Fig. 58-4 Downward dislocation of lens showing elongated zonules with broken zonules attached to lens surface.

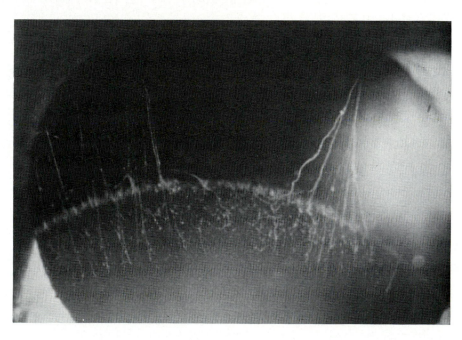

CAUSES OF GLAUCOMA IN THE PRESENCE OF ECTOPIA LENTIS

I. Lens related
   A. Pupillary block by lens
   B. Pupillary block by lens and vitreous
   C. Pupillary block by vitreous
   D. Lens in anterior chamber
   E. Phacolytic glaucoma
   F. Secondary open-angle glaucoma caused by repeated attacks of angle-closure
   G. Peripheral anterior synechiae caused by chronic angle-closure
II. Lens unrelated
   A. Angle recession
   B. Chamber angle anomaly
   C. Coincident primary open-angle glaucoma
   D. Other forms of glaucoma related to an underlying disease process (e.g., ghost cell glaucoma, neovascular glaucoma)

Simple ectopia lentis

Several large pedigrees have been reported in which dislocated lenses exist as an isolated autosomal dominant entity and in which the pupils are normal.[17,19,38] The specific age of onset is unknown, but many patients were under the age of 10 at the time of diagnosis. The condition is usually bilateral and symmetric, with the lenses dislocated upward and laterally. Ocular complications include dislocation of the lens into the anterior chamber, secondary glaucoma, and retinal detachment. The anterior chamber angles have been reported to be normal.[38] Other pedigrees have been described in which dislocation occurs between the ages of 40 and 60.[48,77] Rare recessive inheritance has been reported.[38]

Ectopia lentis et pupillae

In this autosomal recessive, bilateral condition, the lenses and pupils are displaced in opposite directions. The lens tends to be microphakic and often bisects the pupil, resulting in decreased or variable visual acuity or monocular diplopia. In most patients there is also some distortion of the pupil. Patients with lightly pigmented irides and this syndrome have had marked peripheral iris transillumination, poor pupillary dilation, and atrophic sphincters.[69] In a study of patients with densely pigmented irides, there were no transillumination defects, although pupillary dilation was slow, irregular, and incomplete.[28]

Because the iris dilator muscle and zonules are

of neuroectodermal origin, it seems likely that this is a neuroectodermal, rather than mesodermal, syndrome. No systemic anomalies are associated with this disorder. There is commonly a family history of consanguinity,[114] and complications are similar to those of simple lens ectopia. The most common cause of secondary glaucoma appears to be dislocation of the lens into the anterior chamber.

Microspherophakia and the Weill-Marchesani Syndrome

Microspherophakia with ectopia lentis and glaucoma may occur as an isolated familial anomaly and may be inherited in either an autosomal dominant or autosomal recessive pattern[60] and is also occasionally found in association with Marfan's syndrome,[29] homocystinuria,[29] Alport's syndrome,[110] mandibulofacial dysostosis,[70] and Klinefelter's syndrome.[6] The classic associated disorder, however, is the Weill-Marchesani (brachymorphia-brachydactyly) syndrome.

In a 1932 study of Marfan's syndrome, Weill[119] described a patient with brachydactyly and microspherophakia. In 1939 Marchesani[72] recognized this combination as a separate entity. Patients with the syndrome exhibit short stature, stubby hands and feet, brachycephaly, and microspherophakia. There is severe limitation of mobility of the fingers and wrists to both active and passive motion. The presence of both microspherophakia and brachydactyly is essential for the diagnosis.

The size of the globe is usually normal. On dilated examination, the small lens may be seen situated in the center of the pupil, the equator being visible for 360 degrees (Fig. 58-5). In the undilated eye, the anterior chamber may be shallow because of forward displacement of the lens. Gonioscopy often shows a narrowed angle but is otherwise usually unremarkable. In a pedigree in which one member had the typical syndrome, numerous iris processes bridging the meshwork, fraying of the iris root, and anomalous angle vessels were reported.[41] Posterior segment anomalies have not been described.

Secondary myopia caused by the abnormal lens shape occurs early in the second decade. Lens dislocation is common and occurs early. Loss of vision occurs earlier and is more severe among these patients than in other syndromes associated with lens dislocation because of the frequent presence of glaucoma. In one series, 12 lenses of 10 patients were noted to be dislocated at the initial examination (average age 20 years), and 2 dislocated sub-

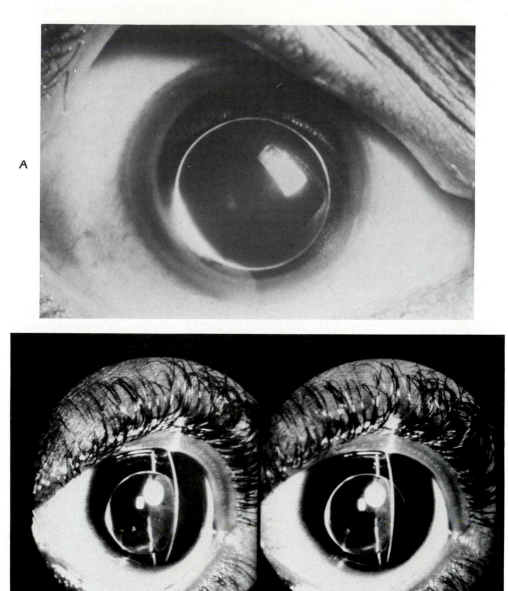

Fig. 58-5 Microspherophakia in Weill-Marchesani syndrome. **A,** Lens periphery is fully visible when pupil is dilated. **B,** Stereoscopic view of microspherophakic lens dislocated anteriorly. (**A** Courtesy Maurice Luntz, MD; **B** courtesy Anthony Caputo, MD.)

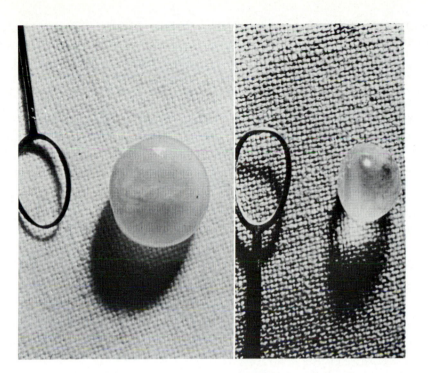

Fig. 58-6   Comparison of normal and microspherophakic lenses. (From Jensen, AD, Cross, HE, and Paton, D: Am J Ophthalmol 77:261, 1974. Copyright by the Ophthalmic Publishing Co)

sequently.[59] One patient without previous evidence of dislocation had subluxation of both lenses into the anterior chambers after dilation.

Genetics and pathophysiology

Consanguinity is present in a large proportion of pedigrees in which microspherophakia and brachymorphia are present.[62] Inheritance appears to be recessive in most, but dominant inheritance has been described.[103,123] Pedigrees exist in which either the brachymorphic habitus[62,68,91,121] or brachydactyly[41,62] occurs as an isolated finding in relatives of patients with the complete syndrome. Brachydactyly and spherophakia may also be inherited independently within a pedigree.[91]

In the microspherophakic lens, the weight and equatorial diameter of the lens are reduced 20% to 25%, whereas the sagittal diameter is increased up to 25%[41,78,81,91] (Fig. 58-6). The zonules have been described as elongated and profuse. Because there is usually no evidence of abnormal zonular development, most authors have considered the defect to be mesodermal, resulting in abnormal ciliary body development.[60] Farnsworth et al.[39] found a decrease of 20% in lens fiber cross-sectional area in a scanning electron microscopic study of a microspherophakic lens. They hypothesized that the increased circumlental space caused by develop-

mental abnormalities of lens fibers places strain on the zonules, leading to the lens subluxation. Jensen et al.[59] suggested that both the lens and zonules might be abnormal as a result of a metabolic defect. As in other syndromes in which patients are categorized by phenotypic criteria and in which the genetic or molecular causes are either poorly understood or appear to be variable, more than one mechanism may eventually be discovered.

Mechanism of glaucoma.   Glaucoma may occur either by forward movement of the lens or by dislocation into the anterior chamber. In the first case, loosening of zonules permits the lens to move forward, increasing its area of contact with the iris. This results in pupillary block, iris bombé, and gradual shallowing of the anterior chamber with angle-closure glaucoma. Prolonged or repeated attacks may result in the formation of peripheral anterior synechiae or permanent damage to the trabecular meshwork, after which elevated intraocular pressure may continue even after iridectomy for the pupillary block component. If treatment is delayed, unrestrained motion of the lens may cause a flat anterior chamber, a condition that does not occur in other forms of angle-closure glaucoma, in which the lens is relatively immobile. Once this occurs, surgical treatment becomes hazardous.

Probert[91] noted that glaucoma could occur either with or without manifest ectopia lentis. In the series of Jensen et al.[59] two eyes had normally positioned lenses and glaucoma.

Angle-closure caused by microspherophakia often becomes worse with miotic therapy, and in 1930 Urbanek[115] coined the term *inverse glaucoma* to describe this phenomenon. Parasympathomimetic agents stimulate contraction of the ciliary muscle and further loosen the zonular support, whereas cycloplegics relax the ciliary muscle, tighten the zonules, and pull the lens more posteriorly. This effect appears to occur only in eyes in which zonular attachments are still present.[7] Patients who do not worsen with miotic treatment may be assumed to have fully dislocated lenses or lack an effect on lens motion by those lens zonules that do remain.

Management

One should be extremely cautious in treating any patient with angle-closure suspected of having an anteriorly subluxed lens. One should also be suspicious when angle-closure occurs in young patients, especially those in whom either the habitus or presence of other congenital anomalies might be suggestive of one of the syndromes associated with lens dislocation. Bilateral acute angle-closure glaucoma has been induced in young patients by middilation of the pupil with cyclopentolate.[122]

One should strongly resist the temptation to try to break the attack through the use of copious instillation of miotics. The cautious use of 2% pilocarpine is reversible by cycloplegics if the anterior chamber shallows further. If this dose of pilocarpine is successful in opening the angle (i.e., does not further shallow the anterior chamber), one should suspect a complete dislocation and use mydriatics cautiously if at all. A reasonable approach in these cases would be to place the patient supine and to give an oral hyperosmotic agent and topical beta blocker. The effect of the hyperosmotic agent in shrinking the volume of the vitreous may permit greater posterior movement of the lens and relief of the pupillary block. Cautious miosis or cycloplegia as outlined above may be used to supplement this therapy. No hard and fast rule can be applied, and treatment must be individualized.

In one series, patients who had grade I (Schaffer) to closed angles after miosis had grade IV angles after mydriasis and after iridectomy.[121] It was suggested that patients refusing iridectomy should be maintained on a regimen of long-term mydriatics. However, this course of treatment may be unwise because of the high incidence of spontaneous dislocation of the lens into the anterior

chamber. Mydriatics should also be avoided in a patient known to have a dislocated lens in the opposite eye to minimize the chance of lens migration into the anterior chamber.

Laser iridectomy is the treatment of choice when angle-closure appears imminent.[100] If the condition is bilateral, the fellow eye should receive laser iridectomy prophylactically. After iridectomy, miotics can be used to constrict the pupil to prevent dislocation into the anterior chamber. Jensen et al.[59] felt that the severe lenticular myopia and subluxation in some cases warranted lens surgery in addition to iridectomy. Surgical complications are common, and vitreous loss more common than in routine iridectomy because of loss of protection of the vitreous face by the lens periphery. One case has been reported in which a successful surgical iridectomy was blocked because of forward movement of the lens.[7]

Dislocation of the lens into the anterior chamber

Dislocation of the lens into the anterior chamber is a therapeutic emergency, since the associated complications can be disastrous to the eye (Fig. 58-7). This situation can arise when dilation in the presence of a dislocated lens permits it to pass through the pupil. Alternatively, the lens may become wedged in the pupil and held there by the iris sphincter, creating pupillary block. The consequent increase in pressure behind the lens may force it through the pupil into the anterior chamber. Alternatively, the chamber may gradually shallow and flatten, the lens remaining within the pupil. Whichever the case, a marked elevation of intraocular pressure ensues because of pupillary block, either by the entrapped lens or by the posterior surface of the lens if it is entirely within the anterior chamber. If the lens remains in the anterior chamber, cataract formation ensues. The lens capsule may become adherent to the corneal endothelium, resulting in corneal decompensation. Glaucomatous damage may progress rapidly.

The two options for treatment consist of replacement of the lens into the posterior chamber or lens removal. If the lens is clear, the former is the more conservative and safer measure. Repositioning may be accomplished in some cases merely by placing the patient in a supine position with a widely dilated pupil,[48] permitting the lens to fall backward. Pressure on the central cornea may facilitate repositioning.[21,64]

If noninvasive measures do not succeed and pupillary block is present, laser iridectomy should

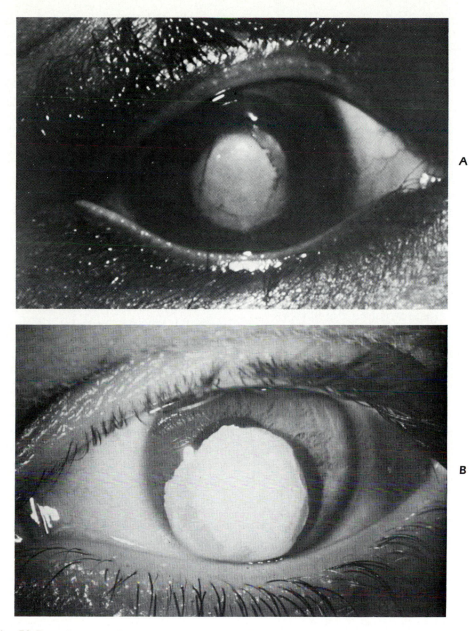

Fig. 58-7 **A,** Long-standing anterior dislocation of lens in Weill-Marchesani syndrome. Lens has opacified and become adherent to cornea. **B,** Dislocation of hypermature lens nucleus into anterior chamber.

be performed. Eliminating pupillary block may deepen the anterior chamber, decrease intraocular pressure, and allow the lens to be reposited more easily.

Once the lens is in the posterior chamber, an iridectomy should be performed if it has not already been done. Anterior dislocation may recur even with the use of miotics if iridectomy is not performed.[37] If the lens repeatedly incarcerates in the pupil, extensive peripheral anterior synechiae

and permanent glaucoma may result.[20,101] After iridectomy, the patient may be treated with miotics to maintain a small pupil and prevent further dislocation. Miotics should not be used in the absence of an iridectomy.

Other authors have favored lens extraction as the primary procedure. Iliff and Kramer[52] preferred aspiration for a lens partially held by zonules and routine incision for a lens completely free in the anterior chamber. They cautioned against attempting to reposit a traumatically dislocated lens. Jaffe[54] has recommended constricting the pupil to trap the lens in the anterior chamber and then removing it by aspiration or phacoemulsification, or intracapsularly via a limbal incision.

We prefer to use conservative methods initially if the lens is clear in cases of simple dislocation into the anterior chamber. If the lens is cataractous, it should be removed. In cases of trauma, if there is additional damage to the eye that requires surgical intervention, the lens should be removed concomitantly. However, conservative measures may be used if the dislocation is the only manifestation of the trauma and if the lens is reposited without much difficulty. Lens extraction can be performed at a later time if cataract formation ensues. If the lens is adherent to the cornea, combined lens extraction and keratoplasty may be required.

Dislocation of the lens into the vitreous

Lenses dislocated into the vitreous cavity may either float free within the vitreous, settle inferiorly, or become attached to the retina. Even when a dense cataract is present, the lens can remain for many years without causing difficulty. Conservative treatment is therefore strongly indicated, and extraction of the lens is not warranted unless phacolytic glaucoma develops. This condition is more difficult to diagnose when the lens is dislocated into the vitreous as opposed to its dislocation into the anterior chamber because of the paucity of cells in the anterior chamber in the former situation.

Attempts to trap the lens in the anterior chamber by placing the patient in a prone position and then constricting the pupil are rarely successful. If the lens is situated in the posterior vitreous, it may be floated into the pupillary space, where it may be grasped by directing a stream of saline into the vitreous. Pars plana lensectomy, which minimizes the possibility of displacing the lens further into the vitreous and permits access to all portions of the lens, is particularly effective.

OTHER HEREDITARY DISORDERS

Marfan's Syndrome

Marfan's syndrome is the most common inherited disorder associated with ectopia lentis. The ocular manifestations were first described by Williams[11] in 1876. In 1896 Marfan[73] described the skeletal abnormalities, and Boerger[9] associated the systemic and ocular findings in 1914.

The disease is characterized by autosomal dominant inheritance with high penetrance. Rarely, patients homozygous for the Marfan gene have been evaluated.[22] The prevalence is about 4 to 6 cases per 100,000,[92] and several clinical varieties exist. Musculoskeletal disturbances consist of arachnodactyly, abnormally long limbs, chest cage deformities, skull anomalies, kyphoscoliosis, hyperextensibility of joints caused by defective joint capsules and ligaments, sparse subcutaneous fat, and poor muscular development. A rare case associated with craniosynostosis has been reported.[42] Cardiovascular anomalies include progressive degenerative changes in the walls of the major vessels, dissecting aortic aneurysm, and cardiac decompensation caused by mitral regurgitation.[65] All patients should have antibiotic prophylaxis for surgical or dental procedures because of the threat of endocarditis from previously damaged cardiac valves. Several cases of neurofibromatosis occurring in conjunction with Marfan's syndrome have been reported,[24,67] as have pedigrees with features of both Marfan's syndrome and the Weill-Marchesani syndrome.[71]

The life expectancy of patients with Marfan's syndrome is reduced when compared with the normal population. Ninety-five percent of these individuals die as a result of cardiac dysfunction.[82]

Ocular abnormalities are numerous. The globe is usually enlarged, often progressively so. Megaloglobus may occur in patients with normal intraocular pressure and is believed to indicate an underlying scleral connective tissue defect. High myopia is common and has an axial as well as a lenticular component.[1] Nearly all patients with the classic syndrome have relatively flat corneas, with keratometry readings several standard deviations below the mean.[92] Axial length measurements vary considerably. The mean axial length of Marfan's patients with retinal detachment may be as high as 28.5 mm.[83]

Transillumination of the iris periphery, hypoplasia of the iris stroma and dilator muscle, and corectopia may be present. The anterior iris surface contains fewer crypts, furrows, and ridges than normal, resulting in a smooth, velvety appearance.[1] Gonioscopy reveals prominent pectinate ligaments, numerous iris processes, peripheral mounds of iris tissue, and vascular anomalies in the angle.[117] Similar gonioscopic findings occur in other systemic connective tissue disorders, such as scolioisis, Legg-Perthes disease, Osgood-Schlatter disease, idiopathic genu varum, and slipped upper femoral epiphysis.[13]

Lens dislocation occurs early in 80% of patients and is virtually always bilateral.[26] The frequency of dislocation varies between pedigrees.[93] Estimates of the age of onset of dislocation range from 50% by 5 years[19] to 70% by 6 years.[51] Maumenee[75] observed progression of ectopia lentis in 7.5% of 193 patient's with Marfan's syndrome. The lens may dislocate in any direction but characteristically moves superiorly or superotemporally. A small percentage dislocate into the anterior chamber or vitreous. Microsperophakia, microphakia, and spherophakia have been reported and may contribute to anterior lens dislocation.

The lens may have an irregular scalloped border, and the zonules are often torn and retracted to the equator[27] and abnormally long.[118] Sufficient zonules may remain intact to prevent lens dislocation and to permit normal accommodation. In marked contrast to homocystinuria, the zonules in Marfan's syndrome have been reported to be normal by light and transmission electron microscopy (Table 58-1).[94] On scanning electron microscopy, however, they are reduced in numbers and malformed, with loss of their regular parallel orientation. The zonules are substantially larger in diameter than those of a normal lens.[40] The zonulocapsular attachments are also abnormally narrow.[94,118]

Lattice degeneration, retinal holes, and retinal detachment are common. Although detachment has been known to follow intraocular surgery,[20,29,55] there does not appear to be an increased risk for retinal detachment after surgery for dislocated lenses in either Marfan's syndrome or homocystinuria.[29] Other ocular findings in Marfan's syndrome include heterochromia, blue sclerae, keratoconus, megalocornea, strabismus, colobomas of the retina and optic nerve, and pigmentary retinopathy.

Glaucoma is present in about 8% of eyes with ectopic lenses and in one third of these is caused by dislocation of the lens into the pupil. Despite the angle anomalies, all proven cases of glaucoma in the largest series were phacogenic.[29]

The ciliary processes are rudimentary, long, and narrow, often extending onto the posterior surface of the iris.[74] The circular and oblique ciliary muscles are hypoplastic,[12] and the longitudinal muscle fibers bypass the scleral spur or pass through it to insert directly onto the trabecular meshwork.[118] The iris root is inserted posteriorly, but the presence of masses of undifferentiated tissue in the angle recess may resemble an anterior insertion on gonioscopy. Schlemm's canal is focally absent and usually discontinuous where present, consisting of small single or multiple endothelium-lined channels bearing a striking resemblance to the chamber angle of the canine eye.[12] Despite the

Table 58-1 *Differential features of Marfan's syndrome and homocystinuria*

	Marfan's syndrome	**Homocystinuria**
Heredity	Autosomal dominant	Autosomal recessive
Skeletal	Arachnodactyly	Occasional arachnodactyly
	Joint laxity	Osteoporosis
	Sternal deformity	Sternal deformity
Vascular	Aortic dissection	Dilation of vessels
	Aortic and mitral valve disease	Frequent thrombosis
		Livedo reticularis
		Malar flush
Skin	Striae distensae	Fair, dry
Amino acids	Hydroxyprolinuria	Homocystinuria
Mental retardation	Rare	60%
Ectopia lentis	80%	90%
	First decade	May occur earlier than in Marfan's syndrome or progress more rapidly
	Usually superiorly	Usually inferiorly
	6% into anterior chamber or vitreous	33% into anterior chamber or vitreous
	Occasional microspherophakia	Occasional microspherophakia
Glaucoma	8% with ectopia lentis	23% with ectopia lentis
	15% with surgical aphakia	
Angle anomalies	Present	None reported
Retinal detachment	12%	9%

frequency of these anomalies, there is little evidence that they are the cause of the associated glaucoma.

Homocystinuria

Homocystinuria comprises three distinct autosomal recessive disorders characterized by increased concentrations of homocystine in blood and urine.

The great majority of patients with homocystinuria have a deficiency or abnormality of the enzyme cystathionine beta-synthase, which catalyzes the condensation of homocysteine and serine to form cystathionine. Excessive homocystine is formed from accumulated homocysteine and is excreted in the urine. Homocysteine reacts with aldehydes to form stable thiazine ring compounds, thus blocking condensation and cross-linking reactions in collagen.[46] The rarer forms are caused by (1) 5,10-methylenetetrahydrofolate reductase deficiency, leading to impaired synthesis of 5-methylatetrahydrofolate, a cofactor in the enzymatic formation of methionine from homocysteine, and (2) a deficiency of methylcobalamin synthesis. Blocks in the remethylation of homocysteine to methionine are associated with reduced levels of serum methionine. Increased serum levels of copper and ornithine have been noted.[86]

Cystathionine beta-synthase deficiency is similar to Marfan's syndrome in that it consists of skeletal, cardiovascular, and ocular abnormalities. It was first described in 1962,[16,43] and prior series of patients with Marfan's syndrome undoubtedly include cases of homocystinuria. In 1973 Cross and Jensen[29] found 142 patients with Marfan's syndrome with negative urine screening tests and 42 chromatographically documented cases of homocystinuria.

The characteristic clinical triad consists of skeletal, cardiovascular, and ocular abnormalities. Mental retardation, which may be progressive, occurs in 50% of patients.[83] The skin is fair and dry; the hair is fair, coarse, and sparse. Many patients are tall and slender, with abnormal upper to lower segment ratios. However, arachnodactyly is usually less marked than in Marfan's syndrome. Other skeletal anomalies are genu valgum, flat feet, kyphoscoliosis, joint laxity, a deformed sternum, generalized osteoporosis with vertebral collapse, and a high, arched palate.

Thromboembolic phenomena occur in about 50% of patients and may be caused by platelet dysfunction. Thrombosis may affect multiple areas of the body, including the central retinal artery. Progressive arterial disease may result in thrombosis in a vital organ. Cerebrovascular thromboses, myocardial infarction, pulmonary emboli, and intermittent claudication may occur at a relatively young age. Premature death occurs in about 40% of patients. Disturbances in the peripheral circulation are evidenced by a malar flush.

Thromboembolic phenomena are more likely to occur after puncture of a vessel during general anesthesia, and patients with homocystinuria are prone to pulmonary emboli after surgery. Indeed, the first patient with known homocystinuria to require surgery for lens extraction died 2 days later from pulmonary embolism.[63] Increased platelet adhesiveness and secondary adhesiveness induced by high blood levels of homocystine and methionine have been implicated.[78] Heterozygous carriers for synthase deficiency (about 1 in 70 to 1 in 200

in the population) may be at increased risk for premature peripheral and cerebral occlusive vascular disease.[10]

The most important ocular finding is lens dislocation, which is present in 90% of cases and is most often inferior or inferotemporal. In about one third of cases the lens is dislocated completely into the vitreous or anterior chamber.[29] In contrast to Marfan's syndrome, the zonules disintegrate, and accommodation is absent.[92] Anterior chamber angle anomalies have not been reported. Whether the zonules are formed abnormally or degenerate more readily because of the metabolic abnormality is unknown.

Histologically, Henkind and Ashton[50] noted the presence of a thickened hyaline membrane overlying an atrophic pigment epithelium of the pars plicata and pars plana. Ramsey et al.[95] found this to be composed of disintegrated zonules. The degree of zonular abnormality was apparently age related.

The incidence of retinal detachment is approximately the same as in Marfan's syndrome and does not appear to be influenced by surgical removal of the lens.[29] Pigmentary retinopathy is more common than in Marfan's syndrome.

Glaucoma is primarily caused by pupillary block. Lens extraction is commonly complicated by vitreous loss. In addition, increased platelet adhesiveness may produce an occlusive vascular disease leading to optic atrophy with cupping resembling glaucomatous optic atrophy in the absence of elevated intraocular pressure.[111]

Supplemental pyridoxine and perhaps a diet low in methionine and high in homocystine may aid in restoring blood levels of the involved metabolites to normal in some patients. Diet control initiated within the first few weeks after birth has been successful in controlling the manifestations of the disease, including lens dislocation, in several patients.[76] Betaine has been used in patients unresponsive to pyridoxine.[109,120] In older children, low-dose aspirin, which must be titrated to minimize both thrombosis and hemorrhage, may reduce vascular manifestations of the disease and surgical complications.[76] Early ambulation after surgery should be encouraged to prevent thrombotic episodes. The use of prophylactic heparin may predispose patients to hemorrhage, and anticoagulants should not be used before surgery.

The sodium nitroprusside test is a simple diagnostic screening test for differentiating homocystinuria from Marfan's syndrome, although false positive and false negative reactions may occur.

The test involves mixing 5 ml of urine with 2 ml of sodium cyanide and, after 10 minutes, adding 2 to 4 drops of 5% sodium nitroprusside. A bright red color develops in the presence of cystine or homocystine. To differentiate cystine, which may be present in the urine in Marfan's syndrome, from homocystine, electrophoresis is necessary.

Other Systemic Disorders with Ectopia Lentis

In the Ehlers-Danlos syndrome, ectopia lentis is not as prominent a feature as in the previously mentioned disorders. Abnormalities of collagen synthesis have been found in the various subtypes.[14,90,105] Gonioscopy has revealed angle anomalies[85] similar to those in Marfan's syndrome, and at least one patient developed glaucoma.[36] Extremely thin sclera has been noted during operative procedures,[85] and the sclera may rupture following relatively minor trauma to the head or globe.[5] Therefore, extreme caution should be taken if one is performing filtering procedures on these patients.

Hyperlysinemia is a rare disorder characterized primarily by mental retardation, hypotonia, and reduced lysine-ketoglutamate reductase.[30] Dislocated lenses also occur.[108,110]

Pfändler reported a pedigree containing three individuals with mental retardation, ectopia lentis, and keratoconus.[89] Each was the offspring of a different consanguineous marriage between normal parents. One patient had unilateral glaucoma.

Sulfite oxidase deficiency is characterized by muscular rigidity, mental retardation, and bilateral ectopia lentis.[53] Increased urinary concentrations of various sulfur-containing compounds may be found.

TRAUMATIC DISLOCATION OF THE LENS

Trauma is the most common cause of dislocated lenses, probably accounting for more than all other causes combined.[49] Dislocation caused by trauma presents additional problems not ordinarily encountered with simple subluxation and dislocation. In addition to the lens, other structures within the eye may be damaged. Hyphema, iridodialysis, angle recession, rupture of the vitreous face, scleral rupture, vitreous hemorrhage, choroidal rupture, and retinal edema, hemorrhage, or detachment may be present. In these cases treatment of the lens is subordinate to or contingent on treatment of the other injuries. The following discussion pertains to treatment of uncomplicated traumatically dislocated lenses.

After contusion injury, severe ciliary spasm may cause forward movement of the lens, shallowing of the anterior chamber, and narrowing of the angle. Angle-closure may be caused by pupillary or ciliary block alone, or by combined pupillary and ciliary block. There is a disparity in the anterior chamber depths and angle configurations between the two eyes. A myopic shift occurs in the involved eye because of forward movement of the lens. These patients are often young, probably because younger patients are more prone to this type of trauma. Treatment with miotics may further shallow the anterior chamber, leading to increased severity of the angle-closure and further elevation of intraocular pressure. Topical mydriatic-cycloplegics in combination with systemic hyperosmotic agents often reverse the condition, decreasing the pupillary block and causing the anterior chamber to deepen. These topical drugs may have to be used on an extended basis to prevent repeated angle-closure.

In other cases there may be breakage of zonules but sufficient integrity of the remaining zonular apparatus to maintain the anatomic connection between the lens and ciliary body. However, ciliary spasm may allow the lens to move forward more than would have occurred were all the zonules intact. One cannot be sure of zonular integrity before dilation, and the examiner should be aware of the possibility of the lens dislocating into the anterior chamber.

If pupillary block persists, argon or Nd:YAG laser iridectomy should be performed. This may be difficult if the pupil is dilated, and miosis should be cautiously attempted just before the procedure.

An additional problem after trauma is lens tilting, causing angle and anterior chamber asymmetry. The vitreous may be herniated between the lens and the pupillary margin, and the vitreous face may be either intact or broken. Angle-closure may occur on the basis of pupillary block by the vitreous or by a combination of the lens and vitreous. In regions of vitreous block, posterior aqueous displacement may occur, resulting in a mixed type of block with pockets of aqueous interspersed with vitreous posterior to the iris. Both miotics and mydriatic-cycloplegics may give variable responses. Occasionally, particularly if the block has a lenticular component, the glaucoma may be relieved by placing the patient in the supine position. The situation is analogous to mixed mechanism block in the presence of an intraocular lens. Laser iridectomy should be performed (see Chapters 30 and 71 for further description).

Vitreous may plug the iridectomy, causing the pupillary block to persist. If all attempts at laser iridectomy are unsuccessful, surgical peripheral iridectomy should be performed over the area of the lens to minimize the chance of vitreous loss. If these measures are insufficient, then surgical vitrectomy and lens extraction should be performed. It should be evident that these cases may be quite difficult to manage, and the above guidelines are not absolute.

A dislocated lens may rarely adhere to the ciliary body. Treatment is as outlined previously with special caution during surgery to prevent cyclodialysis or hemorrhage. If the lens is firmly adherent, it may be better to attempt a modified planned extracapsular cataract extraction in which the peripheral equatorial lens capsule is left adherent to the ciliary body and the remainder of the lens removed.

Jarrett[55] reported that less than 50% of 94 eyes had better vision after the removal of a dislocated lens. The results of lens removal are poorer in traumatic dislocations than in Marfan's syndrome, probably because trauma causes other ocular problems such as angle contusion deformity and retinal damage. The incidence of vitreous loss during the extraction of traumatically dislocated lenses has been reported to be as high as 85%,[102] compared with 21% and 24% in Marfan's syndrome and homocystinuria, respectively.[58]

EXTRACTION OF DISLOCATED LENSES

Techniques of lens removal from various positions of dislocation—anterior chamber, posterior chamber, or vitreous—are beyond the scope of this chapter. These techniques are presented elsewhere and include discission,[20] aspiration,[2,52,54,74,112] cryoextraction[103,124] with aspiration,[33] needling the lens to maintain stability of position during surgery,[3,15] vitrectomy techniques,[88,123] and the use of specifically designed instruments to aid in the extraction of the lens.[8,104]

More recently, pars plana lensectomy has been found to yield promising results.[44,96] Closed-system lensectomy preserves anatomic relationships during lens removal by maintaining intraocular pressure, provides precise control during removal of the lens and vitreous, and offers the flexibility of a bimanual technique. Reese and Weingeist reported excellent results in 12 eyes of 8 patients, 11 of which maintained a visual acuity of 20/40 or better over a mean follow-up time of 5 years without significant surgical complications.[96] Lensectomy and vitrectomy using infusion suction-cutter

techniques are the procedures of choice today.

Criteria for removal of a dislocated lens should be based on the potential for improvement of the condition for which extraction is contemplated. Because of the high incidence of operative complications, a dislocated lens should not be removed merely because it is dislocated. By the same token, a lens in the vitreous should not be removed unless phacolytic glaucoma supervenes.

Legitimate criteria for removal of a dislocated lens include the following:

1. A cataract blocking the visual axis. (If the patient is monocular, this is a stronger indication. If the patient is binocular and has a monocular cataract, the mere presence of the cataract is not sufficient unless the patient has difficulty functioning in the absence of binocular vision.)
2. Decreased visual acuity caused by the dislocated lens (e.g., lens margin in the visual axis) that is uncorrectable with lenses, mydriasis, or photomydriasis[112]
3. Phacolytic glaucoma
4. Pupillary block glaucoma unresponsive to more conservative measures
5. A dislocated lens in the anterior chamber if conservative measures fail or if the lens is cataractous or adherent to the cornea
6. Inadequate visualization of concomitant retinal disease.

REFERENCES

1. Allen, RA, Straatsma, BR, Apt, L, and Hall, MO: Ocular manifestations of the Marfan syndrome, Trans Am Acad Ophthalmol Otolaryngol 71:18, 1967
2. Baikoff, G: Aspiration of ectopia lentis, Dev Ophthalmol 11:157, 1985
3. Barraquer, JI: Surgical treatment of lens displacements, Arc Soc Am Oftal Optom 1:30, 1958
4. Bartholomew, RS: Phakodonesis: a sign of incipient lens displacement, Br J Ophthalmol 54:663, 1970
5. Beighton, P: Serious ophthalmological complications in the Ehlers-Danlos syndrome, Br J Ophthalmol 54:263, 1970
6. Bessière, E, Rivière, J, and Leuret, JP: An association of Klinefelter's disease and congenital anomalies (captodactyly, microphakia), Bull Soc Ophthalmol 54:263, 1970
7. Blaxter, PL: Spherophakia, Trans Ophthalmol Soc UK 88:621, 1969
8. Bode, D, Lloyd, WC, and Griffith, DG: The use of a trochar to fixate a dislocated lens, Ann Ophthalmol 18:14, 1986
9. Boerger, F: Uber zwei Fälle von Arachnodaktylie, Z Kinderheilkd 12:161, 1914

10. Boers, GHJ, et al: Heterozygosity for homocystinuria in premature peripheral and cerebral occlusive arterial disease, N Engl J Med 313:709, 1985

11. Bowers, D: Williams' prior description of Marfan's syndrome, Am J Ophthalmol 50:154, 1960

12. Burian, HM, and Allen, L: Histologic study of the chamber angle of patients with Marfan's syndrome, Arch Ophthalmol 65:323, 1961

13. Burian, HM, von Noorden, GK, and Ponseti, IV: Chamber angle anomalies in systemic connective tissue disorders, Arch Ophthalmol 64:671, 1960

14. Byers, PH, and Holbrook, KA: Molecular basis of clinical heterogeneity in the Ehlers-Danlos syndrome, Ann NY Acad Sci 460:298, 1985

15. Calhoun, FP, Jr, and Jagler, WS: Experience with the Jose Barraquer method of extracting a dislocated lens, Am J Ophthalmol, 50:701, 1960

16. Carson, NAJ, and Weill, DW: Metabolic abnormalities detected in survey of mentally backward individuals in Northern Ireland, Arch Dis Child 37:505, 1962

17. Casper, DS, et al: Familial ectopia lentis: a case study, J Pediatr Ophthalmol Strabismus 22:227, 1985

18. Celichowska, J: Des ectopies et luxations congénitales du cristallin, thesis, Geneva, No. 276, C Zoellner, 1910

19. Chace, RR: Congenital bilateral subluxation of the lens: report of a family, Arch Ophthalmol 34:425, 1945

20. Chandler, PA, and Grant, WM: Choice of treatment is dislocation of the lens, Arch Ophthalmol 71:765, 1964

21. Chandler, PA, and Grant, WM: Glaucoma associated with congenital and spontaneous dislocations of the lens. In Epstein, D, editor: Glaucoma, Philadelphia, 1980, Lea & Febiger

22. Chemke, J, et al: Homozygosity for autosomal dominant Marfan's syndrome, J Med Genet 21:173, 1984

23. Clarke, CC: Ectopia lentis: a pathologic and clinical study, Arch Ophthalmol 21:124, 1939

24. Copeland, T, Tiwary, CM, and Coker, S: Coexistence of neurofibromatosis and Marfan's syndrome, Southern Med J 7a:489, 1986

25. Cotlier, E, and Reinglass, H: Marfan-like syndrome with lens involvement: hyaloideoretinal degeneration with anterior chamber angle, facial, dental, and skeletal anomalies, Arch Ophthalmol 93:93, 1975

26. Cross, HE: Ectopia lentis in systemic heritable disorders, Birth Defects 10:113, 1974

27. Cross, HE: Differential diagnosis and treatment of dislocated lenses, Birth Defects 12:335, 1976

28. Cross, HE: Ectopia lenses et pupillae, Am J Ophthalmol 88:381, 1979

29. Cross, HE, and Jensen, AD: Ocular manifestations in the Marfan syndrome and homocystinuria, Am J Ophthalmol 75:405, 1973

30. Dancis, J, et al: Familial hyperlysinemia with lysine-ketoglutarate reductase insufficiency, J Clin Invest 48:1447, 1969

31. David, R, MacBeath, L, and Jenkins, T: Aniridia associated with microcornea and subluxed lenses, Br J Ophthalmol 62:118, 1978

32. Dinno, ND, Sherer, L, and Weisskopf, B: Familial pseudomarfanism, a new syndrome? Birth Defects 15:179, 1979

33. Douvas, NG: Management of luxated and subluxated lenses, Trans Am Acad Ophthalmol Otolaryngol 73:100, 1969

34. Duke-Elder, S: System of ophthalmology, vol. 3, part 2. Congenital deformities, St. Louis, 1963, The CV Mosby Co

35. Duke-Elder, S: System of ophthalmology, vol. 11 Diseases of the lens and vitreous; glaucoma and hypotony, St. Louis, 1969, The CV Mosby Co

36. Durham, DG: Cutis hyperelastica (Ehlers-Danlos syndrome) with blue scleras, microcornea, and glaucoma, Arch Ophthalmol 49:220, 1953

37. Elkington, AR, Freedman, SS, Jay, B, and Wright, P: Anterior dislocation of the lens in homocystinuria, Br J Ophthalmol 57:325, 1973

38. Falls, HF, and Cotterman, CW: Genetic studies on ectopia lentis: a pedigree of simple ectopia of the lens, Arch Ophthalmol 30:610, 1943

39. Farnsworth, PN, Burke, PA, Blanco, J, and Maltzman, B: Ultrastructural abnormalities in a microspherical ectopic lens, Exp Eye Res 27:399, 1978

40. Farnsworth, PN, Burke, P, Dotto, ME, and Cinotti, AA: Ultrastructural abnormalities in a Marfan's syndrome lens, Arch Ophthalmol 95:1601, 1977

41. Feiler-Ofrey, V, Stein, R, and Godel, V: Marchesani's syndrome and chamber angle anomalies, Am J Ophthalmol 65:862, 1968

42. Furlong, J, Kurcozynski, TW, and Hennessey, JR: New marfanoid syndrome with craniosynostosis, Am J Med Genet 26:599,1987

43. Gerritsen, T, Vaugh, JG, and Waisman, HA: The identification of homocystine in the urine, Biochem Biophys Res Commun 9:493, 1962

44. Girard, LJ: Pars plana lensectomy for subluxated and dislocated lenses, Ophthalmic Surg 12:491, 1981

45. Goltz, RW, Henderson, RR, Hitch, JM, and Ott, JE: Focal dermal hypoplasia syndrome, Arch Dermatol 101:1, 1970

46. Grieco, AJ: Homocystinuria: pathogenetic mechanisms, Am J Med Sci 273:120, 1977

47. Halpern, BL, and Sugar, A: Retinitis pigmentosa associated with bilateral ectopia lentis, Ann Ophthalmol 13:823, 1981

48. Harshman, JP: Glaucoma associated with subluxation of lens in several members of a family, Am J Ophthalmol 31:833, 1948

49. Heath, P: Secondary glaucoma due to the lens, Arch Ophthalmol 25:424, 1941

50. Henkind, P, and Ashton, N: Ocular pathology in homocystinuria, Trans Ophthalmol Soc UK 85:21, 1965
51. Hindle, NW, and Crawford, JS: Dislocation of the lens in Marfan's syndrome: its effect and treatment, Can J Ophthalmol 4:128, 1969
52. Iliff, CE, and Kramer, P: A working guide for the management of dislocated lenses, Ophthalmic Surg 2:251, 1971
53. Irreverre, F, Mudd, SH, Heizer, WD, and Laster, L: Sulfite oxidase deficiency: studies of a patient with mental retardation, dislocated ocular lenses, and abnormal urinary excretion of S-sulfo-L-cysteine sulfite and thiosulfate, Biochem Med 1:187, 1967
54. Jaffe, NS: Subluxation and dislocation of the lens. In Jaffe, NS, editor: Cataract surgery and its complications, ed. 3, St. Louis, 1981, The CV Mosby Co
55. Jarrett, WH: Dislocation of the lens: a study of 166 hospitalized cases, Arch Opthalmol 78:289, 1967
56. Jaureguy, BM, and Hall, JG: Isolated congenital ectopia lentis with autosomal dominant inheritance, Clin Genet 15:97, 1979
57. Jensen, AD: Heritable ectopia lentis. In Goldberg, MF, editor: Genetic and metabolic eye disease, Boston, 1974, Little, Brown & Co
58. Jensen, AD, and Cross, HE: Surgical treatment of dislocated lenses in the Marfan syndrome and homocystinuria, Trans Am Acad Ophthalmol Otolaryngol 76:1491, 1972
59. Jensen, AD, Cross, HE, and Paton, D: Ocular complications in the Weill-Marchesani syndrome, Am J Ophthalmol 77:261, 1974
60. Johnson, VP, Grayson, M, and Christian, JC: Dominant microspherophakia, Arch Ophthalmol 85:534, 1971
61. Kirkham, TH: Mandibulofacial dysostosis with ectopia lentis, Am J Ophthalmol 70:947, 1970
62. Kloepfer, HW, and Rosenthal, JW: Possible genetic carriers in the spherophakia-brachymorphia syndrome, Am J Hum Genet 7:399, 1955
63. Komrower, GM, and Wilson, VK: Homocystinuria, Proc R Soc Med 56:996, 1963
64. Kravits, D: Lens surgery in Marfan's syndrome, Arch Ophthalmol 62:764, 1959
65. Krieg, T, and Muller, PK: The Marfan's syndrome: in vitro study of collagen metabolism in specimens of the aorta, Exp Cell Biol 45:207, 1977
66. Lemmingson, W, and Riethe, P: Beobachtungen bei Dysgenesis mesodermalis corneae et iridis in Kombination mit Oligondontie, Klin Monatsbl Augenheilkd 133:877, 1958
67. Leramo, OB, Fraser, H, and Morgan, OS: Sporadic concurrence of von Recklinghausen's neurofibromatosis and Marfan syndrome, Western Med J 34:131, 1985
68. Levy, J, and Anderson, PE: Marchesani's syndrome, Br J Ophthalmol 45:223, 1961
69. Luebbers, JA, et al: Iris transillumination and variable expression in ectopia lentis et pupillae, Am J Ophthalmol 83:647, 1977
70. Magnasco, A: Unusual malformation association: mandibulofacial dysostosis and bilateral microspherophakia, Ann Ottal 91:489, 1965
71. Manfredi, et al: Etude clinique (oculaire, cardiovasculaire, constitutionelle) et génétique du syndrome de Marfan, J Genet Hum 25(suppl 1), 1977
72. Marchesani, O: Brachydaktylie und angeborene Kugellinse als Systemerkrankung, Klin Monatsbl Augenheilkd 103:392, 1939
73. Marfan, AB: Un cas de déformation congénitale de quatre membres plus prononcée aux extremities characterisé par l'allongement des os avec un certain degré d'émincissement, Bull Mem Soc Hop Paris, 13:220, 1986
74. Maumenee, AE, and Ryan, SJ: Aspiration technique in the management of the dislocated lens, Am J Ophthalmol 68:808, 1969
75. Maumenee, IH: The eye in Marfan syndrome, Trans Am Ophthalmol Soc 79:684, 1981
76. Maumenee, IH: Personal communication, 1988
77. McCulloch, C: Hereditary lens dislocation with angle-closure glaucoma, Can J Ophthalmol 14:230, 1979
78. McGavic, JS: Weill-Marchesani syndrome, Am J Ophthalmol 62:280, 1966
79. McKusick, VA: Primordial dwarfism and ectopia lentis, Am J Hum Gen 7:189, 1955
80. Meyer, ET: Familial ectopia lentis and its complications, Br J Ophthalmol 38:163, 1954
81. Meyer, SJ, and Holstein, T: Spherophakia with glaucoma and brachydactyly, Am J Ophthalmol 24:247, 1941
82. Murdoch, JL, et al: Life expectancy and causes of death in the Marfan syndrome, N Eng J Med 286:804, 1972
83. Nelson, LB, and Maumenee, IH: Ectopia lentis, Surv Ophthalmol 27:143, 1982
84. Nelson, LB, and Szmyd, SM: Aphakic correction in ectopia lentis, Ann Ophthalmol 17:445, 1985
85. Pemberton, JW, Freeman, HM, and Schepens, CL: Familial retinal detachment and the Ehlers-Danlos syndrome, Arch Ophthalmol 76:817, 1966
86. Perry, TL: Mild elevations of plasma ornithine in homocystinuria, Clinica Chimica Acta 117:97, 1981
87. Pesme, P, et al: Dysostose craniofaciale avec ectopie du crystallin, Arch Fr Pediatr 7:348, 1950
88. Peyman, GA, Raichand, M, Goldberg, MF, and Ritacca, D: Management of subluxated and dislocated lenses with the vitrophage, Br J Ophthalmol 63:771, 1979
89. Pfändler, U: Une souche du vallon de St. Imier (Suisse), manifestant par consanguinité, la transmission récessive de malformations oculaires multiples (ectopie du cristallin, keratocone, cataracte congénitale, atrophie du nerf optique), associées à l'oligophrénie: manifestation d'une achromatopsie

totale dans une branche collatérale, Ophthalmologica, 119:103, 1950

90. Pinnel, SR: Molecular defects in the Ehlers-Danlos syndrome, J Invest Dermatol 79:90, 1982

91. Probert, LA: Spherophakia with brachydactyly: comparison with Marfan's syndrome, Am J Ophthalmol 36:1571, 1953

92. Pyeritz, RE, and McKusick, VA: The Marfan syndrome: diagnosis and management, N Engl J Med 300:772, 1979

93. Pyeritz, RE, Murphy, EA, and McKusick, VA: Clinical variability in the Marfan syndrome(s), Birth Defects 15:155, 1979

94. Ramsey, MS, Fine, BS, Shields, JA, and Yanoff, M: The Marfan syndrome: a histopathologic study of ocular findings, Am J Ophthalmol 76:102, 1973

95. Ramsey, MS, Yanoff, M, and Fine, BS: The ocular histopathology of homocystinuria: a light and electron microscopy study, Am J Ophthalmol 74:377, 1972

96. Reese, PD, and Weingeist, TA: Pars plana management of ectopia lentis in children, Arch Ophthalmol 105:1202, 1987

97. Ringelhan, O, and Elschnig, A: Uber die LinsenDislokationen, Arch Augenheilkd 104:325, 1931

98. Ritch, R: Argon laser treatment for medically unresponsive attacks of angle-closure glaucoma, Am J Ophthalmol 94:197, 1982

99. Ritch, R, and Solomon, IS: Glaucoma surgery. In L'Esperance, FA, editor: Ophthalmic lasers, ed 3, St. Louis, 1989, The CV Mosby Co

100. Ritch, R, and Wand, M: Treatment of the Weill-Marchesani syndrome (editorial), Ann Ophthalmol 13:665, 1981

101. Rodman, HI: Chronic open-angle glaucoma associated with traumatic dislocation of the lens, Arch Ophthalmol 69:445, 1963

102. Rosenbaum, LJ, and Podos, SM: Traumatic ectopia lentis: some relationships to syphilis and glaucoma, Am J Ophthalmol 64:1095, 1967

103. Rosenthal, JW, and Kloepfer, HW: The spherophakia-brachymorphia syndrome, Arch Ophthalmol 55:28, 1956

104. Ryan, EH, Jr, and Rosenberg, MT: An instrument to aid ICCE of dislocated lens, Ophthalmic Surg 18:130, 1987

105. Sasaki, T, Arai, K, Ono, M, and Yamaguchi, T: Ehlers-Danlos syndrome, a variant characterized by the deficiency of pro-alpha chain of type I procollagen, Arch Dermatol 123:76, 1987

106. Seetner, AA, and Crawford, JS: Surgical correction of lens dislocation in children, Am J Ophthalmol 91:106, 1981

107. Sichel, J: Ueber die freiwillige Dislocation und Niedersenkung der Crystalllinse, Z Gesamte Med 33:281, 1846

108. Smith, TH, Holland, MG, and Woody, NC: Ocular manifestations of familial hyperlysinemia, Trans Am Acad Ophthalmol Otolaryngol 75:355, 1971

109. Smolin, LA, Benerenga, NJ, and Berlow, S: The use of betaine for the treatment of homocystinuria, J Pediatr 99:467, 1981

110. Sohar, E: Renal disease, inner ear deafness and ocular changes: a new heredofamilial syndrome, Arch Int Med 97:627, 1956

111. Spaeth, GW: Glaucomatous changes in homocystinuria. Discussion of Jay, B: Glaucoma associated with spontaneous displacement of the lens, Br J Ophthalmol 56:258, 1972

112. Straatsma, BR, Allen, RA, Pettit, TH, and Hall, MO: Subluxation of the lens treated with iris photocoagulation, Am J Ophthalmol 61:1312, 1966

113. Thomas, C, Cordier, J, and Alga, B: Une étiologie nouvelle du syndrome de luxation spontanée des cristallins: la maladie d'Ehlers-Danlos, Bull Soc Belge Ophthalmol 100:375, 1952

114. Townes, PL: Ectopia lentis et pupillae, Arch Ophthalmol 94:1126, 1976

115. Urbanek, J: Glaucoma juvenile inversum, Z Augenheilkd, 77:171, 1930

116. Vogt, A: Dislocatio lentis spontanea als erbliche Krankheit, Z Augenheilkd, 14:153, 1905

117. von Noorden, GG, and Schutz, RO: A gonioscopic study of the chamber angle in Marfan's syndrome, Arch Ophthalmol 64:929, 1960

118. Wachtel, JG: The ocular pathology of Marfan's syndrome, Arch Ophthalmol 76:512, 1966

119. Weill, G: Ectopie des cristallins et malformations générales, Ann Ocul 169:21, 1932

120. Wilcken, DEL, et al: Homocystinemia: the effects of betaine in the treatment of patients not responsive to pyridoxine, N Engl J Med 309:448, 1983

121. Willi, M, Kut, L, and Cotlier, E: Pupillary-block in the Marchesani syndrome, Arch Ophthalmol 90:504, 1973

122. Wright, KW, and Chrousos, GA: Weill-Marchesani syndrome with bilateral angle closure glaucoma, J Pediatr Ophthalmol Strabismus 22:129, 1985

123. Young, ID, Fielder, AR, and Casey, TA: Weill-Marchesani syndrome in mother and son, Clin Genet 30:475, 1986

124. Zaidman, MD: The surgical management of dislocated traumatic cataracts, Am J Ophthalmol 99:583, 1985

125. Zuckerman, D, and Lahav, M: A simple method for delivery of a subluxed lens, Am J Ophthalmol 102:537, 1986

Chapter 59

Glaucoma Associated with Retinal Disorders

Andrew M. Prince

This chapter describes the various types of secondary glaucomas that are either caused by or are associated with retinal or vitreoretinal disorders or their treatment. Retinal disorders secondary to glaucoma and its treatment are not included. The principal varieties of glaucoma associated with retinal disorders are listed below. Several of these conditions are described in other chapters of this textbook; to avoid unnecessary repetition, they are not covered in this chapter.

A. Glaucoma caused by retinal disorders
1. Open-angle glaucoma associated with retinal detachment (Schwartz's syndrome)
2. Glaucoma associated with long-standing rhegmatogenous detachment
   a. Angle-closure glaucoma from posterior synechiae and pupillary block caused by detachment-induced iritis (see Chapter 67)
   b. Neovascular glaucoma (see Chapter 60)
3. Hemolytic, ghost cell, and hemosiderotic glaucoma after vitreous hemorrhage (see Chapter 69)
4. Neovascular glaucoma associated with retinal ischemic disorders (see Chapter 60)
5. Angle-closure glaucoma associated with neonatal retinal diseases: retrolental fibroplasia, persistent hyperplastic primary vitreous, Coats' disease, familial exudative vitreoretinopathy, and retinoblastoma (see Chapters 53 and 61)
6. Angle-closure glaucoma, uveal effusion, and retinal detachment associated with nanophthalmos
7. Transient angle-closure glaucoma after central retinal vein occlusion
8. Angle-closure glaucoma in AIDS
9. Iris retraction syndrome
B. Glaucoma caused by treatment of retinal and vitreal disorders
1. Angle-closure glaucoma after retinal photocoagulation
2. Angle-closure glaucoma after scleral buckling procedures
3. Glaucoma after intravitreal gas injection
4. Glaucoma after intraocular silicone injection
5. Glaucoma after pars plana vitrectomy (see Chapter 60)
6. Steroid-induced glaucoma (see Chapter 64)
C. Glaucoma associated with retinal disorders because of a common underlying cause or for unknown reasons
1. Primary open-angle glaucoma and rhegmatogenous retinal detachment
2. Pigmentary glaucoma and retinal detachment
3. Glaucoma and retinitis pigmentosa
4. Open-angle glaucoma and retinal detachment in Stickler's syndrome

5. Traumatic angle-recession glaucoma and retinal detachment (see Chapter 68)
6. Glaucoma (developmental, angle-closure, angle-recession, or phacolytic) and retinal detachment in eyes with displaced lenses (see Chapter 58)
7. Synechial angle-closure glaucoma and retinal detachment in aphakia
8. Other types of glaucoma associated with nonrhegmatogenous detachment
   a. Secondary angle-closure glaucoma in eyes with uveitis and exudative retinal detachment (see Chapter 67)
   b. Neovascular glaucoma in diabetics with traction retinal detachment (see Chapter 60)
   c. Glaucoma in eyes with tumors and secondary retinal detachment (see Chapter 61)

GLAUCOMA CAUSED BY RETINAL DISORDERS

Open-angle Glaucoma Apparently Caused by Retinal Detachment: Schwartz's Syndrome

In most instances, rhegmatogenous retinal detachment reduces intraocular pressure to a level lower than that of the unaffected fellow eye. Intraocular pressure will be decreased from 2 to 3.5 mm Hg in 60% to 74% of eyes, remain unchanged in 20% to 30% of eyes, and become elevated in 6% to 10% of eyes with a retinal detachment.[24,26,36,60,66] The degree of decrease in intraocular pressure directly correlates with the size of the retinal detachment.[36] Several investigators have demonstrated a decrease in outflow facility in eyes with retinal detachment, and it is believed that the mechanism for the intraocular pressure decrease is a reduction in aqueous production rather than an increase in retrograde flow of aqueous.[11,36,60] No difference in ocular rigidity between affected and unaffected eyes of patients with retinal detachments has been found.[60]

In 1973 Schwartz[94] described 11 patients in whom history, postoperative examination, and postoperative course suggested that an untreated rhegmatogenous retinal detachment caused a secondary open-angle glaucoma. Intraocular pressures ranged between 29 and 55 mm Hg and most patients demonstrated an accompanying iridocyclitis. Steroids and antiglaucoma medical therapy were ineffective in reducing the inflammatory reaction or the intraocular pressure. After surgical reattachment of the retina, the glaucoma and iridocyclitis resolved in all patients. Intraocular pressures returned to normal within several days after retinal surgery. Schwartz suggested that the accompanying iridocyclitis may cause a reduction in outflow facility, and despite a decreased aqueous production, this may result in an elevated intraocular pressure. It should be mentioned that 5 of 11 patients gave a history or demonstrated evidence of previous ocular trauma.

Phelps and Burton[81] reported on 817 patients undergoing 863 surgical procedures for repair of a retinal detachment and found 18 (2.1%) patients who fit the criteria for the Schwartz syndrome. Cells were present in the anterior chamber in 11 of the 18 cases, and 6 of the 18 patients had an angle recession. They suggested that the cause of the glaucoma may be a previously damaged aqueous outflow pathway, which may have decompensated when challenged with the retinal detachment-induced inflammation and/or pigment release.

Other investigators have also hypothesized that pigment migration into the anterior chamber with obstruction of the trabecular meshwork may play a role in this intraocular pressure increase.[8,33] Davidorf[33] described four patients with elevated intraocular pressure (range, 24 to 48 mm Hg) and retinal detachment, all of whom had a moderate amount of pigmented cells in the vitreous, cells in the anterior chamber, and increased trabecular meshwork pigmentation when compared with the fellow eye. In all cases, the vitreous and trabecular meshwork pigmentation decreased after reattachment of the retina. He believed that anterior chamber "cells" were actually pigment particles released from the retinal pigment epithelium, which migrated through the retinal hole into the vitreous, and into the anterior chamber where they became trapped in the trabecular meshwork, obstructing outflow.

Matsuo et al.[68] reported on seven patients with this syndrome. In all cases, transmission electron microscopy of the aqueous humor demonstrated many photoreceptor outer segments and few inflammatory cells. They postulated that a retinal break creates a communication between the subretinal space and the anterior chamber, and as a result, photoreceptor outer segments flow into the anterior chamber and obstruct the trabecular meshwork. They also suggested that with a long-standing retinal detachment, a more viscous subretinal fluid may gain access to the anterior chamber and add to the induced decrease in outflow facility.

It is important to be aware that unilateral open-angle glaucoma in an eye with cells or pigment granules in the anterior chamber may be a sign of unsuspected retinal detachment. Also, if the retinal detachment is nonrhegmatogenous, one should think of an underlying choroidal melanoma (see Chapter 61). The peripheral fundus must be examined carefully through a dilated pupil. If a rhegmatogenous retinal detachment is found and successfully treated, the prognosis for the resolution of the glaucoma is quite good.

Angle-closure Glaucoma, Uveal Effusion, and Retinal Detachment in Nanophthalmos

Nanophthalmos is an uncommon developmental ocular anomaly resulting from an arrested development of the globe subsequent to closure of the embryonic fissure, in which the eye is of normal shape but of reduced volume. Both dominant and recessive patterns of inheritance occur. The palpebral fissure is usually narrow, with a deeply set globe in a small orbit.[38] Most nanophthalmic eyes are markedly hyperopic because of their short axial lengths. They are also susceptible to angle-closure glaucoma, which usually begins acutely during the fourth to sixth decade of life.

In one series of 32 eyes in 16 patients with bilateral nanophthalmos, the mean refractive error was +13.60 diopters (range, +7.25 to +20.00 diopters).[99] The mean axial length was 17.00 mm, with an average lens thickness of 5.18 mm (range, 4.20 to 7.26 mm). All eyes demonstrated a marked iris convexity and shallow anterior chamber (mean depth, 1.46 mm). The average corneal diameter was 10.33 mm and the lens-eye volume ratio averaged 12.16%. Ten eyes had grade 1 to 2 angles (Shaffer classification), and 22 of 32 had grade 0 to 1 angles.

In 1974 Brockhurst[20] described five patients with nanophthalmos and angle-closure glaucoma who, after glaucoma surgery or a subsequent cataract operation, were found to have choroidal effusion and nonrhegmatogenous retinal detachment. All five patients were extremely hyperopic, presenting with acute angle-closure in the fourth to sixth decade. Others have described additional patients with this unusual and severe complication.[27,99]

These reports indicated that iridectomy sometimes failed to open the anterior chamber angle, suggesting that relative pupillary block was neither the sole nor the initiating pathogenic mechanism. Brockhurst hypothesized the primary event to be the uveal effusion and suggested that angle-closure resulted when the ciliary body detached and

swelled sufficiently to cause forward rotation of the lens-iris diaphragm. He could not confirm this because the extreme periphery of the fundus was not examined before surgical intervention. Kimbrough et al.[57] described two additional patients with nanophthalmos in whom a peripheral choroidal detachment was identified by ultrasonography before glaucoma surgery, supporting Brockhurst's theory. Spontaneous choroidal detachments have been documented by others.[89,99]

At surgery Brockhurst observed an unusually thick sclera (2.5 mm) in two of his patients, leading Shaffer[96] to suggest that the thick sclera might in some way impede drainage of venous blood through the vortex veins, thus causing the uveal effusion. Kimbrough et al.[57] postulated that thickened sclera, which becomes more sclerotic with age, causes a choroidal effusion by increased resistance to vortex vein outflow, which then results in anterior rotation of the ciliary processes and forward lens movment. This further crowds an already compromised angle resulting in angle-closure glaucoma. Trelstad et al.[104] found the sclera from two nanophthalmic eyes to be thicker than normal and to contain unusually disordered collagen fibrils. Unusual accumulations of perifibrillar aggregates resembling proteoglycans were also found. Yue et al.[110] found collagen fibers twisted, more closely packed, and arranged in irregularly interlacing bundles. Proteins and collagen were synthesized in tissue culture at a rate similar to normals, but the level of glycosaminoglycans produced was significantly reduced, possibly resulting in the abnormal packing of collagen bundles. They suggested that the uveal effusion may result from either a reduced scleral permeability to proteins or from vortex vein compression.

Since these patients often experience serious vision-threatening complications after intraocular surgery, medical and laser therapies are preferred when possible. In the series of Singh et al., surgical iridectomy or glaucoma filtering surgery was performed in 15 eyes.[99] In 13 of 15 patients visual acuity was reduced secondary to postoperative complications. These included malignant glaucoma, retinal and choroidal detachment, and prolonged flat anterior chamber.

Patients with nanophthalmos must be followed closely with regular gonioscopic examinations for evidence of progressive angle-closure. As longstanding appositional closure may result in eventual synechial closure, timely medical and/or laser therapy could prevent the potential serious complications of intraocular surgery.

Medical therapy for angle-closure glaucoma in nanophthalmos should include aqueous suppressants, as well as epinephrine. Miotics may improve some cases but worsen others[99] and should be used cautiously with frequent gonioscopic examination to assess their effect. Laser iridectomy should be employed in cases of angle-closure to eliminate any component of pupillary block. If an angle remains appositionally closed after laser iridectomy and medical therapy, peripheral iridoplasty should be considered. If surgical iridectomy, lensectomy, or glaucoma filtering surgery become necessary, patients should be carefully assessed for the presence of suprachoroidal effusions. It has been suggested that a posterior sclerotomy be performed before entering the anterior segment to prevent choroidal effusion.[89] Brockhurst[21] suggested that the sudden decrease in intraocular pressure during intraocular surgery results in a relative increase in choroidal venous pressure with effusion into the choroid and subretinal space, explaining this common complication in such cases. He performed vortex vein decompression on 10 nanophthalmic eyes with uveal effusion and nonrhegmatogenous retinal detachments with good results.

MacKay et al.[67] described seven related patients with progressive retinal pigmentary degeneration, cystic macular degeneration, nanophthalmos, and angle-closure glaucoma with normal chromosomal analysis. This appears to be a newly recognized, autosomal recessive syndrome.

Transient Angle-closure Glaucoma after Central Retinal Vein Occlusion

Hyams and Neumann[55] were the first to describe the rare condition of transient angle-closure glaucoma after central retinal vein occlusion. Twelve cases have been reported.[15,30,46,55,72] Anterior chamber shallowing without actual angle-closure is likely more common. Characteristically, the shallowing does not occur simultaneously with the vein occlusion. In 11 of the 12 reported cases, the time from the occurrence of symptoms of the vein occlusion to the diagnosis of angle-closure glaucoma ranged from 3 days to 2 months.[15,45,54,72] Some patients have presented with pain, whereas others have complained only of blurred vision.

This condition must be distinguished, both clinically and conceptually, from two other types of angle-closure glaucoma that more often accompany central retinal vein occlusion. In primary angle-closure glaucoma, the high intraocular pressure may occasionally induce a central retinal vein occlusion. Here, the patient's other eye also has a shallow anterior chamber and a narrow anterior

chamber angle. Neovascular glaucoma frequently occurs several weeks or months after the onset of a central retinal vein occlusion (see Chapter 60). Like the transient angle-closure glaucoma developing after central retinal vein occlusion, it is usually unilateral but is distinguished by the presence of rubeosis iridis. Once the angle-closure stage of neovascular glaucoma occurs, it is permanent.

The mechanism of anterior chamber shallowing after central retinal vein occlusion remains obscure. Hyams and Neumann[55] suggested that transudation of fluid from the retinal vessels into the vitreous cavity causes a forward displacement of the lens, pupillary block, and angle-closure glaucoma. However, in two of Grant's patients,[46] iridectomy did not immediately relieve the angle closure. Grant questioned whether blood or edematous fluid in the retina might increase the volume of the posterior segment sufficiently to produce the forward movement of the lens and iris. However, in one patient, no thickening of the retina could be measured by echography.[46] Bloome[15] suggested that swelling of the ciliary body because of spasm, edema, or detachment would cause relaxation of the zonules with displacement of the lens-iris diaphragm anteriorly and resultant crowding and occlusion of the angle by the peripheral iris. Although this would produce the clinical picture observed, he was unable to explain how a retinal vein occlusion could cause the ciliary body to swell. None of these theories explains why the anterior chamber does not shallow in the majority of cases of central retinal vein occlusion.

Whatever the pathogenic mechanism, the prognosis for eventual recovery of normal anterior chamber depth is quite good. In most of the reported cases, the angle gradually widened and the chamber reformed over several weeks. Carbonic anhydrase inhibitors and pilocarpine in some cases appreared to hasten somewhat the resolution of the angle-closure,[46,55] and in three cases, treatment with acetazolamide and cycloplegics produced a rapid and dramatic deepening of the chamber.[15,30] Cycloplegics, in addition to topical steroids and aqueous suppressants, are a logical treatment because the condition resembles malignant glaucoma and angle-closure glaucoma resulting from ciliary body swelling, both of which respond favorably to this treatment regimen. Although the angle-closure eventually resolves, vision is often permanently impaired by retinal damage from the central vein occlusion. In addition, a few of the reported patients developed neovascular glaucoma weeks to months later.[46,55]

Weber et al.[109] described three cases of malignant glaucoma after surgical trabeculectomy for primary open-angle glaucoma in patients with preexisting central retinal vein occlusion. The occlusion had occurred 3 years earlier in one patient, was resolving in another, and was of recent onset in the third. They proposed that the occlusion may have been a factor in the development of malignant glaucoma by causing ciliary body rotation and/or engorgement.

Angle-closure Glaucoma with AIDS

The acquired immune deficiency syndrome (AIDS) is a disorder in which depression of the cellular immune system results in the development of opportunistic infections, as well as Kaposi's sarcoma. The many ocular manifestations include cotton-wool spots, conjunctival Kaposi's sarcoma, retinal periphlebitis and perivasculitis, acute retinal necrosis, herpes zoster ophthalmicus, infectious retinitis, choroiditis and chorioretinitis, cranial nerve paralysis, and papilledema.[77,106]

Bilateral acute angle-closure glaucoma occurring in two homosexual men has been reported. The pathophysiologic mechanism appeared to be anterior rotation of the ciliary body secondary to choroidal effusion. The authors stressed that this mechanism should be differentiated from that of classic pupillary block, as treatment with miotics may worsen this condition. Cycloplegics, by relaxing the ciliary muscle and causing a posterior shift of the lens-iris diaphragm, may open the angle in such cases. If treatment with cycloplegics in combination with aqueous suppressants proves unsuccessful, iridectomy with drainage of suprachoroidal fluid should be considered.[106]

Iris Retraction Syndrome

Campbell[28] described nine patients with rhegmatogenous retinal detachment, hypotony, and iris retraction. Rapid cataract formation was a common finding. All nine patients had secluded pupils. Seven of the patients presented with iris retraction and two with angle-closure glaucoma and iris bombé. The latter two patients converted to the iris retraction configuration with pharmacologic aqueous suppressants. Reversion to iris bombé resulted when therapy was withdrawn. He proposed that the iris retraction was a result of a lower pressure in the posterior than in the anterior chamber, separated by a pressure-sensitive diaphragm (iris), rather than actual posterior traction on the iris. Elimination of pupillary block, either by intracapsular cataract extraction or pharmacologic dilation with disruption of pupillary seclusion, resulted in the resumption of a normal iris configuration. His

findings suggest that the hypotony was due at least in part to aqueous removal behind the iris, supporting the theory of a subretinal pump.

GLAUCOMA CAUSED BY TREATMENT OF RETINAL AND VITREAL DISORDERS

Angle-closure Glaucoma after Retinal Photocoagulation

Intraocular pressure elevations often occur after retinal photocoagulation. At least three pathogenic mechanisms, each occurring at different times after the photocoagulation, may be responsible.

A transient, marked, sharp intraocular pressure elevation may occur at the time of ruby laser or xenon arc photocoagulation.[42,71] These spikes may be as high as 900 mm Hg, particularly with xenon arc photocoagulation, but last less than 1 msec. Significant intraocular pressure rises of this type have not been observed with argon laser therapy.

A second type of intraocular pressure elevation, of more modest magnitude but longer duration, has been observed after extensive argon laser retinal photocoagulation for treatment of diabetic retinopathy.[14,65] Blondeau et al.[14] monitored 18 eyes of 18 patients undergoing panretinal photocoagulation for diabetic retinopathy. Of the 14 eyes exhibiting open-angle intraocular pressure elevations, 12 were found to have increases immediately after the treatment, and 2 had increases 1 to 2 hours later. The maximum pressure elevation averaged 10.2 ± 4.6 mm Hg and was accompanied by a mean decrease in outflow facility of 0.08 μL/min/mm Hg. Because of limited follow-up of some patients and the subsequent development of an angle-closure component in others, the authors were unable to determine the duration of the open-angle portion of this postlaser pressure rise. Liang and Huamonte[65] found a higher incidence of open-angle intraocular pressure elevations in patients whose treatment was performed in two or more sessions over a 3-day period (22%) than in those whose treatment sessions were 2 or more weeks apart (7%). Possibilities for the mechanism of this elevation include a laser-induced decrease in the integrity of the blood-retinal barrier with an increase in intraocular fluid, congestion of the ciliary body with a resulting decrease in uveoscleral outflow, laser damage to the short ciliary nerves causing decreased ciliary muscle tone and outflow facility, and the potential effect of prostaglandin release.[14]

The third type of postlaser intraocular pressure rise results from an angle-closure mechanism. In the series of Blondeau et al.[14] angle-closure glaucoma occurred immediately after treatment in 3 of 18 eyes, whereas partial to complete closure occurred in five of the eyes that initially had had open-angle intraocular pressure elevations within 3 to 48 hours after treatment. The incidence of angle-closure glaucoma after panretinal photocoagulation has been reported to range between 0 and 44%.[14,37,54,65,73] Mensher[73] detected anterior chamber shallowing with angle narrowing in 44 of 45 eyes treated with either argon laser or xenon arc retinal photocoagulation. Fourteen of the 45 eyes (31%) developed angle-closure glaucoma. Doft and Blankenship[37] demonstrated the incidence of angle narrowing and angle closure to be 16% and 12%, respectively, for patients undergoing argon laser panretinal photocoagulation in a single session, whereas for those treated in multiple sessions, the incidences were 12% and 0%, respectively. Liang and Huamonte[65] also found an increased incidence of anterior chamber shallowing in patients undergoing treatment over a shorter period of time. Neither study found a correlation between the incidence of angle narrowing and the extent or type of treatment (argon or xenon arc).

Several mechanisms for anterior chamber shallowing and angle-closure glaucoma after panretinal photocoagulation have been suggested. Mensher[73] hypothesized that photocoagulation-induced choroidal vascular occlusions result in choroidal and ciliary body swelling. Anterior rotation of the ciliary body and resultant forward shifting of the lens-iris diaphragm would explain this clinical picture. Boulton[18] suggested that anterior chamber shallowing was due to a combination of fluid transudation into the vitreous from the choroid and an annular choroidal detachment with resultant anterior displacement of the lens-iris diaphragm.

In cases of angle closure after panretinal photocoagulation, tensions may be as high as 55 mm Hg. Characteristically, patients experience minimal discomfort, often attributed to the trauma of the laser treatment itself. As suggested previously, multiple treatment sessions, separated by 1 to 2 week intervals, may reduce its incidence. Treatment with miotics is not only ineffective but may exacerbate the condition by causing further anterior displacement of the lens-iris diaphragm. Although a controlled therapeutic trial has not yet been performed, treatment with topical cycloplegics and corticosteroids is recomended. Cycloplegics will cause a posterior shift of the lens-iris diaphragm, and corticosteroids lessen the chances of synechial angle closure, as well as reduce any ciliary body inflammation. In addition, the use of aqueous suppressants, as well as hyperosmotic agents, is suggested if the intraocular pressure is considered to be at a dangerous level. Argon laser peripheral iridoplasty is capable of opening the angle in this situation if closure is appositional.

The angle usually reopens with normalization of tension within 2 to 7 days and rarely causes serious long-term sequelae. Although peripheral anterior synechiae may form, intraocular pressure control rarely becomes a long-term problem. A study involving panretinal photocoagulation in normotensive eyes of diabetic patients demonstrated a significant decrease in intraocular pressure (mean 3.1 mm Hg) 1 month after xenon arc photocoagulation. Less of an effect (mean 0.9 mm Hg) was noted after treatment with the argon laser.[92]

Angle-closure Glaucoma after Scleral Buckling Procedures

Temporary shallowing of the anterior chamber often occurs after scleral buckling procedures for the repair of retinal detachments.[41,50,95] Fiore and Newton[41] found anterior chamber shallowing in all of 14 patients 1 week after surgery (mean decrease 0.44 mm). The degree of shallowing is variable, and although it is usually clinically insignificant, angle-closure glaucoma may result.[59,80,95,100]

Smith[98] first described angle-closure glaucoma after scleral buckling for retinal detachment repair. He found this in 4% of 1000 cases. Sebestyn et al.[95] noted angle narrowing in 12% and angle-closure in 4.4% of 160 scleral buckling procedures. Perez et al.[81] reported an incidence of angle-closure of 1.4% in 1558 cases, and Phelps and Burton[81] found a 2% incidence in 817 cases.

These patients most often present within the first several days after surgery with symptoms that are consistent with their recent retinal detachment repair, often resulting in an overlooked diagnosis. Nausea and vomiting associated with a markedly elevated intraocular pressure may be attributed to a common reaction to general anesthesia. Signs include anterior chamber shallowing and corneal edema in cases of extreme tension rises. Applanation pressures usually range between 25 and 55 mm Hg and gonioscopy reveals partial or complete appositional angle closure. There are varying opinions concerning a correlation between the gonioscopic appearance preoperatively of the operative eye or the fellow eye and the predisposition to angle closure.[30,80,95] Choridal detachments (serous and hemorrhagic) are often found in association with this entity.[30,80]

Sebestyn et al.[95] found that the incidence of

angle closure after scleral buckling was increased with a narrow angle preoperatively, an anteriorly placed buckle, and a postoperative ciliochoroidal detachment. Hartley and Marsh[50] found no correlation with the size of the buckle, but permanent shallowing was more common with encircling bands. Perez et al.[80] found no correlation with the preoperative angle configuration, size of the detachment, or size or location of the buckle but did find a higher incidence with episcleral (3.4%) than with intrascleral (0.6%) implants. Simmons[30] suggested that this complication is seen more often after long, complicated cases, in those with large buckles, and when extensive cryotherapy or diathermy are performed. Aaberg and Maggiano[1] have observed that postoperative choroidal detachment, a complication related to postoperative angle-closure, occurs more frequently when the patient is elderly and when the buckle is large.

The anterior chamber is shallow because the lens is shifted forward from its usual position. The contour of the anterior surface of the iris differs from the midperipheral forward convexity seen in pupillary block glaucoma (Fig. 59-1). The iris is pushed forward centrally by the lens but in the midperiphery, it falls away slightly from the cornea. In the angle, the iris root again comes forward toward the cornea to lie against the trabecular meshwork.

Most of the presently available clinical and experimental data suggest that the pathogenic process leading to angle closure is initiated by impedance of venous drainage from the vortex veins by the scleral buckle. As blood from the ciliary body drains into the vortex veins, obstruction leads to congestion and swelling of the ciliary body. This has been demonstrated experimentally in monkeys and rabbits.[35,51] Capillaries of the ciliary processes can enlarge to many times their normal size when their transmural pressure is high.[98] As the ciliary body swells, it resembles, in cross section, a fan unfolding, with its apex attached to the scleral spur and its anterior face rotating toward the trabecular meshwork. If it swells sufficiently, the angle closes.

The frequent finding of peripheral choroidal detachment in eyes with postoperative angle-closure supports the preceding theory. Choroidal detachment in an eye with high intraocular pressure is almost certain evidence of high pressure in the choroidal veins because transudation of fluid from choroidal capillaries to interstitial spaces requires that the capillary pressure be considerably higher than the intraocular pressure. It seems likely that a scleral buckle over or anterior to the vortex ampullae may obstruct or kink the veins draining the choroid and ciliary body.

Several observations have indicated that pupillary block does not have an important role in the pathogenesis of angle-closure after scleral buckling. There is no iris bombé in most cases. This syndrome has been observed in aphakic eyes with a patent iridectomy and a vitreous face well behind the pupil. In two cases treated with an iridectomy, there was no relief.[80] Finally, in experimental models, no clinical or pathologic evidence of pupillary block has been found.[12] Nevertheless, in some cases pupillary block caused by the forward movement of the lens may be partially responsible for the angle-closure.[30]

A third possible mechanism is simple mechanical indentation of the sclera, which, if the buckle is anterior, might rotate the ciliary body forward.[12] This is unlikely to be the sole mechanism because the chamber shallowing and angle-closure resolve with time, even though the buckle seems to maintain its height.

In general, the prognosis for angle-closure glaucoma is good after a scleral buckling operation. In most cases, if left untreated, the chamber gradually deepens after several days, the angle opens, the choroidal detachment flattens, and the intraocular pressure returns to normal. Complete resolution may take from 2 to 4 weeks.

Glaucomatous optic nerve damage from the acute attack is infrequent because the intraocular pressure is usually not exceptionally high, and the pressure elevation usually lasts only 1 to 2 weeks. In some patients, however, peripheral anterior synechiae form, and permanent synechial angle-closure glaucoma may develop.

Iridectomy is of no benefit and miotics worsen the ocular congestion. Drainage of the choroidal detachment may sometimes be effective,[30,59,100] but in other cases the choroidal detachment immediately recurs. Removal of the buckle will quickly deepen the chamber and relieve the angle-closure. Recommended medical treatment includes cycloplegics and phenylephrine to encourage flattening and posterior rotation of the ciliary body. Topical steroids reduce inflammation and peripheral anterior synechia formation. Intraocular pressure is lowered with aqueous suppressants and hyperosmotics, if necessary.

Argon laser peripheral iridoplasty has been used successfully in the treatment of angle-closure after insertion of a scleral buckle.[25,86] The angle was opened easily and effectively, with immediate reduction of intraocular pressure, and the underlying process resolved over time.

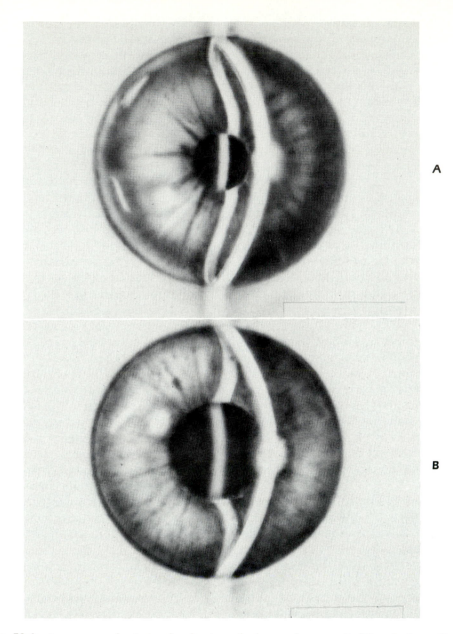

Fig. 59-1 Appearance of anterior chamber in angle-closure glaucoma. **A,** Ciliary body swelling: shallow in center and periphery, with some deepening in midperiphery. **B,** Pupillary block: forward convexity of anterior iris surface. (Courtesy Steven J Vermillion, MD)

Other Glaucomatous Complications of Retinal Detachment Surgery

In 1938, the successful treatment of retinal detachments with retinopexy combined with intraocular gas injection was reported by Rosengren.[87] Despite the advent of the scleral buckling procedure, the use of intraocular gas is still commonly recommended in certain types of detachments.[40,75] The disadvantages of sterile room air are its inability to expand intraocularly and rapid resorption time (5 to 7 days). Sulfur hexafluoride (SF_6), an inert, lipid-soluble gas, can double in volume in 48 hours and can remain within the eye for 11 to 14 days. Both intravitreal SF_6 and perfluorocarbons, commonly used for retinal tamponade, have been associated with early postoperative intraocular pressure elevations.* The incidence of intraocular pressure elevations ≥30 mm Hg after intraocular

---

*References 2, 3, 6, 16, 31, 32, 39, 40, 45, 49, 56, 75, 83, 90.

injection of SF_6 has been reported to be 26% to 45%, with reports of central retinal artery occlusions.[3,90] A significantly higher incidence is found when 100% SF_6 is used, and a 40:60 mixture of SF_6 and air is recomended.[3,56,75] Although Norton[75] suggested that a volume of less than 2 ml of SF_6 reduces the risk of this intraocular pressure rise, Abrams et al.[3] were unable to confirm this finding. They did demonstrate eyes with fibrinous anterior chamber reactions were more likely to have pressure elevations.

After the use of perfluorocarbon gas, Chang et al.[31] found 33 of 56 patients to have postoperative intraocular pressures of >22 mm Hg and 11 >40 mm Hg during the first week. Twelve patients required gas aspiration for intraocular pressure control. They stressed the importance of maintaining the patient in the prone position to prevent forward lens movement and pupillary block secondary to anterior pressure from the gas bubble.

Schiøtz indentation and pneumatic tonometry significantly underestimate the actual intraocular pressure in eyes containing intravitreal gas. Applanation tonometry using either the Goldmann, Perkins, or McKay-Marg tonometers is recommended.[6,83]

Elevated intraocular pressure caused by an expanding gas is usually present within the first postoperative 24 hours and may persist for several days. Although the rise usually responds to aqueous suppressants and hyperosmotic agents, it is occasionally necessary to aspirate some gas.[90] Han et al.[49] described five cases of angle-closure glaucoma with complete iridocorneal apposition in aphakic eyes after vitrectomy and air-fluid exchange and reported success using an anterior chamber deepening procedure with sodium hyaluronate.

Intravitreal silicone oil is also employed as adjuvant treatment in cases of complicated retinal detachments and proliferative vitreoretinopathy and may cause long- and short-term postoperative pressure rises.* However, Watzke[108] was unable to identify any cases of elevated intraocular pressure directly related to the presence of intraocular silicone oil in his series of 33 cases. In an analysis of postoperative intraocular pressure changes occurring in 48 patients having undergone complete vitrectomy with intravitreal silicone oil injection, an intraocular pressure increase (10 mm Hg above preoperative level) was found in 56% of patients (range, 10 to 53 mm Hg; mean increase, 21.6 mm

Hg).[34] The intraocular pressure increases were detected between 6 hours and 60 days after surgery, with 93% of patients showing an increase by postoperative day 2. In 21 of 27 patients, the increase was transient, with 8 requiring no treatment, 7 requiring temporary medical therapy, and 6 requiring removal of the silicone oil. In 6 patients, medical therapy was still required at the time of the data analysis (mean follow-up, 8 months).[34]

Although silicone oil may be found in the trabecular meshwork, evidence suggests that this is not the sole mechanism behind the associated intraocular pressure rise.[22,47,61,62,108] Other possible mechanisms include concomitant neovascular glaucoma, ghost cell glaucoma, hyphema, uveitis, and obstruction of the trabecular meshwork by lens remnants. Cases of pupillary block after silicone oil injection have been reported.[5,76]

A final type of glaucoma occurs in retinal detachment patients who are given corticosteroids in the treatment of ocular inflammation after detachment surgery. Some patients receiving corticosteroids for 2 to 6 weeks develop an elevation of intraocular pressure. In the general population, about 5% of individuals will develop an elevated pressure with prolonged topical corticosteroid use. In retinal detachment populations, the percentages may be higher.[97] Therefore, corticosteroids should be prescribed with caution after retinal detachment surgery.

GLAUCOMA ASSOCIATED WITH RETINAL DISORDERS BECAUSE OF A COMMON UNDERLYING CAUSE OR FOR UNKNOWN REASONS

Primary Open-angle Glaucoma and Rhegmatogenous Retinal Detachment

Primary open-angle glaucoma occurs more commonly in patients with rhegmatogenous retinal detachment than one would expect in the general population. The prevalence of eyes with damage resulting from primary open-angle glaucoma in the general population is somewhat less than 1%.[7,53,64] Open-angle glaucoma was found in 5.8% of 530 retinal detachment patients studied by Becker[11]; Phelps and Burton[81] found primary open-angle glaucoma in 4% and ocular hypertension in 6.5% of 817 retinal detachment patients. Baum and Ruiz[9] found 14% of 451 retinal detachment patients to have intraocular pressures ≥22 mm Hg, but they were not assessed for glaucomatous visual field or disc damage. Others have found reduced outflow facility common in the fellow eyes of patients with unilateral retinal detachment.[11,60] Shammas et al.[97]

*References 22, 29, 34, 47, 62, 69, 70, 74, 76.

found large cup-disc ratios in many of their patients with detached retinas. A large proportion of their patients also developed elevated intraocular pressure after prolonged topical corticosteroid administration. All of these findings suggest that retinal detachment patients are unusually susceptible to open-angle glaucoma.

Why should open-angle glaucoma and retinal detachment be associated? It is unlikely that either of the two disorders causes the other, and each may precede the other. It seems likely that they may be linked by a common underlying predisposing factor.

One possible link is myopia, which occurs frequently in both open-angle glaucoma and retinal detachment patients. However, Phelps and Burton[81] did not find the correlation between the two disorders explainable on this basis.

Another possible link is the miotic treatment of glaucoma. Retinal detachment may develop soon after initiation or increase in strength of miotic therapy.[4,10,63,78] These observations have convinced many clinicians that miotics cause retinal detachment, although no prospective, controlled clinical trial has been undertaken. However, miotics are unlikely to account for more than a small proportion of retinal detachment occurring in patients with open-angle glaucoma. In many patients, glaucoma was unrecognized until the patient presented with the detachment.[11,81] Furthermore, of 30 patients using miotics at the time of detachment, only three had recently begun miotic treatment or had their prescription changed to a higher concentration of miotics.[81] Ciliary muscle spasm may be a factor in miotic-induced detachment.[4]

Whatever the reason for the association of retinal detachment and glaucoma, the concurrence of the two conditions creates special diagnostic and therapeutic problems for the ophthalmologist. The signs of one disease may mask those of the other, and the treatment of one may worsen the other. Diagnosis of a retinal detachment is frequently delayed in a patient who is being treated for glaucoma. The loss of peripheral vision may be mistakenly attributed to the progression of glaucomatous optic nerve damage. Pupillary miosis from treatment of the glaucoma may prevent the ophthalmologist from adequately examining the patient's peripheral retina, and the detachment may be overlooked.

Several simple measures facilitate correct diagnosis. First, of course, one must keep in mind the possibility of the two diseases occurring in the same eye. All patients beginning treatment for glaucoma should have careful peripheral retinal examinations, which should be repeated yearly, as well as when detachment symptoms occur. A sudden change in a patient's peripheral visual field or a sudden drop in intraocular pressure should suggest a detached retina. A retinal tear should be suspected if a glaucoma patient sees flashing lights or new floaters. Floaters beginning after the start of miotic therapy may merely represent enhanced entopic visualization of normal vitreous condensations but sometimes are produced by vitreous hemorrhage from a retinal tear. If permanent miosis or lens opacities prevent adequate fundus examination, ultrasonography may help detect a suspected retinal detachment.

Similarly, the diagnosis of glaucoma in an eye with a detached retina may be difficult. Retinal detachment typically lowers intraocular pressure, even in glaucomatous eyes.[26] The optic disc may be difficult to evaluate if the peripapillary retina is detached or if a bullous detachment overhangs the disc. Glaucomatous cupping is easily missed if the fundus is examined only with an indirect ophthalmoscope, particularly if the examiner is concentrating on the detached retina and not on the disc. Visual fields are difficult to evaluate for glaucomatous damage if the retina is or has previously been detached. It is crucial to assess the intraocular pressure and disc status of the fellow eye, since primary open-angle glaucoma is typically bilateral. Postoperatively, applanation tonometry should be used for the pressure measurements, as retinal detachment surgery often reduces ocular rigidity, which will cause a Schiøtz tonometer to give a falsely low estimate of intraocular pressure.[79,103]

When retinal detachment and glaucoma occur together, the treatment of each condition often must be modified. Because of the possible role of miotics in the pathogenesis of retinal detachment, these drugs should be used with caution in patients who have had retinal detachment or in patients who are susceptible to retinal detachment because of aphakia, lattice degeneration, or a retinal tear. In these patients it is prudent to avoid miotics if possible or to begin with a weak concentration and slowly increase the strength until the desired lowering of pressure has been achieved. Sustained-release miotics (Ocusert or gel) should be considered, as ciliary spasm fluctuates less than with the use of drops.

A patient with retinal detachment and open-angle glaucoma will probably be sensitive to the intraocular pressure-elevating effects of topical corticosteroids, which should be used with caution postoperatively. Patients who have used miotics for many years may have a small and rigid pupil, which prevents adequate visualization of the fundus. Argon laser sphincterotomy of the iris may be used to enlarge the pupil to allow adequate examination.

The presence of glaucoma in an eye with retinal detachment does not adversely affect the chances for a successful reattachment by a scleral buckling operation.[24] It may, however, reduce the visual outcome if the optic nerve has been previously damaged by glaucoma.[26]

In 11 of 12 eyes with preoperative primary open-angle glaucoma, after retinal detachment repair intraocular pressures were controlled without pressure-lowering therapy for 1 to 5.5 years.[43] It was postulated that encircling bands may restrict flow through the long posterior ciliary arteries, reducing blood flow to the ciliary body and aqueous production.

Pigmentary Glaucoma and Retinal Detachment

The pigment dispersion syndrome is described in detail in Chapter 55. Its association with rhegmatogenous retinal detachment warrants mention here.

In 1974 Brachet and Chermet[19] described 19 patients who had both pigmentary glaucoma and retinal detachment. They suggested that the concurrence of the two conditions represented more than simple chance but provided no information about how often either condition occurred with the other. Scheie and Cameron[91] reviewed the case histories of 407 patients with the pigment dispersion syndrome and found 26 (6.4%) who also had retinal detachment. The frequency of detachment was the same whether glaucoma was present (6.0% of 151 patients) or absent (6.6% of 256 patients).

Other studies also suggest that eyes with rhegmatogenous retinal detachment often have pigment dispersion. Sebestyen et al.[95] found marked pigmentation of the angle and glaucoma in 11 of 160 cases of retinal detachment (6.9%). Syrdalen[102] found moderate chamber angle pigmentation in 37 (16.7%) and marked pigmentation in 27 (12.1%) of 223 eyes with retinal detachment. Rodriguez-Gonzales[87] found the pigment dispersion syndrome, with or without glaucoma, in 10% of 1532 eyes with detached retinas.

The association between pigment dispersion and retinal detachment may be secondary to a common degenerative process or, more likely, to the high frequency of myopia in both disorders. It is

unlikely that miotic treatment of pigmentary glaucoma is a primary factor, since the frequency of retinal detachment in the pigment dispersion syndrome appears to be the same whether or not glaucoma is present.

Glaucoma and Retinitis Pigmentosa

An association between glaucoma and retinitis pigmentosa has been described by many investigators during the past century. The reported prevalence of glaucoma in retinitis pigmentosa has ranged from 2% to 12%;[44,58] however, these reports are difficult to evaluate. They rarely define whether the retinitis pigmentosa is hereditary or secondary, and, if inherited, whether the transmission is dominant, recessive, or sex-linked. The type of glaucoma is usually described as primary, but seldom is a distinction made between angle-closure and open-angle mechanisms. In some cases, the glaucoma is described as acute or inflammatory and in others as chronic or simple. Many of the reported case histories and some limited histologic material[44] suggest that the mechanism of glaucoma is often angle-closure.

Little information is available to determine if there is a true association or just a coincidental occurrence. Phelps[82] described three patients whom he treated for both dominantly inherited retinitis pigmentosa and glaucoma. Two had primary angle-closure glaucoma, and the third had congenital glaucoma inherited from the other parent.

Open-angle Glaucoma and Retinal Detachment in Stickler's Syndrome

Stickler's syndrome, an inherited connective tissue disease affecting the eyes, ears, face, and skeleton,[101] remains unfamiliar to many ophthalmologists. However, it is not rare.* In fact, some authorities now think that Stickler's syndrome is the most common of the systemic connective tissue disorders, at least in the North American Midwest.[57] The syndrome is inherited by autosomal dominant transmission.

The more frequent ocular manifestations are high myopia, early cataract, vitreoretinal degeneration, and retinal detachment.[13,51] Strabismus, amblyopia, and glaucoma are found in some patients. The myopia is usually severe, ranging from 8 to 18 or more diopters, and begins in the first decade of life. The vitreous space in the eyes of patients with Stickler's syndrome is optically

---

*References 13, 48, 52, 84, 93, 105.

empty or is crossed only by sparse strands. Pigment accumulates in clumps in the peripheral retina, avascular preretinal membranes are found in the equatorial region, and the retinal vessels have segmental sheathing. Eventually, more than half of the patients with Stickler's syndrome develop a retinal detachment in one or both eyes. Surgical repair may be difficult.

The systemic abnormalities in Stickler's syndrome include orofacial anomalies, skeletal malformations, and neurosensory hearing loss. The orofacial anomaly commonly consists of mandibular hypoplasia, glossoptosis, and palatal defects. These features comprise the well-known Pierre Robin anomaly, which in most cases is probably part of Stickler's syndrome.[52] However, the orofacial anomalies in Stickler's syndrome vary widely in severity, and in some patients the only abnormality may be a bifid uvula, a submucous cleft, or an abnormality in motility of the palate. Skeletal manifestations include hyperextensible fingers, wrists, and knees. Patients often appear marfanoid. Radiographs reveal spondyloepiphysial dysplasia. Degenerative arthropathy may develop and become debilitating.

The ocular manifestations of Stickler's syndrome are easily confused with those of Wagner's disease. In 1938 Wagner[107] described vitreoretinal degeneration and presenile cataracts in a large family with four affected generations. Two other investigators later reexamined members of the same family.[17,85] Although the vitreoretinal degeneration in the family Wagner studied was very similar in appearance to that occurring in Stickler's syndrome; in other respects the two conditions have differed. The myopia in the families Wagner studied was always less than 4 diopters until a cataract developed, and no patient developed retinal detachment. No systemic abnormalities were described in the family members. Although subsequent reports have described patients unrelated to the original family who were thought to have the same syndrome, these patients usually had retinal detachment, and it seems in retrospect that many of them, if not all, had Stickler's syndrome instead.

The glaucoma in Stickler's syndrome has not been well described. Phelps[82] noted that several of his patients with Stickler's syndrome had mild to moderate elevation of intraocular pressure. The anterior chamber angles were open without obvious structural malformation. Some had glaucomatous optic nerve damage. This is not always easily determined because lens opacities and high myopia impair the ophthalmoscopic view of the optic disc.

Furthermore, the discs are often tilted, and cupping when present is shallow. Retinal degeneration may cause visual field defects similar to those of glaucoma, and intraocular pressure, measured by applanation tonometry, may be the only reliable criterion on which to base treatment.

Fortunately, the high intraocular pressure in Stickler's syndrome usually responds well to pressure-lowering medications. It is important to avoid the use of miotics whenever possible. Not only do miotics reduce visual acuity if the eye has an axial lens opacity, but they have the potential to induce retinal detachment in these highly susceptible patients.

REFERENCES

1. Aaberg, TM, and Maggiano, JM: Choroidal edema associated with retinal detachment repair: experimental and clinical correlations, Mod Probl Ophthalmol 20:6, 1979
2. Aaberg, TM, and Van Horn, DL: Late complications of pars plana vitreous surgery, Ophthalmology 85:126, 1978
3. Abrams, GW, Swanson, DE, and Sabates, WI: The results of sulfur hexafluoride gas in vitreous surgery, Am J Ophthalmol 94:165, 1982
4. Alpar, JJ: Miotics and retinal detachment, Ann Ophthalmol 11:395, 1979
5. Ando, F: Intraocular hypertension resulting from pupillary block by silicone oil (correspondence), Am J Ophthalmol 99:87, 1985
6. Aronowitz, JD, and Brubaker, RF: Effect of intraocular gas on intraocular pressure, Arch Ophthalmol 94:1191, 1976
7. Bankes, JL, Perkins ES, Tsolakis, S, and Wright, JE: Bedford glaucoma survey, Br Med J 1:791, 1968
8. Baruch, E, Bracha, R, Godel, V, and Lazar, M: Glaucoma due to rhegmatogenous retinal detachment: Schwartz's syndrome, Glaucoma 3:229, 1981
9. Baum, A, and Ruiz, RS: Intraocular hypertension in retinal detachment, Tex Med 68:104, 1972
10. Beasley, H, and Fraunfelder, FT: Retinal detachments and topical ocular miotics, Ophthalmology 86:95, 1979
11. Becker, B: Discussion of Smith, JL: Retinal detachment and glaucoma, Trans Am Acad Ophthalmol Otolaryngol 67:731, 1963
12. Berler, DK, and Goldstein, B: Scleral buckles and rotation of the ciliary body, Arch Ophthalmol 97:1518, 1979
13. Blair, NP, Albert, DM, Liberfarb, RM, and Hirose, T: Hereditary progressive arthro-ophthalmology of Stickler, Am J Ophthalmol 88:876, 1979
14. Blondeau, P, Pavan, PR, and Phelps, CD: Acute pressure elevation following panretinal photocoagulation, Arch Ophthalmol 99:1239, 1981

15. Bloome, MA: Transient angle-closure glaucoma in central retinal vein occlusion, Ann Ophthalmol 9:44, 1977

16. Blumenkranz, M, Gardner, T, and Blankenship, G: Fluid-gas exchange and photocoagulation after vitrectomy: indications, technique, and results, Arch Ophthalmol 104:291, 1986

17. Bohringer, HR, Dieterle, P, and Landolt, E: Zur Klinik und Pathologie der Degeneration hyaloideoretinalis hereditaria (Wagner), Ophthalmologica 139:330, 1960

18. Boulton, PE: A study of the mechanism of transient myopia following extensive xenon arc photocoagulation, Trans Ophthalmol Soc UK 93:287, 1973

19. Brachet, A, and Chermet, M: Association glaucome pigmentaire et décollement de rétine, Ann Ocul 207:451, 1974

20. Brockhurst, RJ: Nanophthalmos with uveal effusion, Arch Ophthalmol 93:1289, 1975

21. Brockhurst, RJ: Vortex vein decompression for nanophthalmic uveal effusion, Arch Ophthalmol 98:1987, 1980

22. Burke, LL, Shields, MB, Proia, AD, and McCuen, B: Intraocular pressure following intravitreal silicone oil injection, Invest Ophthalmol Vis Sci Suppl 26:159, 1985

23. Burton, TC: Preoperative factors influencing anatomic success rates following retinal detachment surgery, Trans Am Acad Ophthalmol Otolaryngol 83:499, 1977

24. Burton, TC, Arafat, NT, and Phelps, CD: Intraocular pressure in retinal detachment, Int Ophthalmol 1:147, 1979

25. Burton, TC, and Folk, JC: Laser iris retraction for angle closure glaucoma following retinal detachment surgery, Paper presented at the annual meeting of the American Academy of Ophthalmology, Dallas, Nov 10, 1987

26. Burton, TC, and Lambert, RW, Jr: A predictive model for visual recovery following retinal detachment surgery, Ophthalmology 85:619, 1978

27. Calhoun FP, Jr: The management of glaucoma in nanophthalmos, Trans Am Ophthalmol Soc 73:97, 1976

28. Campbell, DG: Iris retraction associated with rhegmatogenous retinal detachment syndrome and hypotony: a new explanation, Arch Ophthalmol 102:1457, 1984

29. Chan, C, and Okun, E: The question of ocular tolerance to intravitreal liquid silicone, Ophthalmology 93:651, 1986

30. Chandler, PA, and Grant, WM: Glaucoma, Philadelphia, Lea & Febiger, 1979

31. Chang, S, et al: Perfluorocarbon gases in vitreous surgery, Ophthalmology 92:651, 1985

32. Crittenden, JJ, deJuan, E, Jr, and Tiedman, J: Expansion of long-lasting gas bubbles for intraocular use: principles and practice, Arth Ophthalmol 103:831, 1985

33. Davidorf, FH: Retinal pigment epithelial glaucoma, Ophthalmol Dig. 38:11, 1976

34. deCorral, LR, Cohen, SB, and Peyman, GA: Effect of intravitreal silicone oil on intraocular pressure, Ophthalmic Surg 18:446, 1987

35. Diddie, KR, and Ernest, JT: Uveal blood flow after 360° constriction in the rabbit, Arch Ophthalmol 98:729, 1980

36. Dobbie, JG: A study of the intraocular fluid dynamics in retinal detachment, Arch Ophthalmol 69:159, 1963

37. Doft, BH, and Blankenship, GW: Single versus multiple treatment sessions of argon laser panretinal photocoagulation for proliferative diabetic retinopathy, Ophthalmology 89:772, 1982

38. Duke-Elder, S, editor: Anomolies in the size of the eye. In System of Ophthalmology, vol 3, pt 2, St Louis, 1964, The CV Mosby Co

39. Faulborn, J, Conway, BP, and Machemer, R: Surgical complications of pars plana vitreous surgery, Ophthalmology 85:116, 1978

40. Fineberg, E, et al: Sulfur hexafluoride in owl monkey vitreous cavity, Am J Ophthalmol 79:67, 1975

41. Fiore, JV, and Newton, JC: Anterior segment changes following the scleral buckling operation, Arch Ophthalmol 84:284, 1970

42. Fraunfelder, F, and Viernstein, LJ: Intraocular pressure variation during xenon and ruby laser photocoagulation, Am J Ophthalmol 71:1261, 1971

43. Friedman, Z, and Neumann, E: Effect of retinal detachment surgery on the course of preexisting open-angle glaucoma, Am J Ophthalmol 80:702, 1975

44. Gartner, S, and Schlossman, A: Retinitis pigmentosa associated with glaucoma, Am J Ophthalmol 32:1337, 1949

45. Ghartey, KN, et al: Closed vitreous surgery. XVII. Results and complications of pars plana vitreous surgery, Arch Ophthalmol 98:1248, 1980

46. Grant, WM: Shallowing of the anterior chamber following occlusion of the central retinal vein, Am J Ophthalmol 75:384, 1973

47. Grey, RHB, and Leaver, PK: Results of silicone oil injection in massive preretinal retraction, Trans Ophthalmol Soc UK 97:238, 1977

48. Hall, JG, and Herrod, H: The Stickler syndrome presenting as a dominantly inherited cleft palate and blindness, J Med Genet 12:397, 1975

49. Han, DP, Lewis, H, and Williams, GA: Management of complete iridocorneal apposition after vitrectomy, Am J Ophthalmol 103:108, 1987

50. Hartley, RE, and Marsh, RJ: Anterior chamber depth changes after retinal detachment, Br J Ophthalmol 57:546, 1973

51. Hayreh, SS, and Baines, JA: Occlusion of the vortex veins: an experimental study, Br J Ophthalmol 57:217, 1973

52. Herrmann, J, et al: The Stickler syndrome (hereditary arthro-ophthalmopathy), Birth Defects 11:76, 1975

53. Hollows, FC, and Graham, PA: Intraocular pressure, glaucoma, and glaucoma suspects in a defined population, Br J Ophthalmol 50:570, 1966

54. Huamonte, FU, et al: Immediate fundus complications after retinal scatter photocoagulation. I. Clinical picture and pathogenesis, Ophthalmic Surg 7:88, 1976

55. Hyams, SW, and Neumann, E: Transient angle-closure glaucoma after retinal vein occlusion, Br J Ophthalmol 56:353, 1972

56. Killey, FP, and Edelhauser, HF, and Aaberg, TM: Intraocular sulfur hexafluoride and octofluorocyclobutane: effect on intraocular pressure and vitreous volume, Arch Ophthalmol 96:511, 1978

57. Kimbrough, RL, Trempe, CS, Brockhurst, RJ, and Simmons, RJ: Angle-closure in nanophthalmos, Am J Ophthalmol 88:572, 1979

58. Kogbe, OI, and Follmann, P: Investigations into aqueous humor dynamics in primary pigmentary degeneration of the retina, Ophthalmologica 171:165, 1975

59. Kreiger, AE, Hodgkinson, BJ, Frederick, AR, and Smith, TR: The results of retinal detachment surgery: analysis of 268 operations with a broad scleral buckle, Arch Ophthalmol 86:385, 1971

60. Langham, ME, and Regan, CDJ: Circulatory changes associated with onset of retinal detachment, Arch Ophthalmol 81:820, 1969

61. Laroche, L, Pavlakis, C, Saraux, H, and Orcel, L: Ocular findings following intravitreal silicone injection, Arch Ophthalmol 101:1422, 1983

62. Leaver, PK, Grey, RHB, and Garner, A: Silicone oil injection in the treatment of massive preretinal retraction. II. Late complications in 93 eyes, Br J Ophthalmol 63:361, 1979

63. Lemcke, HH, and Pischel, DK: Retinal detachments after the use of phospholine iodide, Trans Pac Coast Oto-ophthalmol Soc 47:157, 1966

64. Leske, MC, and Rosenthal, J: Epidemiologic aspects of open-angle glaucoma, Am J Epidemiol 109:250, 1979

65. Liang, JC, Huamonte, FU: Reduction of immediate complications after panretinal photocoagulation, Retina 4:166, 1984

66. Linnér, E: Intra-ocular pressure in retinal detachment, Acta Ophthalmol Suppl 84:101, 1966

67. MacKay, CJ, et al: Retinal degeneration with nanophthalmos, cystic macular degeneration, and angle closure glaucoma, Arch Ophthalmol 105:366, 1987

68. Matsuo, N, et al: Photoreceptor outer segments in the aqueous humor in rhegmatogenous retinal detachment, Am J Ophthalmol 101:673, 1986

69. McCuen, BW, Landers, MB, and Machemer, R: The use of silicone oil following failed vitrectomy for retinal detachment with advanced proliferative vitreoretinopathy, Ophthalmology 92:1029, 1985

70. McCuen, BW, deJuan, E, Jr, Landers, MB, and Machemer, R: Silicone oil in vitreoretinal surgery, part 2: results and complications, Retina 5:198, 1985

71. McNair, J, et al: Acute pressure changes and possible secondary tissue changes due to laser or xenon photocoagulation, Am J Ophthalmol 77:13, 1974

72. Mendelsohn, AD, Jampol, LM, and Shoch, D: Secondary angle-closure glaucoma after central retinal vein occlusion, Am J Ophthalmol 100:581, 1985

73. Mensher, JH: Anterior chamber depth alteration after retinal photocoagulation, Arch Ophthalmol 95:113, 1977

74. Ni, C, Wang, WJ, Albert, DM, and Schepens, CL: Intravitreous silicone injection. Histopathologic findings in a human eye after 12 years, Arch Ophthalmol 101:1399, 1983

75. Norton, EWD: Twenty-ninth Edward Jackson Memorial Lecture: intraocular gas in the management of selected retinal detachments, Trans Am Acad Ophthalmol Otolaryngol 77:85, 1973

76. Okun, E: Intravitreal surgery utilizing liquid silicone: a long term follow-up, Trans Pac Coast Oto-ophthalmol Soc 49:141, 1968

77. Palestine, AG, et al: Ophthalmic involvement in acquired immunodeficiency syndrome, Ophthalmology 91:1092, 1984

78. Pape, LG, and Forbes, M: Retinal detachment and miotic therapy, Am J Ophthalmol 85:558, 1978

79. Pemberton, JW: Schiøtz-applanation disparity following retinal detachment surgery, Arch Ophthalmol 81:534, 1969

80. Perez, RN, Phelps, CD, and Burton, TC: Angle-closure glaucoma following scleral buckling operations, Trans Am Acad Ophthalmol Otolaryngol 81:247, 1976

81. Phelps, CD, and Burton, TC: Glaucoma and retinal detachment, Arch Ophthalmol 95:418, 1977

82. Phelps, CD: Glaucoma associated with retinal disorders. In Ritch, R, and Shields, MB, editors: The secondary glaucomas, St Louis, 1982, The CV Mosby Co

83. Poliner, LS, and Schoch, LH: Intraocular pressure assessment in gas-filled eyes following vitrectomy, Arch Ophthalmol 105:200, 1987

84. Popkin, JS, and Polomeno, RC: Stickler's syndrome (hereditary progressive arthro-ophthalmopathy), Can Med Assoc J 111:1071, 1974

85. Ricci, A: Dégénéresence hyaloideo-rétienne de Wagner, Bull Soc Ophthalmol Fr 9:646, 1961

86. Ritch, R, York, K, and Szmyd, L: Argon laser peripheral iridoplasty, Invest Ophthalmol Vis Sci Suppl 24:94, 1984

87. Rodriguez-Gonzales, A: Personal communication of unpublished data presented at the Pan American Congress of Ophthalmology, Santiago, Chile, 1977, Cited in Phelps, CD: Glaucoma associated with retinal disorders. In Ritch, R, and Shields, MB, editors: The secondary glaucomas, St Louis, 1982, The CV Mosby Co

88. Rosengren, B: Cases of retinal detachment treated with diathermy and injection of air into the vitreous body, Acta Ophthalmol 16:177, 1938

89. Ryan, EA, Zwann, J, and Chylack, LT: Nanophthalmos with uveal effusion, Ophthalmology 89:1013, 1982

90. Sabates, WI, Abrams, GW, Swanson, DE, and Norton, EWD: The use of intraocular gases: the results of sulfur hexafluoride gas in retinal detachment surgery, Ophthalmology 88:447, 1981

91. Scheie, HG, and Cameron, JD: Personal communication, 1980, Cited in Phelps, CD: Glaucoma associated with retinal disorders. In Ritch, R, and Shields, MB, editors: The secondary glaucomas, St Louis, 1982, The CV Mosby Co

92. Schiodte, SN, Changes in eye tension after panretinal xenon arc and argon laser photocoagulation in normotensive diabetic eyes, Acta Ophthalmol 60:692, 1982

93. Schreiner, RL, McAlister, WH, Marshall, RE, and Shearer, WT: Stickler syndrome in a pedigree of Pierre Robin syndrome, Am J Dis Child 126:86, 1973

94. Schwartz, A: Chronic open-angle glaucoma secondary to rhegmatogenous retinal detachment, Am J Ophthalmol 75:205, 1973

95. Sebestyen, JG, Schepens, CL, and Rosenthal, ML: Retinal detachment and glaucoma. I. Tonometric and gonioscopic study of 160 cases, Arch Ophthalmol 67:736, 1962

96. Shaffer, RN: Discussion of Calhoun, FP, Jr: The management of glaucoma in nanophthalmos, Trans Am Ophthalmol Soc 73:97, 1976

97. Shammas, HF, Halassa, AH, and Faris, BH: Variations in intraocular pressure, cup:disc ratio, and steroid responsiveness in the retinal detachment population, Arch Ophthalmol 94:1108, 1976

98. Shimizu, K, and Ujiie, K: Structure of ocular vessels, New York, 1978, Igaku-Shoin

99. Singh, OS, Simmons, RJ, Brockhurst, RJ, and Trempe, CL: Nanophthalmos: a perspective on identification and therapy, Ophthalmology 89:1006, 1982

100. Smith, TR: Acute glaucoma after scleral buckling procedures, Am J Ophthalmol 63:1807, 1967

101. Stickler, GB, et al: Hereditary progressive arthroophthalmopathy, Mayo Clin Proc 40:433, 1966

102. Syrdalen, P: Trauma and retinal detachment: the anterior chamber angle, with special reference to width, pigmentation, and traumatic ruptures, Acta Ophthalmol 48:1006, 1970

103. Syrdalen, P: Intraocular pressures and ocular rigidity in patients with retinal detachment. II. Postoperative study, Acta Ophthalmol 48:1036, 1970

104. Trelstad, RL, Silbermann, NN, and Brockhurst, RJ: Nanophthalmic sclera: ultrastructural, histochemical, and biochemical observations, Arch Ophthalmol 100:1935, 1982

105. Turner, G: The Stickler syndrome in a family with Pierre Robin syndrome and severe myopia, Aust Paediatr J 10:103, 1974

106. Ullman, S, Wilson, RP, and Schwartz, L: Bilateral angle-closure glaucoma in association with the acquired immune deficiency syndrome, Am J Ophthalmol 101:419, 1986

107. Wagner, H: Ein bisher unbekanntes Erbleiden des Auges (Degeneratio hyaloideo-retinitis hereditaria) beobachtet in Kanton Zurich, Klin Monatsbl Augenheilkd 100:840, 1938

108. Watzke, RC: Silicone retinopiesis for retinal detachment: a long-term clinical evaluation, Arch Ophthalmol 77:185, 1967

109. Weber, PA, Cohen, JS, and Baker, ND: Central retinal vein occlusion and malignant glaucoma, Arch Ophthalmol 105:635, 1987

110. Yue, BYJT, et al: Nanophthalmic sclera, Ophthalmology 93:534, 1986

Chapter 60

Neovascular Glaucoma

Martin Wand

HISTORY AND TERMINOLOGY

Until relatively recent times, our knowledge of neovascular glaucoma was rather vague and simplistic. In the absence of any concept of the anatomic changes or the pathophysiology of this disorder, all eyes with elevated pressures and intraocular bleeding were labeled hemorrhagic glaucoma, the term first employed by Pagenstecher in 1871.[266] Subsequently, a confusing array of terms appeared in the literature to identify vastly different disorders with common superfical similarities. Historically, the terms *hemorrhagic glaucoma, thrombotic glaucoma, congestive glaucoma, rubeotic glaucoma,* and *diabetic hemorrhagic glaucoma* all referred to neovascular glaucoma as we now understand it.

Despite scattered earlier clinical reports of new vessels on the irides of eyes with neovascular glaucoma, it was not until the turn of the century that our knowledge of neovascular glaucoma was put on a sound anatomic basis. In 1906, Coats[73] described the histologic finding of new vessels on the irides of eyes with central retinal vein occlusion (CRVO). In 1928, Salus[299] described similar new vessels on the irides of eyes of diabetic patients. After the introduction of clinical gonioscopy in the early 1900's, Kurz[205] correlated his clinical observation of fine, new vessels in the angle with the histologic finding of connective tissue along these vessels. He felt that the contraction of this connective tissue along these new vessels was the cause of synechial angle closure. Because the glaucoma is caused by the new vessels rather than the inconsistently present intraocular bleeding, Weiss and Shaffer[364] proposed the term *neovascular glau-*

coma. This term has since found universal acceptance, although older terms are still occasionally seen in the literature. The term *neovascularization of the iris* would also be more accurate and appropriate than *rubeosis iridis,*[353] but, unfortunately, this term has not found wide acceptance.

Our ability to treat neovascular glaucoma lagged behind our knowledge of its pathophysiology. As late as 1969, Duke Elder said that "the only practical treatment of [neovascular glaucoma] is enucleation."[88] Grant lamented that "no means are known for preventing neovascular glaucoma."[133] However, over the past decade, dramatic strides have been made in our understanding of and ability to treat neovascular glaucoma. We are now on the threshold of elucidating the basic mechanisms of angiogenesis and perhaps being able finally to treat this disorder in a rational manner.

CLINICAL PICTURE

It would be difficult to miss the full-blown picture of neovascular glaucoma (Fig. 60-1). The eye is painful and photophobic. The vision is usually at the counting fingers to hand motion level, and the intraocular pressure may be as high as 60 mm Hg or greater. There is moderate to marked conjunctival congestion frequently associated with a steamy cornea. The new vessels on the iris and the ectropion uveae are visible even through a cloudy cornea. Variable degrees of synechial angle closure are present. The key, however, is to make the diagnosis not at this stage, but to detect it at its earliest stages, so that appropriate preventive measures can be taken.

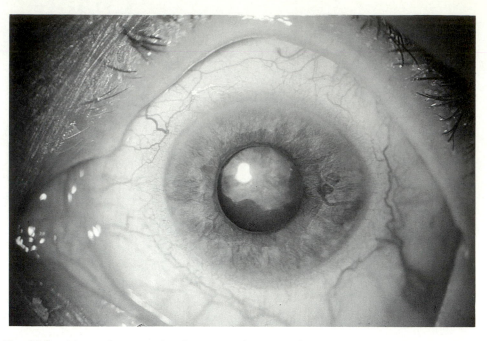

Fig. 60-1 Advanced neovascular glaucoma with congested conjunctival vessels, cloudy cornea, rubeosis iridis, and ectropion uveae.

The first visible signs of incipient neovascular glaucoma are tiny tufts of new vessels at the pupillary margin (Figs. 60-2, *I*, and 60-3 and Plate III, Fig. 7). Histologically, this appears first as aneurysm formation at the bend of a preexisting capillary. These enlarge to become clinically visible knuckles of fine vessels, appearing similar to a glomerulus. Unless one maintains a high index of suspicion and looks carefully under high magnification at the slit-lamp, it is very easy to overlook these vessels and miss the potential opportunity to save the patient's eye. In darkly pigmented irides, it is especially difficult to detect early peripupillary neovascularization. If a contact gonioscopy lens is used at the initial examination, even light pressure on the lens is sufficient to collapse these neovascular tufts and render them clinically invisible.[358] We have not seen rubeosis elsewhere on the iris, or, more significantly, in the angle, without seeing peripupillary rubeosis as well.

It is interesting to note that in 1961 Smith,[322] in discussing various theories of the pathogenesis of neovascularization, said

> With regard to the . . . theory (the transference of a new-vessel-stimulating substance from the retina by the aqueous humour); I wonder if the invariable sites of the earliest new vessels, namely on the extreme margin of the pupil and on the trabecular meshwork, might validly be considered to be due to these sites

being the position of maximum turnover of contact with aqueous humour containing only a very low concentration of the hypothetical substance. I would be particularly interested to hear if any member had a case of rubeosis developing after a peripheral iridectomy. It would be of great significance if the early rubeosis were to develop at the new "pupillary margin" of the iridectomy.

We have observed one such case, namely an elderly man with long-standing diabetes mellitus who had previously had surgical peripheral iridectomies for narrow angles.[358] He was observed to have new vessels around the peripheral iridectomy before any new vessels could be detected at the pupillary margin. In addition, we have recently seen a 15-year-old boy who was struck in his left eye and sustained a peripheral retinal detachment, traumatic cataract, angle recession, and severe iritis. There was a total posterior synechia of the pupil to the lens except for two clock hours, and rubeosis iridis was noted only around this passageway for the aqueous (Fig. 60-4). After a filtration procedure, the posterior synechia became complete, the pupillary rubeosis disappeared, and new vessels appeared at the site of the peripheral iridectomy. Both these cases support the concept of aqueous carrying some angiogenesis factor that stimulates new vessel formation at its primary point of contact with a receptive vascular bed.

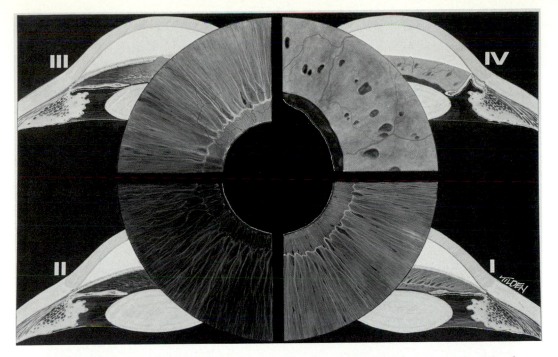

Fig. 60-2   The phases and mechanisms of neovascular glaucoma. I, Early rubeosis iridis. Dilated capillary tufts are present only at pupillary margin; angle is not involved. II, Moderate rubeosis iridis. New vessels extend radially toward angle, sometimes joining a dilated vessel at collarette; angle is still not involved. III, Advanced rubeosis iridis with angle neovascularization. New vessels reach angle and join circumferential ciliary body artery; new vessels emanate from this artery and cross over scleral spur onto trabecular meshwork, where arborization occurs. One area of synechial closure is shown. Pressure can increase at this stage. IV, More advanced neovascular glaucoma. Angle is completely closed; iris is pulled up over whole trabecular meshwork and hides all angle structures posterior to Schwalbe's line; pupil shows ectropion and distortion. A "burned-out" stage can occur later; then there may appear to be little rubeosis iridis, and only an occasional vessel may be seen approaching a completely closed angle. (From Wand, M, Dueker, DK, Aiello, LM, and Grant, WM: Am J Ophthalmol 86:332, 1978. Published with permission from the American Journal of Ophthalmology. Copyright by the Ophthalmic Publishing Co) See also Plate III, Fig. 7.

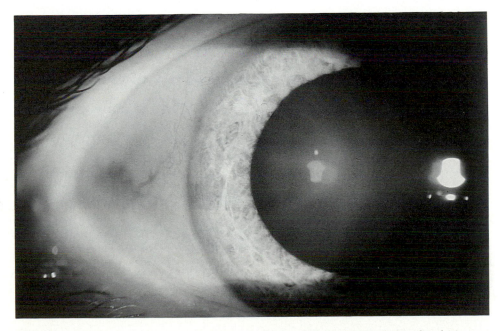

Fig. 60-3   Early rubeosis iridis in patient with diabetes mellitus. Despite light-colored iris, new vascular tufts are barely visible at 8:30 o'clock. See Fig. 60-9 for iris fluorescein angiogram of same eye.

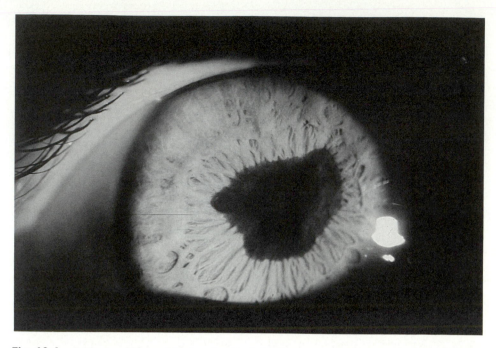

Fig. 60-4 A 15-year-old boy with chronic retinal detachment, traumatic cataract, angle recession, and extensive posterior synechiae. From 9 to 11 o'clock, there are no posterior synechiae and rubeosis iridis is present only in this region.

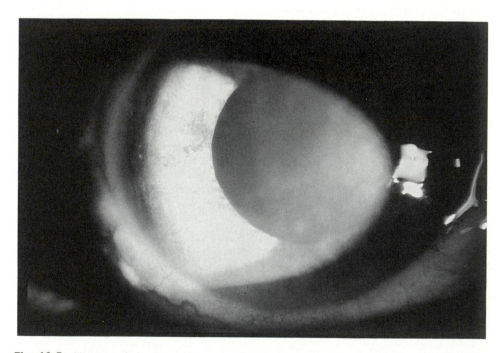

Fig. 60-5 New vessels on iris surface extending from pupillary margin in irregular meandering pattern.

As iris neovascularization progresses, new vessels extend from the pupillary tufts in an irregular, meandering manner (Figs. 60-2, *II*, and 60-5 and Plate III, Fig. 7). New vessels, at least clinically, characteristically appear on the surface of the iris. In elderly people with atrophic irides and those with light irides, normal iris vessels are sometimes visible, but, if one looks carefully, these vessels are really within the stroma of the iris and have a more radial orientation. Occasionally, with inflammation and secondary engorgement, it may be difficult if not impossible to tell if iris vessels are abnormal or not. When new vessels reach the iris collarette, the collarette vessel, which is often normally present but not visible, may become engorged and part of the rubeotic vasculature. At this stage, and more commonly at more advanced stages, it is possible to see effacement of the normal iris surface architecture, resulting in a relatively smooth iris. When these new vessels reach the angle, they cross the ciliary body band and scleral spur onto the trabecular meshwork. (Figs. 60-2, *III*, and 60-6 and Plate III, Fig. 7). Chandler and Grant[66] have long taught that if a blood vessel crosses over the scleral spur onto the trabecular meshwork, it is an abnormal vessel; all normal vessels remain behind the scleral spur.[66] This axiom has withstood the test of time. Occasionally, new vessels seem to arise from the major arterial circle of the iris, and cross onto the trabecular meshwork.

At the angle, the larger vessels, after crossing the scleral spur, will arborize with very fine capillaries over several clock hours of the trabecular meshwork, analogous to a tree trunk with branches overhead. Again, a high index of suspicion and careful examination are necessary to see these early fine angle vessels. The higher magnification and higher light intensity offered by the slit-lamp with the Goldmann goniolens, compared to the Koeppe lens with the Barkan light, generally facilitates this part of the examination. Until new vessels in the angle cover a significant portion of the trabecular meshwork, the intraocular pressure may be completely normal. A fibrovascular membrane, which is invisible on gonioscopy, accompanies these new angle vessels and may block enough of the trabecular meshwork to cause a secondary form of open-angle glaucoma at this time. This fibrovascular membrane along these new angle vessels has a tendency to contract and pull the vessels taut, bridging the angle initially, and then tenting the iris toward the trabecular meshwork (Figs. 60-2, *III*, and 60-7 and Plate III, Fig. 7). As these peripheral anterior synechiae coalesce, synechial angle-

closure occurs. The radial traction along the surface of the iris pulls the posterior pigment layer of the iris around the pupillary margin onto the anterior iris surface, commonly, though inaccurately, known as ectropion uveae. As a corollary, when one sees ectropion uveae in neovascular glaucoma, one can presume that there is synechial angle-closure in the same meridian.

As the scattered areas of synechial closure coalesce, there is total angle-closure. The picture of a very smooth, zippered-up, line of iridocorneal adhesion is almost pathognomonic (Figs. 60-2, *IV*, and 60-8 and Plate III, Fig. 7). After this end stage of neovascular glaucoma is reached, there can be a remarkable decrease in the number of new vessels visible in the angle and on the iris. When a prominent pigmented Schwalbe's line is present, a totally closed angle in neovascular glaucoma can been mistaken by even an experienced gonioscopist as a normal "open" angle.

Attempts have been made to classify and quantitate iris neovascularization.[210,343,364] Such a grading system could be valuable in clinical staging, after progression, in comparing patients, and in evaluating efficacy of therapy. Unfortunately, such a classification has not found wide acceptance.

Having presented this orderly picture of progressive neovascularization, it goes without saying

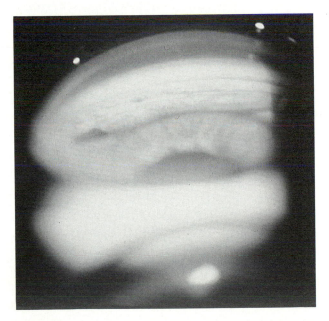

Fig. 60-6 Early neovascularization of angle of a patient who has diabetes mellitus and anterior chamber intraocular lens implant. Rubeosis of pupillary margin and engorgement of major arterial circle of iris are present. Laterally, several new vessels have crossed over scleral spur onto trabecular meshwork.

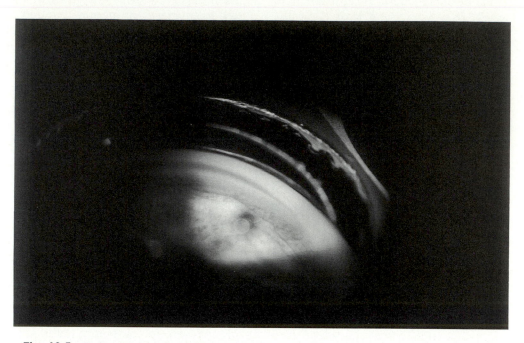

Fig. 60-7 Early synechial angle closure. Note large vessel extending from iris over scleral spur onto trabecular meshwork with tenting of iris toward angle.

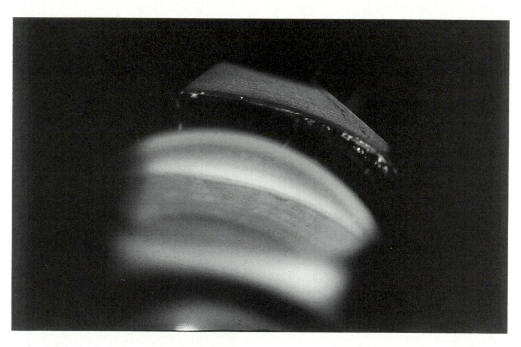

Fig. 60-8 Late neovascular glaucoma with almost total synechial angle closure; only part of rubeotic anterior trabecular meshwork remains visible centrally.

that great variability in the clinical picture and rate of progression is the rule rather than the exception. Usually, the vision is extremely poor because of the edematous cornea and the primary disorder underlying the neovascular glaucoma. Sometimes, the visual acuity can be remarkably good, 20/40 or even better, if the corneal endothelium is healthy and the primary disorder does not significantly involve the macula. The intraocular pressure is usually high, but in some causes of neovascular glaucoma, such as carotid obstructive disease, the intraocular pressure may be normal or even subnormal. If the patient is young and the endothelium is healthy, the cornea may remain clear with intraocular pressures as high as 60 mm Hg. The time sequence is also quite variable.

Rubeosis iridis may progress to total synechial angle-closure within days or it may remain stationary with no angle involvement for years. This quiescent stage may also suddenly become active after years of inactivity. Although the clinical picture of neovascular glaucoma from different primary causes is not distinguishable, and each case of neovascular glaucoma shows its individual pattern of progression, neovascularization from central retinal vein occlusion (CRVO), as a group, seems to be more fulminant in appearance and rapid in course than that from other causes. This clinical impression has been confirmed anatomically by Jocson,[175] who injected liquid rubber into the vasculature of eye bank eyes with neovascular glaucoma and found that the new iris vessels that developed after CRVO were larger, coarser, and more irregular than the new iris vessels that developed from diabetic retinopathy. There does seem to be some correlation between how "angry" these new vessels look and how quickly the neovascularization progresses.

Most important, there may be complete arrest or even total regression of the rubeosis iridis at any stage.[123,226] Parenthetically, any synechial angle closure is, of course, permanent. This unpredictable course of neovascular glaucoma makes the evaluation of various treatment modalities difficult. As a result, only studies with large numbers of patients with proper controls can provide reliable results.

DIFFERENTIAL DIAGNOSIS

As already stressed, the key aim in the treatment of neovascular glaucoma is early diagnosis, so that the currently optimal effective treatment regimen can be instituted. In the differential diagnosis, there are two stages to consider: the early stage, in which only rubeosis iridis is present, and the late stage, in which there is elevated intraocular pressure, a cloudy cornea, and vascular congestion. In both stages, a complete patient history and careful examination of both eyes will usually provide the answer. For true neovascular glaucoma, the history is critical. Diabetes mellitus in the patient or family; history of previous loss of vision, suggesting old CRVO or retinal detachment; or history of hypertension or arteriosclerosis, suggesting possible carotid disease, are all significant. Even a misleadingly benign appearing posterior segment should not deter one from considering one of these major causes of rubeosis iridis.

There are several entities to consider in the differential diagnosis of prominent iris vessels. Rubeosis iridis may be present in Fuchs' heterochromic cyclitis. The eye is usually white and quiet. The iris vessels tend to be extremely fine, thinwalled, and fragile. Spontaneous hyphemas may occur but do so more often with manipulation of the eye, as during gonioscopic examination or after paracentesis. These vessels may cross over the scleral spur onto the trabecular meshwork, but they only rarely cause synechial angle-closure or neovascular glaucoma. Secondary glaucoma may occur but is probably on the basis of the trabeculitis.[273] Histologic studies show localized thickening of the iris vessel walls caused by hyalinization and proliferation of the endothelium, resulting in decreased lumen size and vascular profusion.[121] Recent fluorescein studies have shown leakage from the iris vessels, narrowed radial iris vessels, and ischemic iris sectors, confirming localized areas of iris hypoxia as the cause of the rubeosis iridis.[297]

Rubeosis iridis may also be present in pseudoexfoliation syndrome. Electron microscopic studies have shown endothelial thickening with decreased lumen size and fenestration of vessel walls,[289] accounting for the fluorescein leakage seen in the irides of some eyes.[348] True neovascular glaucoma has not been reported. In all likelihood, the rubeosis iridis occasionally seen after retinal detachment or strabismus surgery is a result of trauma to the anterior ciliary vessels with resultant localized anterior segment hypoxia.[297]

Finally, inflammatory conditions can cause prominent iris vessels, which sometimes are impossible to differentiate clinically from progressive rubeosis iridis. This is especially true in diabetes mellitus after cataract extraction, where a profound iritis and secondary vascular engorgement can simulate fulminant neovascular glaucoma. In view of our current understanding of the pathogenesis of neovascularization and the role of prostaglandins in this process, it is not surprising that inflammation could cause engorgement and dilation of iris vessels, especially in eyes that already have some compromised retinal circulation. In any case, with topical steroid therapy, pseudorubeosis iridis will resolve, but rubeosis iridis will persist.

In the late stages of elevated intraocular pressure with a cloudy cornea, there is another list of differential diagnoses. Although the underlying cause of true neovascular glaucoma is usually of long duration, such as diabetic retinopathy or central retinal vein occlusion, the presenting signs and symptoms are often precipitous. It is not unusual for a patient to present for the first time with an inflamed eye and intraocular pressures 60 mm Hg or higher. Acute angle-closure must be considered high on the differential list. Gonioscopy may be impossible, even with the use of systemic hyperosmotics and topical glycerin. However, it is almost always possible to see the engorged iris vessels through the hazy cornea. More important, gonioscopy of the fellow eye will provide the clue because narrow angles and angle-closure glaucoma tend to be a bilateral disorder. Many surgical or laser iridectomies have been performed inadvertently on eyes with unrecognized neovascular glaucoma. Conversely, we recently examined an elderly woman with all the findings of neovascular glaucoma in one eye and a normal fellow eye with a deep anterior chamber angle. She was found to have an intumescent cataract and secondary angle-closure glaucoma with inflammation. After lens extraction and resolution of the angle closure, the "rubeosis iridis" completely disappeared.

With high pressures, rubeosis iridis, and opaque media preventing any visualization of the posterior segment, the diagnosis may be difficult. Hidden intraocular tumors,[353,377] chronic retinal detachment, and other degenerative conditions,[355] must be considered. Any cause of intraocular bleeding, especially with a hyphema, may be confused with neovascular glaucoma. Ghost cell glaucoma presenting after trauma or surgical procedures should be considered.[58] Usually this diagnosis is easy if there is a khaki-colored hypopyon in the anterior chamber or if there are tiny (4 to 8 μm) khaki-colored ghost cells covering the trabecular meshwork. The difficulty arises when a superimposed hyphema prevents this observation. The history and paracentesis with phase-contrast microscopy of the aspirate will confirm this diagnosis.

FLUORESCEIN STUDIES

Aside from fundus fluorescein angiography, other fluorescein studies have been found to be valuable more in research and in increasing our understanding of neovascular glaucoma than in any practical application at the present time.

The blood-retinal barrier is maintained because of the integrity of the vascular endothelial cells. Normal mature endothelial cells have no fenestration and have very tight intercellular junctions. The luminal face of the endothelium is impermeable to small anionic molecules, such as fluorescein, although it has now been shown that plasmalemmal vesicles can transport anionic molecules into the lumen.[283] This suggests that the endothelial cells form a much more complex barrier then previously thought, and that the initial derangement in angiogenesis may be within the endothelial cells. Experimentally, in nondiabetic rats, when active endothelial cellular transport is inhibited without destruction of the intercellular junctions, fluorescein leakage into the vitreous is similar to that of diabetic rats.[77] Clinically, fluorescein leakage in the vitreous can be seen before any new vessels are visible in diabetes,[174] Fuchs' heterochromic cyclitis,[289] and pseudoexfoliation syndrome.[348] This confirms the hypothesis that a functional change occurs in the endothelium of vessels before any structural changes occur, and certainly before there is visible neovascularization.

As the disease process continues, there are changes in the basement membrane, gaps between endothelial cells, and fenestrations in the endothelial cells, as shown in electron microscopic studies on new iris vessels from diabetics.[340] There seems to be some degree of external control of the presence, numbers, and direction of these fenestrations in health and in various disease states.[21] This is probably a late stage in the breakdown of the blood-retinal barrier.

Clinically, there is not much need for iris fluorescein angiography. Although fluorescein leakage certainly pinpoints early pupillary rubeosis, it is not necessary to detect these new vessels (Fig. 60-9). The fluorescein angiogram is not pathognomonic for any particular underlying disease; whatever its cause, rubeosis iridis has the same fluorescein angiographic pattern.[77] If one examines the eye carefully with a high index of suspicion, pupillary rubeosis can be detected early enough to allow adequate treatment. Studies have not been performed to quantitate how much earlier fluorescein leakage occurs before new vessels are detectable, or to show if it makes any difference in the

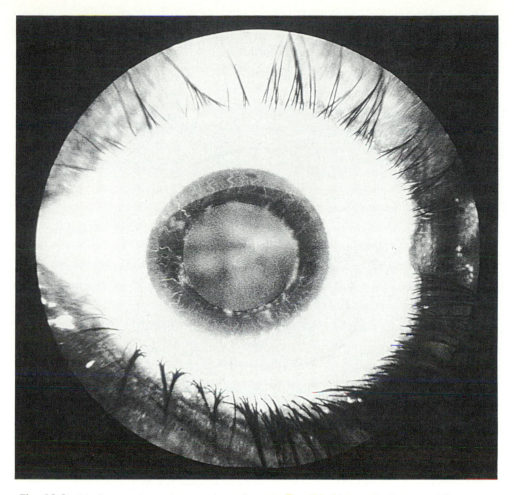

Fig. 60-9   Iris fluorescein angiogram of eye shown in Fig. 60-3. Note multiple areas of fluorescein leakage of pupillary margin, especially at 8:30 o'clock.

visual prognosis. Furthermore, elderly nondiabetic patients without known posterior segment diseases can have pupillary vascular tufts, with or without fluorescein leakage.[15] Eyes in patients with myotonic dystrophy[74] or abnormal insulin secretion[235] can also have pupillary vascular tufts with fluorescein leakage.

High power fluorescein gonioscopy has demonstrated leakage of new angle vessels before they are readily visible.[190] Leakage of fluorescein from the pupillary margin occurs before there is leakage in the angle, confirming clinical observations of new vessel formation at the pupillary margin before angle involvement.[358] Clinically, however, this technique does not seem to be of great value in the diagnosis of neovascular glaucoma.

Of greater potential clinical value is vitreous fluorophotometry. We know that there are functional endothelial abnormalities before there are structural changes.[77] In fact, when the alteration of

the blood-retinal barrier is mild, the only way these abnormalities may be detected is by vitreous fluorophotometry.[77] In diabetics, even when no clinically detectable retinopathy is present, there is a greater concentration of fluorescein in the vitreous than in nondiabetic eyes.[78,352] More significantly, there seems to be a correlation between alteration of the blood-retinal barrier, as detected by vitreous fluorophotometry, and the severity of the retinopathy, duration of diabetes mellitus, and metabolic control of the diabetes.[77,119] The therapeutic implications of this test remains to be seen. As yet there has been no evaluation of any treatment of the early stages of retinopathy detectable by this technique, and the fluorescein studies, at this date, are of greater research value than clinical importance.

PATHOLOGY

It is now generally accepted that the anterior segment histopathology of neovascular glaucoma

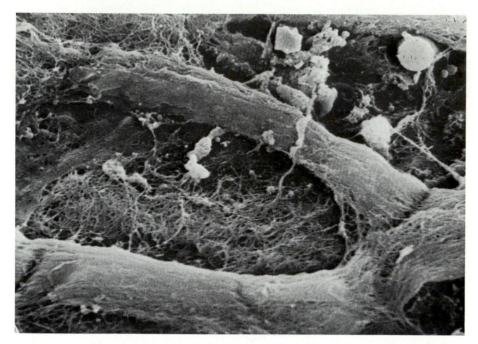

Fig. 60-10 Rubeosis iridis with new vessels that have grown from iris stroma onto surface. (Scanning electron microscopy, ×4000) (Courtesy Thomas M Richardson, MD)

Fig. 60-11 Rubeosis iridis with new, thin-walled vessels in anterior stroma of iris. (Hematoxylin and eosin, ×100.)

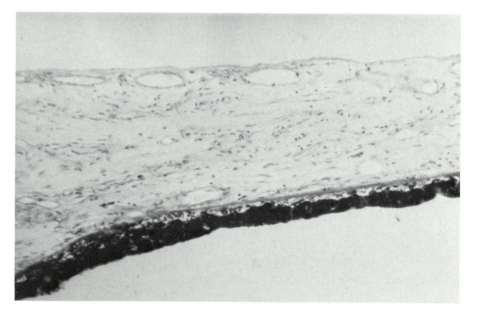

is the same, regardless of the etiology.[119,355] The only exceptions are CRVO, in which the new vessels may be more engorged,[175] and diabetes mellitus, in which there are characteristic iris pigment epithelium cystoid changes from accumulation of glycogen.[119] The neovascularization process begins as endothelial budding from capillaries of the minor arterial circle at the pupil. Clinically, this neovascularization appears to progress sequentially from the pupil to the periphery. However, histologically, once the process starts at the pupillary margin, new endothelial buds may appear from vessels anywhere in the iris, including the major arterial circle in the iris root.[119] These endothelial buds progress to become glomerulus-like vascular tufts. These capillary tufts are not unique to neovascular glaucoma. As mentioned, elderly people without known diseases[15] and people with myotonic dystrophy may have pupillary tufts as well.[74] These tufts leak fluorescein, confirming that they are indeed new vessels.[235] These new vessels are essentially very thin-walled endothelial cells without a muscular layer or much adventitia or supportive tissue. Electron microscopic studies have shown gaps between the endothelial cells,[340] fenestrations in the endothelial cells, and basement membrane changes in new vessels in diabetic eyes.[348] Normal blood vessels in the iris, as in the retina and brain, have nonfenestrated endothelial cells with tight intercellular junctions, called zonula occludens, which prevent leakage of fluorescein and other substances. It is the characteristic of new vessels to leak fluorescein, and presumably, other substances as well.[199] In vivo, these new vessels appear to be on the surface of the iris (Fig. 60-10). Histologically, new vessels have a tendency to be thin walled and to be located toward the surface of the iris, but they can be anywhere within the stroma of the iris[119] (Fig. 60-11).

The existence of a fibrovascular membrane has been known for a long time. This membrane consists of proliferating myofibroblasts, which are fibroblasts with smooth muscle differentiation.[176] These cells are clinically transparent and only hinted at by the aforementioned flattening of the usual iris surface architecture. Scanning electron microscopy shows the uniform presence of this membrane wherever there are new vessels. Anatomically, the new vessels are not on the surface of the iris but actually beneath this layer of myofibroblasts. The pervasiveness of this membrane explains why there can be increased intraocular pressure despite the gonioscopic appearance of a normal open angle or only slight angle neovascularization disproportionate to the degree of pressure elevation. The contractile smooth muscle components explain the effacement of the iris surface, the development of ectropion uveae, formation of peripheral anterior synechiae, and ultimately, synechial angle closure[176] (Fig. 60-12). It is thought that the proliferating new vessels and the myofibroblasts are both primary constituents of granulation tissue and that iris neovascularization may be a reparative process gone awry.

As this membrane continues to contract on the surface of the iris, the posterior pigment layer of the iris is pulled around the pupillary margin onto the anterior surface, causing ectropion uveae and pupillary distortion (Fig. 60-13). The sphincter muscle can also be pulled anteriorly, resulting in ectropion of the sphincter. Contraction may be so extensive that the iris is displaced forward or totally retracted from view (Fig. 60-14). In such cases, the ciliary processes may be visible on gonioscopy. This contraction can also compress and embed the new vessels, hiding them from observation.[119] A fibrotic, nonresponsive iris and a fixed dilated pupil are often seen in late neovascular glaucoma. As mentioned, before total synechial angle-closure, the membrane can obstruct the trabecular meshwork and produce a secondary open-angle glaucoma (Fig. 60-15). Further contraction results in synechial angle-closure with iridocorneal touch (Fig. 60-16). When the neovascularization process is stopped, as with panretinal photocoagulation, the new vessels will regress, but the synechial angle closure cannot be reversed. We do not yet know what happens to the myofibroblast membrane when there is regression of the new vessels.

In some cases of synechial angle-closure of long duration, endothelium and Descemet's membrane may extend from the cornea across the synechiae onto the iris surface[120] (Fig. 60-17). Scanning electron microscopic studies have confirmed this endothelium to be contiguous to and originate from the corneal endothelium.[260] Such endothelialization of the iris is also seen in the iridocorneal endothelial syndrome[59] and after trauma,[120] and may represent a pathogenic mechanism common to violation of the barrier between the cornea and the iris, as with synechial angle closure. This closed angle with few or no visible new vessels and covered with endothelium can easily be mistaken for a normal open angle, and the term *pseudoangle* is most appropriate (Fig. 60-18).

Text continued on p. 1077.

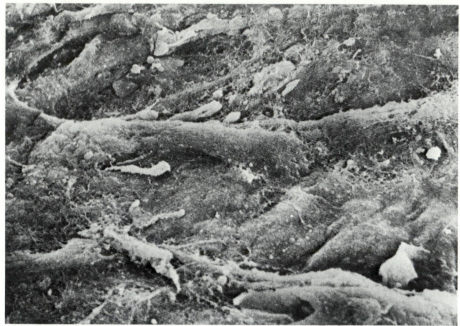

Fig. 60-12 Rubeosis iridis with new vessels on anterior surface of iris. Myofibroblastic membrane covers the new vessels and the iris surface causing effacement of the surface architecture. (Scanning electron microscope, ×2040.) (Courtesy Thomas M Richardson, MD)

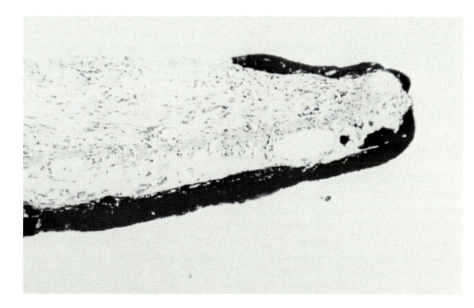

Fig. 60-13 Rubeosis iridis with marked ectropion of iris pigment epithelium. (Hematoxylin and eosin, ×100.)

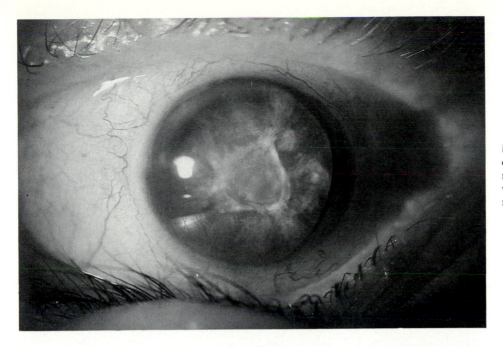

Fig. 60-14 End stage neovascular glaucoma with so much radial contraction of the fibrovascular membrane that almost no iris is visible.

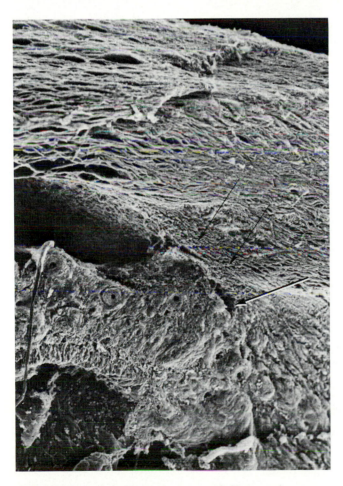

Fig. 60-15 Early angle involvement with fibrovascular membrane partially obstructing trabecular meshwork. True angle, not yet closed, is shown by *single arrow;* posterior trabecular meshwork, with Schlemm's canal superior to it, is shown by *double arrows.* (Scanning electron microscopy, ×108.) (Courtesy Thomas M Richardson, MD)

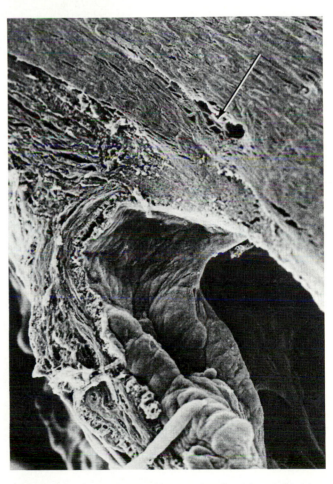

Fig. 60-16 Total synechial closure of angle with atrophic iris pulled anteriorly to Schwalbe's line (not shown). Schlemm's canal is shown by *arrow.* (Scanning electron microscopy, ×172.) (Courtesy Thomas M Richardson, MD)

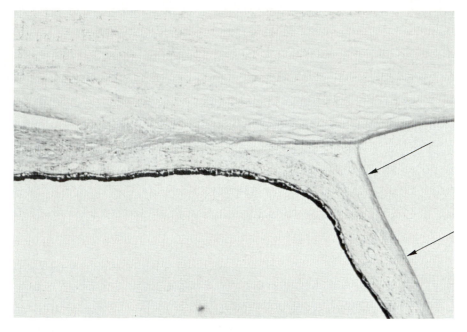

Fig. 60-17 Total synechial closure of angle with corneal endothelium extending onto anterior surface of iris *(arrows)*. (Hematoxylin and eosin, ×40.)

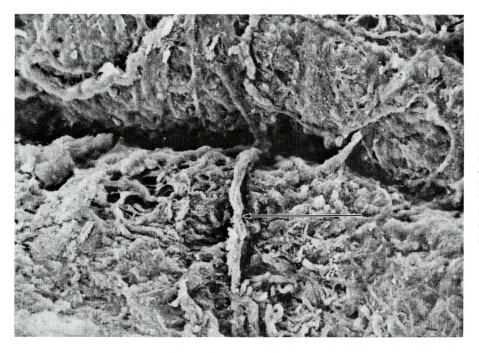

Fig. 60-18 Total synechial closure of angle with formation of pseudoangle. Cornea is on top, and iris is on bottom. There is frequently diminution of new vessels in area of angle-closure. One thin vessel is shown here *(arrow)*. (Scanning electron microscopy, ×960.) (Courtesy Thomas M Richardson, MD)

PATHOGENESIS

Several recent studies on the mechanism of neovascularization have brought our concepts of its pathogenesis almost full circle. In 1948, Michaelson[245] first postulated the existence of a vasoformative factor, "X-factor," which controlled the normal development of new vessels during embryogenesis. Ashton et al.[14] suggested that the retinal ischemia in retrolental fibroplasia might result in excess amounts of this factor, which in turn would lead to retinal neovascularization. Subsequent seemingly divergent studies now are contributing toward a larger, coherent picture.

Greenblatt and Shubick[134] found that a tumor on one side of a Millipore filter could induce new blood vessel formation in tissue on the other side, suggesting that there was a diffusable angiogenesis factor. Folkman et al.[109,111] independently isolated a soluble substance from solid neoplasms capable of stimulating neovascularization and popularized the term "tumor angiogenesis factor."[109,111] Subsequently, members of his laboratory[125,126] and others[105] found that a tumor angiogenesis factor was capable of causing iris neovascularization and retinal neovascularization at a distance from intraocular tumors implanted in various parts of the eye. Extracts from vitreous,[42] cartilage,[212] and retinal pigment epithelial cells[127] were found to inhibit the neovascularization caused by this tumor angiogenesis factor.

On another front, Wise[370] proposed that retinal capillary or venous obstruction resulted in hypoxia of the retinal cells. If the hypoxic cells did not die, he thought they produced a vasoformative factor. Ashton[13] agreed that the prerequisite for neovascularization was hypoxic metabolism. He thought that the vasoformative factor from this hypoxic metabolism could diffuse anteriorly to stimulate iris angiogenesis. Earlier, Ashton had demonstrated that the vaso-obliteration seen in retrolental fibroplasia was comparable to the capillary closure or nonperfusion seen in diabetic retinopathy.[14] Clinically, it has been confirmed that widespread capillary occlusion and chronic tissue hypoxia are almost always present when there is neovascularization.[269] Aqueous and vitreous from human eyes with proliferative neovascularization have vasoproliferative activity in tissue culture studies.[128,136] Angiogenic activity has been demonstrated in the retinal extracts of monkeys,[136] cows, dogs, pigs, lambs, and rabbits.[69] Chen and Chen[69] suggested that this angiogenic activity is normally present in the retina. Angiogenic activity is present in the normal retina of humans, cows, rabbits, and cats[129] and

in damaged rabbit[99] and bovine[284] retina. Whether or not this angiogenic substance comes from normal or damaged retina, several different substances have been isolated.

The number of different angiogenesis factors remains uncertain. Nor is it understood whether these factor(s) cause angiogenesis directly, through some intermediary substances, or are themselves messengers or facilitators in this process. Finally it is not known whether these substances are organ or species specific. A large number of substances have angiogenic activity. Various biogenic amines, such as histamine, acetylcholine, and serotonin, can stimulate corneal neovascularization.[381] Prostaglandins, especially PGE_1, are potent stimulators of neovascularization and might be the common mediating agents of the different angiogenesis factors.[26] Activated leukocytes,[27,118] activated macrophages,[278] and immunocompetent lymphocytes[312] all induce angiogenesis. These cells are components of immunologic and nonimmunologic inflammatory reactions and, like growing tumors, produce prostaglandins.[26] Immunologic ocular inflammation produced by serum albumin[309] and commercial insulin[308] also produces a clinical picture similar to that of proliferative diabetic retinopathy. Inflammation and prostaglandins must play some role in angiogenesis. Supporting this are findings that indomethacin, an antiinflammatory drug that inhibits the effects of prostaglandin;[85] methylprednisolone;[239] and irradiation, which induces leukopenia,[130] all reduce experimental neovascularization.

D'Amore et al.[80] have partially purified and characterized an angiogenic substance from bovine retina. It is a proteoglycan weighing between 50,000 and 100,000 daltons that can be separated into two active components of 50,000 and 70,000 daltons. Other angiogenic substances have been isolated,[104] but none were chemically characterized until the landmark research by Vallee and his group,[104,204,331] who isolated, purified, and characterized the amino acid sequence of a human adenocarcinoma-derived angiogenesis factor, which they termed angiogenin. It is a single chain protein of 14,400 daltons and seems to be extremely potent. They have placed angiogenin in a group of substances called organogenic messenger molecules and suggested that it is only one of a variety of soluble tumor derived mediators.

Finally, two recent reports have brought us back to Michaelson's suggestion that the "X-Factor" controlled normal new vessel development and that disturbances of the normal balance lead to neovascularization. Vascular endothelial cells produce a chemoattractant for retinal pigment epithelial cells.[61] This is a nondialyzable, heat-stable polypeptide that may be identical to other endothelium-derived and platelet-derived growth factors, which have also been shown to be chemoattractants for retinal pigment epithelial cells.[61] Human retinal pigment epithelial cells also release an inhibitor of angiogenesis.[129] The authors speculated that the chorioretinal scars from photocoagulation might be the source of this inhibitor and thus explain the beneficial effects of panretinal photocoagulation.[126] Clearly, there is a finely tuned and intricate interplay between at least two types of cells in the eye to control new vessel formation. Normal development, wound repair, and tumor growth all require orderly development of an adequate blood supply. Michaelson thought, without any experimental evidence, that this "X-factor" was a normal constituent. It has since been shown that some angiogenic substance is present in normal and damaged ocular tissues of various species.[69,99,129,284] This angiogenesis factor may not be a "new moiety, so much as an increase in the stimulus required to maintain existing vessels."[118] Glaser et al.[129] have eloquently illustrated the mechanism by which cell-cell interaction could affect vessel formation in health and disease and have potentially opened new avenues of research in understanding normal development, as well as better treatment of diseases involving neovascularization.

In a completely different theory, Worbarsht and Landers[371] postulated that retinal hypoxia results in chronic dilation of the retinal vessels, which in turn causes angiogenesis.[371] They cite as evidence the beneficial effects of panretinal photocoagulation on rubeosis iridis.

In summary, normal development, tissue repair, and tumor growth, all require orderly angiogenesis. There seems to be a fine balance between factors that stimulate and inhibit blood vessel formation. These factors are either normally present in certain tissues or become rapidly available under appropriate circumstances such as hypoxia. These stimulatory factors may act as messengers, initiators, or mediators of angiogenesis. It is likely that inflammation and its byproducts, especially prostaglandins, are involved. When damage occurs, almost always in the form of hypoxia in the eye, the normal balance is disturbed, and the stimulatory factors predominate over the inhibitory factors.

CAUSES OF NEOVASCULAR GLAUCOMA

Over the past 20 years, there have been comprehensive reviews on neovascular glaucoma every few years.* Each has tried to list the disorders known to cause, or at least be associated with, neovascular glaucoma. The highest count listed 41 different disorders.[119] There have since been more reports of additional entities purportedly causing neovascular glaucoma. However, it has become abundantly clear that wherever rubeosis iridis progresses to neovascular glaucoma, there is almost always widespread posterior segment hypoxia or localized anterior segment hypoxia.

Rather than compiling lists of entities that can cause rubeosis iridis, it now seems more rewarding to review the major groups of disorders that can lead to neovascular glaucoma. In one review of patients with neovascular glaucoma admitted in the 1960s to a Danish hospital, 43% had glaucoma attributed to diabetic retinopathy, 37% to CRVO, and the rest to miscellaneous causes.[225] Surprisingly, despite the widespread use of panretinal photocoagulation, the picture has not changed greatly. Brown et al.[47] reviewed 208 consecutive cases of neovascular glaucoma over 4 years and found 36% caused by CRVO, 32% by diabetic retinopathy, and 13% by carotid artery occlusive disease.[47] At the present time, probably one third of the cases of neovascular glaucoma are attributable to CRVO, one third to diabetic retinopathy, and one third to diverse causes, with carotid occlusive disease being prominent.

Central Retinal Vein Occlusion (CRVO)

It has been known since at least the time of von Graefe[145] (1860s) that CRVO can be associated with neovascular glaucoma. Numerous studies have reported widely varying incidences of this complication, ranging from 15% to 65%, with an average of about 30%.[133] However, there was also a seemingly unpredictable pattern as to which patients with CRVO would develop neovascular glaucoma. Hayreh et al.[139,141,145,146] have brought order to this heretofore confusing picture. They found that CRVO could be divided into two distinct entities, based on the presence or absence of retinal ischemia. The group without retinal ischemia was termed *venous stasis retinopathy*, and the group with retinal ischemia was termed *hemorrhagic retinopathy*. Laatikainen[207,208] confirmed this differentiation using fundus fluorescein angiography. The only unfortunate aspect of Hayreh's work is his original choice of terms; Kearns and Hollenhorst in 1963 had already used the term venous stasis retinopathy to describe the retinopathy of carotid occlusive disease.[184,229] Although this initially led

---

*References 9, 119, 133, 304, 355, 375.

to a great deal of confusion, the terms *ischemic* and *nonischemic* types of CRVO have found wide acceptance in the literature and will be used here.

The natural history of untreated CRVO is that essentially none of the nonischemic eyes progress on to neovascular glaucoma,[145,229,341] whereas 18%[209] to 60%[229] of eyes in the ischemic group do so (Fig. 60-19). At first glance, it would still appear impossible to predict which patients in the ischemic group would subsequently develop neovascular glaucoma. Magargal et al.[231] tried to quantitate the degree of ischemia, which they called the "ischemic index," based on retinal capillary nonperfusion as determined by fluorescein angiogram.[231] Hayreh[145] opted for a more simple classification of mild, moderate, and marked capillary nonperfusion.[145] They and others[197] agreed that the greater the degree of capillary nonperfusion (hence, retinal hypoxia), the greater the chances of developing neovascularization. An overall incidence of 40% for the ischemic type of CRVO is supported by the largest least biased study.[145] With the universal acceptance of the beneficial effects of panretinal photocoagulation on CRVO, it is unlikely that it will again be possible to devise a large, controlled prospective study to confirm these findings. Because neovascular glaucoma can appear anywhere from 2 weeks to 2 years after the initial occlusion,[231] it is logical that the ultimate incidence will be time-related.[145] Neovascular glaucoma has been thought to appear 2 to 3 months after the CRVO[66] (hence the term "100 day glaucoma"). Now that we know there is a time-dependent incidence curve, as well as a quantitative relationship to the extent of the retinal ischemia,[145] it is also easier to understand the variation in the time of appearance of the neovascularization. Nevertheless, in over 80% of the cases, the anterior segment neovascularization and neovascular glaucoma will appear within the first 6 months after the occlusion.[145]

The clinical appearance of the retina can be deceiving in determining the perfusion status. A fluorescein angiogram is imperative in the diagnosis and, ultimately, the treatment of CRVO. Using a multivariate analysis of four different param-

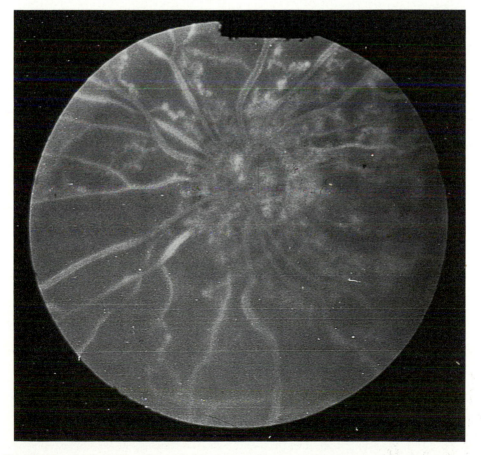

Fig. 60-19   Ischemic type of central retinal vein occlusion with extensive capillary nonperfusion as shown on fluorescein angiogram.

eters obtained on fundus fluorescein angiography, Sinclair and Gragoudas[316] have claimed up to 91% accuracy in predicting which eye would develop rubeosis iridis. Clinically, we have learned that it is sometimes not possible to determine how much capillary nonperfusion there is because retinal hemorrhages block out these areas. Hayreh[145] found that this occurred in 30% of the initial fluorescein angiograms he examined. When retinal hemorrhages prevent adequate visualization of the ischemic retina and it is erroneously interpreted as normal, patients may be falsely reassured only to develop end stage neovascular glaucoma later (Figs. 60-20 and 60-21). When it is not possible to determine the extent of the ischemia on initial fluorescein, the patient must be followed carefully and regularly, and repeat fluorescein studies performed, if necessary, as the retinal hemorrhages clear. Finally, the nonischemic type can convert to the ischemic type,[145] so careful follow-up of patients with any type of CRVO is indicated. We have followed uneventfully for almost 2 years a 55-year-old man with bilateral nonischemic CRVOs noted on routine ocular examination to have early rubeosis iridis (Figs. 60-22 and 60-23). With panretinal photocoagulation, the rubeosis iridis quickly resolved.

When the fluorescein angiogram has not been able to differentiate clearly the two types of the CRVO, electroretinography may do so.[298] Nevertheless, clinically, fluorescein angiogram is still the main diagnostic tool; the place of electroretinopathy has not yet been determined.

Twenty percent of human eyes have a two-trunked central retinal vein,[142] and either of the two trunks may occlude. When that happens, it appears to behave just like CRVO.[145] In general, there needs to be ischemia over at least half of the retina to cause anterior segment neovascularization.[145] For that reason, neovascular glaucoma is extremely rare with branch retinal vein occlusion[233] and macular retinal vein occlusion.[145] However, cases of neovascular glaucoma have been reported after branch retinal vein occlusion.[228]

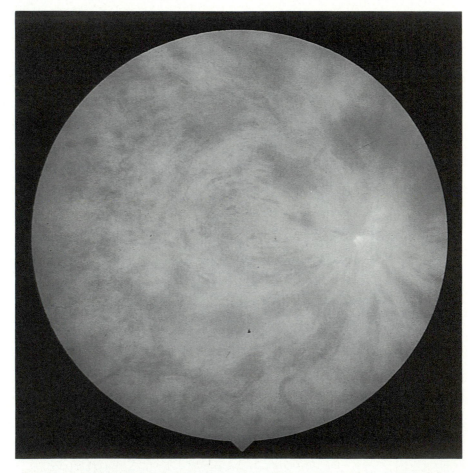

Fig. 60-20 A 48-year-old woman with extensive retinal hemorrhages from a central retinal vein occlusion. Vision was counting fingers.

Verhoeff[350] noted an association between CRVO and preexisting open-angle glaucoma. This relationship has been confirmed in many studies, the incidence ranging from 6% to 66%.[221] In the largest series published, involving 360 patients with CRVO, Hayreh et al.[145] found a 23% incidence of primary open-angle glaucoma or ocular hypertension. The association between CRVO and primary open-angle glaucoma seems to be age related, with up to 75% of patients over 65 years with CRVO having concomitant open-angle glaucoma.[349] The apparent difference between older and younger patients may be partially explained by a recent study by Trope et al.[347] In their series of 12 young (average age 29 years) patients with CRVO, none had daytime intraocular pressure above 21 mm Hg, although 11 of 12 had diurnal fluctuation greater than 21 mm Hg, with some pressures up to 30 mm Hg. In addition, eight patients had a maximum diurnal swing in the intraocular pressure greater than 8 mm Hg.[347] This study supports the feeling that elevated intraocular pressures may play an impor-

tant role in the etiology of CRVO in both young and elderly patients and points out that some cases of open-angle glaucoma, especially in young patients, may be missed if the applanation tension is not taken at different times in the day. However, there is no consensus as to whether the presence of open-angle glaucoma influences the ultimate development of neovascular glaucoma;[145,229] nor is there consensus why open-angle glaucoma should predispose an eye to CRVO. Suggestions have ranged from mechanical pressure on the optic disc and central retinal vein to common vascular abnormalities between CRVO and open-angle glaucoma.[221]

Many authors have noted that, in as many as 80% of eyes with CRVO, the intraocular pressure may be lower in the eye with the occlusion than the fellow eye.[28,143,256] In one series, the reduction was greater in patients with CRVO than branch retinal vein occlusion, greater in the ischemic than the nonischemic type of occlusion, and greater if the fellow eye had high pressures.[143] The mean differ-

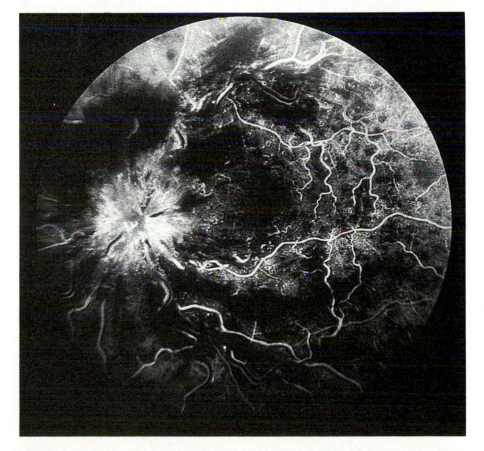

Fig. 60-21   Fluorescein angiogram of eye in Fig. 60-20. The retinal hemorrhages obscure the areas of capillary nonperfusion. As the retinal hemorrhages cleared, nonperfusion was demonstrated on repeat angiograms. She subsequently received panretinal photocoagulation. Her vision improved to 20/80, and she has not developed rubeosis iridis or neovascular glaucoma.

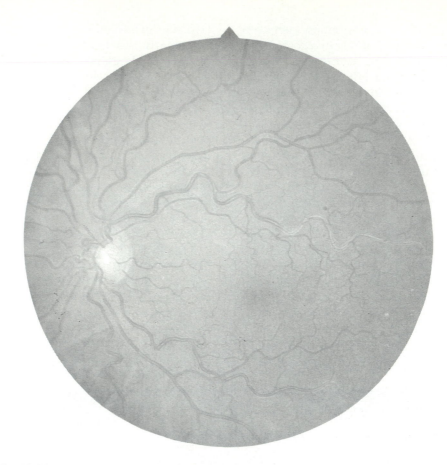

Fig. 60-22   A 55-year-old man with bilateral nonischemic central retinal vein occlusion of 2 years duration who was noted to have early rubeosis iridis.

ence in the intraocular pressures between the two eyes in the ischemic type of occlusion was 4.2 mm Hg, but was as high as 18 mm Hg, and the intraocular pressure may remain lower for up to 2 years.[143] Hayreh thought that retinal ischemia and the resultant anaerobic metabolism produced localized acidosis, which could act similarly to the metabolic acidosis produced by carbonic anhydrase inhibitors to decrease aqueous production.[351] He speculated that the angiogenesis factor may be the same as, or closely related to, this hypotensive factor.[140]

This discussion has important implications in the care of patients with neovascular glaucoma from CRVO. Open-angle glaucoma must be considered a precipitating cause and diligently searched for on the initial and follow-up visits. A patient with CRVO should be considered a glaucoma suspect,[217] and some believe that elderly patients with pressures above 25 mm Hg should be treated with antiglaucoma medication to lower the chance of developing CRVO.[221] We have seen a patient with CRVO in one eye and normal intraocular pressures in both eyes who presented again several years later with advanced open-angle glaucoma and visual field loss in both eyes.

Many studies have found a positive association between CRVO and systemic hypertension,[87,179,229,240] hyperlipidemia,[87,240] and abnormal glucose tolerance test.[229,87,240] Hayreh[145] did not find this correlation, and there is no explanation for this discrepancy.

Diabetes Mellitus

Diabetes mellitus is one of the leading causes of blindness in the United States today.[34,113] In the adult group (approximately age 20 to 60 years), it is *the* leading cause of new blindness and one of the major causes of neovascular glaucoma. Most blindness is caused by diabetic retinopathy, only 5% of the blindness being due to neovascular glaucoma.[113] Despite the 1976 Diabetic Retinopathy Study, which showed the beneficial effects of panretinal photocoagulation in preventing severe visual loss, there has not been a significant decrease in the incidence of neovascular glaucoma from diabetes mellitus.[47,225]

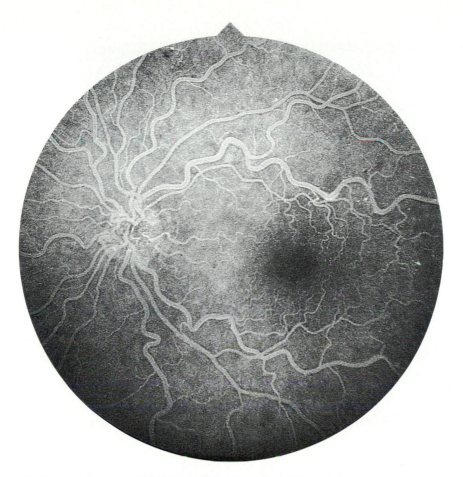

Fig. 60-23 Initial fluorescein angiogram of eye in Fig. 60-22, showing good retinal perfusion. Nonischemic types of central retinal vein occlusion may become ischemic months to years later and cause rubeosis iridis and neovascular glaucoma.

Diabetes mellitus is also a heterogeneous metabolic disorder.[122] This subdivision has made some observations concerning the complications of diabetes mellitus more understandable. The association between rubeosis iridis and diabetes mellitus was first made by Salus in 1928.[299] In 1939, Fehrmann[100] correlated rubeosis iridis with the presence of retinal neovascularization. In subsequent studies on unselected diabetic populations the incidence of rubeosis iridis ranged from 1%[12] to 17%.[225] In eyes with proliferative diabetic retinopathy, the incidence of rubeosis iridis increases to 65%.[267] In a histologic study of eyes removed from patients with diabetes mellitus, Yanoff[376] found that 95% of the eyes had rubeosis iridis, and of these, 90% had retinal neovascularization. It is now well accepted that rubeosis iridis is associated with retinal hypoxia and proliferative diabetic retinopathy.[158] Recently, Isenberg et al.[168] showed that the conjunctival oxygen tension in diabetics with proliferative diabetic retinopathy was significantly

lower than in diabetics with background retinopathy, which in turn was significantly lower than in diabetics with no retinopathy.[168]

Clinically, there can be significant retinal hypoxia with few visible signs of proliferative retinopathy. Fundus fluorescein angiography often is necessary to show capillary nonperfusion. Even then, the posterior pole may appear remarkably benign. It is imperative to examine the peripheral retina on angioscopy and to take peripheral photographs on the angiograms (Figs. 60-24 and 60-25).

There are two major groups of diabetes mellitus.[122] Type I or insulin-dependent diabetes, previously known as juvenile onset diabetes, comprises approximately 15%; and type II or noninsulin dependent diabetes, previously known as maturity or adult-onset diabetes, comprises approximately 80% of the total. The remaining 5% consists of other types of diabetes, such as secondary diabetes mellitus. Type I diabetes is probably caused by autoimmune destruction of islet B

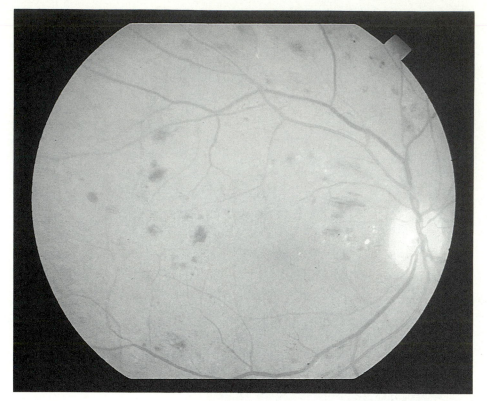

Fig. 60-24 A 51-year-old woman with 10-year history of diabetes mellitus. Fundoscopic examination showed nonproliferative diabetic retinopathy.

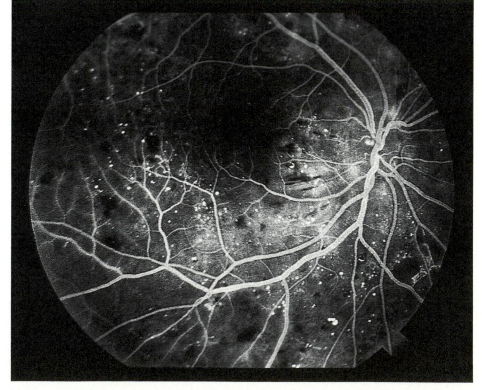

Fig. 60-25 Fluorescein angiogram of eye in Fig. 60-24. Extensive midperipheral areas of capillary dropout and retinal nonperfusion.

cells; the etiology of type II is still unknown. Caird et al.[53] had noted clinically that there seemed to be more blindness from complications of proliferative diabetic retinopathy in type I and more blindness from diabetic maculopathy in type II diabetes mellitus. Bodansky et al.[37] have confirmed this impression. In 100 consecutive diabetic patients referred to a retina clinic, they found a significant association between type I diabetes and initial diagnosis of proliferative diabetic retinopathy and type II diabetes and initial diagnosis of maculopathy.[37] Regardless of the type of diabetes, the major factor in the onset of diabetic retinopathy appears to be the duration of diabetes. In type I diabetes, 10% have retinopathy after 10 years, 50% after 15 years, and 90% after 25 years.[53] In type II diabetes, retinopathy seems to occur sooner than in type I diabetes.[258] After 10 years, up to 50% have retinopathy.[53] The incidence of retinopathy occurring in both types of diabetes appears to be similar.[258]

Despite the difference in the onset of retinopathy between type I and type II diabetes, studies have shown that these long-term complications result from the metabolic derangement (hyperglycemia) rather than from genetic differences between these two types of diabetes.[35,327] However, there has been a great deal of controversy concerning the relationship between control of diabetes and long-term complications.[195] Only recently has there been sufficient evidence for the beneficial effects of good glycemic control. Eschwege et al.[96] showed that the yearly increase in the number of microaneurysms was three times higher in poorly-controlled diabetics using single insulin injections versus well-controlled diabetics using multiple daily insulin injections. Szabo et al.[339] showed that the severity of retinopathy in 324 diabetics increased linearly with an increase in the average fasting blood sugar. In the most impressive study to date, Pirart,[276] who followed 4400 diabetics from 1947 to 1973, noted that after 25 years, in patients with good glycemic control, there was virtually no proliferative diabetic retinopathy compared to a 20% incidence in patients with poor glycemic control. Currently, there are two major ways of achieving near-normal glycemia: continuous subcutaneous insulin infusion (CSII) or multiple daily injections (MDI).[290] Near-normal control is considered to be a blood glucose of 70 to 120 mg/dl preprandially and less than 160 to 180 mg/dl 90 minutes post prandially in nonpregnant diabetic patients.[307]

The most recent prospective studies have shown greater progression of diabetic retinopathy after initiation of intensive insulin therapy than with regular insulin therapy.[275,328] Furthermore, near-normal glucose metabolism does not reverse established diabetic retinopathy.[281] The explanation for these findings is that a decreased blood glucose level decreases retinal blood flow, which in turn results in infarction of the marginally profused areas of the retina.[328] This means that if near-normal glycemia is instituted late, when retinal ischemia is already present, then there may be a period when the retinopathy will worsen before any improvement is noticeable. Individual cases of reversal of retinopathy after institution of CSII have been reported.[342] The theory is that tight metabolic control of diabetes mellitus is important in preventing or delaying the microvascular complications of diabetes and ultimately, therefore, in preventing neovascular glaucoma. The National Institute of Health–sponsored Diabetes Control and Complications Trial (DCCT) is designed to answer this important question.

There is also now convincing evidence that concomitant hypertension in diabetic patients results in greater frequency and greater severity of diabetic retinopathy.[198,339] In a predominantly type II group of diabetic Native Americans, it was found that systolic blood pressure greater than 145 mm Hg was associated with an incidence of retinal exudates twice that of patients with pressure less than 125 mm Hg.[194] Recently, we confirmed the significant association between hypertensive-arteriosclerotic heart disease and complications of diabetic retinopathy.[360] Sixty-two percent of diabetic patients undergoing pars plana vitrectomy for complications of diabetic retinopathy had some form of hypertensive-arteriosclerotic heart disease versus only 19% of patients undergoing vitrectomy for nondiabetes related problems. This is another potential area of early treatment for the ocular complications of diabetes mellitus.

After neovascular glaucoma develops in one eye of a diabetic patient, the natural history without treatment is that the fellow eye will almost inevitably also develop it.[261] Bilateral rubeosis iridis or neovascular glaucoma in an adult is almost always caused by diabetic retinopathy.[119] We know the time interval between the onset of diabetes mellitus and development of retinopathy, but we do not know the time sequence between development of retinopathy and appearance of rubeosis iridis. The time interval between the onset of rubeosis iridis and neovascular glaucoma in untreated cases varies from 1 month to over 3 years.[226] Furthermore, it is unpredictable as to which untreated eyes with rubeosis iridis will ultimately progress to neovascular glaucoma. There are well-documented cases of spontaneous regression of diabetic retinopathy.[123] In up to 26% of eyes, rubeosis iridis may spontaneously disappear over a 5-year span.[226] This unpredictable course of rubeosis iridis and neovascular glaucoma caused by diabetic retinopathy makes the evaluation of any prophylactic treatment for rubeosis iridis difficult at best.

Postcataract Extraction

Capillary dropout and retinal hypoxia make the eye with diabetic retinopathy especially vulnerable to further insult. Surgical procedures, such as cataract extraction and vitrectomy, add considerable risk to the development of neovascular glaucoma in such eyes. Neovascular glaucoma has not been reported as a complication in larger series of intracapsular cataract extraction in unselected populations.[171,344] In 1970, Beasley[18] reported the development of neovascular glaucoma after intracapsular cataract extraction in two diabetic patients. In 1983, we retrospectively reviewed the records of 154 diabetic patients who had undergone intracapsular cataract extraction in one eye, with the fellow eye serving as the unoperated control.[6] Without regard to the preoperative status of the retinopathy, there was a significant incidence of postoperative rubeosis iridis-neovascular glaucoma (7.8% versus 0%). In patients with preoperative proliferative diabetic retinopathy, the risks of developing postoperative rubeosis iridis-neovascular glaucoma was even greater (40% versus 0%). The preoperative presence of proliferative diabetic retinopathy also carries significantly greater risk of developing neovascular glaucoma after vitrectomy.[67,243] It was thought that intracapsular cataract extraction resulted in the removal of a diffusion barrier and allowed easier passage of some angiogenesis factor from the posterior segment to the anterior segment. In any case, after the preoperative status of the diabetic retinopathy had been considered, the seemingly unpredictable postoperative development of neovascular glaucoma became understandable.[6]

Poliner et al.[277] in a follow-up study showed that none of 53 eyes that had undergone extracapsular cataract extraction developed postoperative neovascular glaucoma. Two of 17 eyes (12%) after extracapsular cataract extraction with primary capsulotomy and 13 of 146 eyes (9%) after intracapsular cataract extraction developed postoperative neovascular glaucoma. Proliferative diabetic reti-

nopathy carried with it a significantly higher risk than the presence of background retinopathy (16% versus 3%). They confirmed the feeling that cataract extraction per se does not predispose the diabetic eye to postoperative neovascular glaucoma. Active proliferative diabetic retinopathy is as necessary as a source of some angiogenesis factor as is removal of the diffusion barrier.

There is some question whether the posterior capsule and/or the anterior hyaloid membrane is the critical diffusion barrier.[356] In the development of postoperative cystoid macular edema, the intact posterior capsule and an intact anterior hyaloid seem to provide protection.[172] The posterior capsule exerts a protective effect against passage of *Staphylococcus aureus* from the anterior chamber to the posterior chamber.[95] In experimental malignant glaucoma, the hyaloid membrane acts as a barrier to the passage of aqueous.[29] Thompson and Glaser[345] showed that an intact lens provided a greater barrier than the posterior capsule alone in decreasing the passage of 20,000 and 70,000 dalton dextrans from the vitreous to the aqueous. If a posterior capsulotomy was performed in rabbit eyes, there was even greater passage of dextran from the vitreous to the aqueous. Recently, the importance of the posterior capsule-anterior hyaloid barrier was shown when Weinreb et al.[362] reported three cases of neovascular glaucoma developing after Nd:YAG laser capsulotomy in diabetic patients. The fundus was not visualized before the capsulotomy in their patients; but at the time neovascular glaucoma was noted, two had proliferative diabetic retinopathy and one had background retinopathy. Other concomitant causes of retinal ischemia in that case were not noted.

The posterior capsule-anterior hyaloid barrier is only relative and can be overwhelmed if there is a great amount of angiogenesis factor, since we routinely see neovascular glaucoma in phakic patients with extensive posterior segment ischemia. If this barrier is removed or disrupted, as with intracapsular cataract extraction or extracapsular cataract extraction with capsulotomy, enough angiogenesis factor may then diffuse forward to stimulate neovascularization of the iris. Inflammation from cataract surgery or capsulotomy may contribute as well. Whenever possible, adequate panretinal photocoagulation should be performed in any diabetic patient with early proliferative diabetic retinopathy before cataract extraction is performed.[6] Although no cases have been reported, it would also seem logical that patients who have had ischemic CRVO should have adequate panretinal photocoagulation before cataract surgery. When cataract surgery is performed in a diabetic patient or one who has had CRVO, the procedure should be a planned extracapsular cataract extraction, with or without a posterior chamber intraocular lens implant. We have not seen neovascular glaucoma develop in diabetic patients who have had adequate panretinal photocoagulation before cataract surgery. Diabetics and patients who have had CRVO should be followed carefully after cataract surgery so that rubeosis iridis can be detected early and appropriate treatment started.

Postvitrectomy

Modern pars plana vitrectomy heralded a new era in the treatment of complications of diabetic retinopathy.[223] Initially, concurrent lens surgery was often performed whether or not a cataract was present. It soon became clear that concurrent lensectomy significantly increased the risks of developing postoperative rubeosis iridis and neovascular glaucoma. Recent large series of vitrectomies in diabetic patients showed a twofold[33] to threefold[287] increased risk of developing rubeosis iridis if lensectomy was performed. However, not all studies found this association.[1,71]

Long before the advent of vitrectomy, it had been known that chronic retinal detachment is a significant cause of neovascular glaucoma.[9,119] Several studies have mentioned the importance of retinal detachment as cause of postvitrectomy rubeosis iridis and neovascular glaucoma.[2,62,300] However, the often-cited large studies did not consider the role of postoperative retinal detachment as a cause of postvitrectomy neovascular glaucoma.[287] We reviewed 255 consecutive vitrectomies, 81 of which were performed for complications of diabetic retinopathy and 175 for nondiabetes-related problems that served as controls in the study.[360] Sixty-five different preoperative, intraoperative, and postoperative parameters were statistically analyzed; and only postoperative retinal detachment had a significant correlation with the development of rubeosis iridis and neovascular glaucoma postvitrectomy. In the diabetic group, 83% of the eyes with retinal detachment developed rubeosis iridis/neovascular glaucoma versus 2% of the eyes with an attached retina. In the control group, 19% of the eyes with retinal detachment developed rubeosis iridis and neovascular glaucoma, versus none of the eyes with attached retinas. Aphakia alone did not correlate significantly with the development of rubeosis iridis. However, aphakia combined with ret-

inal detachment was associated with an even greater risk of developing rubeosis iridis and neovascular glaucoma (92%) in the diabetic group.[360]

Several important things can be learned from this study. Both diabetic retinopathy and retinal detachment are important causes of rubeosis iridis and neovascular glaucoma, and when both conditions coexist, there is an even greater stimulus for anterior segment neovascularization. As has been pointed out earlier, the lens–posterior capsule–anterior hyaloid barrier is a relative, but important, diffusion barrier for the anterior passage of the angiogenesis factor.[345,356,362] When the stimulus for neovascularization has not been eliminated, as with reattachment of the retina and adequate panretinal photocoagulation, the presence or absence of a barrier against the angiogenesis factor is of clinical significance. However, if there is no source of this angiogenesis factor, then the presence or absence of this lens-hyaloid barrier is academic. An attached retina does not mean that the stimulus for neovascularization is not present. We also reported cases where rubeosis iridis was present after vitrectomy despite an attached retina. With postvitrectomy retinal photocoagulation, there was regression of the rubeosis iridis.[360] The conclusion is that after a vitrectomy for complications of proliferative diabetic retinopathy, an attached retina with adequate panretinal photocoagulation is of paramount importance in preventing neovascular glaucoma; lensectomy per se is of secondary importance.

Carotid Artery Occlusive Disease

The association between neovascular glaucoma and carotid artery occlusive disease was first noted by Smith in 1962.[321] Numerous subsequent reports on neovascular glaucoma resulting from occlusion of the common carotid, internal carotid, and ophthalmic arteries have been reviewed,[355] and subsequently other cases have been reported.[3,374] Despite these case reports, it had been felt that carotid artery occlusive disease is not a common cause of neovascular glaucoma because enough collateral circulation usually develops to prevent severe retinal ischemia.[133] We now know that carotid artery occlusive disease is the third most common cause of neovascular glaucoma, accounting for at least 13% of the cases.[47] This is probably an underestimate because carotid occlusive disease may also contribute to the more commonly recognized causes of neovascular glaucoma. Demonstrable common or internal carotid artery atherosclerosis was present in 37% of 35 patients with CRVO.[49] The incidence increased to 50% for the ischemic type of CRVO and decreased to 17% for the nonischemic type.[49] Lazzaro[213] found 6 of 12 patients who presented with CRVO to have carotid artery occlusive disease requiring endarterectomy. He also found that 40% of the patients who were ultimately diagnosed with carotid artery occlusive disease initially presented with CRVO. Concomitant hypertension also increases the frequency and severity of diabetic retinopathy.[194,198,339] In a large series of neovascular glaucoma from all causes, over 50% had arterial hypertension.[47] As our diagnostic techniques for carotid occlusive disease improve and as our success in preventing neovascular glaucoma from CRVO and diabetes mellitus increases, carotid occlusive disease will become a more important cause of neovascular glaucoma and a greater therapeutic challenge.

Neovascular glaucoma actually represents only one manifestation of carotid occlusive disease. The spectrum ranges from transient ischemic attack,[159] to hypoperfusion retinopathy,[147] (previously called venous stasis retinopathy[185]), to ocular ischemic syndrome.[193] It has been proposed that the term chronic ocular ischemia be employed for this confusing array of terms.[332] It has been estimated that evidence of chronic ocular ischemia will be found in 4%[92] to 18%[186] of patients with carotid occlusive disease. These patients will usually be seen by an ophthalmologist first, and it is imperative to consider this condition in a patient with neovascular glaucoma.

Neovascular glaucoma resulting from carotid artery occlusive disease has several unique aspects. Decreased perfusion of the ciliary body from carotid artery obstructive disease significantly decreases aqueous production.[16,166,338] Thus, despite extensive synechial angle-closure, the intraocular pressure may be normal or even low.[76,166,338] In every case of neovascular glaucoma with low intraocular pressure disproportionate to the extent of angle-closure, carotid occlusive disease must be considered in the absence of retinal detachment.[76] After endarterectomy or carotid bypass surgery, aqueous production often returns to the normal preischemic level. Intraocular pressure can increase dramatically, despite the seemingly paradoxical regression of the rubeosis iridis.[76,294,378]

Carotid occlusive disease should also be considered when there is markedly asymmetric diabetic retinopathy, when there is no effect on anterior segment neovascularization after adequate panretinal photocoagulation, and whenever there is no apparent cause for the neovascular glaucoma.

Every ophthalmologist should palpate and auscultate the carotid arteries of patients considered likely to have carotid artery occlusive disease. Asymmetric or absent carotid pulses, as well as presence of cervical bruit, deserve further evaluation. Palpebral carotid arteries or absence of cervical bruit, however, do not rule out possible carotid occlusive disease.[288] Unfortunately, none of the currently available noninvasive tests are totally satisfactory. Such well known tests as ophthalmodynamometry, oculoplethysmography, oculopneumoplethysmography, and Doppler imaging are only able to detect occlusions greater than 80%.[232] All patients with signs and symptoms of carotid occlusive disease and who are surgical candidates must have some sort of arteriography. It is beyond the scope of this chapter to review the diagnostic invasive tests for carotid occlusive disease, but intraarterial[41] and intravenous[148] digital subtraction angiography are being used more frequently than the standard four-vessel carotid arteriography. Endarterectomy is not a benign procedure, with a combined stroke and death rate of 5%.[44] Carotid bypass operation may be a bit safer with a 1% mortality.[335] However, bypass procedures do not increase ocular perfusion as much as endarterectomy.[187] For symptomatic patients, these procedures would seem justifiable because resolution of ocular ischemic findings, including neovascular glaucoma, are well documented.[156,187,192,259] We do not recommend endarterectomy in an asymptomatic patient with neovascular glaucoma.

Other vascular disorders, such as aortic arch syndrome (Takayasu's syndrome),[40,246] carotid-cavernous sinus fistula,[333,364] and temporal arteritis,[36,372] have in common decreased blood flow to the ophthalmic and central retinal artery with secondary retinal-ocular ischemia. In general, occlusive vascular diseases involving the eye are probably underdiagnosed as a primary or aggravating cause of neovascular glaucoma.

Central Retinal Artery Occlusion (CRAO)

Loring[219] first associated neovascular glaucoma with CRAO. The incidence has been variously cited as 1%,[24] 5%,[183] and 7%,[46] with a generally accepted figure of 1% to 2%.[119,133,271] Although the histologic picture of neovascular glaucoma from CRAO is the same as from CRVO,[271] others have thought that this is a distinct clinical entity.[160,373] There is almost always concomitant retinal ischemia from another cause. Of 64 eyes in one series with CRAO, 12 had rubeosis iridis and 10 had neovascular glaucoma.[144] Nine of the 10 eyes with neovascular glaucoma had carotid artery obstructive disease.[144] All of 12 eyes with CRAO and neovascular glaucoma in another series had retinal ischemia from some form of arterial obstructive disease.[48] In a study of 31 consecutive patients with CRAO, 45% of the patients with technically acceptable digital subtraction angiography (29 patients) demonstrated carotid stenosis or an atherosclerotic plaque ipsilateral to the involved eye.[310] It is now believed that CRAO is not responsible for ocular neovascularization.[144]

With CRAO, there is destruction of the inner retinal layer and capillary endothelium.[285] This explains why there is generally no retinal neovascularization in CRAO. In addition, with no viable retinal tissue, the eye would not be capable of inducing a neovascular response elsewhere.[149] If this is so, as Coats asked in 1905,[73] why should there be any neovascular glaucoma at all with CRAO? The proposed pathogenic mechanism is that first there is carotid occlusive disease that causes anterior segment ischemia. This leads to rubeosis iridis and secondary neovascular glaucoma. At the same time, the decreased perfusion of the central retinal artery makes it susceptible to occlusion, especially if there is increased intraocular pressure from the already existent neovascular glaucoma.[48,144] In support of this theory, Hayreh[144] found that seven of nine patients with neovascular glaucoma and CRAO (and concomitant carotid artery obstructive disease) either had neovascular glaucoma before the onset of the CRAO or already had neovascular glaucoma when first seen within 1 to 3 weeks after onset of the CRAO. The remaining two patients were seen 3 and 6 months after the CRAO, and neovascular glaucoma was also already present at that time. In a review of the literature, Hayreh[144] found that the reported time interval between the onset of CRAO and neovascular glaucoma was generally between 1 week and 5 months. However, the presence of neovascular glaucoma was determined mostly by appreciable pain, which may occur long after the appearance of anterior segment neovascularization. Thus, rather than CRAO causing neovascular glaucoma, it is more likely that neovascular glaucoma from carotid artery obstructive disease contributes to the CRAO. There are exceptions to this proposed mechanism. Brown[45] has reported one case of neovascular glaucoma associated with CRAO that did not have any concomitant retinal ischemia, as shown by fundus fluorescein angiography, or carotid artery obstructive disease, as shown by digital subtraction angiography.

Intraocular Tumor

Ellett[91] first noted the association between neovascular glaucoma and untreated malignant melanoma. The incidence in subsequent studies has ranged from 0.5% to 15%. Makley and Teed[234] found that 0.5% of the eyes had rubeosis iridis clinically diagnosed before enucleation for malignant melanoma. That this was a postenucleation review of clinical records without histologic examination may explain this low incidence. In histopathologic studies, Yanoff[375] found that 4% of eyes with malignant melanoma had neovascular glaucoma. Schulze[304] found that 9% of eyes with rubeosis iridis had malignant melanoma. Cappin,[63] in a histopathologic study of 308 eyes with malignant melanoma, found an incidence of rubeosis iridis of 15%. The occurrence of rubeosis iridis correlates with increased tumor size, tumor necrosis, and/or extent of overlying retinal detachment.[52,63,189] With newer treatment modalities for uveal melanomas, Kim et al.[189] found that 13% of 169 patients with uveal melanomas treated with helium ion irradiation developed neovascular glaucoma. Most of their patients with neovascular glaucoma had large tumors and none of them had small tumors. Because the incidence of rubeosis iridis and neovascular glaucoma in untreated malignant melanoma varies from 0.5% to 15%, it is difficult to know if the neovascular glaucoma in this study was from the treatment of the tumor, from the tumor itself, or both. Furthermore, various forms of irradiation had been known to cause neovascular glaucoma.[132,180,265] Lewis et al.[216] reported two eyes with malignant melanoma developing neovascular glaucoma after photoradiation with hematoporphyrin derivative. It was not possible to determine if this neovascularization was caused by the tumor, the irradiation, or the secondary tumor necrosis. In any case, it is clear that the larger the tumor and the greater the retinal involvement, the greater the chances of developing rubeosis iridis and neovascular glaucoma. Associated retinal detachment and tumor necrosis, either spontaneous or radiation induced, are certainly contributory factors. All of these factors have in common production of some degree of retinal hypoxia.

The incidence of neovascular glaucoma with malignant melanoma is not high, and malignant melanoma as a cause of neovascular glaucoma is relatively low on the list of differential diagnoses. Nevertheless, in an eye with neovascular glaucoma in which the posterior segment is not visible because of opaque media, malignant melanoma must be considered, especially in the absence of diabetic retinopathy in the fellow eye or a past history of CRVO.

Howard and Ellsworth[165] had noted the association between retinoblastoma and glaucoma in 1965 but did not elaborate on the incidence of neovascular glaucoma. Walton and Grant[353] found 38 of 56 children with rubeosis iridis to have retinoblastoma. They reviewed 88 eyes enucleated for retinoblastoma and found that 39 eyes (44%) had histologically confirmed rubeosis iridis. Yoshizumi et al.[377] examined 149 eyes enucleated for retinoblastoma and found rubeosis iridis in 30% of the eyes. Gartner and Henkind[119] found an incidence of 72%. Walton and Grant found a significant association between the presence of rubeosis iridis and choroidal involvement by the tumor. Yoshizumi found a significant correlation between rubeosis iridis and tumor involvement of the posterior pole. All of these tumors involved the central or large retinal vessels, or there was diffuse intraretinal infiltration by the tumor. The posterior pole involvement was so consistent that they could predict the presence or absence of rubeosis iridis by histologic examination of the posterior pole only. Walton and Grant found that the duration of retinoblastoma was associated with the development of rubeosis iridis. In children who present with opaque media and rubeosis iridis or neovascular glaucoma, one must consider occult retinoblastoma high on the list. Ultrasound, CT scan, and other appropriate studies must be performed. Rubeosis iridis has also been described in eyes with metastatic tumors[103] and reticulum cell sarcoma.[334]

Postretinal Detachment Surgery

Chronic retinal detachment is a well-known cause of neovascular glaucoma.[9,119,382] Schulze found retinal detachment as the second most common cause (23%) of rubeosis iridis in his series of 105 enucleated eyes with neovascular glaucoma.[304] In children under 5 years of age, Walton and Grant also found that retinal detachment was the second most common cause (32%) of rubeosis iridis.[353] As previously mentioned, persistent retinal detachment is the major cause of postvitrectomy rubeosis iridis and neovascular glaucoma.[360] Several conditions thought to cause neovascular glaucoma may,

in fact, act through a common pathway of secondary retinal detachment. Neovascular glaucoma associated with Coats' disease is also often associated with retinal detachment.[72,304,353] Other reported causes such as X-linked juvenile retinoschisis[167] and laser coreoplasty in Marfan's syndrome[64] also had retinal detachment as a common denominator. Retinal detachment must be considered if an obvious cause of neovascular glaucoma cannot be found since the retina must be reattached, if possible, as the first step in the treatment of neovascular glaucoma.

Miscellaneous Causes

It no longer seems instructive to compile a long list of conditions found to be associated with anterior segment neovascularization. Now that we have a better understanding of the pathophysiology of this condition, we know that there are several common pathways, such as chronic retinal detachment and extensive capillary nonperfusion with resultant retinal hypoxia. In addition to CRVO, sickle cell retinopathy[38,117] and Stickler's syndrome[379] produce neovascular glaucoma by the latter pathway. Decreased ocular perfusion, as with carotid artery obstructive disease, is yet another common pathway. For instance, reported cases of optic disc glioma causing neovascular glaucoma probably result from the enlarging tumor compressing ciliary and retinal vessels with resultant retinal hypoxia.[51] More localized anterior segment perfusion compromise has been shown to be the cause of rubeosis iridis in Fuchs' heterochromic iridocyclitis[273,397] and pseudoexfoliation syndrome.[289] There has not been any documented case of neovascular glaucoma from these two entities, perhaps because the vascular occlusion and secondary hypoxia is so limited. The association between scleritis and neovascular glaucoma is also probably the result of secondary vascular occlusion.[367] As more ocular conditions associated with neovascular glaucoma are found, a careful search should be made for chronic diffuse retinal and/or anterior segment hypoxia, which must be resolved before we can attempt to treat the secondary glaucoma.

MANAGEMENT

As recently as 1974, no means were known to prevent or treat neovascular glaucoma.[133,163] Since 1974, many review articles have appeared on the management of neovascular glaucoma,[31,55,296,361] but preventive treatment has received little attention.[55,357]

Prophylactic Treatment

In 2600 BC, Huang Ti said "the superior physician helps before the early budding of the disease . . . the inferior physician begins to help when disease has already developed." Nowhere else in ophthalmology is this more valid than with neovascular glaucoma. All patients with central retinal vein occlusion should undergo fluoroescein angiography. If it is of the ischemic type, panretinal photocoagulation should be performed as soon as possible. If retinal hemorrhage prevents photocoagulation, the patient should be followed carefully, and treated as soon as the hemorrhage clears. Nonischemic CRVO should also be followed carefully. Without panretinal photocoagulation, approximately 40% of the ischemic type of central retinal vein occlusion will progress to neovascular glaucoma.[145] In several early studies involving small numbers of patients with xenon arc photocoagulation, none of the patients with central retinal vein occlusion treated with panretinal photocoagulation developed neovascular glaucoma.[196,206,237,238] The untreated control patients developed neovascular glaucoma at the expected incidence. Similar results were noted in a small study using the argon and xenon arc coagulator.[164] The largest and most convincing study to date is a series of 100 eyes with ischemic-type central retinal vein occlusion treated by Magargal et al.[230] All eyes received early argon panretinal photocoagulation and none developed neovascular glaucoma. In general, the visual outcome is unchanged whether or not panretinal photocoagulation is performed because the visual acuity has been determined by the primary vascular accident.[196] However, the majority of the treated patients will show some improvement in the visual acuity.[293] Open-angle glaucoma should also be well controlled, especially in the higher risk elderly patients. Because there is frequently a low intraocular pressure in eyes after a CRVO, all eyes with CRVO should be considered suspect and followed accordingly.

For neovascular glaucoma to develop in diabetes mellitus, there must be retinal hypoxia associated with proliferative diabetic retinopathy.[158] It has been well documented that the major factor in the onset of diabetic retinopathy is the duration of the diabetes mellitus.[53,258] However, recent evidence suggests that near-normal glycemia is associated with later development and lesser severity of diabetic retinopathy.[96,276,339] Recent studies in patients started on intensive insulin therapy have shown initial worsening of the retinopathy.[201,245,328] The feeling is that these patients already had advanced diabetic retinopathy and the decreased blood sugar levels resulted in decreased retinal blood flow, which subsequently caused infarction of the marginally perfused retina.[328] One of the most important things we can do is to encourage a diabetic patient to achieve as near normal glycemia as possible. Once diabetic retinopathy is present, many studies have shown panretinal photocoagulation to effectively cause regression of rubeosis iridis.[170,206,218] Only one large study has shown that panretinal photocoagulation in diabetic patients prevents the later development of rubeosis iridis, angle neovascularization, and neovascular glaucoma.[358] In a retrospective study of 93 patients who had received panretinal photocoagulation for proliferative diabetic retinopathy in one eye with the fellow untreated eye serving as control, we found that after an average follow-up of 7 years, there was a significantly lower incidence of anterior segment neovascularization in the treated eye.[358] Finally, another important prophylaxis against neovascular glaucoma is to control hypertension in all diabetic patients.

Prophylactic therapy in carotid occlusive disease is not aimed at preventing anterior segment neovascularization, which is generally not possible, but rather at considering this diagnosis as a cause of neovascular glaucoma. Carotid occlusive disease should always be considered if there is asymmetric severity of diabetic retinopathy between two eyes, in any case of neovascular glaucoma where the intraocular pressure is normal or subnormal, where adequate panretinal photocoagulation has not caused regression of the rubeosis iridis, or when there is no other apparent cause. If unsuspected carotid occlusive disease is detected, and appropriate therapy instituted, potential stroke or death could be averted.

Therapeutic: Early Stage

In the therapy of neovascular glaucoma, the critical aspect is early detection of rubeosis iridis. For that reason, every patient with diabetes, regardless of duration, as well as every patient who has had a CRVO, should have a careful high-powered slit-lamp examination of the iris, especially the pupillary margin. Once rubeosis is discovered, and there is little or no angle involvement, the mainstay in early therapy is panretinal photocoagulation.

Panretinal photocoagulation

Photocoagulation was introduced by Meyer-Schwickerath[241] in 1955 to treat diabetic retinopathy. It was not until 1967 that photocoagulation as we now employ the technique was introduced by Beetham et al.[4] Their observation that other causes of retinal suppression, including photocoagulation, resulted in the arrest of proliferative diabetic retinopathy led them to consider ruby laser photocoagulation as a treatment for diabetic retinopathy.[4] In a large number of unilaterally treated patients, 80% of the treated eyes had definite improvement of the retinopathy versus none of the untreated eyes.[5,20]

How panretinal photocoagulation produces its beneficial effects remains unclear. Since retinal ischemia is critical to the development of anterior segment neovascularization, panretinal photocoagulation must somehow eliminate the source and/or antagonize the effects of the angiogenesis factor. The effectiveness of various lasers is more dependent on the amount of retina treated than on the type of laser employed.[150] This is in agreement with studies showing that other forms of retinal destruction such as xenon arc photocoagulation,[86] retinal diathermy,[11] and retinal cryotherapy* also have beneficial effects on preventing and causing regression of anterior segment neovascularization.

Wolbarsht and Landers[371] believe that retinal hypoxia causes chronic dilation of the retinal vessels, which in turn is the cause of new vessel formation. When panretinal photocoagulation is performed, the destruction of the rods and cones allows more choroidal oxygen to reach the inner retina and constrict the blood vessels.[371] They note that two thirds of the total retinal oxygen consumption is in the outer photoreceptor-retinal pigment epithelium complex[365] and that photocoagulation, at least by the argon laser, selectively damages this outer higher oxygen consuming layer.[191,280] Retinal vessels show autoregulation by dilating with low ambient oxygen levels and constricting with high oxygen levels.[10] Studies in animals have shown increased preretinal oxygen concentration after photocoagulation,[250,325,326] and laser Doppler studies have confirmed retinal vessel constriction and decreased retinal blood flow after photocoagulation.[102]

Despite appealing aspects of this theory, many questions remain unanswererd. Outside the macula, there is no difference in the retinal lesions produced by argon green, argon blue-green, and krypton red lasers.[319,320] Recent studies have shown that krypton and argon lasers produce damage to the choroidal vessels and that this damage may persist

up to 14 months.[178,369] If there is persistent choriocapillaris damage after photocoagulation, an increased oxygen supply from the choroid might not be expected after photocoagulation.[369] Perry and Risco[272] have shown that there is repair of the choriocapillaris after photocoagulation, but that if the intensity of the photocoagulation was increased, this damage was permanent.[329] Further studies comparing the integrity of the choriocapillaris after photocoagulation with the preretinal oxygen levels are necessary to confirm the validity of the Wolbarsht-Landers theory. Glaser et al.[61] have shown that vascular endothelial cells can produce a chemoattractant for retinal pigment epithelial cells and that human retinal pigment epithelial cells can release an inhibitor of vascular endothelial cell proliferation and neovascularization.[127] When the normal single layer of retinal pigment epithelial cells is altered in vitro, there is increased production of this inhibitor.[126,268] It is now thought that the alteration of the retinal pigment epithelial layer after laser photocoagulation may induce release of this inhibitor.[126] These studies open exciting areas of research and will certainly help elucidate the mechanisms of angiogenesis, as well as how photocoagulation exerts its beneficial effects.

In practice, the most common cause of "failed" panretinal photocoagulation is inadequate photocoagulation.[224] According to the guidelines of the Diabetic Retinopathy Study, a total of 1200 to 1600 500μm burns should be applied randomly over the peripheral retina.[10] More than this number of photocoagulation burns may be necessary to effect regression of neovascularization.[317] Twelve hundred spots represents less than one fourth of the total confluent 500 μm spots that can be placed on the average extramacular retinal area of a human eye.[17] Many retinal specialists feel a minimum of 1500 to 2000 800 μm spots using the Rodenstock wide-angle fundus contact lens is necessary to constitute adequate panretinal photocoagulation[224] (Fig. 60-26). The Rodenstock lens produces an 800 μm size retinal lesion, so a correspondingly greater number of lesions must be produced if the Goldmann lens is employed.[17] It is still not certain whether the argon or krypton laser is clinically better, but if there is some opacity in the media, or if there are retinal hemorrhages present, the krypton laser will frequently be more effective than the argon laser.

When adequate panretinal photocoagulation is performed early in the course of rubeosis iridis, there is ample documentation that there is regres-

---

*References 43, 157, 169, 236, 249, 270, 301.

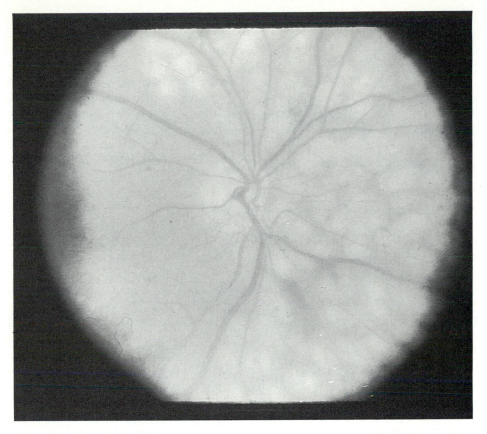

Fig. 60-26   Example of adequate panretinal photocoagulation in a patient with proliferative diabetic retinopathy. Photocoagulation marks are confluent and should number 1500 to 2000 if the Rodenstock lens (800 μm spot size) is employed.

sion of the iris vessels in central retinal vein occlusion,[39,56,200,218] and diabetes mellitus.[170,218] Even with carotid occlusive disease, where the hypoxia may not be limited to the retina alone, panretinal photocoagulation can still produce a diminution of iris vessels until more definitive therapy can be instituted.[65,89] Thus, panretinal photocoagulation is the most important early treatment for rubeosis iridis. Obviously, if the cause is a detached retina or an ocular tumor, the therapy must be directed at these primary causes.

Endophotocoagulation

In some situations it is not possible to perform preoperative panretinal photocoagulation in an eye with rubeosis iridis, and intraocular surgery, such as cataract extraction or vitrectomy, must be performed. Increased postoperative risks of developing neovascular glaucoma in such a situation have already been noted, and postoperative vitreous hemorrhages could prevent postoperative photocoagulation. Charles[67] used a xenon arc photocoagulator with a fiberoptic probe intraoperatively in 60 eyes undergoing vitrectomy for complications of proliferative diabetic retinopathy. Thirteen percent developed postoperative neovascular glaucoma, compared with 7 of 12 similar eyes (58%), that did not receive any photocoagulation. There are major problems with the xenon endophotocoagulator. The tip of the probe must be extremely close (0.1 to 0.5 mm) to the retina, and iatrogenic retinal tears are sometimes unavoidable. The long cooling-off period between each application means that at least 30 minutes is required to perform adequate xenon endophotocoagulation.[357] The argon endophotocoagulator overcomes these disadvantages because the argon probe can be effective from the middle of the vitreous cavity, and there is no cooling-off period.[107] Recently, a method for performing endophotocoagulation with indirect ophthalmoscopy has been described; this technique allows better visualization of the fundus.[138] Histologic studies in monkeys[211] and rabbits[274] have shown primarily outer retinal layer damage, comparable to argon laser lesions via the standard slit-lamp delivery system. One human eye, which had received argon endophotocoagulation when the vitreous cavity was filled with air, showed full-thickness retinal involvement.[177] We know that endophotocoagulation can be just as effective as standard photocoagulation, and this procedure is now used extensively, especially during vitrectomy.[50,68,177,242] In high risk eyes, endophotocoagulation is valuable in providing a "head-start" on retinal photocoagulation. In many cases, further photocoagulation needs to be performed via the slit-lamp at a later time.[357]

Panretinal cryotherapy

In cases where the cornea, lens, or vitreous is too hazy to allow adequate retinal photocoagulation, there is a role for panretinal cryotherapy.* May et al.[236] perform a 360-degree peritomy with isolation of the four rectus muscles. A 2.5 mm retinal cryoprobe is employed, with the first row of applications just anterior to the equator, three spots between each rectus muscle. Two additional rows of cryoapplications are placed posteriorly so that the third row is just outside the major vascular arcades, for a total of 32 applications. This is accomplished under direct visualization, and the tip is in contact with the sclera until − 70° C is achieved (approximately 5 to 10 sec, depending on the probe). Pavan and Folk[270] perform a total of 54 applications in separate sessions 2 weeks apart with one half of the eye being treated at each session. As might be expected, cryopexy over an area of retinal detachment has no effect because the retina is not touched by the freezing. This is a major operation producing significantly more inflammation and blood-retinal barrier breakdown than panretinal photocoagulation, as shown by vitreous fluorophotometry.[169] Potential complications include traction and exudative retinal detachment and vitreous hemorrhage. The reported results have been encouraging,[43] and there seems to be an added, though as yet unexplained, benefit of facilitating the clearance of existing vitreous blood.[257,264,306] We have employed this technique on occasion with some success, but a prospective controlled study is necessary to show its real role in the therapy of neovascular glaucoma.

Goniophotocoagulation

In 1966, when the use of lasers in ophthalmology was still fairly new, Farnarier et al.[97] considered direct laser treatment of the new iris vessels before neovascular glaucoma developed. In 1973, DalFiume et al.[79] used the argon laser to treat 10

eyes at various stages of rubeosis iridis. He treated the pupillary margin, the peripheral iris, and the angle. Of the four glaucomatous eyes, there was no reduction of the intraocular pressure. One normotensive eye had an acute rise in intraocular pressure. The remaining five eyes did not develop synechial angle closure, but there was never total obliteration of the new vessels. Follow-up was only a few months.

Direct treatment of the new iris vessels was attempted again by Simmons et al.[313,314] They reported a total of 88 eyes treated with direct laser applications to the angle vessels, with a 73% overall success rate as defined by elimination of angle vessels in the treated area, prevention of further angle-closure in the treated area, and maintenance of intraocular pressure below 25 mm Hg. However, 38% of their eyes also had concurrent panretinal photocoagulation or panretinal cryotherapy, and they did not break down the success rate with and without this adjuvant therapy. The natural history of untreated diabetic retinopathy is rather unpredictable, and spontaneous arrest and even regression of rubeosis iridis is well known.[123,226] Up to one third of eyes with rubeosis iridis have shown spontaneous regression.[146] Unfortunately, the only way to determine the efficacy of this treatment is through a prospective randomized study. One study has evaluated the effect of preoperative goniophotocoagulation on the success of filtration surgery. Allen et al.[8] did not find any beneficial effects of goniophotocoagulation, but their patient population was small, and it was not possible to fully evaluate their data.

When goniophotocoagulation was first introduced in 1977, the role and efficacy of panretinal photocoagulation in the treatment of neovascular glaucoma was still being evaluated. It was believed that there might be cases where goniophotocoagulation might provide "a period of grace to delay imminent synechial angle closure until the definitive effect of the panretinal photocoagulation can manifest itself."[357] However, since then, in a limited number of patients in whom it was not possible to perform panretinal photocoagulation, goniophotocoagulation alone has not proven beneficial in preventing synechial angle-closure and, at times, has caused increased inflammation and seemingly more rapid progression of angle neovascularization. At this stage, until a prospective randomized study is performed, the role of goniophotocoagulation in the treatment of neovascular glaucoma remains unclear.

---

*References 43, 157, 236, 249, 257, 264, 270, 301.

Medical therapy

Before synechial angle-closure has occurred, it is possible to have a secondary open-angle glaucoma caused by the fibrovascular membrane accompanying the angle vessels. Of course, there can be a concomitant open-angle glaucoma component in patients with diabetic retinopathy or CRVO anyway. Under these circumstances, all of the standard antiglaucoma medications will be effective to some degree in lowering the intraocular pressure, but one should not be lulled into a false sense of security regarding medical therapy. Unless panretinal photocoagulation is performed, the angle can relentlessly close. The two medications that are probably of the greatest use during this period are topical atropine 1% twice per day to decrease ocular congestion[60,355] and topical steroids four times per day to decrease ocular inflammation.[30,355]

Therapeutic: Late Stage

Panretinal photocoagulation

When synechial angle-closure has already occurred, this is considered the late stage. If possible, panretinal photocoagulation or panretinal cryotherapy should still be performed to eliminate the stimulus for new vessel formation. Synechial angle-closure cannot be reversed with panretinal photocoagulation, but further closure can be prevented. We have seen remarkable regression of rubeosis iridis within days of completed photocoagulation. Without elimination of the stimulus for new vessel formation, any filtration surgery is doomed to failure. After panretinal photocoagulation has been completed, it is most important to allow adequate time for as much regression of the new vessels as possible and for the eye to quiet down. At least 1 week, and preferably 3 to 4 weeks, should elapse between completed photocoagulation and filtration surgery. Generally, eyes with neovascular glaucoma do not have as compromised optic nerve heads as in advanced chronic open-angle glaucoma, and can tolerate pressures below 50 mm Hg for this time span.[359] If possible, adequate disc perfusion should be confirmed by observing for the absence of central retinal artery pulsation.[359]

Medical therapy

With extensive synechial angle-closure, any of the medications acting on aqueous outflow, such as pilocarpine or phospholine iodide, are useless, and, in fact, contraindicated because of the hyperemia they produce. For the same reasons, epinephrine and dipivefrin should not be used. Medications that decrease aqueous production, such as topical beta-blockers and carbonic anhydrase inhibitors, are beneficial but may not lower the intraocular pressure to a normal range in the face of a closed angle. Osmotic agents can be used intermittently to clear the cornea enough for treatment and/or diagnosis. The most important medications remain topical atropine and topical steroids to decrease congestion and inflammation and prepare the eye for definitive surgery.

Conventional surgery

If there are engorged iris vessels at the time of surgery, intraoperative and postoperative hemorrhages are major complications. The presence of active neovascularization leads to late bleb failure through conjunctival scarring at the filtration site. With the advent of panretinal photocoagulation to eliminate the neovascularization stimulus, surgical treatment of neovascular glaucoma has entered a new era. The surgical treatment before the widespread use of panretinal photocoagulation, such as employing electrocautery iridotomy,[93] diathermy iridotomy,[227] bipolar microcautery,[151,152,267] nonpenetrating cyclodiathermy,[214] or even removing the superior half of the iris to eliminate the source of bleeding,[70] had been directed toward controlling bleeding during surgery. Carbon dioxide laser, because of its ability to cauterize and cut simultaneously, has been employed to perform trabeculotomy in a relatively bloodless manner;[19,215,346] and the whole anterior segment has been bypassed in a pars plana filtration technique.[315] To prevent postoperative scarring of the filtration bleb, beta-irradiation has been tried.[57] There have been many other interesting and even novel surgical techniques, but the number of cases involved are small and the follow-up too short to provide any meaningful information. These reports have been reviewed[133,355] and are of historical interest only. It is well accepted now that whatever the surgical procedure, preoperative panretinal photocoagulation should be performed whenever possible.[8,106,202,253]

Filtration technique. After adequate panretinal photocoagulation, administration of topical atropine and steroids, and enough time for the eye to quiet down, the patient is ready for surgery. If the pressure is very high, osmotic agents may be employed preoperatively, if the general medical status permits, to avoid sudden surgical decompression of a hard eye. Retrobulbar anesthesia with epinephrine plus orbital massage is preferred to soften the eye further and reduce vascular congestion. A preplaced paracentesis incision into the anterior chamber is performed at the temporal limbus to allow for slow decompression of a firm eye, to irrigate blood from the anterior chamber if necessary, and to allow reformation of the anterior chamber and filtration bleb at the end of the procedure.

Microsurgical techniques are mandatory, with special emphasis on delicate handling of tissue and meticulous hemostasis. A limbus-based conjunctival flap is made at least 10 mm posterior to the limbus in the superior nasal quadrant so that the temporal nasal quadrant will be available for additional filtration surgery if necessary. The dissection to the limbus is made between conjunctiva and Tenon's capsule to minimize bleeding and to provide a thin flap. The final dissection to the limbus is carried to the peripheral cornea with a combination of blunt dissection with a spatula, and sharp dissection with a Beaver 67 blade or equivalent. Cautery is applied to even the smallest bleeding point, with care taken to avoid heating the conjunctival flap. Tenon's capsule is carefully removed with smooth curve scissors, avoiding the episcleral vessels.

At this point, a full-thickness procedure, such as a trephine or posterior lip sclerectomy, or a guarded procedure, such as a trabeculectomy, may be performed, depending on the surgeon's choice. The results appear to be the same regardless of which procedure is employed.[8] When the peripheral iridectomy is performed, if some new vessels remain on the iris, preiridectomy cautery to the iris is possible when the iris is lifted by the forceps. Not infrequently, even with this precaution, some bleeding will occur with the iris surgery. Irrigation of the anterior chamber with balanced saline solution via the previously made paracentesis incision will usually keep the anterior chamber clear until the bleeding stops spontaneously. Occasionally, topical epinephrine may be necessary, but postiridectomy cautery to the iris or ciliary body is to be avoided. After hemostasis is achieved, the conjunctival flap is closed with 8-0 vicryl sutures, approximating the conjunctival flap edges and incorporating the posterior edge of Tenon's capsule to help prevent the incision from migrating anteriorly toward the filtration area. The anterior chamber and bleb are formed with balanced saline solution through the paracentesis opening. Topical steroids and antibiotics are applied and a single eye patch and protective shield placed over the eye.

Postoperative medications include topical atropine two to three times per day, topical steroids four to six times per day, and topical antibiotics four times per day.

Using this technique, Allen et al.[8] achieved a success rate of 67% in patients with neovascular glaucoma. Success was defined as intraocular pressures less than 25 mm Hg with the patient on no more than on one medication. True failure (no light perception vision) was only 17%. The average follow-up was over 22 months.

Postoperatively, the filtration bleb tends to be more limited in size, appears less succulent, and often has a characteristic ring of conjunctival and episcleral vessels, which delineate the base of the bleb[355,359] (Fig. 60-27). Because panretinal photocoagulation would not be expected to ablate all of the ischemic retina, it is logical that some angiogenesis factor would still be present. The base of the filtration bleb is probably the new main interface between the aqueous (and the angiogenesis factor) and the potential vascular bed. The intraocular pressure in successful filtration with neovascular glaucoma tends to be somewhat higher than with open-angle glaucoma, but because the optic nerve is usually not as compromised in neovascular glaucoma, a slightly higher postoperative pressure may be tolerable.

Valve implant surgery. Because one of the major problems with filtration surgery in neovascular glaucoma is failure of the filtration bleb through conjunctival–Tenon's capsule–episcleral scarring, a natural idea would be to employ some physical means to maintain an opening between the anterior chamber and the subconjunctival space. Countless different materials have been tried, including many kinds of sutures, metals, and plastics in various sheet, tube, or wire forms. None of them worked very well, and their history has been reviewed.[94,324,355] With the development of newer nonallergenic plastics, and the knowledge of how previous stents and valves have failed, new implants have been developed for use with neovascular glaucoma and other refractory glaucomas.

Filtration surgery in neovascular glaucoma should be reserved for eyes that have useful vision, bearing in mind that almost any vision is worth preserving in eyes with proliferative diabetic retinopathy. Honrubia et al.[161,162] have used a simple silicone tube connecting the anterior chamber to a trabeculectomy flap. Molteno[255] uses a drainage implant that has undergone several modifications. Initially, it was a translimbal silicone tube connecting the anterior chamber to a methacrylate

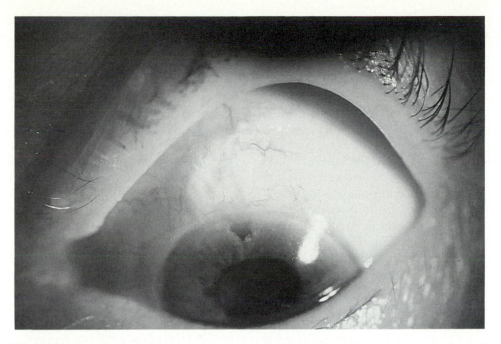

Fig. 60-27   Successful trabeculectomy in a patient with neovascular glaucoma from central retinal vein occlusion. Panretinal photocoagulation was performed several weeks before the surgery. Note the characteristic ring of conjunctival-episcleral vessels delineating the filtration bleb.

plate placed beneath Tenon's capsule posterior to the equator to form an unilocular cavity for aqueous drainage. Because of the large surface area of this cavity, scarring of the surrounding conjunctiva did not affect the drainage from the anterior chamber. Postoperative hypotony was an early complication, with resultant choroidal detachment and intraocular hemorrhages.[251] A two-stage procedure was then developed whereby the plate and tube were placed in position, but the tube was not put into the anterior chamber initially. After 6 to 8 weeks, when enough connective tissue had formed around the plate to form a defined cavity, the silicone tube was inserted into the anterior chamber.[253] This has been modified once more so that now the tube is placed into the anterior chamber primarily along with the plate, but the tube is closed off with a 5-0 vicryl suture. When the vicryl suture absorbs in 3 to 5 weeks, enough fibrosis has occurred around the plate to prevent severe hypotension.[254]

Schocket et al.[302] used a silicone tube connecting the anterior chamber to a subconjunctival encircling equatorial silicone band to serve as the drainage cavity. To decrease postoperative hypotony, they have subsequently added a viscoelastic agent into the anterior chamber at the end of the procedure.[305] Another way to avoid the problem of

postoperative hypotony is the Krupin-Denver implant, which employs a Silastic valve that opens at 11 to 14 mm Hg.[57,202] White,[366] and Joseph et al.[181] have developed similar valve devices to prevent hypotony. The number of patients involved in some of these studies are too small to adequately evaluate.[366] Honrubia at el.[161,162] reported 63% success in controlling intraocular pressure (25 mm Hg or less) in 59 eyes using the simple silicone tube. Molteno and Haddad[253] reported 83% success in controlling the intraocular pressure (20 mm Hg or less) in 24 patients using variations of his implant in his initial series of eyes with neovascular glaucoma; in his second series of 24 eyes with neovascular glaucoma, he did not report the success rate regarding the intraocular pressure control. The largest reported series of valve implant surgery used the Krupin-Denver valve. Seventy-nine eyes with neovascular glaucoma were operated on, with a 67% success in controlling intraocular pressure (24 mm Hg or less); mean follow-up was 23 months. This success rate was exactly the same as reported by Forestier and Salvenet-Bonccara[112] using the Krupin-Denver valve in nine eyes with neovascular glaucoma.

The problems with all these stent and valve procedures remain the same: early postoperative hypotony, blockage of the internal fistula, and blockage of the external filtration site. Postoperative hypotony and flat anterior chamber, with all its attendant complications, are problems common to all filtration procedures but are certainly more frequent with a drainage device. Obstruction of the internal fistula is unique to the usage of a drainage device, and there appears to be no way currently available to prevent this. A recent report noted an intense foreign body-giant cell reaction around the Supramid portion of the Krupin-Denver valve and raises the question of tolerance to these intraocular devices.[108] The problem of conjunctival scarring is also common to all filtration procedures. In a small series of 10 patients, Sutton et al.[337] had nine failures (intraocular pressure 29 mm Hg or greater, or phthisis) using the Krupin-Denver valve. They felt that valves do not eliminate the fibrosis of the posterior subconjunctival drainage site. In experimental studies in monkeys, a new type of valve draining the vitreous cavity through the sclera, choroid, and retina into the retrobulbar space ultimately failed also because of fibrous incapsulation of the outflow system.[137] Molteno[252] employed systemic steroids, fluphenamic acid (a prostaglandin inhibitor) and colchicine, as well as topical steroids, atropine, and epinephrine for 6 weeks postoperatively. With this regimen, it is difficult to separate the effects of the drainage device from the antiinflammatory regimen.

There is greater promise at the moment in the employment of 5-fluorouracil, an antimetabolite with antifibroblastic activity, which seems to decrease the incidence of bleb failures.[154,155] Subconjunctival injections of 5-fluorouracil seem to be less toxic than topical administration.[153] Rockwood et al.[292] employing subconjunctival 5-fluorouracil, reported a 2 year success rate of 62% in 29 eyes with neovascular glaucoma. The real key in the ultimate success of filtration surgery in neovascular glaucoma is the prevention of filtration bleb scarring. Whether preoperative elimination of the angiogenesis factor through panretinal photocoagulation, the postoperative use of antifibroblastic agents, or the use of various mechanical devices is the answer to successful filtration remains to be seen. Only prospective studies comparing these different methods will give us the answer. Until then, the primary thrust of surgical intervention in neovascular glaucoma must begin with adequate panretinal photocoagulation and/or panretinal cryotherapy.

End Stage Neovascular Glaucoma

When there is total synechial angle-closure and no useful vision remaining, there is no indication for surgical intervention, and control of pain becomes the primary therapeutic aim.

Medical

Most often, the combination of topical atropine 1% twice a day, and topical steroids four times a day, provides enough symptomatic relief, despite pressures as high as 60 mm Hg, to eliminate the need for other treatment. When there is corneal microcystic edema, the combination of these drops with a bandage soft contact lens is frequently effective.

Cyclocryotherapy

When medical therapy does not provide relief, cyclocryotherapy should be considered. Cyclocryotherapy was introduced in 1950 by Bietti.[30] This procedure probably produces its hypotensive effect by destruction of the secretory ciliary epithelium.[282,323] DeRoetth[82,84] revived this method of therapy in 1966 when he treated several large series of glaucoma patients with high success and low complication rates.[82,84] In 1972, Goldstein and Ide[131] reported the results of cyclocryotherapy in three patients with neovascular glaucoma. All three eyes had transient (months) lowering of the intraocular pressure, aggravation of the rubeosis iridis, and relief of ocular pain. Faulborn and Hoster[98] and Boniuk[38] also achieved high success in the control of pain with cyclocryotherapy. The relief of pain is one of the major benefits of cyclocryotherapy and may occur despite persistent corneal edema and high intraocular pressures. Grant[133] attributed the beneficial effects to partial freezing of the corneal sensory nerves. Feibel and Bigger[101] presented the first large series of cyclocryotherapy on neovascular glaucoma. In 38 patients with neovascular glaucoma, they achieved 63% success in controlling the intraocular pressure, but almost 40% had posttreatment hypotony. Krupin et al. confirmed this high complication rate.[203] They found that 34% achieved intraocular pressures 25 mm Hg or less, 34% developed phthisis, and 57% lost all light perception. Their study employed 360 degrees of cyclocryotherapy, and the other studies all employed different techniques. Bellows and Grant[23] introduced a protocol that standardized the treatment regimen and allowed sensible comparison of data between studies. Essentially, they treated only 180 degrees of the ciliary body at one time, employing six spots of freezing, 2.5 mm posterior to the limbus. The 3.5 mm probe reached −60°C to −80°C and was left in place for one minute. Employing this technique, the complication rate was lower, but still higher than acceptable.[22] Bellows[22] found that 45% of 43 eyes with neovascular glaucoma had good intraocular pressure control, but 33% lost all light perception and another 25% had a significant decrease in vision.[22] At this time, we believe that cyclocryotherapy should be reserved for achieving comfort in the treatment of neovascular glaucoma. If saving functional vision is not a factor and relief of pain is the main consideration, cyclocryotherapy is a useful technique.

Other cyclodestructive procedures

Other forms of cyclodestructive procedures have been tried. DeRoetth[83] employed cyclodiathermy on two eyes with neovascular glaucoma, but both eyes developed phthisis. Subsequently, others tried cyclodiathermy with good results, but the number of eyes was small.[11,92] Walton and Grant[354] performed 100 penetrating cyclodiathermy procedures on 53 eyes with various refractory glaucomas. They had a success rate of 5% in lowering the intraocular pressure (25 mm Hg or less for greater than 4 months), and produced phthisis in another 5%. They concluded that the beneficial effects of cyclodiathermy was low. Recently, attempts have been made to treat the ciliary body under direct visualization through a scleral flap.[25,135] Riaskoff and Pameyer[286] presented a series of 21 eyes with neovascular glaucoma treated with direct diathermy of the dissected ciliary body. All

eyes had intraocular pressures below 30 mm Hg, but 10 eyes also received cyclocryotherapy. In addition, 17 eyes lost more vision, 7 eyes had postoperative hyphema, and "a number of eyes" developed postoperative hypotony. At this stage, cyclodiathermy appears to be more destructive than cyclocryotherapy, without offering any real advantages.

Several newer methods of cyclodestruction appear promising. Transpupillary argon cyclophotocoagulation allows the direct visualization of the ciliary processes.[248] This procedure is possible only if there is marked pupillary dilation from ectropion uveae or if a large sector iridectomy is already present so that the ciliary processes are visible with a goniolens. Of course, the cornea also must be clear enough to allow adequate visualization. The major problem with the procedure is that only the anterior aspect of the ciliary processes are accessible to treatment. Our argon laser settings have been 100 μm 0.1 sec, and approximately 500 to 1000 mW to produce confluent whitening of all visible ciliary processes (Fig. 60-28). We have obtained some success in transiently lowering the intraocular pressure, but the patient population is too small to report. Because this is a relatively benign procedure, where possible, it should be tried before surgical intervention. Shields[311] has developed an endoscopic argon photocoagulator that would allow di-

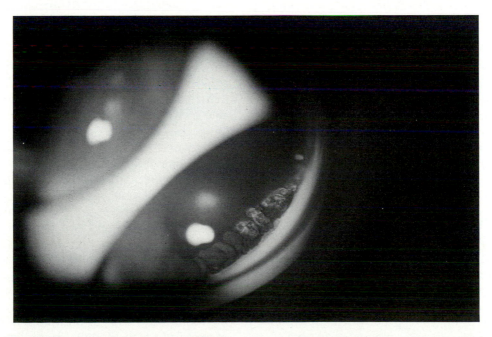

Fig. 60-28 Goniophotograph of aphakic eye with sector iridectomy that has undergone partial transpupillary argon cyclophotocoagulation. Right half of ciliary processes are white and confluent after adequate treatment.

rect visualization of all surfaces of the ciliary processes; this appears to be a promising approach to quantitate the amount of ciliary ablation. Blacharski and Charles[32] have reported preliminary results (average follow-up 7.3 weeks) on four eyes that received endocyclophotocoagulation. More definitive studies are needed to assess the role of this technique. Intraocular carbon dioxide photocautery is another procedure being evaluated.[247] Finally, transscleral cyclophotocoagulation with the Nd: YAG laser is another potential method of controlled cyclodestruction.[182,305]

Pituitary ablation

For historical interests only, pituitary ablation as a treatment for diabetic retinopathy should also be mentioned. In 1953, Poulson[279] reported regression of diabetic retinopathy in a woman who developed postpartum pituitary necrosis. Unfortunately, the patient had only background diabetic retinopathy, which is known to frequently undergo spontaneous regression.[123,226] Based on this one case report, numerous studies have been published,[54,220,295] but all had been faulted, either by being uncontrolled or by having too few patients to achieve statistical significance.[113] Pituitary ablation is a destructive procedure with high morbidity and mortality and without clear evidence that it is beneficial. With the current availability of other high benefit-low risk prophylactic and therapeutic treatments for diabetic retinopathy, pituitary ablation should be relegated to the realm of medical history.

Alcohol injection

We have not found any case where pain could not be controlled with a combination of topical atropine and steroid or, infrequently, cyclocryotherapy. However, others have used retrobulbar alcohol injection with long-lasting relief of pain.[244] The major complications are temporary blepharoptosis or external ophthalmoplegia.[263] Rarely, enucleation may have to be performed for intractable pain.

Future Prospects

Since the last review on neovascular glaucoma just 5 years ago,[355] there has been a geometric growth in our knowledge about angiogenesis and the clinical conditions initiating this neovascularization process and in our ability to translate this knowledge into effective prophylactic and therapeutic regimens. There is no question that our knowledge will continue to expand at this rapid

rate because many recent studies point to imminent major breakthroughs. Abnormal accumulation of sorbitol, a sugar alcohol product of the sorbitol pathway mediated by the enzyme aldose reductase, has been implicated in the pathogenesis of several diabetic complications. In diabetic and galactosemic rats, the intracellular accumulation of the sugar alcohols, sorbitol and galactolol, have been shown to initiate cataract formation,[116] delay reepithelization of the cornea,[81] and decrease motor nerve conduction velocity.[380] One of the hallmarks of early diabetic retinopathy is selective loss of retinal mural cells.[75] Thickening of the capillary basement membrane is another characteristic of diabetes mellitus.[188] It has now been shown that the enzyme aldose reductase is in the cytoplasm of human retinal mural cells[7] and that galactose-induced retinal capillary basement membrane thickening is prevented by Sorbinil, an aldose reductase inhibitor.[114,291] In diabetic rats, Sorbinil has been shown to reduce sciatic nerve sorbitol concentration and improve motor nerve conduction velocity.[380] In a preliminary study, 8 of 11 patients with painful diabetic neuropathy, unresponsive to other medications, had moderate to marked relief of symptoms with corresponding improved autonomic nerve function.[173] In the near future, aldose reductase inhibitors may be able to prevent the complications of diabetes mellitus, including neovascular glaucoma.

On another front, inhibitors of neovascularization have been found in the bovine aorta,[90] bovine vitreous,[222] human lens,[368] and human retinal pigment epithelial cells.[127] Undoubtedly, we will witness the isolation and characterization of various inhibitors of the angiogenesis process, with clinical applications not far behind. To aid this research, an in vitro angiogenesis assay is now available to detect and quantitate angiogenesis. Most important, this test now offers the possibility to differentiate between direct and indirect angiogenesis factors.[110] In the future, the genetic basis of diabetes mellitus and other predisposing conditions of neovascular glaucoma may be elucidated and all the information presented here will be of historical interest only.

To end on a sobering note, despite what we are now capable of doing to prevent and treat neovascular glaucoma, this knowledge is not being disseminated. Eighteen months after the publication of the Diabetic Retinopathy Study, 72% of family physicians and 54% of internists were not aware of this study or its therapeutic implications.[330] Even more frightening, Sussman et al[336] found that in examining eyes of diabetic patients, proliferative diabetic retinopathy was missed by 52% of internists, 50% of medical residents, 33% of diabetologists, and 9% of general ophthalmologists! We cannot use what we have not learned.

REFERENCES

1. Aaberg, TM: Pars plana vitrectomy for diabetic traction retinal detachment, Am Acad Ophthalmol 88:639, 1981
2. Aaberg, TM, and Van Horn, DL: Late complications of pars plana vitreous surgery, Ophthalmology 85:126, 1978
3. Abedin, S, and Simmons, RJ: Neovascular glaucoma in systemic occlusive vascular disease, Ann Ophthalmol 14:284, 1982
4. Aiello, LM, et al: Ruby laser photocoagulation and treatment of diabetic proliferating retinopathy. In: Goldberg, MF, and Fine, SL, editors: Symposium on the treatment of diabetic retinopathy, Pub No 1890, Washington, DC, 1969, US Public Health Service
5. Aiello, LM, and Briones, JC: Ruby laser photocoagulation of proliferating diabetic retinopathy: fifth year follow-up, Int Ophthalmol Clin 16:15, 1976
6. Aiello, LM, Wand, M, and Liang, G: Neovascular glaucoma and vitreous hemorrhage following cataract surgery in patients with diabetes mellitus, Ophthalmology 90:814, 1983
7. Akagi, Y, et al: Aldose reductase localization in human retinal mural cells, Invest Ophthalmol Vis Sci 24:1516, 1983
8. Allen, RC, et al: Filtration surgery in the treatment of neovascular glaucoma, Ophthalmology 89:1181, 1982
9. Anderson, DM, Morin, DJ, and Hunter, WS: Rubeosis iridis, Can J Ophthalmol 6:183, 1971
10. Anderson, F, Jr, Saltzman, HA, and Frayser, R: Changes in arterial pCO_2 and retinal vessel size with oxygen breathing, Invest Ophthalmol 6:416, 1967
11. Ando, A, and Kyu, N: Surgical treatment of hemorrhagic glaucoma (peripheral retinal diathermy), Folia Ophthalmol Jpn 24:113, 1973
12. Armaly, MF, and Baloglou, PJ: Diabetes and the eye. I. Changes in the anterior segment, Arch Ophthalmol 77:485, 1967
13. Ashton, N: Retinal vascularization in health and disease, Am J Ophthalmol 44:7, 1957
14. Ashton, N, Ward, B, and Serpell, G: Effect of oxygen on developing retinal vessels with particular reference to the problem of retrolental fibroplasia, Br J Ophthalmol 38:397, 1954
15. Bagessen, LH: Fluorescein angiography of the iris in diabetics and nondiabetics, Acta Ophthalmol 47:449, 1969
16. Barany, E: Influence of local arterial blood pressure on aqueous humor and intraocular pressure, Acta Ophthalmol 24:337, 1946
17. Barr, CC: Estimation of the maximum number of argon laser burns possible in panretinal photocoagulation, Am J Ophthalmol 97:697, 1984
18. Beasley, H: Rubeosis iridis in aphakic diabetics, JAMA 213:128, 1970
19. Beckman, H, and Fuller, TA: Carbon dioxide laser scleral dissections and filtering procedure for glaucoma, Am J Ophthalmol 88:73, 1979
20. Beetham, WP, et al: Ruby laser photocoagulation of early diabetic neovascular retinopathy, Arch Ophthalmol 83:261, 1970
21. Bellhorn, RW: Control of blood vessel development, Trans Ophthalmol Soc UK 100:328, 1980
22. Bellows, AR: Cyclocryotherapy for glaucoma, Int Ophthalmol Clin 21:99, 1981
23. Bellows, AR, and Grant, WM: Cyclocryotherapy in advanced inadequately controlled glaucoma, Am J Ophthalmol 75:679, 1973
24. Benedict, WL: The clinical significance of closure of the retinal vessels, JAMA 38:423, 1949
25. Benedikt, O, and Hiti, H: Die Ziliarkorperfreilegung. Eine neue Operationsmethode zur Behandlung des irreversiblen Winkelblockglaukoms und des Aphakieglaukoms, Klin Mbl Augenheilkd 169:711, 1976
26. Ben Ezra, D: Neovasculogenic ability of prostaglandins, growth factors, and synthetic chemoattractants, Am J Ophthalmol 86:455, 1978
27. Ben Ezra, D: Neovasculogenesis: triggering factors and possible mechanisms, Surv Ophthalmol 24:167, 1979
28. Bertelsen, TI: The relationship between thrombosis in the retinal vein and primary glaucoma, Acta Ophthalmol 39:603, 1961
29. Beyer, TL, et al: Protective barrier effect on the posterior lens capsule in exogenous bacterial endophthalmitis, Invest Ophthalmol Vis Sci 25:108, 1984
30. Bietti, G: Surgical intervention on the ciliary body: new trends for the relief of glaucoma, JAMA 142:889, 1950
31. Blach, RK, Hitchings, RA, and Laatikainen, L: Thrombotic glaucoma: prophylaxis and management, Trans Ophthalmol Soc UK 97:275, 1977
32. Blacharski, PA, and Charles, S: Endocyclophotocoagulation, Ophthalmic Laser Surg 2:13, 1987
33. Blankenship, G, Cortez, R, and Machemer, R: The lens and pars plana vitrectomy for diabetic retinopathy complications, Arch Ophthalmol 97:1263, 1979
34. Blankenship, GW, and Skyler, JS: Diabetic retinopathy: a general survey, Diabetes Care 1:127, 1978
35. Bloodworth, JMB, Jr, and Engerman, RL: Diabetic microangiopathy in the experimentally-diabetic dog and its prevention by careful control with insulin, Diabetes 22:290, 1973
36. Boberg-Ans, J, and Vesti Nielsen, N: Neovascular glaucoma as the primary ocular complication in temporal arteritis, Glaucoma 8:138, 1986
37. Codansky, HJ, et al: Diabetic retinopathy and its relation to type of diabetes: review of a retinal clinic population, Br J Ophthalmol 66:596, 1982

38. Boniuk, M: Cryotherapy in neovascular glaucoma, Trans Am Acad Ophthalmol Otolaryngol 78:337, 1974

39. Bouchon, JDG, et al: Traitement du glaucome secondaire à néovascularisation de l'iris (rubeose de l'iris), par la photocoagulation, Ann Ocul 209:439, 1976

40. Bouzas, MA: Les manifestations oculaires de la maladie de Takayasu avant et après l'opération, Bull Soc Ophthalmol Fr 69:560, 1969

41. Brant-Zawadzki, M, et al: Digital subtraction cerebral angiography by intraarterial injection: comparison with conventional angiography, AJNR 3:593, 1982

42. Brem, S, et al: Inhibition of neovascularization by an extract derived from vitreous, Am J Ophthalmol 84:323, 1977

43. Brodell, LP, et al: Neovascular glaucoma: a retrospective analysis of treatment with peripheral panretinal cryotherapy, Ophthalmic Surg 18:200, 1987

44. Brott, TG, Labutta, RJ, and Kempczinski, RF: Changing patterns in the practice of carotid endarterectomy in a large metropolitan area, JAMA 255:2609, 1986

45. Brown, GC: Isolated central retinal artery obstruction in association with ocular neovascularization, Am J Ophthalmol 96:110, 1983

46. Brown, GC, Magargal, LE, and Federman, JL: Ischaemia and neovascularization, Trans Ophthalmol Soc UK 100:377, 1980

47. Brown, GC, et al: Neovascular glaucoma: etiologic considerations, Ophthalmology 91:315, 1984

48. Brown, GC, et al: Arterial obstruction and ocular neovascularization, Ophthalmology 89:139, 1982

49. Brown, GC, et al: Central retinal vein obstruction and carotid artery disease, Ophthalmology 91:1627, 1984

50. Brucker, AJ, et al: New instrumentation for fluid-air exchange, Retina 3:135, 1983

51. Buchanan, TAS, and Hoyt, WF: Optic nerve glioma and neovascular glaucoma: report of a case, Br J Ophthalmol 66:96, 1982

52. Buiera, K: Necrotic malignant melanomas of the choroid and ciliary body: a clinicopathological and statistical study, Graefes Arch Clin Exp Ophthalmol 291:40, 1982

53. Caird, RI, Pirie, A, and Ramsell, TG: Diabetes and the eye, Oxford, England, 1968, Blackwell Scientific Publications, Ltd

54. Caird, FI, Pirie, A, and Ramsell, TG: Diabetes and the eye, Oxford, England, 1969, Blackwell Scientific Publications, Ltd

55. Cairns, JE: Rationale for therapy in neovascular glaucoma, Trans Ophthalmol Soc UK 101:184, 1981

56. Callahan, MA, and Hilton, GF: Photocoagulation and rubeosis iridis, Am J Ophthalmol 78:873, 1974

57. Cameron, ME: Thrombotic glaucoma successfully treated, Trans Ophthalmol Soc UK 93:537, 1973

58. Campbell, DG, Simmons, RJ, and Grant, WM: Ghost cells as a cause of glaucoma, Am J Ophthalmol 81:441, 1976

59. Campbell, DG, Shields, MB, and Smith, TR: The corneal endothelium and the spectrum of essential iris atrophy, Am J Ophthalmol 86:317, 1978

60. Campinchi, R, and Haut, J: Traitement exceptionnel de cértains glaucomes absolus par l'atropine, Bull Soc Ophthalmol Fr 66:10, 1966

61. Campochiaro, PA, and Glaser, BM: Endothelial cells release a chemoattractant for retinal pigment epithelial cells in vitro, Arch Ophthalmol 103:1876, 1985

62. Canny, CLB, O'Hanley, GP, and Wells, GA: Pars plana vitrectomy for the complications of diabetic retinopathy: a report on 131 cases, Can J Ophthalmol 20:11, 1985

63. Cappin, JM: Malignant melanoma and rubeosis iridis, Br J Ophthalmol 57:815, 1973

64. Carroll, RP, and Landers, MB: Pinwheel rubeosis iridis following argon laser coreoplasty, Ann Ophthalmol 7:357, 1975

65. Carter, JE: Panretinal photocoagulation for progressive ocular neovascularization secondary to occlusion of the common carotid artery, Ann Ophthalmol 16:572, 1984

66. Chandler, PA, and Grant, WM: Lectures on glaucoma, Philadelphia, 1965, Lea & Febiger

67. Charles, S: Endophotocoagulation, Retina 1:117, 1981

68. Charles S, and Wang, C: A motorized gas injector for vitreous surgery, Arch Ophthalmol 99:1398, 1981

69. Chen, CH, and Chen, SC: Angiogenic activity of vitreous and retinal extract, Invest Ophthalmol Vis Sci 19:596, 1980

70. Christensen, RL, and Meyer, SL: Neovascular glaucoma: a new surgical approach, Trans Am Acad Ophthalmol Otolaryngol 75:372, 1975

71. Chu, KM, Chen, TT, and Lee, PF: Clinical results of pars plana vitrectomy in posterior segment disorders, Ann Ophthalmol 17:686, 1985

72. Coats, G: Forms of retinal disease with massive exudation, Royal London Ophthalmic Hosp Rep 17:440, 1908

73. Coats, G: Further cases of thrombosis of the central vein, Royal London Ophthalmic Hosp Rep 16:516, 1906

74. Cobb, B, Shilling, JS, and Chisholm, IH: Vascular tufts at the pupillary margin in myotonic dystrophy, Am J Ophthalmol 69:573, 1970

75. Cogan, DG, Toussaint, D, and Kuwabara, T: Retinal vascular patterns, IV. Diabetic retinopathy, Arch Ophthalmol 66:366, 1961

76. Coppeto, J, and Wand, M: Neovascular glaucoma and carotid vascular occlusion, Am J Ophthalmol 99:567, 1985

77. Cunha-Vaz, JG: Blood-retinal barriers in health and disease, Trans Ophthalmol Soc UK 100:337, 1980

78. Cunha-Vaz, JG, et al: Early breakdown of the blood-retinal barrier in diabetes, Br J Ophthalmol 59:649, 1975

79. Dalfiume, E, Saccol, G, and Verzella, F: Rubeosis iridea trattamento mediante fotocoagulatore laser di argon, Arch Rass Ital Ottal 3:19, 1973

80. D'Amore, PA, et al: Angiogenic activity from bovine retina: partial purification and characterization, Proc Natl Acad Sci 78:3068, 1981

81. Datiles, MB, et al: Corneal re-epithelialization in galactosemic rats, Invest Ophthalmol Vis Sci 24:563, 1983

82. DeRoetth, A: Cryosurgery for the treatment of glaucoma, Am J Ophthalmol 61:443, 1966

83. DeRoetth, A: Cyclodiathermy in treatment of glaucoma due to rubeosis iridis diabetica, Arch Ophthalmol 35:20, 1946

84. DeRoetth, A: Cryosurgery for treatment of advanced chronic simple glaucoma, Am J Ophthalmol 66:1034, 1968

85. Deutsch, TA, and Hughes, WF: Suppressive effects of indomethacin on thermally induced neovascularization of rabbit corneas, Am J Ophthalmol 87:436, 1979

86. Diabetic Retinopathy Study Research Group: Preliminary report on effects of photocoagulation therapy, Am J Ophthalmol 81:383, 1976

87. Dodson, PM, et al: Retinal vein occlusion and the prevalence of lipoprotein abnormalities, Br J Ophthalmol 66:161, 1982

88. Duke-Elder, S: System of ophthalmology, vol 2, Diseases of the lens and vitreous; glaucoma and hypotony, St Louis, 1969, The CV Mosby Co

89. Eggleston, TF, et al: Photocoagulation for ocular ischemia associated with carotid artery occlusion, Ann Ophthalmol 12:84, 1980

90. Eisenstein, R, et al: The inhibition of corneal vascularization with aortic extracts in rabbits, Am J Ophthalmol 88:1005, 1979

91. Ellett, EC: Metastatic carcinoma of choroid. III. Rubeosis iridis with melanoma of the choroid and secondary glaucoma, Am J Ophthalmol 27:726, 1944

92. Ellis, PP: Regression of rubeosis iridis following cyclodiathermy, Am J Ophthalmol 40:253, 1955

93. Ellis, PP, Thompson, RL, and Tyner, GS: A modified filtering operation for hemorrhagic glaucoma, Am J Ophthalmol 50:733, 1960

94. Ellis, RA: Reduction of intraocular pressure using plastics in surgery, Am J Ophthalmol 50:733, 1960

95. Epstein, DL, et al: Experimental perfusions through the anterior and vitreous chambers with possible relationships to malignant glaucoma, Am J Ophthalmol 88:1078, 1979

96. Eschwege, E, et al: Delayed progression of diabetic retinopathy by divided insulin administration: a further follow-up, Diabetologia 16:13, 1979

97. Farnarier, G, Rampin, S, and Lancon, M: La rubeose iriénne diabetique, Ann Ocul 199:574, 1966

98. Faulborn, J, and Hoster, K: Ergebnisse der Zyklokryotherapie beim haemorrhagischen Glaukom, Klin Monatsbl Augenheilkd 162:513, 1973

99. Federman, JL, et al: Experimental ocular angiogenesis, Am J Ophthalmol 89:231, 1980

100. Fehrmann, H: Uber Rubeosis iridis diabetica and ihre allegemein-medizinische Bedeutung; mit anatomischem Befund, v Graefe's Arch Ophthalmol Klin Exp 140:354, 1939

101. Feibel, RM, and Bigger, JF: Rubeosis iridis and neovascular glaucoma, Am J Ophthalmol 74:862, 1972

102. Feke, GT, et al: Laser doppler measurements of the effect of panretinal photocoagulation on retinal blood flow, Ophthalmology 89:757, 1982

103. Ferry, AP, and Font, RL: Carcinoma metastatic to the eye and orbit, Arch Ophthalmol 93:472, 1975

104. Fett, JW, et al: Isolation and characterization of angiogenin, an angiogenic protein from human carcinoma cells, Biochemistry 24:5480, 1985

105. Finkelstein, D, et al: Experimental retinal neovascularization induced by intravitreal tumors, Am J Ophthalmol 83:660, 1987

106. Flanagan, DW, and Blach, RK: Place of panretinal photocoagulation and trabeculectomy in the management of neovascular glaucoma, Br J Ophthalmol 67:526, 1983

107. Fleischman, JA, Swartz, M, and Dixon, JA: Argon laser endophotocoagulation: an intraoperative trans-pars plana technique, Arch Ophthalmol 99:1610, 1981

108. Folberg, R, et al: Filtering valve implant for neovascular glaucoma in proliferative diabetic retinopathy, Ophthalmology 89:286, 1982

109. Folkman, J: The vascularization of tumors, Sci Am 234:59, 1976

110. Folkman, J, and Haudenschild, C: Angiogenesis by capillary endothelial cells in culture, Trans Ophthalmol Soc UK 100:346, 1980

111. Folkman, J, et al: Isolation of a tumor factor responsible for angiogenesis, J Exp Med 133:275, 1971

112. Forestier, F, and Salvanet-Bouccara, A: An evaluation of the Krupin-Denver valve implant in glaucoma, Glaucoma 8:92, 1986

113. Frank, RN: Diabetic retinopathy. In Ryan, ST, and Smith, RE, editors: Selected topics on the eye in systemic disease, New York, 1974, Grune and Stratton, Inc

114. Frank, RN, et al: Galactose-induced retinal capillary basement membrane thickening: prevention by Sorbinil, Invest Ophthalmol Vis Sci 24:1519, 1983

115. Fromer, CH, and Klintworth, GK: An evaluation of the role of leukocytes in the pathogenesis of experimentally induced corneal vascularization, Am J Pathol 82:157, 1976

116. Fukushi, S, Merola, LO, and Kinoshita, JH: Altering the course of cataracts in diabetic rats, Invest Ophthalmol Vis Sci 19:313, 1980

117. Galinos, S, et al: Hemoglobin SC disease and iris atrophy, Am J Ophthalmol 75:421, 1973

118. Garner, A, and Kissun, RD: Ocular angiogenesis in disease states, Trans Ophthalmol Soc UK 100:381, 1980

119. Gartner, S, and Henkind, P: Neovascularization of the iris (rubeosis iridis), Surv Ophthalmol 22:291, 1978

120. Gartner, S, Taffet, S, and Friedman, AH: The association of rubeosis iridis with endothelialisation of the anterior chamber: report of a clinical case with histopathological review of 16 additional cases, Br J Ophthalmol 61:267, 1977

121. Georgiades, G: Les lesions de l'iris heterochromique en general, Bulletins et memoires de la Societe Francaise d'Ophthalmologie 77:465, 1964

122. Gerich, JE: Insulin-dependent diabetes mellitus: pathophysiology, Mayo Clin Proc 61:787, 1986

123. Gerritzen, FM: The course of diabetic retinopathy: a longitudinal study, Diabetes 22:122, 1973

124. Gimbrone, MA, et al: Tumor angiogenesis: iris neovascularization at a distance from experimental intraocular tumors, J Natl Cancer Inst 50:219, 1973

125. Gimbrone, MA, et al: Tumor growth and neovascularization: an experimental model using rabbit cornea, J Natl Cancer Inst 52:413, 1974

126. Glaser, BM: Angiogenesis and inhibitors of neovascularization, Ophthalmology (In press)

127. Glaser, BM, et al: Retinal pigment epithelial cells release an inhibitor of neovascularization, Arch Ophthalmol 103:1870, 1985

128. Glaser, BM, D'Amore, PA, and Michels, RG: The effect of human intraocular fluid on vascular endothelial cell migration, Ophthalmology 88:986, 1981

129. Glaser, BM, et al: The demonstration of angiogenic activity from ocular tissues, Ophthalmology 87:440, 1980

130. Glatt, HJ, et al: Effect of irradiation on vascularization of corneas grafted onto chorioallantoic membranes, Invest Ophthalmol Vis Sci 26:1533, 1985

131. Goldstein, AL, and Ide, CH: Cyclocryotherapy for secondary glaucoma due to rubeosis iridis, Mo Med 69:736, 1972

132. Gragoudas, ES, et al: Current results of proton beam irradiation of uveal melanomas, Ophthalmology 92:284, 1985

133. Grant, WM: Management of neovascular glaucoma. In Leopold, IH, editor: Symposium on ocular therapy, vol 7, St Louis, 1974, The CV Mosby Co

134. Greenblatt, M, and Shubik, P: Tumor angiogenesis: transfilter diffusion studies in the hamster by the transparent chamber technique, J Natl Cancer Inst 41:111, 1968

135. Grote, P, and Harms, H: Erste Ergebnisse der direkten Ziliarkorperfreilegung bei sekundarem Winkelblockglaukom. II. Histologische Befunde, Klin Mbl Augenheilk 173:625, 1978

136. Gu, QX, et al: Ocular neovascularization, Arch Ophthalmol 103:111, 1985

137. Haas, JS, Peyman, GA, and Lim, J: Experimental evaluation of a posterior drainage system, Ophthalmic Surg 14:494, 1983

138. Hampton, GR: Argon endophotocoagulation with indirect ophthalmoscopy, Arch Ophthalmol 105:132, 1987

139. Hayreh, SS: Occlusion of the central retinal vessels, Br J Ophthalmol 49:626, 1965

140. Hayreh, SS: Ocular neovascularization, Arch Ophthalmol 98:574, 1980

141. Hayreh, SS: Classification of central retinal vein occlusion, Ophthalmology 90:458, 1983

142. Hayreh, SS, and Hayreh, MS: Hemi-central retinal vein occlusion, Arch Ophthalmol 98:1600, 1980

143. Hayreh, SS, March, W, and Phelps, CD: Ocular hypotony following retinal vein occlusion, Arch Ophthalmol 96:827, 1978

144. Hayreh, SS, and Podhajsky, P: Ocular neovascularization with retinal vascular occlusion. II. Occurence in central and branch retinal artery occlusion, Arch Ophthalmol 100:1585, 1982

145. Hayreh, SS, et al: Ocular neovascularization with retinal vascular occlusion. III. Incidence of ocular neovascularization with retinal vein occlusion, Ophthalmology 90:488, 1983

146. Hayreh, SS, van Heuven, WAJ, and Hayreh, MS: Experimental retinal vascular occlusion. I. Pathogenesis of central retinal vein occlusion, Arch Ophthalmol 96:311, 1978

147. Hedges, TR: Ophthalmoscopic findings in internal carotid artery occlusion, Johns Hopkins Med J 111:89, 1962

148. Hedges, TR, Giliberti, OL, and Magargal, L: Intravenous digital subtraction angiography and its role in ocular vascular disease, Arch Ophthalmol 103:666, 1985

149. Henkind, P, and Wise, GN: Retinal neovascularization, collaterals, and vascular shunts, Br J Ophthalmol 58:413, 1974

150. Hercules, B, et al: Peripheral retinal ablation in the treatment of proliferative diabetic retinopathy: a three-year interim report of a randomized, controlled study using the argon laser, Br J Ophthalmol 61:555, 1977

151. Hersch, SB, and Kass, MA: Iridectomy in rubeosis iridis, Ophthalmic Surg 7:19, 1976

152. Herschler, J, and Agness, D: A modified filtering operation for neovascular glaucoma, Arch Ophthalmol 97:2339, 1979

153. Heuer, DK, et al: Topical fluorouracil. II. Postoperative administration in an animal model of glaucoma filtering surgery, Arch Ophthalmol 104:132, 1986

154. Heuer, DK, et al: 5-Fluorouracil and glaucoma filtering surgery, Ophthalmology 91:384, 1984

155. Heuer, DK, et al: 5-Fluorouracil and glaucoma filtering surgery. III. Intermediate follow-up of a pilot study, Ophthalmology 93:1537, 1986

156. Higgins, RA: Neovascular glaucoma associated with ocular hypoperfusion secondary to carotid artery disease, Australian J Ophthalmol 12:155, 1984

157. Hilton, G: Panretinal cryotherapy of diabetic rubeosis, Arch Ophthalmol 97:776, 1979

158. Hohl, RD, and Barnett, DM: Diabetic hemorrhagic glaucoma, Diabetes 19:994, 1970

159. Hollenhorst, RW: Ocular manifestations of insufficiency or thrombosis of the internal carotid artery, Trans Am Ophthalmol Soc 56:472, 1958

160. Holm, A, Sachs, J, and Wilson, A: Glaucoma secondary to occlusion of the central retinal artery, Am J Ophthalmol 48:530, 1959

161. Honrubia, FM, et al: Long-term results of silicone tube in filtering surgery for eyes with neovascular glaucoma, Am J Ophthalmol 97:501, 1984

162. Honrubia, FM, et al: Surgical treatment of neovascular glaucoma, Trans Ophthalmol Soc UK 99:89, 1979

163. Hoskins, HD: Neovascular glaucoma: current concepts, Trans Am Acad Ophthalmol Otolaryngol 78:330, 1974

164. Hovener, G: Photocoagulation for central retinal vein occlusion, Klin Monatsbl Augenheilkd 173:392, 1978

165. Howard, GM, and Ellsworth, RM: Differential diagnosis of retinoblastoma, Am J Ophthalmol 60:618, 1965

166. Huckman, MS, and Haas, J: Reversed flow through the ophthalmic artery as a cause of rubeosis iridis, Am J Ophthalmol 74:1094, 1972

167. Hung, E, and Hilton, GF: Neovascular glaucoma in a patient with X-linked juvenile retinoschisis, Ann Ophthalmol 12:1054, 1980

168. Isenberg, SJ, McRee, WE, and Jedrzynski, MS: Conjunctival hypoxia in diabetes mellitus, Invest Ophthalmol Vis Sci 27:1512, 1986

169. Jaccoma, EH, Conway, BP, and Campochiaro, PA: Cryotherapy causes extensive breakdown of the blood-retinal barrier, Arch Ophthalmol 103:1728, 1985

170. Jacobson, DR, Murphy, RP, and Rosenthal, AR: The treatment of angle neovascularization with panretinal photocoagulation, Ophthalmology 86:1270, 1979

171. Jaffe, NS: Cataract surgery and its complications, St Louis, 1972, The CV Mosby Co

172. Jaffe, NS: Cystoid macular edema: a fluorescein angiographic study. In. Emergy, JM, and Jacobson, AC, editors: Current concepts in cataract surgery; selected proceedings of the sixth Biennial Cataract Surgical Congress, St Louis, 1980, The CV Mosby Co

173. Jaspan, J, et al: Treatment of severely painful diabetic neuropathy with an aldose reductase inhibitor: relief of pain and improved somatic and autonomic nerve function, The Lancet 2:758, 1983

174. Jensen, VA, and Lundbock, K: Fluorescein angiography of this iris in recent and long-term diabetes: preliminary communication, Acta Ophthalmol 46:584, 1968

175. Jocson, VL: Microvascular injection studies in rubeosis iridis and neovascular glaucoma, Am J Ophthalmol 83:508, 1977

176. John, T, Sassani, JW, and Eagle, RC: The myofibroblastic component of rubeosis iridis, Ophthalmology 90:721, 1983

177. Johnson, RN, Irvine, AR, and Wood, RS: Endolaser, cryopexy, and retinal reattachment in the air-filled eye, Arch Ophthalmol 105:231, 1987

178. Johnson, RN, Irvine, AR, and Wood, IS: Histopathology of krypton red laser panretinal photocoagulation: a clinicopathologic correlation, Arch Ophthalmol 105:235, 1987

179. Johnston, RL, et al: Risk factors of branch retinal vein occlusion, Arch Ophthalmol 103:1831, 1985

180. Jones, RF: Glaucoma following radiotherapy, Br J Ophthalmol 42:636, 1958

181. Joseph, NH, et al: A one-piece drainage system for glaucoma surgery (In press)

182. Kankhauser, F, et al: Transscleral cyclophotocoagulation using a neodymium YAG laser, Ophthalmic Surg 17:94, 1986

183. Karjalainen, K: Occlusion of the central retinal artery and retinal branch arterioles: a clinical, tonographic and fluorescein angiographic study of 175 patients, Acta Ophthalmol Suppl 109:9, 1971

184. Kearns, TP: Differential diagnosis of central retinal vein obstruction, Ophthalmology 90:475, 1983

185. Kearns, TP, and Hollenhorst, RW: Venous-stasis retinopathy of occlusive disease of the carotid artery, Mayo Clin Proc 38:304, 1963

186. Kearns, TP, Siekert, RG, and Sundt, TM: The ocular aspects of bypass surgery of the carotid artery, Mayo Clin Proc 54:3, 1979

187. Kearns, TP, Young, BR, and Piepgras, DG: Resolution of venous stasis retinopathy after carotid artery bypass surgery, Mayo Clin Proc 55:342, 1980

188. Kilo, C, Vogler, N, and Williamson, JR: Muscle capillary basement membrane changes related to aging and to diabetes mellitus, Diabetes 21:881, 1972

189. Kim, MK, et al: Neovascular glaucoma after helium ion irradiation for uveal melanoma, Ophthalmology 93:189, 1986

190. Kimura, R: Fluorescein goniophotography, Glaucoma 2:359, 1980

191. Kincaid, MD, et al: An ocular clinicopathologic correlative study of six patients from the diabetic retinopathy study, Retina 3:21, 1983

192. Kiser, WD, et al: Recovery of vision following treatment of the ocular ischemic syndrome, Ann Ophthalmol 15:305, 1983

193. Knox, DL: Ischemic ocular inflammation, Am J Ophthalmol 60:995, 1965

194. Knowles, WC, Bennett, PH, and Ballentine, EJ: Increased incidence of diabetic retinopathy and elevated blood pressure, N Engl J Med 302:645, 1980

195. Knowles, HC, Jr: The problem of the relation of the control of diabetes to the development of vascular disease, Trans Am Clin Climatol Assoc 76:142, 1964

196. Kohner, EM, Laatikainen, L, and Oughton, J: The management of central retinal vein occlusion, Ophthalmology 90:484, 1983

197. Kohner, EM, Shilling, JS, and Hamilton, AM: The role of avascular retina in new vessel formation, Metabolic Ophthalmol 1:15, 1976

198. Kornerup, T: Blood pressure and diabetic retinopathy, Acta Ophthalmol 35:163, 1957

199. Kottow, MW: Anterior segment fluorescein angiography, Baltimore, 1978, The Williams & Wilkins Co

200. Krill, AE, Archer, D, and Newell, FW: Photocoagulation in complications secondary to branch vein occlusion, Arch Ophtahlmol 85:48, 1971

201. The KROC Collaborative Study Group: Blood glucose control and the evolution of diabetic retinopathy and albuminuria: a preliminary multicenter trial, N Engl J Med 311:365, 1984

202. Krupin, T, et al: Long-term results of valve implants in filtering surgery for eyes with neovascular glaucoma, Am J Ophthalmol 95:775, 1983

203. Krupin, T, Mitchell, KB, and Becker, B: Cyclocryotherapy in neovascular glaucoma, Am J Ophthalmol 86:24, 1978

204. Kurachi, K, et al: Sequence of the cDNA and gene for angiogenin, a human angiogenesis factor, Biochemistry 24:5494, 1985

205. Kurz, O: Zur Rubeosis iridis diabetica, Arch Augenheilkd 110:284, 1937

206. Laatikainen, L: Preliminary report on effect of retinal photocoagulation on rubeosis iridis and neovascular glaucoma, Br J Ophthalmol 61:278, 1977

207. Laatikainen, L., and Blach, RK: Behavior of the iris vasculature in central retinal vein occlusion: a fluorescein angiographic study of the vascular response of the retina and the iris, Br J Ophthalmol 61:272, 1977

208. Laatikainen, L, and Kohner, EM: Fluorescein angiography and its prognostic significance in central retinal vein occlusion, Br J Ophthalmol 64:411, 1976

209. Laatikainen L, et al: Panretinal photocoagulation in central retinal vein occlusion: a randomised controlled clinical study, Br J Ophthalmol 61:741, 1977

210. Laatinkainen, L: Development and classification of rubeosis iridis in diabetic eye disease, Br J Ophthalmol 63:156, 1979

211. Landers, MB, et al: Argon laser intraocular photocoagulation, Ophthalmology 89:785, 1982

212. Langer, R, et al: Isolation of a cartilage factor that inhibits tumor neovascularization, Science 183:70, 1976

213. Lazzaro, EC: Retinal-vein occlusions: carotid artery evaluation indicated, Ann Ophthalmol 18:116, 1986

214. Lee, P, Shihab, ZM, and Fu, Y: Modified trabeculectomy: a new procedure for neovascular glaucoma, Ophthalmic Surg 11:181, 1980

215. L'Esperance, FA, Jr, and Mittl, RN: Carbon dioxide laser trabeculostomy for the treatment of neovascular glaucoma, Trans Am Ophthalmol Soc 80:262, 1982

216. Lewis, RA, et al: Neovascular glaucoma after photoradiation therapy for uveal melanoma, Arch Ophthalmol 102:839, 1984

217. Linnér, E: Discussion of Bertelsen, TI: The relationship between thrombosis in the retinal vein and primary glaucoma, Acta Ophthalmol 39:603, 1961

218. Little, HL, et al: The effect of panretinal photocoagulation on rubeosis iridis, Am J Ophthalmol 81:804, 1976

219. Loring, EG: Remarks on embolism, Am J Med Sci 67:313, 1874

220. Lundback, K, et al: Hypophysectomy for diabetic angiopathy. In Goldberg, MF, and Fine, SC, editors: Symposium on the treatment of diabetic retinopathy, Washington, DC, 1969, U.S. Government Printing Office

221. Luntz, M, and Schenker, HI: Retinal vascular accidents in glaucoma and ocular hypertension, Survey Ophthalmol 25:163, 1980

222. Lutty, GA, et al: Vitreous: an inhibitor of retinal extract–induced neovascularization, Invest Ophthalmol Vis Sci 24:52, 1983

223. Machemer, R, et al: Vitrectomy: a pars plana approach, Trans Am Acad Ophthalmol Otolaryngol 75:813, 1971

224. Madigan, JC, and Gaudio, AR: Personal communication

225. Madsen, PH: Haemorrhagic glaucoma: comparative study in diabetic and non-diabetic patients, Br J Ophthalmol 55:444, 1971

226. Madsen, PH: Rubeosis of the iris and haemorrhagic glaucoma in patients with proliferative diabetic retinopathy, Br J Ophthalmol 55:369, 1971

227. Madsen, PH: Experiences in surgical treatment of haemorrhagic glaucoma, Acta Ophthalmol Suppl 120:88, 1973

228. Magargal, LE, et al: Neovascular glaucoma following branch retinal vein obstruction, Glaucoma 3:333, 1981

229. Magargal, LE, et al: Neovascular glaucoma following central retinal vein obstruction, Ophthalmology 88:1095, 1981

230. Magargal, LE, et al: Efficacy of panretinal photocoagulation in preventing neovascular glaucoma following ischemic central retinal vein obstruction, Am Acad Ophthalmol 89:780, 1982

231. Magargal, LE, Donoso, LA, and Sanborn, GE: Retinal ischemia and risk of neovascularization following central retinal vein obstruction, Ophthalmology 89:1241, 1982

232. Magargal, LE, and Sanborn, GE: The ocular ischemic syndrome: carotid artery disease and the eye, Geriatr Ophthalmol 2:38, 1986

233. Magargal, LE, et al: Temporal branch retinal vein obstruction: a review. Ophthalmic Surg 17:240, 1986

234. Makley, TA, and Teed, RW: Unsuspected intraocular malignant melanoma, Arch Ophthalmol 60:475, 1950

235. Mason, GI: Iris neovascular tufts: relationship to rubeosis, insulin, and hypotony, Arch Ophthalmol 97:2346, 1979

236. May, DR, et al: Treatment of neovascular glaucoma with transcleral panretinal cryotherapy, Ophthalmology 87:1106, 1980

237. May, DR, Klein, ML, and Peyman, GA: A prospective study on xenon arc photocoagulation for central retinal vein occlusion, Br J Ophthalmol 60:816, 1976

238. May, DR, et al: Xenon arc panretinal photocoagulation for central retinal vein occlusion: a randomised prospective study, Br J Ophthalmol 63:725, 1979

239. McAuslan, BR, and Gole, GA: Cellular and molecular mechanisms in angiogenesis, Trans Ophthalmol Soc UK 100:354, 1980

240. McGrath, MA, et al: Systemic factors contributory to retinal vein occlusion, Arch Intern Med 138:216, 1978

241. Meyer-Schwickerath, G: Lichtkoagulation, Stuttgart, Germany, 1959, Enke Verlang

242. Michaels, RG; Vitrectomy techniques in retinal reattachment surgery, Ophthalmology 86:556, 1979

243. Michaels, RG: Vitrectomy for complications of diabetic retinopathy, Arch Ophthalmol 96:237, 1978

244. Michaels, RG, and Maumenee, AE: Retrobulbar alcohol injection in seeing eyes, Trans Am Acad Ophthalmol Otolaryngol 77:164, 1973

245. Michaelson, IC: The mode of development of the vascular system of the retina with some observations of its significance in certain retinal diseases. Trans Ophthalmol Soc UK 68:137, 1948

246. Milan, B, and Josip, K: Maniféstations oculaires dans le syndrome de l'arc de l'aorte, Ann Ocul 200:1168, 1967

247. Miller, JB, Smith, MR, and Boyer, DS: Intraocular carbon dioxide laser photocautery, Ophthalmology 87:1112, 1980

248. Mochizuki, M: Transpupillary cyclophotocoagulation in hemorrhagic glaucoma: a case report, Jpn J Ophthalmol 19:191, 1975

249. Mohan, V, and Eagling, EM: Peripheral retinal cryotherapy as a treatment for neovascular glaucoma, Trans Ophthalmol Soc UK 98:93, 1978

250. Molnar, I, et al: Effect of laser photocoagulation on oxygenation of the retina in miniature pigs, Invest Ophthalmol Vis Sci 26:1410, 1985

251. Molteno, ACB: Advanced buphthalmos treated by implants, S Afr Arch Ophthalmol 1:55, 1973

252. Molteno, ACB: Mechanisms of intraocular inflammation, Trans Ophthalmol Soc NZ 32:69, 1980

253. Molteno, ACB, and Haddad, PJ: The visual outcome in cases of neovascular glaucoma, Aust NZ J Ophthalmol 13:329, 1985

254. Molteno, ACB, Polkinghorne, PJ, and Bowbyes, JA: The vicryl tie technique for inserting a draining implant in the treatment of secondary glaucoma (In press)

255. Molteno, ACB, Van Rooyen, MB, and Bartholomew, RS: Implants for draining neovascular glaucoma, Br J Ophthalmol 61:120, 1977

256. Moore, RF: Some observations on the intraocular tension in cases of thrombosis of the retinal veins, Trans Ophthalmol Soc UK 42:115, 1922

257. Mosier, MA, Del Piero, E, and Gheewala, SM: Anterior retinal cryotherapy in diabetic vitreous hemorrhage, Am J Ophthalmol 100:440, 1985

258. Nathan, DM, et al: Retinopathy in older type II diabetics: association with glucose control, Diabetes 35:797, 1986

259. Neupert, JR, et al: Rapid resolution of venous stasis retinopathy after carotid endarterectomy, Am J Ophthalmol 81:600, 1976

260. Nomura, T: Pathology of anterior chamber angle in diabetic neovascular glaucoma: extension of corneal endothelium onto iris surface, Jpn J Ophthalmol 27:193, 1983

261. Ohrt, V: Glaucoma due to rubeosis iridis diabetica, Ophthalmologica 142:356, 1961

262. Ohrt, V: The frequency of rubeosis iridis in diabetic patients, Acta Ophthalmol 49:301, 1971

263. Olurin, O, and Osuntokun, O: Complications of retrobulbar alcohol injections, Ann Ophthalmol 10:474, 1978

264. Oosterhuis, JA, and Bijlmer-Gorter, H: Cryotreatment in proliferative diabetic retinopathy, Ophthalmologica 181:81, 1980

265. Packer, S, Rotman, M, and Salanitro, P: Iodine-125 irradiation of choroidal melanoma: clinical experience, Ophthalmology 91:1700, 1984

266. Pagenstecher, M: Beitrage zur Lehre vom hämorrhagischen Glaucom, v Graefes Arch Klin Exp Ophthalmol 17:98, 1871

267. Parrish, R, and Herschler, J: Eyes with end-stage neovascular glaucoma: natural history following successful modified filtering operation, Arch Ophthalmol 101:745, 1983

268. Patz, A: A new look at the retinal pigment epithelium and its neighbors, Arch Ophthalmol 103:1794, 1985

269. Patz, A, et al: Branch retinal venous occlusion, Trans Am Acad Ophthalmol Otolaryngol 83:373, 1977

270. Pavan, PR and Folk, JC: Anterior neovascularization, Int Ophthalmol Clinic 24:61, 1984

271. Perrault, E, and Zimmerman, LW: The occurrence of glaucoma following occlusion of the central retinal artery, Arch Ophthalmol 61:845, 1959

272. Perry, DD, and Risco, JM: Choroidal microvascular repair after argon laser photocoagulation, Am J Ophthalmol 93:787, 1982

273. Perry, HD, Yanoff, M, and Scheie, HG: Rubeosis in Fuchs' heterochromic iridocyclitis, Arch Ophthalmol 93:337, 1975

274. Peyman, GA, Grisalono, JM, and Palacio, MN: Intraocular photocoagulation with the argon-krypton laser, Arch Ophthalmol 98:2062, 1980

275. Phelps, RL, et al: Changes in diabetic retinopathy during pregnancy: correlation with regulation of hyperglycemia, Arch Ophthalmol 104:1806, 1986

276. Pirart, J: Diabetes mellitus and its degenerative complications: a prospective study of 4400 patients observed between 1947 and 1973, Diabetes Care 1:168, 1978

277. Poliner, LS, et al: Neovascular glaucoma after intracapsular and extracapsular cataract extraction in diabetic patients, Am J Ophthalmol 100:637, 1985

278. Polverini, PJ, et al: Activated macrophages induce vascular proliferation, Nature 269:804, 1977

279. Poulsen, JE: The Houssay phenomenon in man: recovery from retinopathy in a case of diabetes with Simmonds' disease, Diabetes 2:7, 1953

280. Powell, JO, et al: Ocular effects of argon laser radiation: histopathology of chorioretinal lesions, Ophthalmology 71:1267, 1971

281. Puklin, JE, et al: Influence of long-term insulin infusion pump treatment of type I diabetes on diabetic retinopathy, Ophthalmology 89:735, 1982

282. Quigley, HA: Histologic and physiologic studies of cyclocryotherapy in primate and human eyes, Am J Ophthalmol 82:722, 1976

283. Raviola, G, and Butler, JM: Asymmetric distribution of charged domains on the two fronts of the endothelium of iris blood vessels, Invest Ophthalmol Vis Sci 26:597, 1985

284. Raymond, L, and Jacobson, B: Isolation and identification of stimulatory and inhibitory cell growth factors in bovine vitreous, Exp Eye Res 34:267, 1982

285. Reinecke, RD, et al: Retinal vascular patterns. V Experimental ischemia of the cat eye, Arch Ophthalmol 67:470, 1962

286. Riaskoff, S, and Pameyer, JH: Results of the treatment of neovascular glaucoma by diathermy of the dissected ciliary body, Documenta Ophthalmologica 48:277, 1979

287. Rice, TA, et al: The effect of lensectomy on the incidence of iris neovascularization and neovascular glaucoma after vitrectomy for diabetic retinopathy, Am J Ophthalmol 85:1, 1983

288. Riles, TS, et al: Symptoms, stenosis, and bruits: interrelationships in carotid artery disease, Arch Surg 116:218, 1981

289. Ringvold, A, and Davanger, M: Iris neovascularisation in eyes with pseudoexfoliation syndrome, Br J Ophthalmol 65:138, 1981

290. Rizza, RA: Treatment options for insulin-dependent diabetes mellitus: A comparison of the artificial endocrine pancreas, continuous subcutaneous insulin infusion, and multiple daily insulin injections, Mayo Clin Proc 61:796, 1986

291. Robinson, WG, Jr, Kador, PF, and Kinoshita, JH: Retinal capillaries: basement membrane thickening by galactosemia prevented with aldose reductase inhibitor, Science 1177, 1983

292. Rockwood, EJ, et al: Life-table analysis of filtering surgery with 5-fluorouracil, Ophthalmology (In press)

293. Romem, M, and Isakow, I: Photocoagulation in retinal vein occlusion, Ann Ophthalmol 13:1057, 1981

294. Rosenberg, PR, Walsh, JB, and Zimmerman, RD: Neovascular glaucoma and carotid bruits, J Clin Neuro-ophthalmol 4:459, 1984

295. Rucker, CW, Gastineau, CF, and Svien, HJ: Effect of section of pituitary stalk on diabetic retinopathy, Mayo Clinic Proc 42:409, 1967

296. Ryan, SJ: An approach to the management of neovascularization of the iris and secondary glaucoma, Trans Am Ophthalmol Soc 78:107, 1980

297. Saari, M, Vuorre, I, and Nieminen H: Fuchs's heterochromic cyclitis: a simultaneous bilateral fluorescein angiographic study of the iris, Br J Ophthalmol 62:715, 1978

298. Sabates, R, Hirose, T, and McMeel, JW: Electroretinography in the prognosis and classification of central retinal vein occlusion, Arch Ophthalmol 101:232, 1983

299. Salus, R: Rubeosis iridis diabetica, eine bisher unbekannte diabetische Irisveranderung, Med Klin 24:256, 1928

300. Scader, JJ, Blumenkranz, MS, and Blankenship, G: Regression of diabetic rubeosis iridis following successful surgical reattachment of the retina by vitrectomy, Retina 2:193, 1982

301. Schimek, RA, and Spencer, R: Cryopexy treatment of proliferative diabetic retinopathy, Arch Ophthalmol 97:1276, 1979

302. Schocket, SS, Lakhanpal, V, and Richards, RD: Anterior chamber tube shunt to an encircling band in the treatment of neovascular glaucoma, Ophthalmology 89:1188, 1982

303. Schocket, SS, et al: Anterior chamber tube shunt to an encircling band in the treatment of neovascular glaucoma and other refractory glaucomas: a long-term study, Ophthalmology 92:553, 1985

304. Schulze, RR: Rubeosis iridis, Am J Ophthalmol 63:487, 1967

305. Schwartz, DM, Quigley, MA, and Thomas, B: Transscleral cyclophotocoagulation, Scientific poster, annual meeting of the American Academy of Ophthalmology, 1986

306. Segato, T, et al: Retinal cryotherapy in the management of proliferative diabetic retinopathy, Am J Ophthalmol 98:240, 1984

307. Service, FJ: What is "tight control" of diabetes? Goals, limitations, and evaluation of therapy, Mayo Clin Proc, 61:792, 1986

308. Shabo, AL, and Maxwell, DS: Insulin-induced immunogenic retinopathy resembling retinitis proliferans of diabetes, Trans Am Acad Ophthalmol Otolaryngol 81:497, 1976

309. Shabo, AL, and Maxwell, DS: Experimental immunogenic proliferative retinopathy in monkeys, Am J Ophthalmol 83:471, 1977

310. Shah, HG, Brown, GC, and Goldberg, RE: Digital subtraction carotid angiography and retinal arterial obstruction, Ophthalmology 92:68, 1985

311. Shields, MB: Cyclodestructive surgery for glaucoma: past, present, and future, Trans Am Ophthalmol Soc 23:285, 1985

312. Sidkey, YA, and Auerbach, R: Lymphocyte-induced angiogenesis: a quantitative and sensitive assay of the graft-vs-host reaction, J Exp Med 141:1084, 1975

313. Simmons, RJ, Depperman, SR, and Dueker, DK: The role of goniophotocoagulation in neovascularization of the anterior chamber angle, Ophthalmology 87:79, 1980

314. Simmons, RJ, et al: Goniophotocoagulation for neovascular glaucoma, Trans Am acad Ophthalmol Otolaryngol 83:80, 1977

315. Sinclair, SH, Aaberg, TM, and Meredith, TA: A pars plana filtering procedure combined with lensectomy and vitrectomy for neovascular glaucoma, Am J Ophthalmol 93:185, 1982

316. Sinclair, SM, and Gragoudas, ES: Prognosis for rubeosis iridis following central retinal vein occlusion, Br J Ophthalmol 63:735, 1979

317. Singerman, L, and Weaver, D: High-risk proliferative diabetic retinopathy in juvenile onset diabetes, Retina 1:18, 1981

318. Skyler, JS: Complications of diabetes mellitus: relationship to metabolic dysfunction, Diabetes Care 2:499, 1979

319. Smiddy, WE, et al: Clinicopathologic correlation of krypton red, argon blue-green, and argon green laser photocoagulation in the human fundus, Retina 4:15, 1984

320. Smiddy, WE, et al: Comparison of krypton and argon laser photocoagulation: results of simulated clinical treatment of primate retina, Arch Ophthalmol 102:1086, 1984

321. Smith, JL: Unilateral glaucoma in carotid occlusive disease, JAMA, 182:683, 1962

322. Smith, R: Neovascularization in ocular disease, Trans Ophthalmol Soc UK 81:125, 1961

323. Smith, RS, Boyle, E, and Rudt, LA: Cyclocryotherapy: a light and electron microscopic study, Arch Ophthalmol 95:284, 1977

324. Spaeth, GL: A new old procedure for glaucoma, Ophthalmic Surg 14:479, 1983

325. Stefansson, E, et al: Panretinal photocoagulation and retinal oxygenation in normal and diabetic cats, Am J Ophthalmol 101:657, 1986

326. Stefansson, E, Landers, MB, III, and Wolbarsht, ML: Increased retinal oxygen supply following panretinal photocoagulation and vitrectomy and lensectomy, Trans Am Ophthalmol Soc 79:307, 1981

327. Steffes, MW, et al: Studies of kidney and muscle biopsy specimens from identical twins discordant for type I diabetes mellitus, N Engl J Med 312:1282, 1985

328. Steno Study Group: Effect of 6 months of strict metabolic control on eye and kidney function in insulin-dependent diabetics with background retinopathy, Lancet 1:121, 1982

329. Stratas, BA, et al: Observations on the microvascular repair process after confluent argon laser photocoagulation, Arch Ophthalmol 104:126, 1986

330. Stross, JK, and Harlan, WR: The dissemination of new medical information, JAMA 241:2622, 1979

331. Strydom, DJ, et al: Amino acid sequence of human tumor derived angiogenin, Biochemistry 24:5486, 1985

332. Sturrock, GD, and Mueller, HR: Chronic ocular ischaemia, Br J Ophthalmol 68:716, 1984

333. Sugar, HS: Neovascular glaucoma after carotid-cavernous fistula formation, Am Ophthalmol 11:1667, 1979

334. Sullivan, ST, and Dallow, RL: Intraocular reticulum cell sarcoma, Ann Ophthalmol 9:401, 1977

335. Sundt, TM, et al: Results, complications, and follow-up of 415 bypass operations for occlusive disease of the carotid system, Mayo Clin Proc 60:230, 1985

336. Sussman, EJ, Tsiaras, WG, and Soper, KA: Diagnosis of diabetic eye disease, JAMA 242:3231, 1982

337. Sutton, GE, Popp, JC, and Records, RE: Krupin-Denver valve and neovascular glaucoma, Trans Ophthalmol Soc UK 102:119, 1982

338. Swan, KC, and Raff, J: Changes in the eye and orbit following carotid ligation, Trans Am Ophthalmol Soc 49:435, 1951

339. Szabo, AJ, Stewart, AG, and Joron, GE: Factors associated with increased prevalence of diabetic retinopathy, Can Med Ass J 97:286, 1967

340. Tamura, T: Electron microscopic study on the small blood vessels in rubeosis iridis diabetica, Jpn J Ophthalmol 13:65, 1969

341. Tasman, W, Magargal, LE, and Augsberger, JJ: Effects of argon laser photocoagulation on rubeosis iridis and angle neovascularization, Ophthalmology 87:400, 1980

342. Tchobroutsky, G: Relation of diabetes control to development of microvascular complications, Diabetologia 15:143, 1978

343. Teich, SA, and Walsh, JB: A grading system for neovascularization: Prognostic implications for treatment, Ophthalmology 88:1102, 1981

344. Theodore, FH, editor: Complications after cataract surgery, Boston, 1965, Little, Brown & Co

345. Thompson, JT, and Glaser, BM: Role of lensectomy and posterior capsule in movement of tracers from vitreous to aqueous, Arch Ophthalmol 103:420, 1985

346. Ticho, U, et al: Carbon dioxide laser filtering surgery in hemorrhagic glaucoma, Glaucoma 1:114, 1979

347. Trope, GE, Chew, EY, and Mitchell, BJ: Diurnal intraocular pressure in young patients with central retinal vein occlusion, Ophthalmology. (In press)

348. Vannas, A.: Fluorescein angiography of the vessels of the iris in pseudo-exfoliation of the lens capsule, capsular glaucoma, and some other forms of glaucoma, Acta Ophthalmol Suppl 105:9, 1969

349. Vannas, S: Discussion of Bertelsen, TI: The relationship between thrombosis in the retinal vein and primary glaucoma, Acta Ophthalmol 39:603, 1961

350. Verhoeff, FH: Effect of chronic glaucoma on central retinal vessels, Arch Ophthalmol 42:145, 1913

351. Virdi, PS, and Hayreh, SS: Ocular neovascularization with retinal vascular occlusion, Arch Ophthalmol 100:331, 1982

352. Waltman, SR, et al: Quantitative vitreous fluorophotometry: a sensitive technique for measuring early breakdown of the blood-retinal barrier in young diabetic patients, Diabetes 27:85, 1978

353. Walton, DS, and Grant, WM: Retinoblastoma and iris neovascularization, Am J Ophthalmol 65:598, 1968

354. Walton, DS, and Grant, WM: Penetrating cyclodiathermy for filtration, Arch Ophthalmol 83:47, 1970

355. Wand, M: Neovascular glaucoma. In Ritch, R, and Shields, MB, editors: The secondary glaucomas, St Louis, 1982, The CV Mosby Co

356. Wand, M: Hyaloid membrane vs posterior capsule as a protective barrier, Arch Ophthalmol 103:1112, 1985

357. Wand, M: Treatment of neovascular glaucoma. In Jakobiec, FA, and Sigelman, J, editors: Advanced techniques in ocular surgery, Philadelphia, 1984, WB Saunders Co

358. Wand, M, et al: Effects of panretinal photocoagulation on rubeosis iridis, angle neovascularization, and neovascular glaucoma, Am J Ophthalmol 86:332, 1978

359. Wand, M, and Hutchinson, BT: The surgical management of neovascular glaucoma, Perspect Ophthalmol 4:147, 1980

360. Wand, M, et al: Rubeosis iridis and neovascular glaucoma following pars plana vitrectomy for complications of diabetic vitrectomy, Ophthalmology 93(Suppl):73, 1986

361. Weber, PA: Neovascular glaucoma, current management, Surv Ophthalmol 25:149, 1981

362. Weinreb, RN, Wasserstrom, JP, and Parker, W: Neovascular glaucoma following neodymium-YAG laser posterior capsulotomy, Arch Ophthalmol 104:730, 1986

363. Weiss, DI, and Gold, D: Neofibrovascularization of iris and anterior chamber angle: a clinical classification, Ann Ophthalmol 10:488, 1978

364. Weiss, DI, Shaffer, RN, and Nehrenberg, TR: Neovascular glaucoma complicating carotid-cavernous fistula, Arch Ophthalmol 69:304, 1963

365. Weiter, JJ, and Zuckerman, R: The influence of the photoreceptor–RPE complex on the inner retina: an explanation for the beneficial effects of photocoagulation, Ophthalmology 87:1133, 1980

366. White, TC: A new implantable ocular pressure relief device: a preliminary report, Glaucoma 7:289, 1985

367. Wilhelmus, KR, Grierson, I, and Watson, PG: Histopathologic and clinical associations of scleritis and glaucoma, Am J Ophthalmol 91:697, 1981

368. Williams, GA, et al: Inhibitor of vascular endothelial cell growth in the lens, Am J Ophthalmol 92:366, 1984

369. Wilson, DJ, and Green WR: Argon laser panretinal photocoagulation for diabetic retinopthy: scanning electron microscopy of human choroidal vascular casts, Arch Ophthalmol 105:239, 1987

370. Wise, GN: Retinal neovascularization, Trans Am Ophthalmol Soc 54:729, 1956

371. Wolbarsht, ML, and Landers, MB, III: A rationale of photocoagulation therapy for proliferative diabetic retinopathy: a review and a model, Ophthalmic Surg 11:235, 1980

372. Wolter, JR: Secondary glaucoma in cranial arteritis, Am J Ophthalmol 59:625, 1965

373. Wolter, JR, and Liddicoat, DA: Secondary glaucoma following occlusion of the central artery of the retina, Am J Ophthalmol 46:182, 1958

374. Yablonski, ME, Jacobson, J, and Goldfarb, M: Glaucoma and bilateral carotid artery occlusion, Glaucoma 7:19, 1985

375. Yanoff, M: Mechanisms of glaucoma in eyes with uveal melanoma, Int Ophthalmol Clin 12:51, 1972

376. Yanoff, M, and Fine, BS: Ocular pathology: a text and atlas, New York, 1975, Harper & Row, Publishers

377. Yoshizumi, MO, Thomas, JV, and Smith, TR: Glaucoma-inducing mechanisms in eyes with retinoblastoma, Arch Ophthalmol 96:105, 1978

378. Young, LHY, and Appen, RE: Ischemic oculopathy: a manifestation of carotid artery disease, Arch Neurol 18:358, 1981

379. Young, NJA, et al: Stickler's syndrome and neovascular glaucoma, Br J Ophthalmol 63:826, 1979

380. Yue, DK, et al: The effect of aldose reductase inhibition on motor nerve conduction velocity in diabetic rats, Diabetes 31:789, 1982

381. Zauberman, H, et al: Stimulation of neovascularization of the cornea by biogenic amines, Exp Eye Res 8:77, 1969

382. Zollinger, R: Klinische Untersuchungen uber Gafassneubildungen auf der Iris, Ophthalmologica 123:215, 1952

Chapter 61

Glaucomas Associated with Intraocular Tumors

Jerry A. Shields
Carol L. Shields
M. Bruce Shields

GENERAL CONSIDERATIONS

A number of intraocular tumors can produce secondary glaucoma.[6,13] In such instances, clinical recognition of the underlying neoplasm may be delayed while the patient is being treated for glaucoma. In cases of malignant tumors, a delay in diagnosis may have serious consequences.

In contrast to the primary glaucomas, which are generally bilateral, tumor-induced secondary glaucomas are almost always unilateral. Mechanisms of the secondary glaucoma vary with the type, size, and extent of the tumor. More posteriorly located intraocular neoplasms may produce anterior displacement of the lens-iris diaphragm with angle-closure; may induce iris and angle neovascularization; or may liberate tumor cells into the anterior chamber angle, blocking aqueous outflow. Tumors in the iris and ciliary body are more likely to obstruct aqueous outflow by infiltrating the trabecular meshwork directly.

This chapter covers the clinical features, pathology, and mechanisms of glaucoma, as well as the differential diagnoses, diagnostic approaches, and management of glaucoma secondary to intraocular tumors. Much of the information in this chapter is based on a study of 126 eyes with secondary glaucoma among 2704 eyes with intraocular tumors in patients evaluated on the Ocular Oncology Service at Wills Eye Hospital between 1974 and 1986.[4]

TUMORS OF THE UVEAL TRACT

Uveal Melanoma

Iris melanoma

In the Wills Eye Hospital series, there were 102 eyes with iris melanoma, seven of which had secondary glaucoma (7%).[4] Clinically, iris melanomas are usually well circumscribed, variably pigmented, stationary or slowly growing lesions that do not produce significant alterations in the intraocular pressure. In rare instances, a circumscribed iris melanoma can occupy enough of the trabecular meshwork to produce glaucoma (Fig. 61-1).[6] The diffuse iris melanoma, which is considerably less common than the circumscribed type, produces a classic clinical syndrome of unilateral acquired hyperchromic heterochromia and ipsilateral glaucoma. In such cases, one sees a diffuse pigmented thickening of the iris stroma with tumor invasion of the trabecular meshwork (Fig. 61-2). Pathologically, the great majority of iris melanomas have relatively low grade malignant features, consisting of spindle melanoma cells with epithelioid melanoma cells being less common.

The most common mechanism of glaucoma caused by large circumscribed iris melanomas and diffuse iris melanomas is direct invasion of the trabecular meshwork by tumor tissue (Fig. 61-3). Circumscribed or diffuse iris melanomas may occasionally bleed spontaneously, leading to hyphema and obstruction of aqueous outflow by blood, producing increased intraocular pressure. A circum-

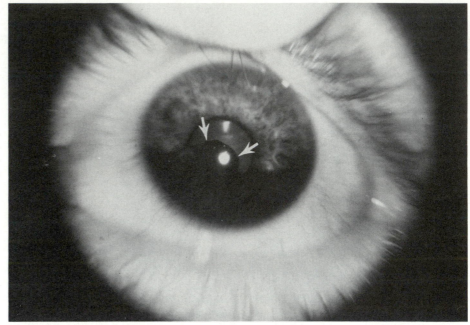

Fig. 61-1 Large inferior iris melanoma *(arrows)* with extensive involvement of anterior chamber angle, producing secondary glaucoma.

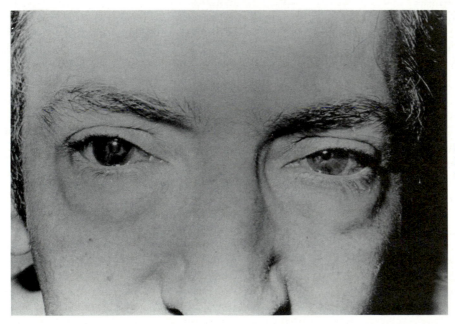

Fig. 61-2 Acquired hyperchromic heterochromia in right eye secondary to diffuse iris melanoma.

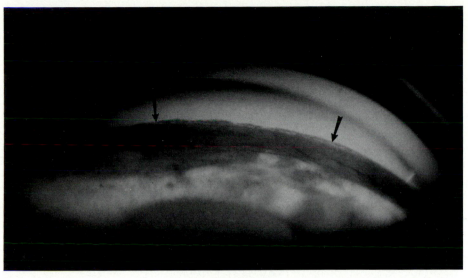

Fig. 61-3 Diffuse angle involvement by iris melanoma (*arrows*) shown in goniophotograph.

scribed iris melanoma has also been reported to cause neovascular glaucoma, which resolved after total excision of the tumor.[15]

The differential diagnosis of circumscribed iris melanoma includes iris cysts, benign iris tumors, and iris atrophy.[12] The differential diagnosis of the diffuse iris melanoma includes conditions that produce acquired hyperchromic heterochromia, such as hemosiderosis, siderosis, congenital melanocytosis, and the iris nevus syndrome.

The diagnosis of iris melanoma is best made by recognizing the typical features seen with slit-lamp biomicroscopy. In questionable cases, we have employed fine-needle aspiration biopsy or a sector or peripheral iridectomy to confirm the diagnosis.

Most melanocytic iris tumors should be managed initially by periodic observation, and any associated glaucoma should be managed medically. If the tumor shows evidence of growth or if the glaucoma cannot be controlled, surgical intervention should be considered. In cases of circumscribed tumors, excision of the tumor by a partial iridectomy, sometimes with laser or surgical trabeculectomy to control the glaucoma, should be undertaken. In the case of a diffuse iris melanoma with secondary glaucoma, enucleation is generally necessary. We have found that biopsy of the iris tumor or surgery to control the glaucoma in such cases can predispose to extrascleral extension of the tumor. Patients with iris melanomas generally have an excellent systemic prognosis, although we recently managed a patient who developed clinical evidence of liver metastasis 16 years after enucleation for a diffuse spindle-cell melanoma of the iris.

Ciliary body melanoma

In the Wills Eye Hospital series, there were 96 eyes with ciliary body melanomas, 16 (17%) of which had secondary glaucoma.[4]

In contrast to iris melanomas, ciliary body melanomas tend to attain a fairly large size before diagnosis. The tumor appears as a circumscribed mass posterior to the iris, sometimes with anterior displacement of the peripheral iris. In rare instances, a ciliary body melanoma may grow circumferentially around the ciliary body (ring melanoma). Ring melanomas tend to be more malignant, produce secondary glaucoma, and often extend extrasclerally in the ciliary body region (Fig. 61-4).

On gross examination, the ciliary body melanoma appears as a circumscribed mass that replaces the ciliary body (Fig. 61-5). Microscopically, the tumor may contain both spindle and epithelioid melanoma cells, but there is a greater proportion of epithelioid cells than found in iris melanomas.

Ciliary body melanomas can produce secondary glaucoma by causing anterior displacement of the iris with secondary angle-closure, or by growing anteriorly into the trabecular meshwork and obstructing aqueous outflow (Fig. 61-5).[14] Less commonly, they can produce a hyphema, undergo necrosis with macrophage response (melanomalytic glaucoma), or cause iris neovascularization.

The differential diagnosis of ciliary body melanoma includes iris or ciliary body cysts, ciliochoroidal detachment, and other tumors.[6,10] The differentiation from other adult-onset ciliary body tumors such as leiomyoma, adenoma of the ciliary pigmented or nonpigmented epithelium, and me-

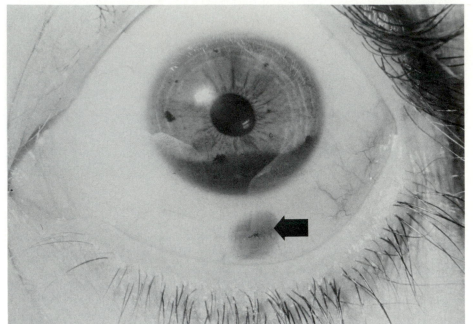

Fig. 61-4 Extraocular extension of ciliary body malignant melanoma *(arrow)*.

Fig. 61-5 Gross pathology of ciliary body malignant melanoma in angle.

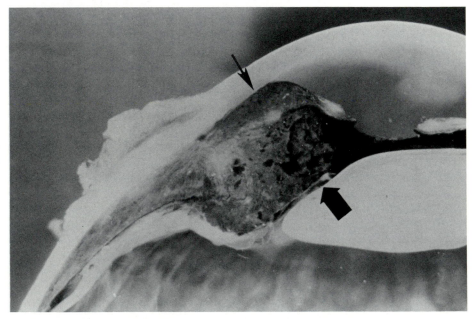

lanocytoma of the ciliary body may be quite difficult. When a ciliary body melanoma produces a cataract or otherwise causes opaque ocular media, the tumor cannot be visualized clinically. In such instances, several ancillary diagnostic procedures may assist in the diagnosis.[11]

The diagnosis of ciliary body melanoma can usually be made on the basis of biomicroscopy, indirect ophthalmoscopy, ultrasonography, and/or a radioactive phosphorus uptake (^{32}P) test.[6] In recent years, we have frequently employed transocular fine-needle aspiration biopsy to help establish a cytologic diagnosis.[1] In cases with opaque media, transillumination, ultrasonography, and a ^{32}P test may be necessary to make the diagnosis.[11] Small ciliary body melanomas can be managed by simple periodic observation until growth is documented before initiating treatment. Somewhat larger tumors can be managed by local resection or episcleral plaque radiotherapy. Most tumors that are large or infiltrative enough to produce secondary glaucoma are generally best managed by enucleation. Careful medical evaluation and follow-up are warranted because of the relatively high risk of metastatic disease in cases of ciliary body melanomas with secondary glaucoma. In the Wills Eye Hospital series, 50% of patients with ciliary body

melanoma and secondary glaucoma died as a result of metastatic melanoma within 2 years of the diagnosis.[4]

Choroidal melanoma

In the Wills Eye Hospital series, there were 1913 eyes with choroidal melanoma, only 32 (2%) of which had secondary glaucoma. The fact that the incidence of secondary glaucoma has been higher in most earlier series, probably reflects the earlier clinical recognition of choroidal melanomas in recent years.[4]

A choroidal melanoma clinically appears as a variably pigmented mass that can produce a secondary nonrhegmatogenous retinal detachment. The many variations are well described in the literature[6] and are beyond the scope of this chapter. A rather specific clinical feature in many cases is the mushroom shape caused by the tumor's breaking through Bruch's membrane.

On gross examination, a choroidal melanoma that has produced secondary glaucoma may be quite large, occupying a large portion of the vitreous cavity (Fig. 61-6). Microscopically, choroidal melanomas can be composed of spindle cells, epithelioid cells, or any combination of the two.

Choroidal melanomas can produce secondary

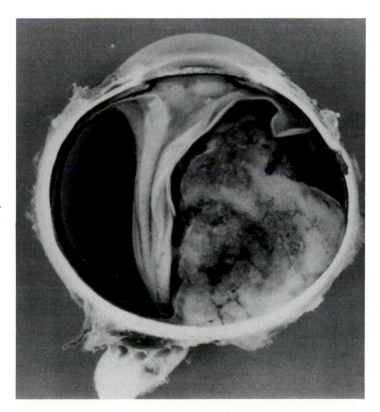

Fig. 61-6 Large malignant melanoma of choroid producing total retinal detachment and secondary glaucoma.

glaucoma by causing iris and angle neovascularization (56%) or by causing anterior displacement of the lens-iris diaphragm and secondary angle-closure (Fig. 61-6). Large necrotic choroidal melanomas can occasionally produce intraocular inflammation or hemorrhage, which can further contribute to secondary glaucoma.[16]

The differential diagnosis for choroidal melanoma is similar to that for ciliary body melanoma. Also important in the differential diagnosis of choroidal melanoma are retinal detachment, choroidal effusion syndrome, disciform macular degeneration, and hypertrophy of the retinal pigment epithelium.[10]

The diagnosis of choroidal melanoma can usually be made on the basis of indirect ophthalmoscopy and a knowledge of the typical clinical features. When the diagnosis is uncertain, fine-needle aspiration biopsy has been employed to establish the diagnosis in selected cases.[1] Larger tumors, which have produced secondary glaucoma, are often associated with opaque ocular media. In these cases, ancillary procedures such as transillumination, ultrasonography, and the ^{32}P test can establish the correct diagnosis in the majority of cases.[11]

The options in management of choroidal melanomas are well outlined in the literature and include simple observation, photocoagulation, radiotherapy, local resection, enucleation, and even exenteration.[5,6] Unfortunately, choroidal melanomas that have produced secondary glaucoma are generally so large that enucleation is necessary.

Uveal Nevus

Uveal nevi are benign lesions that rarely produce secondary glaucoma. Occasionally, however, localized or diffuse uveal nevi can lead to secondary glaucoma. This most often occurs with a specific variant of localized nevus called a melanocytoma or with a diffuse nevus of the iris.

The melanocytoma is a specific variant of nevus that usually occurs in the optic disc, but that can arise anywhere in the uveal tract. Those located in the optic disc or choroid rarely produce secondary glaucoma, whereas those that occur in the ciliary body or iris are more likely to produce secondary glaucoma.

The localized iris melanocytoma appears as a dark brown or black circumscribed but often irregular lesion[7] (Fig. 61-7, *A*). This tumor has an unusual tendency to undergo necrosis and fragmentation, liberating pigment into the anterior chamber and trabecular meshwork (Fig. 61-7, *B*).

Histopathologically, the uveal melanocytoma consists of deeply pigmented cells that, after bleaching, are seen to be large round to oval cells with abundant cytoplasm and small round nuclei without mitoses. Areas of necrosis are commonly present in those tumors that come to histopathologic evaluation.

Melanocytomas of the iris and ciliary body can undergo necrosis and liberate pigment into the trabecular meshwork, obstructing aqueous outflow (Fig. 61-7, *B*). Large ciliary body melancytomas can apparently grow very slowly through the iris root to involve the trabecular meshwork.[9] Rarely, large melanocytomas of the choroid or optic nerve can liberate pigment into the vitreous cavity and anterior chamber angle to produce secondary glaucoma.

The differential diagnosis of melanocytoma of the iris, ciliary body, and choroid is the same as for malignant melanomas of the uvea. In general, the melanocytoma is more deeply pigmented clinically and is somewhat more likely to undergo necrosis.

The diagnostic techniques for uveal melanocytoma are the same as for uveal melanomas. In many cases, the differential from melanoma cannot be made clinically, and histopathologic studies are necessary to establish a definitive diagnosis.

The management of uveal melanocytoma is generally the same as for other uveal nevi and consists of simple periodic observation and photographs to document growth. Glaucoma caused by uveal melanocytomas should initially be managed medically but, when it cannot be controlled, surgical treatment may be necessary. In the case of iris melanocytomas, the liberated pigment in the trabecular meshwork may gradually disappear following excision of the main tumor by iridectomy.[6,7] On occasion, an iris nevus may assume a diffuse pattern with a number of rather typical clinical features (iris nevus syndrome).[6] It is commonly associated with secondary glaucoma and has been considered to be in the spectrum of the iridocorneal endothelial syndrome (see Chapter 54).

Metastatic Tumors

Metastatic tumors from distant primary sites can metastasize to the uveal tract via hematogenous routes. Retinal and optic nerve metastases are rather rare. Choroidal metastases produce secondary glaucoma only when they attain a large size,

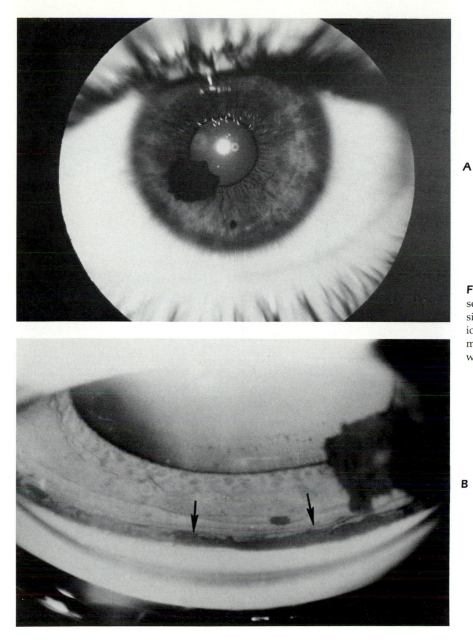

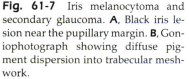

Fig. 61-7 Iris melanocytoma and secondary glaucoma. **A,** Black iris lesion near the pupillary margin. **B,** Goniophotograph showing diffuse pigment dispersion into trabecular meshwork.

whereas iris and ciliary body metastases often produce secondary glaucoma because of their tendency to involve the angle structures. In the Wills Eye Hospital Oncology Service series, secondary glaucoma was found in 64% of iris metastases, 67% of ciliary body metastases, and 2% of choroidal metastases.[4] Metastatic tumors to the intraocular structures most commonly occur from primary sites in the breast and lung, and less often from the gastrointestinal tract, kidney, thyroid, cutaneous melanoma, and other primary sites. In many cases, the location of the primary lesion is never determined clinically.

Iris and ciliary body metastasis

Iris and ciliary body metastases can occur as solitary or as diffuse multinodular lesions. Such metastases to the anterior uveal structures are composed of cells that are frequently loosely cohesive and friable. As a result, they may seed into the aqueous humor, producing a pseudohypopyon consisting of tumor cells layered inferiorly (Fig. 61-8). Ciliary body metastases may be extremely difficult to detect clinically because of their position posterior to the iris.

The pathology of iris and ciliary body metastases varies with the primary lesion. In some cases,

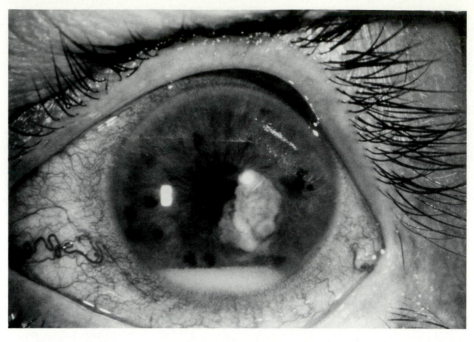

Fig. 61-8 Metastatic carcinoma to iris with shedding of tumor cells, producing pseudohypopyon and secondary glaucoma.

the cells are so poorly differentiated that the primary tumor cannot be determined on pathologic examination. In many cases cords or shells of mucin-containing cells can suggest a primary site in the gastrointestinal tract or breast. Metastatic small cell carcinoma, thyroid carcinoma, or renal cell carcinoma can also have typical features. In other cases, histochemistry, immunohistochemistry, and electron microscopy may provide help in recognizing the primary site.

Iris and ciliary body metastases usually produce secondary glaucoma by seeding into the anterior chamber angle and trabecular meshwork, mechanically blocking aqueous outflow. In some cases, a solid growth of tumor cells can assume a ring-type infiltration of the trabecular meshwork, resulting in intractable glaucoma.

The differential diagnosis of iris and ciliary body metastases includes granulomatous iritis, iris melanoma, intraocular lymphoma, and other tumors. When tumor cells form a pseudohypopyon, metastases can be clinically confused with purulent endophthalmitis. The typical appearance of a fleshy yellow, often vascularized nodule, particularly in a patient with evidence of lung or breast cancer, should be helpful in making the correct diagnosis.

Detailed slit-lamp biomicroscopy, gonioscopy, and clinical awareness of the condition can usually suggest the diagnosis of iris or ciliary body metastasis, particularly if the patient has a known primary tumor. When the diagnosis is uncertain, fine-needle aspiration biopsy with cytologic analysis can be diagnostically helpful.[1] If necessary, an iris or ciliary body biopsy can be done for a more definitive diagnosis. When the patient with a typical anterior uveal lesion has a well-established diagnosis of systemic metastases, however, biopsy is not generally necessary.

The primary management of iris and ciliary body metastases should be chemotherapy or other systemic management that the patient is receiving for the primary tumor. If the ocular tumor continues to proliferate, then external beam ocular radiotherapy, giving 3500 to 4000 R to the affected eye in divided doses over a 4-week period should be initiated. If secondary glaucoma does not resolve following chemotherapy and radiotherapy, medical therapy should be continued. In many instances, the glaucoma progresses relentlessly, and filtering surgery may be considered. In many of these cases, the glaucoma may ultimately require cyclocryotherapy, retrobulbar alcohol injection, or even enucleation. Since most affected patients have a poor systemic prognosis, such aggressive treatment should be avoided if possible.

Choroidal metastasis

Metastatic tumors to the choroid appear as single or multiple elevated or diffuse lesions often associated with a secondary nonrhegmatogenous retinal detachment.[6] They typically have a characteristic cream-yellow color, except for metastatic melanoma, which can appear brown or gray. In

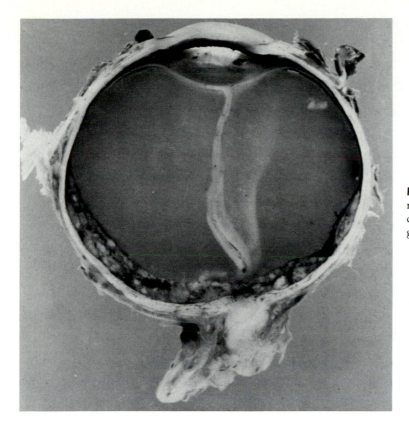

Fig. 61-9 Diffuse metastatic carcinoma of choroid, producing total retinal detachment, anterior displacement of lens-iris diaphragm, and secondary glaucoma.

contrast to iris and ciliary body metastases, choroidal metastases rarely produce secondary glaucoma. The pathology of metastatic tumors to the choroid is the same as that for metastatic tumors to the iris and ciliary body described previously.

As mentioned, only about 2% of metastatic carcinomas to the choroid produce secondary glaucoma.[4] When the tumors become quite elevated or when they diffusely involve the entire posterior uvea, however, they can produce severe uncontrollable glaucoma. The most common mechanism is angle-closure caused by anterior displacement of the lens-iris diaphragm secondary to total retinal detachment (Fig. 61-9). It is also feasible that neovascular glaucoma could occur in advanced cases with total retinal detachment.

The differential diagnosis of and diagnostic approach to choroidal metastases are the same as for choroidal melanoma described earlier. Fine-needle aspiration biopsy has a role in cases in which there is reasonable uncertainty as to whether the tumor represents a primary melanoma or a metastatic carcinoma.[1] If cytologic study of the aspirate indicates the diagnosis of melanoma, enucleation or radioactive plaque therapy may be justified. If it sug-gests the diagnosis of metastatic carcinoma, external beam radiotherapy is generally more appropriate.

In general, eyes with choroidal metastases are best managed by external beam radiotherapy combined with any chemotherapy that the patient may be receiving for associated systemic metastases. In rare instances, the associated glaucoma can produce such severe pain that palliative enucleation is necessary.

Other Tumors of the Uveal Stroma

Other rare uveal tumors such as neurilemmomas, leiomyomas, neurofibromas, and perhaps choroidal osteomas can theoretically produce secondary glaucoma.[1] The mechanism of glaucoma is the same as seen with uveal melanomas of similar size and location.

TUMORS OF THE SENSORY RETINA

Tumors of the sensory retina include retinoblastoma, vascular tumors, glial tumors, and other rare benign and malignant tumors. Retinoblastoma is the only tumor of the sensory retina that is clinically important with regard to secondary glaucoma.

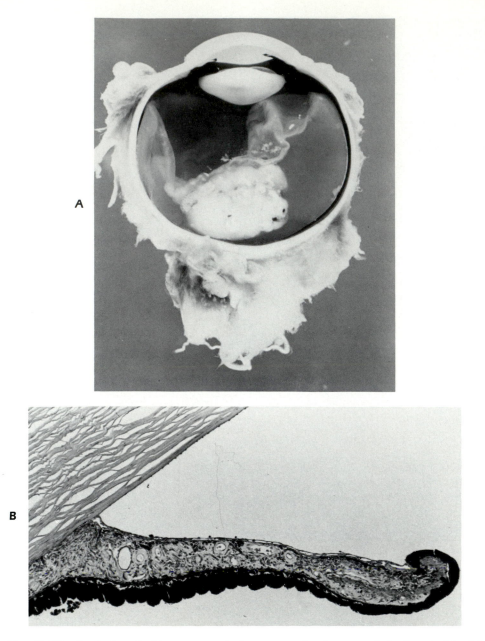

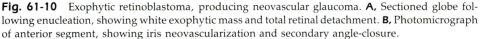

Fig. 61-10 Exophytic retinoblastoma, producing neovascular glaucoma. **A,** Sectioned globe following enucleation, showing white exophytic mass and total retinal detachment. **B,** Photomicrograph of anterior segment, showing iris neovascularization and secondary angle-closure.

Retinoblastoma

Retinoblastoma is the most common malignant intraocular tumor of childhood. Advanced cases can produce secondary glaucoma. The various clinical aspects of retinoblastoma are well known and are not discussed in detail here.[6,8] Early retinoblastomas appear as white, elevated lesions in the sensory retina, with prominent afferent and efferent blood vessels. More advanced tumors produce a white pupillary reflex, or leukocoria. The tumor may assume an endophytic growth pattern in which the loosely cohesive tumor cells break free into the viteous and sometimes into the anterior chamber. In other cases, the tumor may assume an exophytic growth pattern, in which it grows outward into the subretinal space, producing a retinal detachment with a clear vitreous. Both types of growth pattern can be associated with secondary glaucoma.

Pathologically, in the grossly sectioned eye, a retinoblastoma appears as a chalky white mass within the globe (Fig. 61-10, *A*). Microscopically,

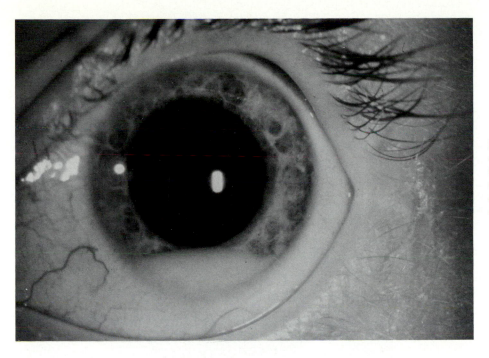

Fig. 61-11 Pseudohypopyon caused by endophytic retinoblastoma. Glaucoma presumably occurred secondary to both tumor cells in the angle and iris neovascularization.

the tumor is composed of well-differentiated to poorly differentiated neuroblastic cells, often with areas of calcification and necrosis. The well-differentiated tumors are characterized by Flexner-Wintersteiner rosettes. The loosely cohesive tumor cells can migrate into the aqueous and sometimes settle in the anterior chamber angle.

In the Wills Eye Hospital Oncology Service series of 248 patients with retinoblastoma, about 17% of 303 affected eyes had secondary glaucoma. The secondary glaucoma was caused by iris neovascularization in 72% (Fig. 61-10, *B*), angle-closure secondary to anterior displacement of the lens-iris diaphragm in 26%, and tumor seeding into the anterior chamber in 2% (Fig. 61-11). In cases with iris neovascularization, secondary hyphema contributed to the mechanism of glaucoma in some cases.

The differential diagnosis of retinoblastoma includes any white fundus lesion in a child; these are listed in detail in the literature.[6] The conditions that can simulate retinoblastoma most closely include persistent hyperplastic primary vitreous (PHPV), nematode endophthalmitis, and Coats' disease.

Proper diagnosis of retinoblastoma requires that the physician be familiar with the clinical variations of the tumor and perform a complete ophthalmologic examination including indirect ophthalmoscopy. Ancillary studies such as ultrasonography, computed tomography, and fluorescein angiography can assist in the diagnosis. The selected management of retinoblastoma should de-

pend on the overall clinical findings and can include enucleation, methods of radiotherapy, cryotherapy and photocoagulation.[6,8] In cases with secondary glaucoma, the tumor is usually quite advanced, and enucleation is considered the treatment of choice. In most cases of retinoblastoma associated with secondary glaucoma, the optic disc cannot be visualized ophthalmoscopically. Therefore, it is particularly important in these cases to obtain a long section of optic nerve stump along with the globe at the time of enucleation, since the most important route of extraocular extension of this tumor is through the optic nerve to the central nervous system.

Other Retinal Tumors

Other than retinoblastoma, most tumors of the sensory retina do not produce secondary glaucoma. In rare instances, advanced retinal capillary hemangiomas may produce secondary glaucoma in association with a total retinal detachment. Cavernous and racemose hemangiomas and astrocytic tumors of the retina almost never become large enough to cause secondary glaucoma.

TUMORS OF THE NONPIGMENTED CILIARY EPITHELIUM

Tumors of the nonpigmented epithelium of the ciliary body can be congenital (medulloepithelioma) or acquired (adenoma and adenocarcinoma).

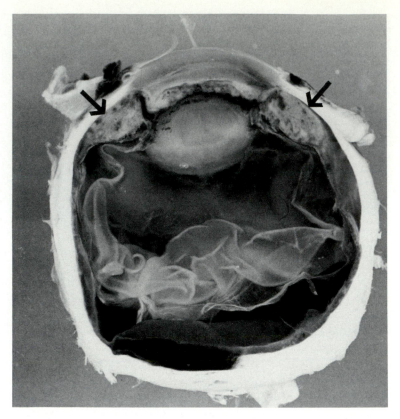

Fig. 61-12   Section of enucleated eye showing diffuse thickening of anterior uveal tract *(arrows)* by large cell lymphoma in this 46-year-old woman with acute congestive glaucoma.

Medulloepithelioma

The medulloepithelioma (previously called diktyoma) is an embryonic ciliary body tumor that becomes clinically apparent in the first few years of life.[2,6] Intraocular medulloepithelioma can have a variety of clinical manifestations. The child may have a solid or cystic ciliary body mass extending into the anterior chamber or have signs and symptoms of secondary glaucoma caused by the large ciliary body mass. Leukocoria or hyphema can also be presenting features. In the Wills Eye Hospital Oncology Service series, both patients with medulloepithelioma had secondary glaucoma.[4] In a large series from the Armed Forces Institute of Pathology, glaucoma occurred in 46% of patients.[2]

On gross examination, the medulloepithelioma appears as a yellow or pink, solid or cystic mass, which can be confined to the ciliary region or extend to occupy a large portion of the globe. Microscopically, the tumor can show only cordlike proliferation of nonpigmented ciliary epithelium (nonteratoid type), or it can show elements of cartilage, skeletel muscle, and other heterotopic elements (teratoid type). Either type can be classified as benign or malignant, depending on cytologic features.

In cases of medulloepithelioma, glaucoma may occur secondary to iris neovascularization or from direct invasion of the anterior chamber angle structures by the tumor. In some instances, hyphema or cysts in the anterior chamber may also contribute to obstruction of aqueous outflow.

The differential diagnosis of intraocular medulloepithelioma includes virtually all congenital ocular malformations, inflammations, and conditions that cause leukocoria, particularly in children. The diagnostic techniques are the same techniques that are described in the section on retinoblastoma.

Since most intraocular medulloepitheliomas are relatively benign, an attempt at local resection by cyclectomy is generally appropriate for smaller tumors. Unfortunately, it is extremely difficult to completely remove such tumors, and recurrence is common, eventually requiring enucleation. In cases with glaucoma, enucleation is usually necessary because of pain or because malignancy cannot be excluded clinically.

Adenoma and Adenocarcinoma

Acquired tumors of the nonpigmented ciliary epithelium are rare, slow-growing, benign or lowly malignant lesions that have clinical features similar to those of malignant melanoma of the ciliary body.[6] They rarely produce secondary glaucoma, but the mechanisms of glaucoma are the same as those that occur with malignant melanomas of the ciliary body. Of four patients seen on the Ocular Oncology Service at Wills Eye Hospital, none had secondary glaucoma.

LYMPHOID TUMORS AND LEUKEMIAS

Lymphoid tumors and leukemias are grouped together here because they can produce a similar infiltration of the uveal tract and retina. The most important lymphoid tumors of the intraocular structures include benign reactive lymphoid hyperplasia (BRLH) of the uvea and malignant lymphoma, particularly large cell lymphoma (histiocytic lymphoma, reticulum cell sarcoma).

Clinical Features

Lymphoid tumors and leukemias can involve the eye by producing a localized or (more commonly) a diffuse infiltration of the uveal tract with the neoplastic cells. Thus, they can simulate clinically a diffuse uveal tumor or uveitis.

On pathologic examination, the uveal tract may be diffusely thickened by the involved cells. In the case of BRLH, the tumor is composed of uniform lymphocytes and plasma cells. In the case of large cell lymphoma and leukemias, there is a uniform infiltration by the characteristic malignant cells.

In cases of intraocular involvement with lymphoid tumors and leukemias, secondary glaucoma most often occurs from direct infiltration of the anterior chamber angle and thickening of the iris and ciliary body by tumor cells[3] (Fig. 61-12). This results in blockage of aqueous outflow and secondary elevation of intraocular pressure.

As mentioned earlier, the differential diagnosis includes all causes of diffuse tumors of the uveal tract, including diffuse melanoma, metastatic carcinomas, and the various causes of uveitis. In patients with intraocular lymphoma or leukemia, the history or general evaluation will often reveal evidence of the systemic disease, thus facilitating the diagnosis. In the case of BRLH, the systemic history and findings are usually normal because the condition is generally confined to the eye. In most cases, fluorescein angiography and ultrasonography are not particularly helpful in the diagnosis. In difficult cases, however, fine-needle aspiration biopsy and cytologic analysis may help establish the correct diagnosis.[1]

The appropriate management of intraocular lymphoid tumors and leukemia is ocular radiotherapy combined with the chemotherapy that the patient may be receiving for the systemic disease. In the case of BRLH, about 2000 R is generally sufficient, whereas in the case of malignant tumors, about 3000 to 4000 R may be necessary to bring about good resolution of the intraocular tumor. In cases with severe glaucoma, radiotherapy may not help, and enucleation of the eye, if it is blind and painful, may be necessary.

TUMORS OF THE PIGMENTED EPITHELIUM

Primary tumors of the pigmented epithelium (adenoma and adenocarcinoma) of the iris, ciliary, and retina are rare lesions. They may be difficult to impossible to differentiate clinically from malignant melanomas of the uveal tract. The mechanisms of glaucoma are the same as those of malignant melanomas.

SYSTEMIC HAMARTOMATOSES (PHAKOMATOSES)

The classic phakomatoses include encephalofacial hemangiomatosis, neurofibromatosis, retinocerebellar capillary hemangiomatosis, and tuberous sclerosis. The two that are more likely to be associated with either infantile or juvenile glaucoma include encephalofacial hemangiomatosis (Sturge-Weber syndrome) and neurofibromatosis. The clinical features, mechanisms of glaucoma, and treatment of the glaucoma associated with these conditions are discussed in Chapter 52.

REFERENCES

1. Augsburger, JJ, et al: Fine needle aspiration biopsy in the diagnosis of intraocular cancer: cytologic-histologic correlations, Ophthalmology 92:39, 1985
2. Broughton, WL, and Zimmerman, LE: A clinicopathologic study of 56 cases of intraocular medulloepitheliomas, Am J Ophthalmol 85:407, 1978
3. Duker, JS, Shields, JA, and Ross M: Intraocular large cell lymphoma presenting as massive thickening of the uveal tract, Retina 7:41, 1987
4. Shields, CL, Shields, JA, Shields, MB, and Augsburger, JJ: Prevalence and mechanisms of secondary intraocular pressure elevation in eyes with intraocular tumors, Ophthalmology 94:839, 1987
5. Shields, JA: Current approaches to the diagnosis and management of choroidal melanomas, Surv Ophthalmol 21:443, 1977
6. Shields, JA: Diagnosis and management of intraocular tumors, St Louis, 1983. The C V Mosby Co
7. Shields, JA, Annesley, WH, and Spaeth, GL: Necrotic melanocytoma of iris with secondary glaucoma, Am J Ophthalmol 84:826, 1977

8. Shields, JA, and Augsburger, JJ: Current approaches to the diagnosis and management of retinoblastoma, Surv Ophthalmol 25:347, 1981

9. Shields, JA, et al: Melanocytoma of the ciliary body and iris, Am J Ophthalmol 89:6332, 1980

10. Shields, JA, Augsburger, JJ, Brown, GC, and Stephens, RF: The differential diagnosis of posterior uveal melanomas, Ophthalmology 87:543, 1980

11. Shields, JA, McDonald, PR, Leonard, BC, and Canny, CLB: The diagnosis of uveal malignant melanoma in eyes with opaque media, Am J Ophthalmol 83:95, 1977

12. Shields, JA, Sanborn, GE, and Augsburger, JJ: The differential diagnosis of iris melanomas, Ophthalmology 90:716, 1983

13. Shields, MB: Textbook of glaucoma, ed. 2, Baltimore, 1986, Williams & Wilkins

14. Shields, MB, and Klintworth, GK: Anterior uveal melanomas and intraocular pressure, Ophthalmology 87:503, 1980

15. Shields, MB, and Proia, AD: Neovascular glaucoma associated with an iris melanoma: a clinicopathologic report, Arch Ophthalmol 105:672, 1987

16. Yanoff, M: Glaucoma mechanisms in ocular malignant melanomas, Am J Ophthalmol 70:898, 1970

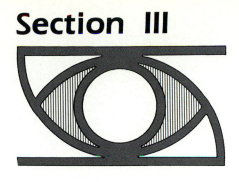

Glaucomas Associated with Systemic Disease and Drugs

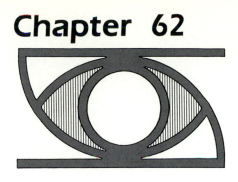

Chapter 62

Glaucoma Secondary to Elevated Episcleral Venous Pressure

Robert N. Weinreb
Shyun Jeng
Bruce J. Goldstick

HISTORICAL BACKGROUND

In 1923, Seidel[90] showed that India ink injected into the anterior chamber of a rabbit soon appeared in episcleral veins. He postulated that the driving force for aqueous flow out of the eye was the hydrostatic pressure difference between the anterior chamber and episcleral veins. It was not until 1942 that Ascher[4-6] observed clear aqueous laminated with blood in a vessel (aqueous vein of Ascher). This confirmed the presence of an anatomic connection between Schlemm's canal and the episcleral veins, which had been demonstrated previously in human eyes. Initially, it was thought that study of these veins might provide useful information concerning the diagnosis and treatment of glaucoma. Ascher postulated that there were fundamental differences in the appearance of these veins in glaucomatous eyes as compared with veins in normal eyes. Although a number of studies have reported subsequently that the appearance of aqueous veins can be altered pharmacologically,[4,5] the clinical significance of these observations remains unclear.[35,52,62,107] Nevertheless, the measurement of episcleral venous pressure continues to be of interest and is useful both in physiologic studies of ocular circulation and in the diagnosis of several secondary glaucomas described in this chapter.

ANATOMY OF THE VENOUS SYSTEM

The venous drainage of the orbit occurs by three principal routes: the superior ophthalmic vein, the inferior ophthalmic vein, and the facial veins, all of which are interanastomosed.[106] The main route of blood flow from the eye is via the superior ophthalmic vein, which drains intracranially through the superior orbital fissure into the cavernous sinus. From here, blood is drained primarily by the superior and inferior petrosal sinuses into the internal jugular vein.[2] A relatively small amount is drained by the external jugular veins and still less by the suboccipital plexus into the vertebral and deep cervical veins.[2,75] The cavernous sinus also has connections with the ipsilateral pterygoid plexus and the contralateral cavernous sinus.

The inferior ophthalmic vein communicates with the larger superior ophthalmic vein and also sends branches through the inferior orbital fissure to the pterygoid plexus, which drains into the deep veins of the neck.

The facial veins communicate with the superior ophthalmic vein via the nasofrontal, lacrimal, and lid veins and communicate with the inferior ophthalmic vein via the infraorbital vein. The facial veins drain mainly in the external jugular veins.

Because of the numerous interconnections between the orbital venous drainage routes and the lack of venous valves, blood can be diverted from one system to the other with blood flow in any direction, depending on the hydrostatic pressure gradient.[26,94]

The venous distribution of the eye has several

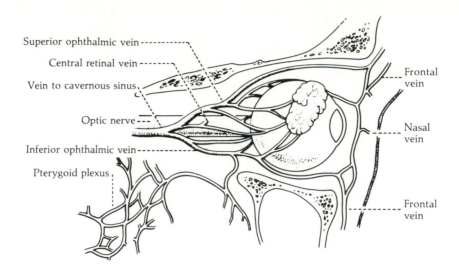

Fig. 62-1   Venous drainage of the orbit. Superior ophthalmic vein, inferior ophthalmic vein, and facial veins are the three principal routes of orbital venous drainage.

drainage routes: retinal veins, vortex veins, anterior ciliary veins, and posterior ciliary veins. Variable connections exist between them. These are diagrammed in Fig. 62-1.

The retinal veins drain into the central retinal vein, which passes into the axial portion of the optic nerve for approximately 10 mm and eventually joins the superior (rarely, the inferior) ophthalmic vein or passes directly into the cavernous sinus.

The vortex veins provide the main venous drainage for the choroid, ciliary body, and iris. The superior vortex veins drain into the superior ophthalmic vein, and the inferior vortex veins open into the inferior ophthalmic vein.[48]

The outer region of the ciliary body is drained by the anterior ciliary venous system (see Chapter 3). As these vessels traverse the sclera, they anastomose with the efferent vessels emanating from Schlemm's canal and eventually pass into the episcleral venous plexus.[34] Schlemm's canal is connected to the episcleral and conjunctival veins by intrascleral aqueous vessels (aqueous veins of Ascher).

The intrascleral vessels can usually be divided into two systems (direct and indirect). The direct vessels have a short intrascleral course and drain directly into the episcleral veins. The indirect vessels form a plexus of fine channels before eventually joining the episcleral venous system.

The aqueous vessels either pass posteriorly and directly drain into the episcleral or conjunctival veins, or they pass anteriorly and run parallel to the limbus (or into the cornea) before eventual anastomosis.[43]

The episcleral vessels drain into the cavernous sinus via the anterior ciliary and superior ophthalmic veins, and the conjunctival vessels either drain into the superior ophthalmic vein or into the facial veins via the angular and palpebral veins.

Under conditions in which central venous pressure is abnormally high, anastomotic channels are found between the retinal venous system and the vortex system.[3] In humans, there are no appreciable connections between the vortex veins and the episcleral veins.

MEASUREMENT OF EPISCLERAL VENOUS PRESSURE

Since Seidel[90] first used a pressure chamber technique to measure episcleral venous pressure, many other methods have been evaluated.[66] Goldmann[41] employed a torsion balance technique, Podos et al.[85] designed an isometric force-displacement transducer, and Krakau et al.[57,58] used a jet of air to measure episcleral venous pressure. These instruments have not been employed widely and are not convenient to use. More recently, two other devices to measure episcleral venous pressure have been described. Zeimer et al.[115] developed an instrument, an episcleral venomanometer, which is attached to a slit-lamp biomicroscope and is operated like a Goldmann tonometer. Friberg et al.[32] designed a portable device that attaches to a sphygmomanometer. These devices have been discussed in Chapter 10 and are reviewed only briefly here.

All methods used to measure episcleral venous pressure involve the external application of a known pressure to an episcleral vessel. The external pressure is increased until there is collapse of the vessel walls. Implicit in these techniques is the assumption that venous walls have little inherent rigidity, so that as soon as the external pressure exceeds the intraluminal pressure, the wall of the vein should begin to collapse. These methods, however, neglect the inherent tension caused by smooth muscle contraction in an episcleral vein and, hence, may underestimate episcleral venous pressure.[84]

There has been considerable debate as to whether the first detectable change in vessel caliber or complete collapse of the vein should be used as the endpoint for measuring episcleral venous pressure.[36,57,68,76] Using the complete collapse of the vein as an endpoint may give falsely elevated measurements.[68] Phelps and Armaly[84] reported a difference of 2 to 3 mm Hg between the pressure required to indent the blood column slightly and that required to obliterate the vessel completely. They described an endpoint whereby the width of the blood column was unchanged, but appeared "blanched." Brubaker,[21] in a study with rabbits, reported that the point at which some portion of a preselected vessel collapsed correlated best with cannulated pressure. However, Gaasterland and Pederson[36] and Mims and Holland[76] suggested that the earliest perceptible change in venous caliber is the most accurate endpoint compared with cannulation measurements. They also found a difference of 5 to 7 mm Hg between slight indentation and complete obliteration of the episcleral vein.

Methods of Measurement and Normal Values

The pressure chamber method was first described by Seidel[90] in 1923. This method uses a device with a chamber in which the pressure can be altered to any desired level. One side of the chamber is formed by a thin, transparent elastic membrane, which is placed against the eye. The opposite side of the chamber is rigid and transparent, enabling one to view the episcleral vein against which the membrane is applied. The pressure in the chamber required to cause the desired venous endpoint is recorded as the episcleral venous pressure.

Goldmann[41] used a torsion balance to apply a variable force over a constant area of conjunctiva overlying the episcleral vein under study.[21,39] Epi-scleral venous pressure was determined by dividing the force of the torsion balance required to reach the desired endpoint by the area of the probe tip.

Krakau et al.[57] directed a jet of air against an episcleral vein and measured the pressure needed to collapse the vein. One advantage of this method is that local anesthetics are not required.

The venomanometer, described by Zeimer et al.,[115] is an instrument that can be mounted on a slit-lamp in a similar fashion to a Goldmann tonometer. A flexible transparent tip is connected to an air chamber. A rotating dial controls the position of an air-sealed piston, and the position of the piston determines the volume and, therefore, pressure of the air chamber. The pressure at which there is half blanching of the vessel is recorded as the episcleral venous pressure.

Recently, Friberg et al.[32] have described a device that attaches to a sphygmomanometer to measure episcleral venous pressure. The advantage of this device is that it is portable and does not need to be used in conjunction with a slit-lamp.

Numerous methods have been used to determine episcleral venous pressure in the eyes of normal subjects. Phelps and Armaly,[84] using the air chamber technique, reported a mean episcleral venous pressure of 9.0 ± 1.6 mm Hg in 56 eyes. Podos et al,[87] using a lucite cone connected to a displacement transducer (modified Goldmann device), noted a mean value of 9.0 ± 1.4 mm Hg in 39 eyes. Talusan and Schwartz[96] obtained a mean episcleral venous pressure of 9.1 mm Hg in 20 eyes. Zeimer et al.,[115] using the venomanometer, found a mean value of 7.6 ± 1.3 mm Hg. Zeimer attributed this low value to the sensitivity of his device for detecting small amounts of blanching of an episcleral vessel.

Results of episcleral venous pressure measurement in glaucomatous eyes have been variable. Linnér,[67] Leith,[65] and Podos et al.[85] did not find a significant difference in episcleral venous pressure between normal and glaucomatous eyes. However, Lohlein and Weigelin,[70] Rickenbach and Werner,[88] and Goldmann[42] observed a lower mean episcleral venous pressure in eyes with primary open-angle glaucoma. Similarly, Talusan and Schwartz[96] found that episcleral venous pressure correlates negatively with intraocular pressure. They postulated that intraocular venous and aqueous channels are compressed in eyes with high intraocular pressure, resulting in a decrease in aqueous outflow, and this could lead to a decrease in episcleral venous pressure.

Clinical Implications

In the steady state, the dependence of intraocular pressure on episcleral venous pressure is approximated by the modified Goldmann equation[41] P_0 - F/C + P_{ev}, where P_0 = intraocular pressure, P_{ev} = episcleral venous pressure, F = aqueous inflow, and C = outflow facility. According to this formula, a rise in episcleral venous pressure, unless compensated by a fall in the rate of aqueous inflow or an increase in outflow facility,[13,14] will cause an equal rise in intraocular pressure. Although this relationship has led many investigators to speculate that elevated episcleral venous pressure could be an important factor in primary open-angle glaucoma, this has not been demonstrated to be the case.[85,96] However, a rise in episcleral venous pressure may be important in several secondary types of glaucoma, including those associated with carotid-cavernous sinus fistula,[104] orbital venous cavernous sinus thrombosis, dural arteriovenous shunts,[45] thyroid endocrine exophthalmos,[56] superior vena cava syndrome,[8,20] and Sturge-Weber syndrome.[85,109] Rarely, episcleral venous pressure is elevated idiopathically in eyes with open-angle glaucoma.[12,77,86,95] Positional variation of intraocular pressure also may be related to changes of episcleral venous pressure.[37,61,98]

PATHOPHYSIOLOGY

Precise relationships between elevated episcleral venous presure and increased intraocular pressure are difficult to predict. If outflow facility and aqueous inflow remain constant, Goldmann's equation indicates that there should be a direct correlation between intraocular pressure and episcleral venous pressure. However, when the episcleral venous pressure was artificially elevated by tightening a cuff around the neck of human subjects, intraocular pressure increased only 80% of the measured rise of episcleral venous pressure.[63,64] Several hypotheses have been proposed to explain this relationship. Aqueous humor may drain from the anterior chamber by other pathways (e.g., uveoscleral outflow), or the elevation of intraocular pressure may result in a coincident decrease in the rate of aqueous inflow (pseudofacility).[63,64,112] Using fluorophotometry, Brubaker[22] could not confirm an effect of increased intraocular pressure on aqueous inflow,[22] and Moses et al.[79] have questioned the existence of pseudofacility.

Besides the direct effect of elevated episcleral venous pressure on intraocular pressure, there are times when dilated episcleral veins are present but are not the direct cause of the glaucoma. If elevated venous pressure involves the vortex venous system, then congestion and edema of the choroid may produce forward displacement of the lens-iris diaphragm, resulting in a shallow anterior chamber and possibly secondary angle-closure glaucoma.* Also, carotid-cavernous sinus fistulae can produce elevated venous pressure and reduce arterial supply, which may lead to ocular ischemia and central retinal vein occlusion. This can lead to the development of rubeosis iridis and neovascular glaucoma.[89,94,107]

Chronic elevation of intraocular pressure caused by elevated venous pressure may cause glaucomatous optic nerve damage similar to that produced by primary open-angle glaucoma. The increased venous pressure decreases the perfusion pressure to the nerve head, making it more susceptible to damage.[86,89,94,107] Moses[78] provided a mechanical model to study the effect of increased venous pressure and demonstrated an increase in intraocular pressure and an increased tendency for intraocular veins to collapse, retarding intraocular blood flow.

EFFECT OF POSTURAL CHANGE ON EPISCLERAL VENOUS PRESSURE

Intraocular pressure varies with body position. As posture changes from upright to sitting to supine, corresponding increases of intraocular pressure have been documented.† Intraocular pressure in normal eyes may increase twofold when one changes from a sitting to an inverted position.[32,105] Krieglstein et al.[61] evaluated postural effects on intraocular pressure and speculated that they correlated with changes of episcleral venous pressure. This was confirmed by Friberg et al.[32] They measured both intraocular pressure and episcleral venous pressure during postural inversion and concluded that increases in the latter, in large part, contributed to elevations of intraocular pressure.[32] In addition, they noted that retinal arteriolar caliber decreases and central retinal artery pressure increases during inversion[33]; this can cause impairment of vascular perfusion of the eye.

EFFECT OF PHARMACOLOGIC AGENTS ON EPISCLERAL VENOUS PRESSURE

The effects of a number of pharmacologic agents on episcleral venous pressure have been evaluated.

Initially, Thomassen[99] reported that pilocar-

---

*References 15, 42, 43, 46, 93, 110.
†References 33, 40, 51, 54, 60, 91, 98.

pine decreases episcleral venous pressure. In retrospect, his measurements of episcleral venous pressure were high (30 mm Hg) and probably unreliable. Bain[7] found that topical pilocarpine caused a decrease in episcleral venous pressure, which preceded the fall in intraocular pressure. Linnér,[68] however, found that pilocarpine and acetazolamide have no effect on episcleral venous pressure. Recent studies[35,38,52] have reported that pilocarpine causes an initial transient rise in episcleral venous pressure followed by a return to normal.

Wilke[109] and Kupfer et al.[62] have shown that topical epinephrine has no effect on episcleral venous pressure. In contrast, Kaskel et al.[52] reported that episcleral venous pressure was reduced significantly within 45 minutes in association with corresponding changes in intraocular pressure. Wettrell et al.[108] reported that orally administered beta-adrenergic agonists and antagonists have no net effect on episcleral venous pressure.

Clonidine,[59] an alpha-adrenergic agonist, has been reported to decrease episcleral venous pressure. However, the changes were too small to account for the observed concomitant decrease in intraocular pressure. In other studies,[52] clonidine caused a transient reduction of episcleral venous pressure that persisted for approximately 15 minutes. Although episcleral venous pressure returned to baseline levels within 1 hour, the associated reduction of intraocular pressure persisted.

The sustained decrease of intraocular pressure in rabbits exposed to oxygen reported by Yablonski et al.[111] has been postulated to be caused by a decrease in episcleral venous pressure.

INCREASED EPISCLERAL VENOUS PRESSURE

Clinical Characteristics

Generally, patients with elevated episcleral venous pressure have dilated and tortuous episcleral veins. However, a "caput-medusa" appearance of the vessel may not be pathognomonic and may occur in other types of long-standing glaucoma.[30]

The site at which the underlying disease process interferes with the venous drainage determines whether elevated episcleral venous pressure is unilateral or bilateral. If it is localized near the eye, the glaucoma is unilateral. For example, orbital varices and Sturge-Weber syndrome characteristically produce unilateral elevated episcleral venous pressure. If venous obstruction occurs in the neck, as in the superior vena cava syndrome, the eyes are generally affected bilaterally. If the venous disturbance is located in the head, such as with a

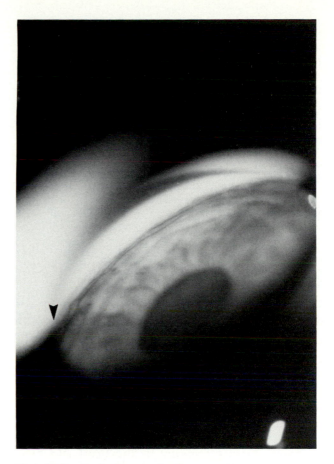

Fig. 62-2 Goniophotograph demonstrating open anterior chamber angle with reflux of blood into Schlemm's canal *(arrow)* in patient with idiopathic elevated episcleral venous pressure.

carotid-cavernous sinus fistula, ocular involvement may be either unilateral or bilateral, depending on the size of the fistula and its specific anatomic communications.[18,94]

In patients with elevated episcleral venous pressure, the anterior chamber angle is usually open and appears normal except for the possible presence of blood in Schlemm's canal (Fig. 62-2). Tonography usually is normal, except in long-standing cases when outflow facility may be decreased.[101] This may persist after episcleral venous pressure is normalized.[77] Rarely, decreased ocular perfusion may lead to relative ischemia and, possibly, neovascular glaucoma.[47,92] Increased venous stasis in the posterior segment may cause congestion of the uvea, push the lens diaphragm forward, and cause angle-closure glaucoma.[46]

Specific Clinical Entities

These are summarized in the box on p. 1130.

**CLASSIFICATION OF ELEVATED EPISCLERAL
VENOUS PRESSURE**

Venous obstruction
1. Retrobulbar tumor[9,81]
2. Thyroid ophthalmopathy
3. Superior vena cava syndrome (mediastinal tumor)
4. Congestive heart failure[10]
5. Thrombosis of cavernous sinus or orbital vein[19]
6. Vasculitis involving episcleral vein or orbital vein
7. Jugular vein obstruction

Arteriovenous anomalies
1. Carotid cavernous sinus fistula[18,26]
2. Orbital varix[73,101]
3. Sturge-Weber syndrome[83,106]
4. Orbital-meningeal shunts[22]
5. Carotid jugular venous shunts
6. Intraocular vascular shunts[81]

Idiopathic elevation of episcleral venous pressure[12,77,86]
1. Sporadic
2. Familial

Orbital varices

Orbital varices are typically found in young persons with a history of intermittent unilateral proptosis dating from birth or early childhood. Proptosis may be provoked or worsened by increasing venous pressure in the head and neck such as following a Valsalva maneuver or bending over.[56,73,110] Between episodes, the involved eye may become enophthalmic.[56] Patients may present with dilated veins in the eyelid and anterior orbit, acute orbital hemorrhage, or thrombophlebitis.[72,74,110] Approximately 50% may have other systemic venous anomalies involving the scalp, palate, and forehead and, rarely, it may be associated with the Klippel-Trenaunay-Weber syndrome.[74,87] The conjunctiva may show multiloculated cysts, which may be misdiagnosed as orbital lymphangioma.[110]

Orbital x-ray films may reveal orbital phleboliths and an enlarged orbit,[72,73,110] whereas ultrasonography and computed tomography may demonstrate a soft tissue mass.[56] B-scan ultrasonography may show retroocular fluid-filled spaces that enlarge during a Valsalva maneuver.[56] Venography usually reveals an abnormal venous pattern. Theoretically, glaucomatous damage to the optic nerve may result if the varix causes a persistent or a large transient elevation of episcleral venous pressure. However, since venous pressure is normal between attacks and the rise in episcleral venous pressure is small and transient, glaucoma is uncommon. Vision is seldom affected unless the varix compresses the optic nerve directly; most patients continue to

have stable vision throughout life.[17,56] Surgical intervention for an orbital varix is generally performed for cosmetic reasons[110] and is virtually never needed for the treatment of glaucoma, which usually responds to medical therapy.

Carotid-cavernous sinus and other arteriovenous fistulae

Fistulae between the carotid artery and cavernous sinus, whether traumatic or spontaneous in origin, cause ocular manifestations that may include a bruit, pulsating exophthalmos, conjunctival and orbital vessel engorgement from reversal of blood flow into the orbital venous system, diplopia from traumatic paresis or orbital compression, blurred vision, and orbital pain[26,29,49,80,89] (Fig. 62-3). There may be a subjective sensation of a pulsating sound. Spontaneous choroidal detachments, papilledema, and retinal hemorrhage occur rarely.[45] Because of intracranial connections between the two cavernous sinuses, a unilateral fistula may result in bilateral ocular symptoms or signs.[18,94] Carotid-cavernous fistulae produce elevated venous pressure and reduced arterial pressure and may result in ischemic ocular necrosis.[92]

Visual impairment and diplopia are present in about 50% of cases.[49,62] Visual loss can be caused by corneal exposure, hypoxic-ischemic eye syndrome or glaucoma.[62,89] The intraocular pressure is elevated in 60% to 70% of patients.[62,94]; however, characteristic glaucomatous optic disc damage is much less common.[74,89,94] Elevated episcleral venous pressure is the most common reason for elevated intraocular pressure in the presence of arteriovenous fistulae.[44,89,94,104] Madsen[74] reported one case of absolute glaucoma out of 18 patients with arteriovenous fistulae, and Kupersmith et al.[62] reported a case of central retinal artery occlusion caused by elevated intraocular pressure. Other signs may include a low ophthalmic artery pressure on the involved side,[23,49,89] dilated ocular veins, and large intraocular pressure pulsations noted during tonometry or tonography. Initially, patients have a normal outflow facility, and therefore miotic therapy is usually of little value. In cases of long-standing episcleral venous pressure elevation, outflow facility may become impaired. With time, routine x-ray films may show widening of the superior orbital fissure and erosion of the adjacent sella and sphenoid sinus. The diagnosis is confirmed using carotid arteriography.[97]

Carotid-cavernous fistulae may be associated with rarer causes of elevated intraocular pressure. The decrease in arterial flow and venous stasis can

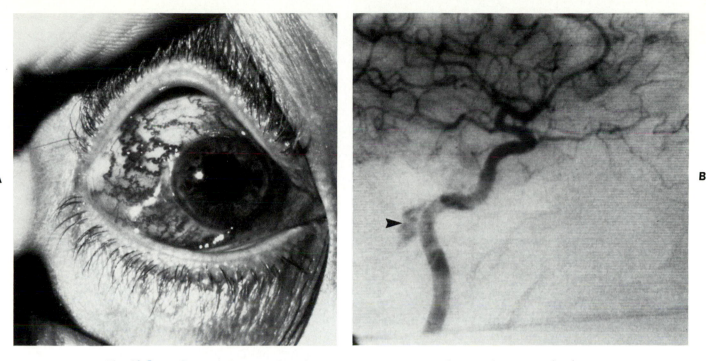

Fig. 62-3 **A,** Caput-medusa vascular enlargement seen in a patient with a carotid-cavernous fistula. **B,** Fistula *(arrow)* is demonstrated angiographically.

reduce ocular perfusion pressure, resulting in ischemia and neovascularization of the optic disc and rubeosis iridis. Neovascular glaucoma may result.[50,89,92,107] Ophthalmodynamometry shows decreased ophthalmic artery pressure on the involved side. A carotid-cavernous sinus fistula can cause elevated venous pressure in the vortex veins, the central retinal vein, and the episcleral veins. Harris and Rice[46] reported a case of angle-closure glaucoma caused by a carotid-cavernous sinus fistula. He proposed that the pressure in the vortex veins caused engorgement of the choroidal vessels, increasing the volume of the posterior segment and producing a forward shift of the iris-lens diaphragm with subsequent angle-closure. In some cases, choroidal detachments may be caused by the same mechanism.

The decision to operate on patients with carotid-cavernous fistulae is often difficult.[67] Although secondary glaucoma and ischemic optic atrophy may be indications for surgery, potential surgical complications are severe,[102] including vascular accidents and ocular ischemia.[89,107] Additionally, in a study of 18 patients, Madsen[74] demonstrated spontaneous closure of the fistulae in 18% of patients, a significant improvement in 43%, no change in 33% and death from an underlying disease in 6%. Both the favorable prognosis in some patients and

the potential for serious surgical complications have resulted in a conservative approach to many patients with this problem.[89,102] Recently, Kupersmith et al.[62] were able to close 97% of traumatic carotid-cavernous sinus fistulae without complication using a transvascular approach and superselective angiographic demonstrations of the fistulae. This and other new techniques need further evaluation.

Sturge-Weber syndrome

Hemangiomas of the lid either without intracranial involvement or with intracranial involvement (Sturge-Weber syndrome) are associated with increased episcleral venous pressure and secondary glaucoma.[28,83,106] Several theories have been proposed to explain the pathogenesis of glaucoma in Sturge-Weber syndrome including (1) the presence of a congenital-like angle structure with anterior insertion of the iris root and a thick uveoscleral meshwork[24,31]; (2) the presence of a choroidal hemangioma leading to transudation of fluid and a hypersecretion type of glaucoma; (3) choroidal hemangioma leading to shallow anterior chamber and subsequent angle-closure glaucoma; and (4) elevated episcleral venous pressure.[83,106]

Phelps[83] examined episcleral venous pressure in 16 patients with Sturge-Weber syndrome and glaucoma and found that all but one had markedly elevated episcleral venous pressure. All glaucomatous eyes were noted to have an episcleral hemangioma, and he proposed that the hemangioma, with its arteriovenous shunts, may elevate episcleral venous pressure and, subsequently, intraocular pressure.

The glaucoma is characteristically ipsilateral to the hemangioma (Fig. 62-4). Glaucoma may occur in newborns, children, or adults. In general, the more extensive the hemangioma, the more severe the glaucoma, and the earlier it is diagnosed.[83] The episcleral hemangioma may be difficult to detect except by careful biomicroscopic examination.

If glaucoma is diagnosed, a trial of medical therapy should be initiated. Many patients respond poorly to medical therapy, and surgery may become necessary. Because nitroglycerin causes potent dilation of the venous capacitance system, it has been suggested that it may be useful in Sturge-Weber syndrome.[114] In the few reported cases, laser trabeculoplasty has been ineffective in lowering intraocular pressure in these eyes. Goniotomy has been reported to be ineffective in those with a congenital type of glaucoma. During trabeculectomy,[53,83] a sudden uveal effusion with detachment of the choroid and ciliary body may occur when the anterior chamber is entered. Bellows et al.[9] have suggested that a prophylactic posterior sclerotomy may prevent this complication.

Idiopathic elevation of episcleral venous pressure

Although most eyes with elevated episcleral venous pressure are associated with local or systemic causes, idiopathic elevation has been reported to occur sporadically[9,12,86,85] and in families.[77] Various medical and neurologic examinations may be necessary to exclude other causes. Episcleral venous pressure in these cases is approximately 20 mm Hg. Some patients demonstrate an intraocular pressure that is higher than the corresponding elevation of episcleral venous pressure, accompanied by decreased outflow facility.[9,86,95] Idiopathic elevation of episcleral venous pressure may occur in all age groups. The anterior chamber angle appears open with or without blood in Schlemm's canal. Although a satisfactory explanation has not been offered for this phenomenon, the right eye is involved in a disproportionate number of unilateral cases (Fig. 62-5) and is more severely damaged in bilateral cases.[95] The clinical course is similar to primary open-angle glaucoma. Although many eyes can be controlled with topical medication, surgery is indicated if medical therapy is unsuccessful.

Superior vena cava syndrome

Obstruction of the superior vena cava results in increased venous pressure in those areas in which it provides venous drainage. It is associated with edema and cyanosis of the head, neck, and upper extremities and dilated, engorged veins of the chest wall resulting from the development of collateral circulation.[100] Increased intracranial pressure may cause headache, visual distortion, and altered consciousness. Ocular findings include eyelid edema,[82] papilledema, prominent conjunctival, episcleral, and retinal veins, elevated episcleral venous pressure,[1,2] and increased intraocular pressure, particularly in the supine position.[8,20] The optic discs usually do not show glaucomatous cupping, presumably because of an opposing effect of increased intracranial pressure.[113]

Before the advent of antibiotics, the superior

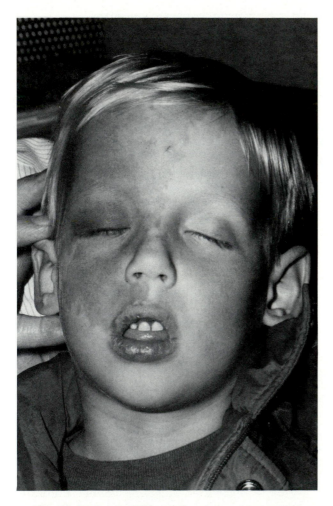

Fig. 62-4 Sturge-Weber syndrome in 6-year-old boy.

vena cava syndrome was commonly caused by mediastinitis secondary to pulmonary infections (syphilis or tuberculosis). Today, malignancy is the cause of 97% of all cases of the superior vena cava syndrome.[71] Other causes include aortic aneurysm, enlarged hilar nodes, and thyroid disease. Treatment of the superior vena cava syndrome must be directed to the underlying disease processes, and the prognosis depends on the underlying cause.

Thyroid ophthalmopathy

Thyroid ophthalmopathy is a common cause of exophthalmos (Fig. 62-6). Pathologically, there is infiltration of the orbit with lymphocytes, mast cells, and plasma cells. This may lead to secondary glaucoma by several mechanisms:

1. Elevated episcleral venous pressure may result from the retrobulbar infiltration process. The congestion and edema of the orbit may compromise the orbital venous system (i.e., superior and inferior ophthalmic veins) and raise episcleral venous pressure. Rarely, thrombosis of the orbital veins can result in increased episcleral venous pressure.
2. The contraction of extraocular muscles may cause abnormally high intraocular pressure in some specific directions of gaze.[16] Usually, fibrosis of the inferior rectus muscle causes significantly increased intraocular pressure during upward gaze.
3. Idiopathic decreased outflow facility may occur.

4. Corneal exposure and secondary infection may lead to peripheral anterior synechiae and secondary glaucoma.

In cases of glaucoma caused by orbital infiltration, steroids have been used successfully. Occasionally, radiation or surgical orbital decompression becomes necessary in patients suffering from visual impairment caused by direct compression of the optic nerve, corneal exposure, or rarely secondary glaucoma.

Treatment of Glaucoma Secondary to Elevated Episcleral Venous Pressure

Medical treatment

Medical therapy should be employed initially to treat glaucoma secondary to increased episcleral venous pressure. Theoretically, if glaucoma is entirely the result of elevated episcleral venous pressure, parasympathomimetic agents, such as pilocarpine, should have little effect in lowering intraocular pressure. However, pilocarpine is effective in lowering intraocular pressure if outflow facility is decreased.[1,5,49,95] Drugs that decrease aqueous inflow, such as carbonic anhydrase inhibitors and beta-blocking agents, decrease intraocular pressure in some eyes.[76] Medical therapy cannot lower intraocular pressure below the abnormally elevated episcleral venous pressure.

Surgical treatment

When glaucoma secondary to elevated episcleral venous pressure is not controlled by maximal tolerated medical therapy, surgical interven-

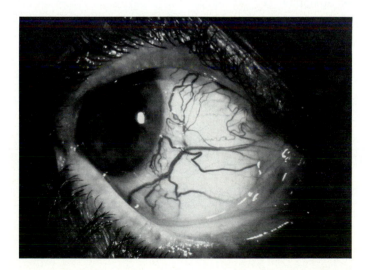

Fig. 62-5 Enlarged episcleral veins in the right eye of a patient with idiopathic elevated episcleral venous pressure.

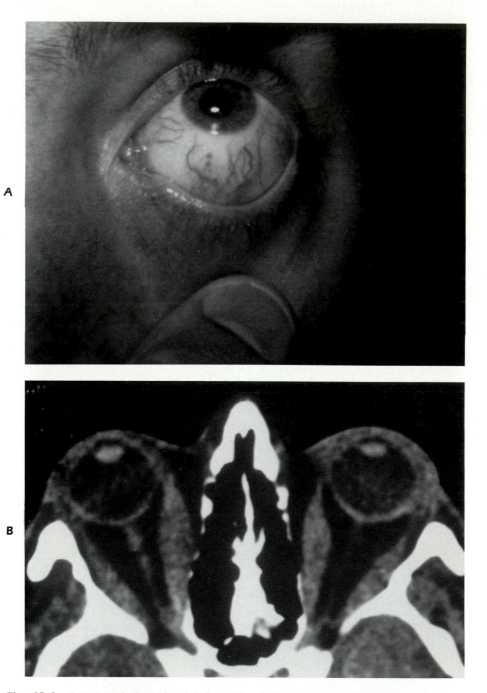

Fig. 62-6 Patient with thyroid ophthalmopathy demonstrating exophthalmos, and hyperemia overlying the inferior rectus muscle, **A,** and enlarged rectus muscles (with characteristic sparing of tendons) on CT scanning, **B.**

tion is indicated. Laser trabeculoplasty may be attempted. Other than isolated reports, there is no consensus whether this is a predictably effective treatment modality in these eyes.

Filtration surgery provides a pathway for aqueous humor to bypass the elevated episcleral venous pressure. However, filtering surgery in these eyes can be associated with untoward events that are unusual following similar procedures in eyes with primary open-angle glaucoma. Bellows et al.[9] reported marked intraoperative choroidal effusion during glaucoma surgery in eyes with prominent episcleral veins. When episcleral venous pressure is elevated, a substantial increase in the pressure differential across the capillary membranes of uveal tissue exists when the eye is entered during surgery and intraocular pressure is lowered to atmospheric pressure. The increased transcapillary pressure favors the rapid transudation of fluid from the intravascular to the extravascular space. This can be marked in the choroid and ciliary body. To void this complication, Bellows recommended performing a posterior sclerotomy before opening the anterior chamber and advised leaving the sclerotomy patent after surgery to prevent postoperative formation of choroidal effusion.

Bigger[12] believes that ocular surgery in these patients is associated with an increased incidence of hemorrhage because of the dilated veins and hyperemic tissue. Christensen and Records[25] reported a case of expulsive hemorrhage during surgery for Sturge-Weber syndrome, presumably secondary to elevated capillary pressure and a choroidal hemangioma.

If neovascular glaucoma is concurrently present, then the prognosis is poor. This represents a sign of severe ocular ischemia in patients with carotid-cavernous fistulae, and surgical intervention for the fistula has a poor prognosis.[102] Harris et al.[47] have reported good response to panretinal photocoagulation in a patient with proliferative retinopathy caused by a carotid-cavernous fistula.

REFERENCES

1. Alfano, JE: Glaucoma following ligation of the superior vena cava, Am J Ophthalmol 60:412, 1965
2. Alfano, JE, and Alfano, PA: Glaucoma and the superior vena caval obstruction syndrome, Am J Ophthalmol 42:685, 1956
3. Anderson, DR: Vascular supply to the optic nerve of primates, Am J Ophthalmol 70:341, 1970
4. Ascher, KW: Aqueous veins, Am J Ophthalmol 25:31, 1942
5. Ascher, KW: The aqueous veins: physiologic importance of the visible elimination of intraocular fluid, Am J Ophthalmol 25:1174, 1942
6. Ascher, KW: Aqueous veins: local pharmacologic effects on aqueous veins; glaucoma and aqueous veins, Am J Ophthalmol 25:1301, 1942
7. Bain, WES: Variations in the episcleral venous pressure in relation to glaucoma, Br J Ophthalmol 38:129, 1954
8. Bedrosian, EH: Increased intraocular pressure secondary to mediastinal syndrome, Arch Ophthalmol 47:641, 1952
9. Bellows, RA, Chylack LT, Epstein, DL, and Hutchinson, T: Choroidal effusion during glaucoma surgery in patients with prominent episcleral vessels, Arch Ophthalmol 97:493, 1979
10. Bettelheim, H: Der episklerale Venendruck bei pulmonar Hypertension: ein Beitrag zur Frage des kardiogenen Glaukoms, v Graefe's Arch Klin Exp Ophthalmol 177:108, 1969
11. Bietti, GB, and Vanni, V: Glaucoma secondaire à une obstruction veineuse extra-oculaire, Ophthalmologica 142:227, 1961
12. Bigger, JF: Glaucoma with elevated episcleral venous pressure, South Med J 68:1444, 1975
13. Bill, A: Aspects of the drainage of aqueous humor in cats, Arch Ophthalmol 67:148, 1962
14. Bill, A: Early effects of epinephrine on aqueous humor dynamics in vervet monkeys (Cercopithecus ethiops), Exp Eye Res 8:35, 1969
15. Bloome, MA: Transient angle-closure glaucoma in central retinal vein occlusion, Ann Ophthalmol 9:44, 1977
16. Bock, VJ, and Stepanik, J: Glaukom bei thyreogenem Exophthalmus, Ophthalmologica 142:365, 1961
17. Brauston, BB, and Norton, EWD: Intermittent exophthalmos, Am J Ophthalmol 55:701, 1963
18. Brismar, G, and Brismar, J: Spontaneous carotid-cavernous fistulas: clinical symptomatology, Acta Ophthalmol 54:542, 1976
19. Brismar, G, and Brismar, J: Aseptic thrombosis of orbital veins and cavernous sinus, Acta Ophthalmol 55:9, 1977
20. Brolin, ES: Ocular tension changes imposed by rapid, intentionally varied venous pressure in a case of pulmonary tumor, Acta Ophthalmol 27:394, 1949
21. Brubaker, RF: Determination of episcleral venous pressure in the eye, Arch Ophthalmol 77:110, 1967
22. Brubaker RF: Physiology of aqueous humor formation. In Drance, S, and Neufeld, A, editors: Applied pharmacology in the medical treatment of glaucoma, New York, 1984, Grune & Stratton, Inc
23. Burton, CV, and Goldberg, MF: Exophthalmos from ruptured intracavernous carotid aneurysm without pulsation, bruit or murmur, Am J Ophthalmol 70:830, 1970
24. Chandler, P, and Grant, WM: Lecture notes on glaucoma, Philadelphia, 1968, Lea & Febiger
25. Christensen, GR, and Records, RE: Glaucoma and expulsive hemorrhage mechanisms in the Sturge-Weber syndrome, Ophthalmology 86:1360, 1979

26. DeKeiyer, RJW: Spontaneous carotico-cavernous fistulas: the importance of the typical limbal vascular loops for the diagnosis, the recognition of glaucoma and the uses of conservative therapy in this condition, Doc Ophthalmol 46:403, 1979

27. Duke-Elder, S, and McFaul, PA: The ocular adenexa. II. Lacrimal orbital and paraorbital disease, System of ophthalmology, vol 13, St. Louis, 1974, The CV Mosby Co

28. Dunphy, EB: Glaucoma accompanying nevus flammeus, Am J Ophthalmol 18:709, 1935

29. Elliot, AJ: Ocular manifestations of carotid-cavernous fistulas, Postgrad Med 15:191, 1954

30. Epstein, DL: Chandler and Grant's glaucoma, Philadelphia, 1986, Lea & Febiger

31. Font, RL, and Ferry, AP: The phakomatoses, Int Ophthalmol Clin 12:1, 1972

32. Friberg, TR, Sandborn, G, and Weinreb, RN: Episcleral venous pressure and intraocular pressure elevation during inverted posture, Am J Ophthalmol 103:523, 1987

33. Friberg, TR, and Weinreb, RN: Ocular manifestations of gravity inversion, JAMA 253:1755, 1985

34. Gaasterland, DE, Jocson, VL, and Sears, ML: Channels of aqueous outflow and related blood vessels. III. Episcleral arteriovenous anastomoses in the rhesus monkey eye (Macaca mulatta), Arch Ophthalmol 84:770, 1970

35. Gaasterland, D, Kupfer, C, and Ross, K: Studies of aqueous humor dynamics in man. IV. Effects of pilocarpine upon measurements in young normal volunteers, Invest Ophthalmol Vis Sci 14:848, 1975

36. Gaasterland, DE, and Pederson, JE: Episcleral venous pressure: a comparison of invasive and noninvasive measurement, Invest Ophthalmol Vis Sci 24:1417, 1983

37. Galin, MA, McIvor, JW, and Magruder, GB: Influence of position on intraocular pressure, Am J Ophthalmol 55:720, 1963

38. Gallin, PF, Yablonski, ME, Shapiro, D, and Podos, SM: Oxygen effects on aqueous flow and episcleral venous pressure, Invest Ophthalmol Vis Sci 19:43, 1980

39. Gartner, S: Blood vessels of the conjunctiva, Arch Ophthalmol 32:464, 1944

40. Gartner, S, and Beck, W: Ocular tension in the Trendelenburg position, Am J Ophthalmol 51:1040, 1965

41. Goldmann, H: Die Kammerwasservenen und das poiseulle'sche Gesetz, Ophthalmologica 118:496, 1949

42. Goldmann, H: Der Druck im Schlemmschen Kanal bei Normalen und Glaucoma simplex, Experientia 6:110, 1950

43. Graffin, AL, and Corddry, EG: Studies of the peripheral blood vascular beds in the bulbar conjunctiva of man, Bull Johns Hopkins Hosp 93:275, 1953

44. Grant, WM: Shallowing of the anterior chamber following occlusion of the central retinal vein, Am J Ophthalmol 75:384, 1973

45. Harbison, JW, Guerry, D, and Wiesinger, H: Dural arteriovenous fistula and spontaneous choroidal detachment: new cause of an old disease, Br J Ophthalmol 62:483, 1978

46. Harris, GJ, and Rice, PR: Angle closure in carotid cavernous fistula, Ophthalmology 86:1521, 1979

47. Harris, MJ, Fine, SL, and Miller, NR: Photocoagulation treatment of proliferative retinopathy secondary to carotid-cavernous fistula, Am J Ophthalmol 90:515, 1980

48. Hayreh, SS, and Baines, JAB: Occlusion of the vortex veins: an experimental study, Br J Ophthalmol 57:217, 1973

49. Henderson, JW, and Schneider, RC: The ocular findings in carotid-cavernous fistula in a series of 17 cases, Am J Ophthalmol 48:585, 1959

50. Holman, E, Gerbode, F, and Richards, V: Communications between the carotid artery and cavernous sinus, Angiology 2:311, 1951

51. Jain, MR, and Marmion, VJ: Rapid pneumatic and Mackay-Marg applanation tonometry to evaluate the postural effect on intraocular pressure, Br J Ophthalmol 68:687, 1976

52. Kaskel, D, Becker, H, and Rudolf, H: Fruhwirkungen von Clonidin, Adrenalin, und Pilocarpin auf den Augeninnendruck und Episkleralvenendruck des gesunden menschlichen Auges, v Graefes Arch Klin Exp Ophthalmol 213:251, 1980

53. Keverline, PO, and Hiles, DA: Trabeculectomy for adolescent onset glaucoma in the Sturge-Weber syndrome, J Pediatr Ophthalmol 13:144, 1977

54. Klatz, RM, et al: The effects of gravity inversion procedures on systemic blood pressure, intraocular pressure, and central retinal arterial pressure, J Am Optometric Assoc 82:853, 1983

55. Kolker, AE, and Hetherington, J: Diagnosis and treatment of glaucoma, ed 5, St. Louis, 1984, The CV Mosby Co

56. Kollarits, CR, et al: Management of a patient with orbital varices, visual loss and ipsilateral glaucoma, Ophthalmic Surg 8:54, 1977

57. Krakau, CE, Widakowich, J, and Wilke, K: Measurement of the episcleral venous pressure by means of an airjet, Acta Ophthalmol 51:185, 1973

58. Krakau, CE, and Wilke, K: Effects of loading of the eye on intraocular pressure and on the episcleral venous pressure, Acta Ophthalmol 52:107, 1974

59. Krieglstein, GK, Langham, ME, and Leydhecker, W: The peripheral and central neural actions of clonidine in normal and glaucomatous eyes, Invest Ophthalmol Vis Sci 17;149, 1978

60. Krieglstein, GK, and Langham, ME: Influence of body position on the intraocular pressure of normal and glaucomatous eyes, Ophthalmologica 171:132, 1975

61. Krieglstein, GK, Waller, WK, and Leydhecker, W: The vascular basis of the positional influence on the intraocular pressure, v Graefes Arch Klin Exp Ophthalmol 206:99, 1978

62. Kupersmith, MJ, Berenstein, A, Flamm, E, and Ransohoff, J: Neuro-ophthalmology abnormalities and intravascular therapy of traumatic carotid cavernous fistulas, Ophthalmology 93:906, 1986

63. Kupfer, C, Gaasterland, D, and Ross, K: Studies of aqueous humor dynamics in man. II. Measurements in young normal subjects using acetazolamide and L-epinephrine, Invest Ophthalmol 10:523, 1971

64. Kupfer, C, and Ross, K: Studies of aqueous humor dynamics in man. I. Measurements in young normal subjects, Invest Ophthalmol 19:518, 1971

65. Leith, AB: Episcleral venous pressure in tonography, Br J Ophthalmol 47:271, 1963

66. Linnér, E: Measurement of pressure in Schlemm's canal and in the anterior chamber of the human eye, Experientia 5:451, 1949

67. Linnér, E: The outflow pressure in normal and glaucomatous eyes, Acta Ophthalmol 33:101, 1955

68. Linnér, E: Further studies of the episcleral venous pressure in glaucoma, Am J Ophthalmol 41:646, 1956

69. Linnér, E, Rickenbach, C, and Werner, H: Comparative measurements of pressure in the aqueous veins and the conjunctival veins using different methods, Acta Ophthalmol 33:101, 1955

70. Lohlein, H, and Weigelin, E: Uber den Abfluss des Kammerwassers am normalen und glaukomkranken Augen, Dtsch Ophthalmol Geselsch 55:170, 1949

71. Lokich, JJ, and Goodman, R: Superior vena cava syndrome, JAMA 231:58, 1975

72. Lloyd, GAS: Phleboliths in the orbit, Clin Radiol 16:339, 1965

73. Lloyd, GAS: Wright, JE, and Morgan, G: Venous malformations in the orbit, Br J Ophthalmol 55:505, 1971

74. Madsen, PH: Carotid cavernous fistulae: a study of 18 cases, Acta Ophthalmol 48:731, 1970

75. Meyer, O: Inflammatory jugular phlebostenosis as the cause of glaucoma exogenicum, Br J Ophthalmol 30:682, 1946

76. Mims, JL, and Holland, MG: Applanation and Schiøtz tonometer standardizations for the owl monkey eye with a new technique for measuring episcleral venous pressure, Invest Ophthalmol 10:190, 1971

77. Minas, TF, and Podos, SM: Familial glaucoma associated with elevated episcleral venous pressure, Arch Ophthalmol 80:201, 1968

78. Moses, RA, and Grodzki, WJ: Mechanism of glaucoma secondary to increased venous pressure, Arch Ophthalmol 103:1701, 1985

79. Moses, RA, Grodzki, WJ, and Carras, PL: Pseudofacility: where did it go? Arch Ophthalmol 103:1653, 1985

80. Newton, TH, and Cronqvist, S: Involvement of dural arteries in intracranial arteriovenous malformation, Radiology 93:1071, 1969

81. Nordmann, J, et al: A propos de 14 cas de glaucome par hypertension veineuse d'origine extraoculaire, Ophthalmologica 142(suppl):501, 1961

82. Pecora, JL, and Patel, AJ: Eyelid edema as the presenting sign in superior vena cava syndrome, Ann Ophthalmol 12:1161, 1980

83. Phelps, CD: The pathogenesis of glaucoma in Sturge-Weber syndrome, Trans Am Acad Ophthalmol Otolaryngol 85:276, 1978

84. Phelps, CD, and Armaly, MF: Measurement of episcleral venous pressure, Am J Ophthalmol 85:33, 1978

85. Podos, SM, Minas, TF, and Macri, JT: A new instrument to measure episcleral venous pressure: comparison of normal eyes and eyes with primary open angle glaucoma, Arch Ophthalmol 80:209, 1968

86. Radius, RL, and Maumenee, AE: Dilated episcleral vessels and open angle glaucoma, Am J Ophthalmol 86:31, 1978

87. Rathbun, JE, Hoyt, WF, and Beard, C: Surgical management of orbitofrontal varix in Klippel-Trenaunay-Weber syndrome, Am J Ophthalmol 70:109, 1970

88. Rickenbach, K, and Werner, H: Scheinbarer Abflussdruck: Tension und Druck, in Kammerwasservenen, Ophthalmologica 120:22, 1950

89. Sanders, M, and Hoyt, W: Hypoxic ocular sequelae of carotid-cavernous fistulae: study of the causes of visual failure before and after neurosurgical treatment in a series of 25 cases. Br J Ophthalmol 53:82, 1969

90. Seidel, E: Weitere experimentelle Untersuchungen uber die Quelle und den Verlauf der intraokularen Saftsrommung. XX. Uber die Messung des Blutdruckes in dem episcleral Venengeflecht, den vorderen ciliar-und den Wirbelvenen normaler Augen, v Graefes Arch Klin Exp Ophthalmol 112:252, 1923

91. Shapiro, A: The physiological changes that may affect intraocular pressure, Ann Ophthalmol 15:895, 1983

92. Spencer, WH, Thompson, HS, and Hoyt, WF: Ischemic ocular necrosis from carotid-cavernous fistula, Br J Ophthalmol 57:145, 1973

93. Stolpman, E: Doppelseitige nicht-traumatische carotid sinus cavernosis Fistel, v Graefes Arch Klin Exp Ophthalmol 185:83, 1972

94. Sugar, HS, and Meyer, SJ: Pulsating exophthalmos, Arch Ophthalmol 23:1288, 1939

95. Talusan, ED, Fishbein, SL, and Schwartz, B: Increased pressure of dilated episcleral veins with open-angle glaucoma without exophthalmos, Ophthalmology 90:257, 1983

96. Talusan, ED, and Schwartz, B: Episcleral venous pressure: difference between normal, ocular hypertensive and primary open angle glaucoma, Arch Ophthalmol 99:824, 1981

97. Taniguchi, RM, Goree, JA, and Odom, Gl: Spontaneous carotid-cavernous shunts presenting diagnostic problems, J Neurosurg 35:384, 1971

98. Tarkkanen, A, and Leikola, J: Postural variations of the intraocular pressure as measured with the Mackay-Marg tonometer, Acta Ophthalmol 45:569, 1967

99. Thomassen, TL: The venous tension in eyes suffering from simple glaucoma, Acta Ophthalmol 25:221, 1947

100. Urschel, HC, and Paulson, DL: Superior vena cava canal obstruction, Dis Chest 49:155-164, 1966

101. Walsh, FB, and Dandy, WE: The pathogenesis of intermittent exophthalmos, Trans Am Ophthalmol Soc 42:334, 1944

102. Walsh, TJ: Neuro-ophthalmology clinical signs and symptoms, Philadelphia, 1985, Lea & Febiger

103. Warwick, R: Eugene Wolff's anatomy of the eye and orbit, Philadelphia, 1976, WB Saunders

104. Weekers, R, and Delmarcelle, Y: Pathogenesis of intraocular hypertension in cases of arteriovenous aneurysm, Arch Ophthalmol 48:338, 1952

105. Weinreb, RN, Cook, J, and Friberg, T: Effect of inverted body position on the intraocular pressure, Am J Ophthalmol 98:784, 1984

106. Weiss, DL: Dual origin of glaucoma in encephalotrigeminal hemangiomatosis, Trans Ophthalmol Soc UK 93:477, 1971

107. Weiss, DI, and Shaffer, RN: Neovascular glaucoma complicating carotid-cavernous fistula, Arch Ophthalmol 69:60, 1963

108. Wettrell, K, Wilke, K, and Pandolfi, M: Effect of beta-adrenergic agonists and antagonists on repeated tonometry and episcleral venous pressure, Exp Eye Res 24:613, 1977

109. Wilke, K: Early effects of epinephrine and pilocarpine on the intraocular pressure and the episcleral venous pressure in the normal human eye, Acta Ophthalmol 52:231, 1974

110. Wright, JE: Orbital vascular anomalies, Trans Am Acad Ophthalmol Otolaryngol 78:OP606, 1974

111. Yablonski, ME, Gallin, P, and Shapiro, D: Effect of oxygen on aqueous humor dynamics in rabbits, Invest Ophthalmol Vis Sci 26:1781, 1985

112. Yablonski, ME, Ritch, R, and Pokorny, K: Effect of decreased intracranial pressure on optic disc, Invest Ophthalmol Vis Sci Suppl 20:165, 1979

113. Yablonski, ME, and Podos, SM: Glaucoma secondary to elevated episcleral venous pressure. In Shields, MB, and Ritch, R, editors: The secondary glaucomas, St. Louis, 1982, The CV Mosby Co

114. Zalta, AH, Karlin, KM, Ziegler, L, and Zimmerman, TJ: The effect of nitroglycerin ointment on the external ocular structures of rabbits, J Ocular Pharmacol 1:71, 1985

115. Zeimer, RC, et al: A practical venomanometer, Arch Ophthalmol 101:1447, 1983

Chapter 63

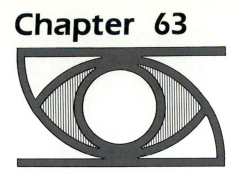

Systemic Diseases Associated with Elevated Intraocular Pressure and Secondary Glaucoma

Richard A. Stone

The relationship between systemic disease and secondary glaucoma is complex. Many of these relationships are discussed elsewhere in this text. For instance, a number of systemic conditions have well-defined ocular complications, such as uveitis and rubeosis, that produce an elevated intraocular pressure and secondary glaucoma. There also is an association of several systemic disorders with primary open-angle glaucoma and with low-tension glaucoma. Although review of all these associations is beyond the scope of this chapter, some are discussed particularly when the distinction between primary and secondary glaucoma is not clear.

ENDOCRINE DISORDERS

The possibility that endocrine mechanisms may have a role in the regulation of intraocular pressure in the normal eye and may explain the abnormalities in aqueous humor dynamics that occur in glaucoma has stimulated many investigations. To date, no study has demonstrated convincingly that primary open-angle glaucoma is related to an abnormality in endocrine function.[64] Glaucoma does occur, however, in association with several endocrine disorders.

Pituitary Disease

Many authors have reported an association of glaucoma with pituitary tumors. The glaucoma occurring in these cases resembles primary open-angle glaucoma.

Several investigators have reported an association of glaucoma with acromegaly arising from eosinophilic pituitary adenomas. Howard and English[55] found that 7 of 70 patients with acromegaly had glaucoma, although in one case there was a previous history of fibrinous iritis and peripheral anterior synechiae. The diagnosis of glaucoma was made 6 to 34 years after the onset of acromegaly. These patients had cupping of the optic disc and visual field defects, and tonography showed decreased facilities of outflow. The intraocular pressures of five of these patients were controlled with topical medication, but two required filtering surgery. Forty-five of the 70 patients in this series, however, did not have intraocular pressures recorded in their charts, and Howard and English stressed that the true prevalence of elevated intraocular pressures in this series of patients may well have been higher than that reported. Smaller series also have noted an association of elevated intraocular pressure or glaucoma with acromegaly.

The coexistence of glaucoma and chromophobe pituitary adenomas also has been noted. Van Bijsterveld and Richards[110] found three cases of open-angle glaucoma among 14 patients with chromophobe adenomas. All three of these patients had decreased outflow facility and optic nerve head cupping. Although field loss occurred in all three patients, in one and perhaps both of the patients without frank optic nerve cupping the field loss may have been related to the pituitary tumor rather than to the elevated intraocular pressure. The concurrence of glaucoma and basophilic pituitary adenomas has also been reported.[95]

The above studies indicate that the association of glaucoma with pituitary tumor, although unusual, does appear to occur more frequently than by chance. Although this concurrence may be accidental, a possible causative role for pituitary disease in the development of these glaucomas cannot be excluded at present.[41] The strongest clinical evidence for association occurs with acromegaly, and these patients may have an increased incidence of low outflow facilities and elevated intraocular pressures. Although there is as yet no conclusive evidence linking growth hormone with the control of intraocular pressure in normal patients or with the development of primary open-angle glaucoma, a hormonal mechanism may be present. For instance, although patients with primary open-angle glaucoma have normal baseline plasma growth hormone levels, they show an exaggerated elevation of growth hormone levels after intravenous arginine administration.[48] In acromegaly, however, central corneal thickness is increased as a result of the disease.[16] In humans, increased corneal thickness induces an artifactual small elevation in the applanation reading of intraocular pressure.[33] When corrected for the increased corneal thickness, the intraocular pressure of 27 patients with acromegaly was no different from a control group.[16] Thus, although true glaucoma may occur with increased frequency among patients with acromegaly, the relationship of this condition with abnormal aqueous humor dynamics requires further evaluation.

The treatment of patients with pituitary disease and elevated intraocular pressures is identical to that for patients with primary open-angle glaucoma. Visual field changes can occur because of glaucoma or pituitary disease, and it is important to follow these patients with careful perimetry so that the cause of any progressive field change can be identified. This association of glaucoma with pituitary disease underscores the need for careful scrutiny of the visual fields of all glaucoma patients to detect coexisting disease in the visual pathways, particularly when the pattern of visual field loss is not typical of glaucoma or when the amount of field loss is disproportionate to the degree of cupping. In addition, patients with pituitary disease should be screened for glaucoma.

Cushing's Syndrome

Cushing's syndrome is a metabolic disorder caused by a chronic excess of glucocorticoids. It can arise from adrenocortical tumors that secrete cortisol or from certain nonpituitary tumors that secrete adrenocorticotropic hormone (ACTH) and cause adrenal hyperplasia. In those cases where the pituitary gland secretes excessive ACTH, typically from a basophilic adenoma, the specific term *Cushing's disease* is applied.

Abnormalities in intraocular pressure have been reported in patients with Cushing's syndrome either from adrenal adenoma or from excessive ACTH production. Krasnovid[67] found both elevations of intraocular pressure and increased diurnal variations in intraocular pressure in patients with Cushing's syndrome, and both he and Linnér[75] found decreased diurnal fluctuations in intraocular pressure in patients with adrenal or pituitary insufficiency.

Some patients with Cushing's syndrome develop increased intraocular pressure and may develop optic nerve cupping and visual field loss. In one series, 7 of 29 patients with Cushing's syndrome had intraocular pressures above 23 mm Hg.[84] Three of these patients had visual field defects, but only one had a true glaucomatous defect. The facility of outflow generally is reduced in such cases, and following adrenalectomy the increased intraocular pressure and the reduced facility of outflow may return to normal.[5,64] Haas and Nootens[49] reported a patient with Cushing's syndrome caused by a benign adrenal adenoma who had marked bilateral intraocular pressure elevations, reduced aqueous outflow facilities, and optic nerve head cupping in one eye. Following adrenalectomy, the patient's intraocular pressures and outflow facilities returned to normal. Topical steroid testing showed that the patient, both of his parents, and one sister were high corticosteroid responders. Haas and Nootens postulated that a genetic sensitivity to the intraocular pressure effects of corticosteroids causes the rise in intraocular pressure found in some patients with Cushing's syndrome.

The relationship between corticosteroids, intraocular pressure, and glaucoma is discussed in greater detail in Chapter 64.

Diabetes Mellitus

The relationship between diabetes and open-angle glaucoma has been studied extensively. Although not all series are in agreement,[3,4] primary open-angle glaucoma appears to be more prevalent among patients with diabetes,* and the intraocular pressures of both adult and juvenile diabetic patients appear to be higher than in the nondiabetic population.[94,106] In addition, secondary glaucomas can develop as a direct or indirect consequence of diabetes mellitus. These conditions are discussed elsewhere in this text.

Several recent observations also suggest a possible relationship of diabetes mellitus and angle-closure glaucoma. Patients with narrow angles or angle-closure glaucoma tend to have abnormal responses to an oral glucose tolerance test, compared with open-angle glaucoma patients and a control group.[78] A high proportion of non-insulin-dependent diabetes mellitus also is observed in patients with angle-closure glaucoma.[22] It has been suggested that acute angle-closure glaucoma may be a symptom of diabetes, perhaps because of autonomic dysfunction.[78] Lens swelling from hyperglycemia may also precipitate angle-closure glaucoma in susceptible individuals.[102]

Thyroid Disease

Graves' disease is characterized by hyperthyroidism with diffuse goiter, dermopathy, and ophthalmopathy. All of these need not occur, and the clinical course of any one of the manifestations may proceed independent of the others. The disorder may occur at any age, but the incidence is highest between the ages of 30 and 50 years. Women are affected more frequently than men. The cause of the ophthalmic manifestations of this disease is uncertain.

A nonuniform and sometimes confusing terminology has been applied to the ophthalmopathy of Graves' disease, but most authors separate the thyrotoxic, or noninfiltrative, form from the thyrotropic, or infiltrative, form. This distinction is useful for purposes of discussion, but clinically there is often overlap.

Thyrotoxic ophthalmopathy occurs in 50% to 75% of patients with Grave's disease. Affected patients are usually between 20 and 40 years of age,

and there is a marked female preponderance. The eye findings consist of a characteristic stare with lid retraction and lid lag that is most marked in downward gaze. Mild exophthalmos, although uncommon, may occur, but the proptosis may be more apparent than real because of the lid retraction. The globe retrodisplaces normally. With correction of the hyperthyroidism, the eye signs generally resolve spontaneously.

Thyrotropic ophthalmopathy (Fig. 63-1) occurs less frequently, but some evidence of infiltrative ophthalmopathy occurs in 10% to 20% of patients with Grave's disease. About 2% develop severe "malignant" exophthalmos. Thyrotropic ophthalmopathy usually occurs with the onset of the hyperthyroidism and subsides with its treatment. However, it may occur in euthyroid patients or may develop after the hyperthyroidism has been treated.

Secondary glaucoma can occur in thyrotropic ophthalmopathy by means of several mechanisms. The retrobulbar inflammatory process can compromise the orbital venous system and raise the episcleral venous pressure. In some instances thrombosis of the orbital veins has been documented.[31] An impaired outflow facility can also contribute to intraocular pressure elevation. Contraction of the extraocular muscles against intraorbital adhesions may caused marked variations in intraocular pressure in different positions of gaze. Usually fibrosis affects the inferior muscles, and a significant increase in intraocular pressure may occur in upward gaze.[116] Because of these gaze-related changes in intraocular pressure, tonometry should be performed on these patients in several positions of gaze. Scleral rigidity shows wide variability in patients with thyroid disease.[50] In the management of these patients, it is best to use applanation rather than indentation tonometry to avoid this potential problem.

In patients with thyrotropic ophthalmopathy and normal outflow facilities, intraocular pressure elevations in isolated fields of gaze usually require no therapy. With significantly impaired outflow facilities, sustained pressure elevations may be present in all fields of gaze but exaggerated in certain gaze positions. Whether this latter condition represents a concurrence of primary open-angle glaucoma and thyrotropic opthalmopathy or a true secondary glaucoma generally cannot be determined on clinical grounds, but the treatment of such patients is analogous to the treatment of patients with primary open-angle glaucoma. Visual acuity and visual field studies are important in following these

*References 2, 6, 64, 66, 85, 100.

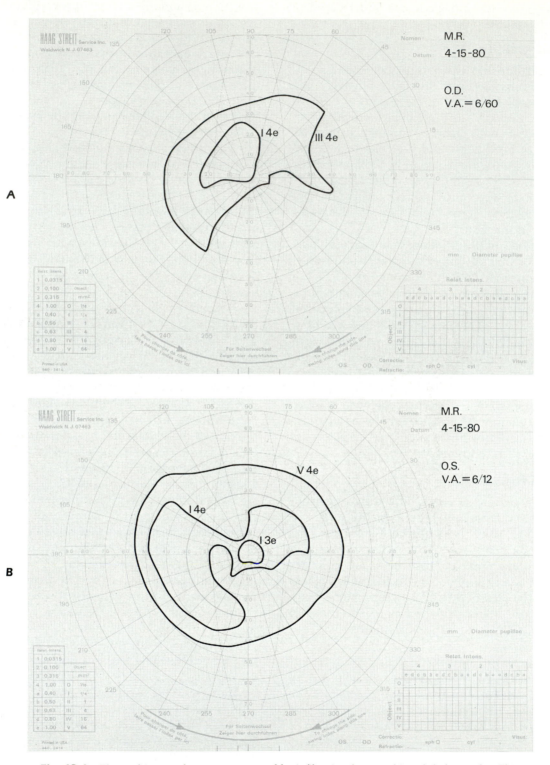

Fig. 63-1 Elevated intraocular pressure caused by infiltrative thyrotrophic ophthalmopathy. This 53-year-old woman underwent radioactive iodide treatment for hyperthyroidism 1 year before rapid onset of bilateral exophthalmos, motility limitation, and blurred vision. **A,** Visual acuity in right eye measured 20/200 with marked visual field deficit and afferent pupillary defect. **B,** Her left eye had visual acuity of 20/40 with less marked visual field defect. Intraocular pressures measured in mid 20s bilaterally with eyes in primary position and increased to low to mid 30s on attempted upward gaze. Optic discs showed no significant cupping in either eye.

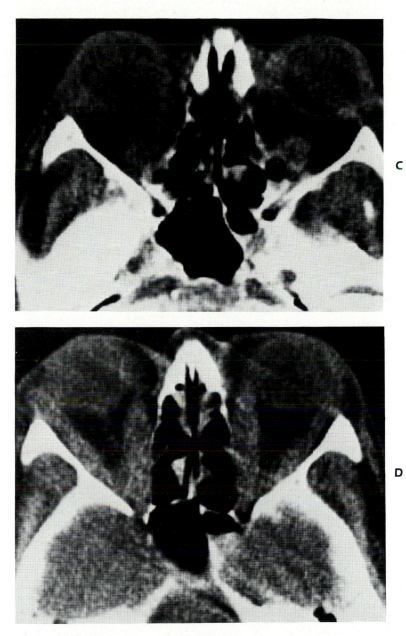

Fig. 63-1, cont'd   C, CT scan without contrast illustrates bilateral proptosis. **D,** With contrast, muscles appear thickened and show slight enhancement on CT scan. Patient received high-dose oral steroids, resulting in some improvement in motility and some lessening of orbital congestion.

Continued.

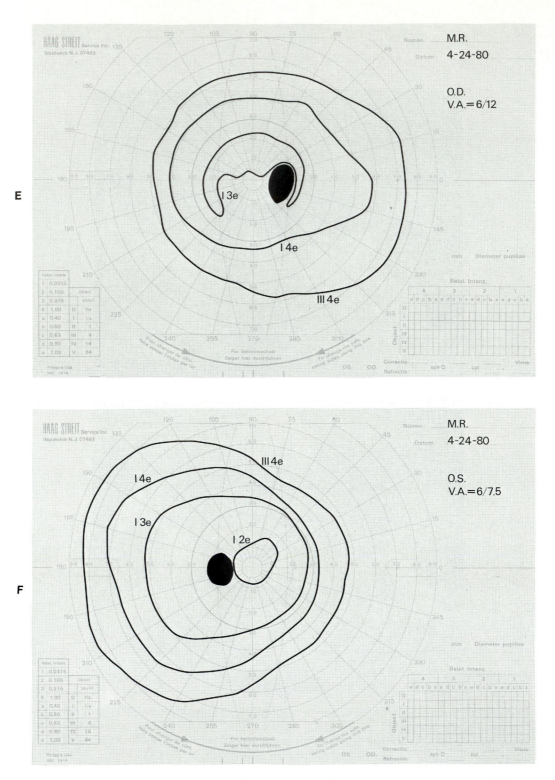

Fig. 63-1, cont'd   Visual acuity improved to 20/40 in right eye and 20/25 in left eye with corresponding improvement in both right, **E,** and left, **F,** visual fields. Intraocular pressure was normal in primary position but still rose as high as low 30s bilaterally in attempted upward gaze. No specific antiglaucoma therapy was advised. (Courtesy Irving M. Raber, M.D.)

patients. It sometimes can be difficult to determine the cause of visual loss because the infiltrative optic neuropathy may cause visual field defects similar to those seen in glaucoma. After a period of several years the orbital disease often goes into remission with some reduction in orbital congestion, but the glaucoma may persist. The prognosis for vision in many of these patients may be poor.

Corneal exposure and secondary infection also can occur as a result of thyrotropic ophthalmopathy. A severe anterior chamber reaction may develop leading to peripheral anterior synechiae and secondary glaucoma. In such cases the corneal disease should be treated primarily and glaucoma therapy instituted as necessary.

Efforts to correlate abnormalities of thyroid function with primary open-angle glaucoma have yielded inconclusive findings. Although some studies have reported a high incidence of elevated intraocular pressure in patients with hyperthyroidism,[88] most studies are unable to substantiate such a relationship.[21] Patients with hypothyroidism have been noted to have elevated intraocular pressures as well, and low protein-bound iodine values and low radioiodide uptakes have been reported in patients with open-angle glaucoma.[7] A subsequent study, however, has demonstrated that the thyroxine (T4), thyrotropin (TSH), and triiodothyronine (T3) resin uptake levels of glaucoma patients do not differ from those of normal controls.[68] In patients with hypothyroidism and elevated intraocular pressures, systemic thyroid medication has been reported to lower the intraocular pressure.[86,88] Much of the experimental data are contradictory, but it appears that pharmacologic doses of thyroid hormone may decrease intraocular pressure by increasing outflow facility.[64] Nevertheless, thyroid hormone currently has no therapeutic role in treating glaucoma.

In summary, current evidence does not conclusively demonstrate that abnormalities in thyroid function directly affect elevated intraocular pressure. Only in thyrotropic ophthalmopathy, where an elevated intraocular pressure may develop from complications of the orbital disease, does a true secondary glaucoma arise from thyroid dysfunction.

VASCULAR DISEASE

Ocular Ischemia

Local ocular ischemia, including central retinal vein occlusion and, rarely, central retinal artery occlusion, can lead to the development of rubeosis iridis and hemorrhagic glaucoma.[17,53] About 25% of patients experiencing central retinal vein occlusion develop rubeosis iridis. Rubeosis iridis is discussed in detail in Chapter 60.

Retinal Vein Occlusion
(Figs. 63-2 and 63-3)

In addition to the development of rubeosis iridis, there is a striking association between central retinal vein occlusion and preexisting glaucoma,[36,111] including the occurrence of retinal vascular accidents after acute glaucoma.[101] Estimates of the prevalence of preexisting open-angle glaucoma among patients with central retinal vein occlusion vary considerably and have been reported in the broad range of 9% to 69%.[28] As association of branch retinal vein occlusion and elevated intraocular pressure or open-angle glaucoma is less certain[61,76] but has been observed in some studies.[11,60] Presumably, elevated intraocular pressure impairs venous drainage from the eye. Typically, there is coexisting atherosclerotic disease in the central retinal artery; elevated intraocular pressure lowers the perfusion pressure in the central retinal artery, permitting mechanical occlusion or thrombosis of the central retinal vein. Increased intraocular pressure also may cause mechanical distortion of the lamina cribrosa and further compromise flow through the central retinal vein.[9] An eye with a recent vein occlusion often is relatively hypotonous,[91] and the underlying abnormality in intraocular pressure in that eye may not be immediately apparent. Therefore, it is imperative to examine the contralateral eye for evidence of elevated intraocular pressure. Because an elevation of intraocular pressure is a predisposing factor to the development of a retinal vein occlusion, an elevated intraocular pressure in either eye of such a patient should be treated appropriately.

Occasionally occlusion of the central retinal vein causes a shallowing of the anterior chamber, and in some cases acute angle-closure glaucoma.[12,20,47,57,81] Two mechanisms have been postulated: anterior displacement of the lens-iris diaphragm by posterior segment blood or edema, and marked swelling or vascular congestion of the ciliary body. One or both may occur in individual cases. This glaucoma usually has been noted within 2 to 3 weeks after the occurrence of the vein occlusion. With absorption of the fluid in the posterior segment, or with resolution of the ciliary body congestion, the anterior chamber depth returns to normal, often within several weeks.

Gonioscopy of the uninvolved eye may help distinguish this unusual form of secondary angle-

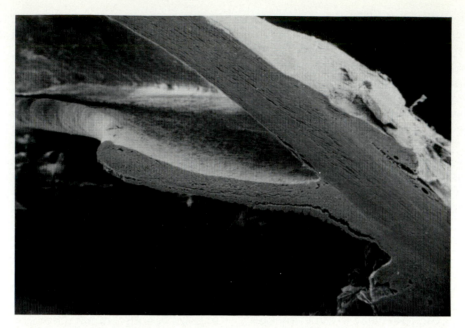

Fig. 63-2   Neovascular glaucoma caused by central retinal vein occlusion. Broad peripheral anterior synechiae and early ectropion uveae are present. Normal contours of anterior iris surface are effaced by fibrovascular membrane. (Scanning electron microscope; ×25.) (Courtesy Ralph C. Eagle, Jr., M.D.)

closure glaucoma from primary angle-closure glaucoma. If the contralateral eye has an open angle, one must consider a secondary angle-closure mechanism. If the contralateral eye has a narrow, potentially occludable angle, one must consider a primary angle-closure mechanism. The diagnostic distinction is important because of the therapy. In primary angle-closure glaucoma with a pupillary block mechanism, iridectomy is necessary. In this form of secondary angle-closure glaucoma associated with central vein occlusion, surgical iridectomy fails to deepen the anterior chamber acutely and may not immediately normalize the intraocular pressure. Because of the self-limited nature of this form of secondary angle-closure glaucoma, medical therapy is the preferred treatment, and iridectomy should be reserved for nonresponsive cases. Pilocarpine has been reported to control the intraocular pressure in most patients sufficiently for spontaneous resolution of the chamber shallowing to occur.[47,57] Use of topical steroids and drugs to supress aqueous secretion, such as topical beta-adrenergic blockers or carbonic anhydrase inhibitors, and treatment with cycloplegics to tighten the lens zonules and to displace the lens-iris diaphragm posteriorly may produce a more dramatic and consistent therapeutic response[12] and appear to be a rational therapeutic approach.[20,81] Argon laser peripheral iridoplasty is often useful (see Chapter 30). There

is no apparent association between this unusual form of angle-closure glaucoma and the subsequent development of rubeosis iridis.[20]

Cerebrovascular Disease

Elevated episcleral venous pressure and secondary glaucoma may arise from arteriovenous malformations or from carotid-cavernous fistulas, as discussed in Chapter 62. Ocular ischemia and rubeosis iridis may develop as a complication of a variety of systemic vascular diseases, including carotid occlusive disease, Takayasu's (pulseless) disease, and temporal arteritis. The occurrence of a central retinal artery occlusion or a central retinal vein occlusion in association with systemic vascular disease also can result in the development of rubeosis and secondary glaucoma.[1,23,40] These conditions are discussed elsewhere in this text.

Rapid progression of visual field loss has been noted in some glaucoma patients with low systemic or low ophthalmic artery blood pressures,[26,27,70,93] and occlusive carotid artery disease has been cited as an etiologic factor in low-tension glaucoma. It should be emphasized, however that these findings are by no means invariable. For instance, Jampol and Miller[59] have reported five patients with occlusive carotid artery disease and untreated intraocular pressure elevations who did not develop glaucomatous disc or field changes over a 3- to 12-year follow-up period.

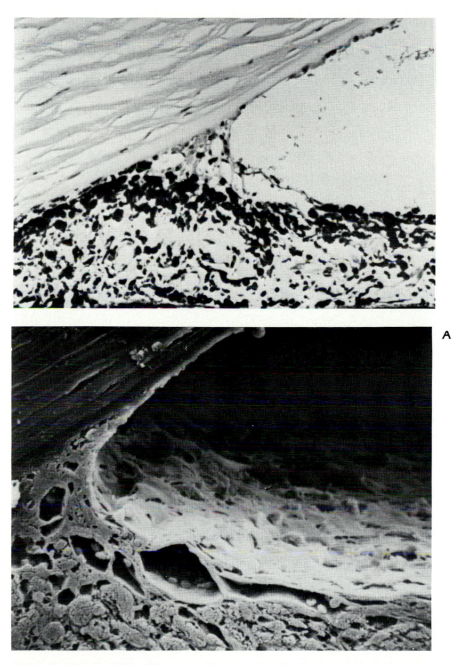

Fig. 63-3   Neovascular glaucoma caused by central retinal vein occlusion. Eye illustrated in Fig. 63-2 is examined at higher magnification by light *(top)* and scanning electron microscopy *(bottom).* **A,** Peripheral iris is adherent to Descemet's membrane. Membrane of fibroblasts covers new blood vessels in pseudoangle and on anterior iris surface. *(Top:* Hematoxylin and eosin; ×125. *Bottom:* Scanning electron microscope; ×256.) (Courtesy Ralph C. Eagle, Jr., M.D.)

Continued.

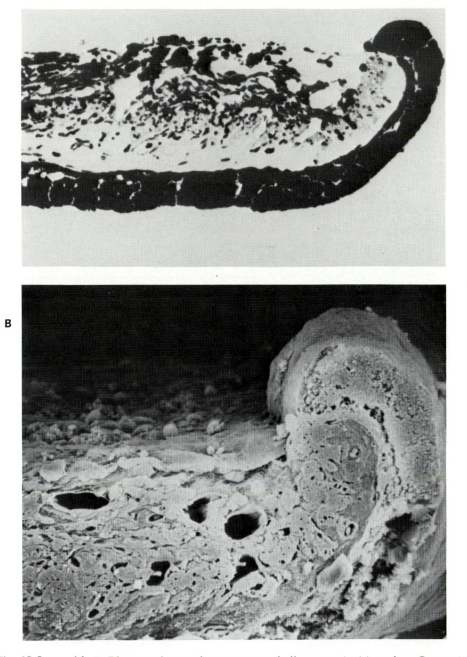

Fig. 63-3, cont'd **B,** Fibrovascular membrane covers and effaces anterior iris surface. Contraction of membrane has led to eversion of pigment epithelium and sphincter muscle (ectropion uveae). (*Top:* Hematoxylin and eosin; × 125. *Bottom:* Scanning electron microscope; × 256.) (Courtesy Ralph C. Eagle, Jr., M.D.)

Blood Pressure and Intraocular Pressure

There tends to be a positive correlation between intraocular pressure readings and blood pressure measurements.[10,39,98] The Framingham study furthermore has demonstrated an association between ocular hypertension and systemic blood pressure.[63] The two disorders, however, do not necessarily occur in the same patient, and systemic hypertension does not appear to be an etiologic factor in the development of glaucoma. Sudden lowering of an elevated systemic blood pressure in patients with established glaucoma may precipitate acute visual field loss in susceptible individuals,[34,52,93] presumably because of a sudden drop in the perfusion pressure at the optic nerve head. Considering the large number of glaucoma patients undergoing treatment for systemic hypertension and the small number of these reported cases, it is not clear whether the visual loss described in these reports is causally or coincidentally related to lowering of the systemic blood pressure. Nevertheless, the high prevalence of both disorders makes the suggestion that sudden blood pressure control in glaucoma patients may result in visual field loss an important concern.

In the absence of controlled prospective clinical studies, it appears wisest to monitor glaucoma patients carefully when medication for systemic hypertension is given and to recommend gradual control of the systemic blood pressure in glaucoma patients, particularly if the glaucoma is not well controlled.

During extracorporeal circulation when there is a controlled systemic hypotension, intraocular pressure during cardiopulmonary bypass has been reported to increase,[104] to decrease,[72] or to be unchanged.[74] The reasons for the conflicting findings are unclear but may relate to different cardiopulmonary bypass techniques.

COLLAGEN VASCULAR DISORDERS

Secondary glaucoma can arise from the uveitis or may occasionally be associated with the episcleritis or scleritis that accompanies some of these disorders. Corticosteroid-induced glaucoma—either from topical or, less commonly, from systemic steroid administration—is another problem in these patients. These disorders are discussed in detail in other chapters of this text.

RENAL DISEASE AND HEMODIALYSIS

Elevated intraocular pressures occur in patients after renal transplantation with a reported incidence as high as 33%.[54,119] Frequently the intraocu-

lar pressure elevation appears to be related to the intake of systemic steroids because the intraocular pressure elevation parallels the steroid use. The intraocular pressures usually respond well to conventional topical antiglaucoma therapy.

During hemodialysis in patients with renal failure, fluctuations in intraocular pressure occur. During the first 2 hours of hemodialysis, a small fall in intraocular pressure has been noted.[92] After more prolonged hemodialysis, however, the intraocular pressure rises in most patients. The degree of elevation is variable but averages 7 mm Hg or less in those patients experiencing an intraocular pressure rise.[18,92,99] Serum osmolality falls during hemodialysis, and a lag in the equilibration of the osmolality of the intraocular fluids to the changing serum osmolality may result in the osmotic transfer of free water into the eye and contribute to the elevation of intraocular pressure.[71] Additional factors, perhaps related to central nervous system mechanisms, might mediate this response.[92] Generally, these swings in intraocular pressure are not of sufficient magnitude or duration to be of clinical significance in patients with normal outflow facilities. In patients with impaired outflow facilities or with narrow anterior chamber angles, however, a marked rise in intraocular pressure may occur. Prevention of large changes in serum osmolality during hemodialysis will help stabilize intraocular pressure in such cases, and long-term therapy with acetazolamide may be necessary.[58] It has been recommended that the intraocular pressure of patients beginning hemodialysis be monitored during the procedure.[58]

Cystinosis, a rare autosomal recessive metabolic disease, results in the accumulation of cystine crystals in many tissues; renal involvement is common. In the eye, characteristic iridescent crystal deposits in the cornea and conjunctiva are prominent clinical features. Peripheral pigmentary retinopathy has been observed in the childhood but not the adult form of the disease. Cystine crystals also have been observed histologically in other ocular tissues, including the uvea. A single report describes the occurrence of acute angle-closure glaucoma requiring trabeculectomy in a 19-year-old woman with childhood cystinosis.[114] Because of the extensive cystine crystal deposition observed histologically in the iridectomy specimen, it was postulated that the crystal deposition caused iris thickening and stiffening, which resulted in the pupillary block. Cystine deposition may have occurred in the anterior chamber angle tissues, but this was not confirmed histologically.

HEMATOLOGIC DISORDERS

Blood Composition

Abnormalities in serum protein, chloride, cholesterol, the potassium/calcium ratio, pH, and osmolality in patients with open-angle glaucoma have been reported but have not been found consistently.[29] Hyperlipoproteinemias also have been found associated with elevated intraocular pressure.[120] There is no definite evidence, however, for a causal or prognostic relationship between any of these blood constituents and the development of elevated intraocular pressure or glaucoma.

Hyperviscosity Syndromes

Diseases such as polycythemia and the dysproteinemias are associated with increased serum viscosity and decreased blood flow velocity, resulting in dilation, tortuosity, and possible thrombosis of the retinal veins. If thrombosis of the central retinal vein occurs, neovascular glaucoma may develop.

In hyperviscosity syndromes, an acute rise in intraocular pressure may occur without the presence of rubeosis iridis but with an open-angle and blood in Schlemm's canal. Presumably, the glaucoma in these cases develops because of an acute thrombosis within Schlemm's canal. Medical treatment of the increased intraocular pressure is the preferred therapeutic approach, although the intraocular pressure may be difficult to control.[46]

Platelet Dysfunction

A higher incidence of spontaneous platelet aggregation occurs in patients with primary open-angle glaucoma compared with similar-aged glaucoma suspects having elevated intraocular pressure but normal optic discs and normal visual fields.[56] Further work will be necessary to demonstrate whether platelet function contributes to the development of glaucomatous optic atrophy or whether tests of platelet function have predictive value when applied to glaucoma suspects.

Sickle Cell Hemoglobinopathies

The sickle cell hemoglobinopathies arise from the substitution of a single amino acid in normal adult hemoglobin A to form hemoglobin S. Erythrocytes containing hemoglobin S may develop a sickle configuration under certain conditions, such as hypoxia. Sickled erythrocytes are less pliable than normal red blood cells and can therefore occlude small blood vessels. Some 10% of North American blacks have hemoglobin S. The hemoglobin mutation is inherited directly from either parent and can occur as the sickle cell trait (AS

hemoglobin) or sickle cell anemia (SS disease). Hemoglobin S also can occur in sickle cell thalassemia (SThal) and sickle cell C disease (SC disease). SS disease causes the most severe systemic problems, with chronic anemia and recurrent episodes of hemolysis and painful crises. The SC and SThal hemoglobinopathies cause less severe anemia and milder symptoms. The sickle cell trait causes the least severe symptoms of these disorders.

The predominant ocular complication of the sickle cell hemoglobinopathies is sickle cell retinopathy,[73,118] which can be classified into proliferative and nonproliferative forms.[44] The proliferative retinopathy is characterized by peripheral arteriolar-venous anastomoses, peripheral neovascularization, vitreous hemorrhage, and retinal detachment. These ocular complications, particularly retinal neovascularization, vitreous hemorrhage, and retinal detachment, appear to be most prevalent in SC and SThal disease. The nonproliferative sickle cell retinopathy has venous tortuosity, "black sunbursts," refractile fundus deposits, "silver wire" changes in the arterioles, and salmon-patch hemorrhages. Central retinal artery occlusions and central retinal vein occlusions have been observed, particularly in patients with SS disease. Patients with the other forms of sickle cell hemoglobinopathies, however, are not immune from the vaso-occlusive ocular complications. Angioid streaks have been described in all types of sickle cell hemoglobinopathies. Sickle cell trait itself is not a risk factor for the development of open-angle glaucoma.[103]

Secondary glaucoma can occur as a complication of the retinal vascular disease (Fig. 63-4). As in other conditions characterized by ocular ischemia, rubeosis iridis and neovascular glaucoma can develop. Only a small number of cases of rubeosis iridis have been reported as a complication of sickle cell hemoglobinopathies, however, and the association appears strongest with SC disease.[45] The development of rubeosis has been noted in patients with the sickle cell trait, but these patients also had coexisting diabetes mellitus[14] or central retinal vein occlusion[122] that may have accounted for the rubeosis.

Vitreous hemorrhage that occurs in sickle cell retinopathy may cause a hemolytic glaucoma analogous to the hemolytic glaucoma occurring after any intraocular hemorrhage, as discussed in Chapter 60.

Shapiro and Baum[97] reported a patient with the sickle cell trait who developed an acute rise in intraocular pressure. The angle was open, but Schlemm's canal was filled with blood. They pos-

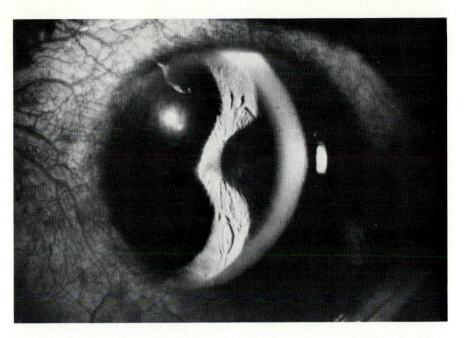

Fig. 63-4   Secondary glaucoma and sickle cell hemoglobinopathy. This 41-year-old black woman with sickle cell disease developed sudden visual acuity drop to 20/40 in her left eye. Initial findings included neovascularization of temporal retina extending into vitreous cavity, superior traction retinal detachment, and vitreous and subretinal hemorrhage. Small fibrovascular tuft was also noted temporally in right eye. No retinal therapy was recommended at that time. Over next 4 years, left eye developed uveitis, rubeosis iridis, secluded pupil, and secondary glaucoma. Right eye has maintained good vision, but vision in left eye has deteriorated to no light perception. Photograph illustrates secluded pupil with iris bombé in left eye.

tulated that low-grade asymptomatic iritis, which was also present in the contralateral eye, created ocular hypotony and allowed blood to reflux into Schlemm's canal. Then hemostasis with resulting hypoxia and pH alterations may have produced sickling and occlusion of Schlemm's canal. In this patient normalization of the intraocular pressure and outflow facility paralleled the disappearance of the blood from Schlemm's canal. Friedman et al.[35] also reported a patient with sickle cell trait, spontaneous hemorrhage into the trabecular meshwork, blood in Schlemm's canal, and an elevated intraocular pressure, but no iritis. The elevated intraocular pressure was treated medically. After the trabecular hemorrhage and blood in Schlemm's canal reabsorbed, the intraocular pressure remained normal without medication.

Patients with sickle cell hemoglobinopathies, even the sickle cell trait, may develop significant intraocular pressure elevations in response to the occurrence of relatively small hyphemas.[35,43] Anterior chamber aspirates from AS and SC patients with hyphemas reveal a higher percentage of sickled erythrocytes in the aqueous humor than in the plasma.[42] This sickling may arise from the reducing properties of the high ascorbate in the aqueous

humor or perhaps from a drop in aqueous pH and a fall in P_{O_2} associated with the occurrence of the hyphema, all of which would contribute to increased sickling. The sickled erythrocytes may significantly impair aqueous outflow and cause the intraocular pressure elevation.[42]

The medical treatment for hyphema-induced glaucoma in patients with sickle cell hemoglobinopathies may adversely affect the sickling process or the ocular circulation.[42,43,90] Acetazolamide administration can cause hemoconcentration and systemic acidosis, the latter of which may exacerbate erythrocyte sickling. Acetazolamide also increases the aqueous concentration of ascorbic acid, and this may cause further sickling in the aqueous humor. Methazolamide may be a safer carbonic anhydrase inhibitor to use because it tends to cause less systemic acidosis than acetazolamide and may slightly raise aqueous humor pH. Hyperosmolar agents may increase hemoconcentration and viscosity and thus further compromise the microcirculation in the eye, particularly in the central retinal artery and the small vessels of the optic nerve and perifoveal region. Topical epinephrine, if it induces vasoconstriction, may further compromise the local ocular circulation.[42] Although no clinical or laboratory studies exist that directly provide clinical guidance, it appears that topical beta-adrenergic blockers may be the agent of choice in such situations.

Acute intraocular pressure elevations in patients with sickle cell hemoglobinopathies are of concern because of associated retinal vascular complications, particularly central retinal artery occlusions, at normal or moderately elevated intraocular pressures.[42] Although the blood flow in the small vessels of the optic nerve or central retinal artery can be compromised by an elevated intraocular pressure in any patient, several reports suggest that patients with sickle cell hemoglobinopathies are particularly susceptible.[90,115]

Goldberg[42] has emphasized that the clinical management of black patients with hyphemas requires reassessment because of the high incidence of sickle cell hemoglobinopathies among this group. Black patients with hyphemas should be screened immediately for sickle cell hemoglobin, followed by a hemoglobin electrophoresis if positive. In addition, 24-hour monitoring of the intraocular pressure and visual function are important. According to Goldberg, paracentesis may be indicated in such circumstances with only a slight intraocular pressure elevation of "perhaps 25 mm Hg or greater, for more than one day, despite judicious use of anti-glaucomatous medications, and even if the hyphema is less than total." A prospective clinical trial of patients with sickle cell hemoglobinopathy and hyphemas is currently underway to provide more precise guidelines for management of these patients.

INTRAOCULAR NEOPLASTIC DISEASE

Malignant intraocular tumors, such as retinoblastoma, leukemic infiltration of the eye, and neoplastic disease metastatic to the eye, can produce secondary glaucoma. Nonmalignant neoplastic conditions, such as neurofibromatosis or juvenile xanthogranuloma, can also result in secondary glaucoma when they involve intraocular structures. Such conditions are discussed elsewhere in this text.

PRIMARY FAMILIAL AMYLOIDOSIS

The hereditary systemic amyloidoses are a group of generalized disorders, the systemic manifestations of which include weakness, peripheral neuropathy, and gastrointestinal, cardiovascular, renal, and endocrine abnormalities consistent with the widespread deposition of amyloid. The predominant inheritance pattern is autosomal dominant. Ocular involvement includes the accumula-

tion of characteristic cotton-like amyloid vitreous capacities, bilateral severe secondary open-angle glaucoma, lid abnormalities, extraocular muscle weakness, proptosis, conjunctival microaneurysms, internal ophthalmoplegia, irregularity of the pupil margin, anisocoria, and retinal perivasculitis. The vitreous opacification can progress to impair vision and prevent fundus visualization.[19,65,87]

Patients who develop glaucoma have open angles, pigment in the trabecular meshwork, pigment on the corneal endothelium, and abnormal iris transillumination. Powdery white flakes also may occur on the pupillary margin of the iris and on the anterior lens capsule in patients with glaucoma. Amyloid vitreous opacities are present in these cases. Although primary familial amyloidosis is a rare disease, up to one fourth of the patients may be at risk to develop glaucoma. The longer the disease has been present, the greater appears to be the risk of developing glaucoma.[107]

Widespread deposition of amyloid in ocular structures occurs in this condition. Using light microscopy, Paton and Duke[87] demonstrated amyloid deposition within the trabecular meshwork of a glaucomatous eye from a patient with primary familial amyloidosis but found no amyloid deposition within the trabecular meshwork in the contralateral nonglaucomatous eye. With the use of electron microscopy, amyloid accumulation and other degenerative changes have been observed in the trabecular meshwork of trabeculectomy specimens from patients with primary systemic amyloidosis and glaucoma.[38,96,107] This trabecular amyloid deposition presumably accounts for the aqueous outflow abnormality.

The exfoliation syndrome clinically has similar deposits in the anterior segment that are composed of an amyloid-like substance.[25,69,83] Patients with primary familial amyloidosis, however, also have vitreous opacities, systemic manifestations of generalized amyloid deposition, a strong family history, and a greater likelihood of bilateral glaucoma, all of which help differentiate this disorder from the exfoliation syndrome. Other ocular conditions with vitreous opacities, such as asteroid hyalosis, posterior uveitis, and intraocular neoplastic disease, are not likely to be confused with amyloidosis.

Meretoja[82] described another group of patients with familial amyloidosis, cranial neuropathy, and lattice corneal dystrophy who also appeared at risk to develop a secondary open-angle glaucoma. However, none had vitreous opacities.

The therapy for glaucoma associated with primary systemic amyloidosis should follow the general guidelines for treating primary open-angle glaucoma. Visual fields and optic discs can become difficult to follow in patients with advanced vitreous opacities. Filtering surgery may be necessary, but Chandler and Grant[19] have noted the deposition of what appears to be amyloid within the bleb and a resulting gradual failure of filtration. Cyclodialysis also may be effective in controlling intraocular pressure.[19]

IRRADIATION

Ocular radiotherapy may cause difficult-to-control elevations of intraocular pressure by a variety of mechanisms. An iridocyclitis with or without an associated hyphema may produce an elevation of intraocular pressure,[29,30] or peripheral anterior synechiae may obliterate the angle structures.[37] Atrophy and depigmentation of the ciliary processes also may occur, with marked pigment deposition in the outflow channels and a subsequent rise in intraocular pressure.[15] Interstitial keratitis and scleral necrosis have been noted to occur following radiation[30]; and in theory radiation injuries may cause direct obliteration of the outflow channels, although histologic evidence for such a mechanism is lacking.

Glaucoma also may develop in response to irradiation-induced changes in the ocular blood vessels. Conjunctival telangiectases can develop after ocular irradiation. When localized, such conjunctival telangiectases are of little consequence, but if generalized, may result in a rise in intraocular pressure.[8] Radiation-induced thrombosis of the iris and ciliary body vessels with degeneration of the ciliary epithelium and an associated glaucoma has been described.[30] Generalized retinal ischemia, central retinal artery occlusions, and central retinal vein occlusions occur as sequelae of high doses of ocular radiation, and rubeosis iridis may develop in this context. Rubeosis iridis with angle neovascularization and secondary glaucoma also has occurred after irradiation in an eye with an ophthalmoscopically normal fundus.[62]

ORBITAL DISEASE

Any orbital condition causing obstruction or thrombosis of the venous system draining the eye can produce a secondary glaucoma. Such conditions include orbital hemorrhage, orbital cellulitis, orbital abscess, orbital tumors and pseudotumors, thyrotropic ophthalmopathy, and Paget's disease involving the bones of the orbit. In some instances, aqueous outflow facility may be impaired without an elevation of episcleral venous pressure.

SYSTEMIC VIRAL INFECTIONS
Nephropathia Epidemica

Nephropathia epidemica, a Scandanavian form of hemorrhagic fever with renal syndrome, is a viral disease characterized by fever, malaise, nausea and vomiting, hypertension, hematuria, albuminuria, oliguria, and uremia. Hemorrhagic phenomena occur because of capillary dsyfunction and the deficiency of multiple blood coagulation factors suggesting disseminated intravascular coagulation. Mortality is as high as 10%. About the tenth day after the onset of symptoms, diuresis begins and clinical improvement occurs.

Eye findings during the acute period include lid edema, conjunctival injection and hemorrhage, retinal hemorrhages, and transient myopia. Matti Saari[79] described three patients with this disease who developed acute bilateral glaucoma characterized by a sudden increase in intraocular pressure and marked shallowing of the anterior chamber. Bilateral iridectomies in one patient did not result in immediate deepening of the anterior chambers, suggesting that pupillary block was not the underlying mechanism. Matti Saari attributed the chamber shallowing to vascular congestion, edema, and hemorrhage into the ciliary body accompanied by relaxation of the lens zonules, forward displacement of the lens-iris diaphragm, and occlusion of the trabecular meshwork by the peripheral iris. This mechanism explains the myopia as well as the acute glaucoma. Mydriatics and topical steroids resulted in more rapid improvement than treatment with miotics and appeared to be the more suitable therapeutic regimen. The use of systemic antiglaucomatous medications may have to be curtailed because of the severe renal failure in these patients. In all three patients studied, the anterior chambers deepened after the onset of the diuretic phase of the disease. Medical rather than surgical therapy is to be recommended in this condition because of the self-limited nature of the disorder. Matti Saari has emphasized that acute glaucoma rarely may occur with other infectious diseases, also causing acute tubulointerstitial nephritis.[80]

Herpes Zoster

Two forms of secondary glaucoma can occur with herpes zoster. Glaucoma usually develops as a consequence of acute iridocyclitis.[121] Rarely, an acute unilateral glaucoma can occur on the affected side, characterized by pupillary dilation, limbal injection, severe pain, and the absence of iridocyclitis. This latter form of glaucoma usually follows the skin eruption but occasionally may precede it. Duke-Elder and Perkins[32] have postulated a mechanism involving the affected ophthalmic division of the trigeminal nerve.

Mumps

Polland and Thorburn[89] noted the occurrence of transient bilateral acute open-angle glaucoma in an adult during convalescence from mumps. Although the superficial periocular tissues were injected, there was no sign of episcleritis or iritis in this patient. Polland and Thorburn attributed the intraocular pressure elevation to trabecular edema and recommended treatment with oral acetazolamide and topical steroids. They suggested that a transient rise in intraocular pressure during convalescence from mumps may be overlooked or misinterpreted as conjunctivitis in a young person and that this complication may be more common than is currently appreciated.

Influenza

Acute angle-closure glaucoma has been noted to occur occasionally in association with influenza.[24] It is not certain whether these observations represent the coincidental occurrence of the two disorders or whether influenza causes ocular changes such as vascular congestion of the ciliary body that further compromise an already narrow angle.

Acquired Immune Deficiency Syndrome

The ocular manifestations of acquired immune deficiency syndrome (AIDS) include cotton-wool spots, infectious retinitis, retinal periphlebitis, papilledema, perivasculitis, Roth spots, and cranial nerve palsies. Two cases of acute angle-closure glaucoma have been reported in this condition, both associated with choroidal effusions and secondary anterior rotation of the ciliary body.[109] Treatment with cycloplegics and aqueous suppressants is recommended, followed by iridectomy and drainage of the choroidal effusion if medical therapy is unsuccessful.[109]

Congenital Rubella

The ocular complications of congenital rubella include cataracts, pigmentary retinopathy, microphthalmos, and congenital glaucoma. Boger has reported late-onset glaucoma in a series of patients with congenital rubella.[13] Age at diagnosis of glaucoma ranged between 3 and 21 years. Almost all eyes were microphthalmic. All had cataracts, either surgically removed or spontaneously absorbed. Fluctuating keratic precipitates were observed in some patients but did not seem to correlate with the glaucoma; there were no other signs of active inflammation. The etiology of the glaucoma in these cases was not clear. Perhaps it was caused by inflammation, anterior chamber angle anomalies, or persistent viral replication in these eyes. Diagnosis, because of microphthalmia and nystagmus, was difficult. Therapy, both medical and surgical, similarly was difficult.[13]

PARASITIC DISEASE

Involvement of the eye by parasitic disease, such as onchocerciasis or river blindness, can cause uveitis and secondary glaucoma.

DERMATOLOGIC DISORDERS

Glaucoma may occur in association with certain dermatologic disorders. For instance, acne rosacea or erythema multiforme may be accompanied by keratitis. An associated uveitis or inflammation of the outflow pathways may result in secondary glaucoma.[117] Secondary open-angle glaucoma also has been noted in poikilodermatomyositis with uveitis and retinal hemorrhages.[108] Heterochromia and pigmentary glaucoma may occur in association with periocular linear scleroderma (morphea).[105] A unilateral secondary glaucoma, presumably on a vascular basis, has also been noted with generalized scleroderma.[51] The phakomatoses are discussed in Chapter 52, and juvenile xanthogranuloma is discussed in Chapter 61.

NEUROLOGIC DISORDERS

The mechanisms that control intraocular pressure are incompletely understood; but a possible role for the central nervous system has been studied extensively, and a possible neural etiology for glaucoma has occasionally been proposed. Electroencephalographic abnormalities in patients with glaucoma have been used as evidence for possible diencephalic dysfunction; autonomic dysfunction also has been postulated.[77] At the present time such hypotheses are speculative.[112] Ocular hypotony commonly occurs in patients with myotonic dystrophy, but the aqueous flow rate appears normal as measured by fluorophotometry,[113] and the mechanism for this hypotony is uncertain.

REFERENCES

1. Abedin, S, and Simmons, RJ: Neovascular glaucoma in systemic occlusive vascular disease, Ann Ophthalmol 14:284, 1982
2. Armaly, MF, and Baloglou PJ: Diabetes mellitus and the eye. II. Intraocular pressure and aqueous outflow facility, Arch Ophthalmol 77:493, 1967
3. Armstrong, JR, Daily, RK, Dobson, HL, and Girard, LJ: The incidence of glaucoma in diabetes mellitus: a comparison with the incidence of glaucoma in the general population, Am J Ophthalmol 50:55, 1960
4. Bankes, JLK: Ocular tension and diabetes mellitus, Br J Ophthalmol 61:557, 1967
5. Bayer, JM, and Neuner, HP: Cushing-Syndrom und erhohter Augeninnendruck, Dtsch Med Wochenschr 92:1792, 1967
6. Becker, B: Diabetes mellitus and primary open-angle glaucoma, Am J Ophthalmol 71:1, 1971
7. Becker, B, Kolker, AE, and Ballin, N: Thyroid function and glaucoma, Am J Ophthalmol 61:997, 1966
8. Bedford, MA: The corneal and conjunctival complications following radiotherapy, Proc R Soc Med 59:529, 1966
9. Behrman, S: Retinal vein obstruction, Br J Ophthalmol 46:336, 1962
10. Bengtsson, B: Some factors affecting the distribution of intraocular pressures in a population, Acta Ophthalmol 50:33, 1972
11. Blankenship, GW, and Okun, E: Retinal tributary vein occlusion, Arch Ophthalmol 89:363, 1973
12. Bloome, MA: Transient angle-closure glaucoma in central retinal vein occlusion, Ann Ophthalmol 9:44, 1977
13. Boger, WP: Late ocular complications in congenital rubella syndrome, Ophthalmology 87:1244, 1980
14. Boniuk, M, and Burton, GL: Unilateral glaucoma associated with sickle-cell retinopathy, Trans Am Acad Ophthalmol Otolaryngol 68:316, 1964
15. Bothman, L: Glaucoma following irradiation, Arch Ophthalmol 23:1198, 1940
16. Bramson, T, Klauber, A, and Bjerre, P: Central corneal thickness and intraocular tension in patients with acromegaly, Acta Ophthalmol 58:971, 1980
17. Brown, GC, Magargal, LE, Schachat, A, and Shah, H: Neovascular glaucoma: etiological considerations, Ophthalmology 91:315, 1984
18. Burn, RA: Intraocular pressure during haemodialysis, Br J Ophthalmol 57:511, 1973
19. Chandler, PA, and Grant, WM: Amyloidosis and open-angle glaucoma. In Glaucoma, ed. 2, Philadelphia, 1979, Lea & Febiger
20. Chandler, PA, and Grant, WM: Angle closure glaucoma secondary to occlusion of the central retinal vein. In Glaucoma, Philadelphia, 1979, Lea & Febiger
21. Cheng, H, and Perkins, ES: Thyroid disease and glaucoma, Br J Ophthalmol 51:547, 1967
22. Clark, CV, and Mapstone, R: The prevalence of diabetes mellitus in the family history of patients with primary glaucoma, Doc Ophthalmol 62:161, 1986
23. Coppeto, JR, Wand, M, Bear, L, and Sciarra, R: Neovascular glaucoma and carotid artery obstructive disease, Am J Ophthalmol 99:567, 1985
24. Daniele, S: Primary closed-angle glaucoma and influenza: report of three cases, Ann Ottal 95:961, 1969
25. Dark, AJ, Streeten, BW, and Cornwall, CC: Pseudoexfoliative disease of the lens: a study in electron microscopy and histochemistry, Br J Ophthalmol 61:462, 1977
26. Drance, SM: Some factors in the production of low tension glaucoma, Br J Ophthalmol 56:229, 1972
27. Drance, SM, Sweeney, VP, Morgan, RW, and Feldman, F: Studies of factors involved in the production of low tension glaucoma, Arch Ophthalmol 89:457, 1973
28. Dryden, RM: Central retinal vein occlusions and chronic simple glaucoma, Arch Ophthalmol 73:659, 1965
29. Duke-Elder, S: System of ophthalmology, vol 11, Diseases of the lens and vitreous: glaucoma and hypotony, St. Louis, 1969, The CV Mosby Co
30. Duke-Elder, S, and McFaul, PA: Injuries, part 2, non-mechanical injuries, vol 14. In Duke-Elder, S, editor: System of ophthalmology, St. Louis, 1972, The CV Mosby Co
31. Duke-Elder, S, and McFaul, PA: The ocular adnexa, part 2, Lacrimal, orbital and para-orbital diseases, vol 13. In Duke-Elder, S, editor: System of ophthalmology, St Louis, 1974, The CV Mosby Co
32. Duke-Elder, S, and Perkins, ES: Diseases of the uveal tract, vol 9. In Duke-Elder, S, editor: System of ophthalmology, St. Louis, 1966, The CV Mosby Co
33. Ehlers, N, Bramsen, T, and Sperling, S: Applanation tonometry and central corneal thickness, Acta Ophthalmol 53:34, 1975
34. François, J, and Neetens, A: The determination of the visual field in glaucoma and the blood pressure, Doc Ophthalmol 28:70, 1970
35. Friedman, AH, et al: Transient open-angle glaucoma associated with sickle cell trait: report on four cases, Br J Ophthalmol 63:832, 1979
36. Frucht, J, Shapiro, A, and Merin, S: Intraocular pressure in retinal vein occlusion, Br J Ophthalmol 68:26, 1984
37. Fry, WE: Secondary glaucoma, cataract and retinal degeneration following irradiation, Trans Am Acad Ophthalmol Otolaryngol 56:888, 1952
38. Futa, R, et al: Familial amyloidotic polyneuropathy: ocular manifestations with clinicopathological observation, Jpn J Ophthalmol 28:289, 1984
39. Ganly, JP: Epidemiological aspects of ocular hypertension, Surv Ophthalmol 25:130, 1980

40. Gartner, S, and Henkind, P: Neovascularization of the iris (rubeosis iridis), Surv Ophthalmol 22:291, 1978

41. Godtfredsen, E: Glaucoma and pituitary tumour, Acta Ophthalmol 46:600, 1968

42. Goldberg, MF: The diagnosis and treatment of sickled erythrocytes in human hyphemas, Trans Am Ophthalmol Soc 76:481, 1978

43. Goldberg, MF: The diagnosis and treatment of secondary glaucoma after hyphema in sickle cell patients, Am J Ophthalmol 87:43, 1979

44. Goldberg, MF: Sickle cell retinopathy. In Duane, TD, editor: Clinical ophthalmology, vol 3, Diseases of the retina, New York, 1979, Harper & Row, Publishers

45. Goldberg, MF, and Tso, MOM: Rubeosis iridis and glaucoma associated with sickle cell retinopathy: a light and electron microscopic study, Ophthalmology 85:1028, 1978

46. Gorin, G: Clinical glaucoma, New York, 1977, Marcel Dekker, Inc

47. Grant, WM: Shallowing of the anterior chamber following occlusion of the central retinal vein, Am J Ophthalmol 75:384, 1973

48. Greco, AV, et al: GH secretion in open-angle glaucoma, Ophthalmologica 179:168, 1979

49. Haas, JS, and Nootens, RH: Glaucoma secondary to benign adrenal adenoma, Am J Ophthalmol 78:497, 1974

50. Haddad, HH: Tonography and visual fields in endocrine exophthalmos, Am J Ophthalmol 64:63, 1967

51. Halmay, VO, Bajan, OM, and Felden, E: Halbeseitiges mit Skleroderma assoziiertes Glaukom, Klin Monatsbl Augenheilkd 152:558, 1968

52. Harrington, DO: The pathogenesis of the glaucoma field, Am J Ophthalmol 47(part 2):177, 1959

53. Hayreh, SS, and Podhajsky, P: Ocular neovascularization with retinal vascular occlusion. II. Occurrence in central and branch retinal artery occlusion, Arch Ophthalmol 100:1585, 1982

54. Hovland, KE, and Ellis, PP: Ocular changes in renal transplant patients, Am J Ophthalmol 63:283, 1967

55. Howard, GM, and English, FP: Occurrence of glaucoma in acromegalics, Arch Ophthalmol 73:765, 1965

56. Hoyng, PFJ, et al: Platelet aggregation and glaucoma, Doc Ophthalmol 61:167, 1985

57. Hyams, SW, and Neumann, E: Transient angle closure glaucoma after retinal vein occlusion, Br J Ophthalmol 56:353, 1972

58. Jaeger, PH, Morisod, L, Wauters, JP, and Faggioni, R: Prevention of glaucoma during hemodialysis by mannitol and acetazolamide, N Engl J Med 303:702, 1980

59. Jampol, LM, and Miller, NR: Carotid artery disease and glaucoma, Br J Ophthalmol 62:324, 1978

60. Joffe, L, Goldberg, RE, Magargal, LE, and Annesley, WH: Macular branch vein occlusion, Ophthalmology 87:91, 1980

61. Johnston, RL, et al: Risk factors of branch retinal vein occlusion, Arch Ophthalmol 103:1831, 1985

62. Jones, RF: Glaucoma following radiotherapy, Br J Ophthalmol 42:636, 1958

63. Kahn, HA, et al: The Framingham eye study. II. Association of ophthalmic pathology with single variables previously measured in the Framingham heart study, Am J Epidemiol 106:33, 1977

64. Kass, MA, and Sears, ML: Hormonal regulation of intraocular pressure, Surv Ophthalmol 22:153, 1977

65. Kaufman, HE: Primary familial amyloidosis, Arch Ophthalmol 60:1036, 1958

66. Klein, BEK, Klein, R, and Moss, SE: Intraocular pressure in diabetic persons, Ophthalmology 91:1356, 1984

67. Krasnovid, TA: A new hypothesis on the mechanism of diurnal variations in intraocular tension, Oftalmol Zh 21:185, 1966

68. Krupin, T, Jacobs, LS, Podos, SM, and Becker, B: Thyroid function and the intraocular pressure response to topical corticosteroids, Am J Ophthalmol 82:643, 1977

69. Layden, WE, and Shaffer, RN: Exfoliation syndrome, Am J Ophthalmol 78:835, 1974

70. Leighton, DA, and Phillips, CI: Systemic blood pressure in open-angle glaucoma, low tension glaucoma, and the normal eye, Br J Ophthalmol 56:447, 1972

71. Lentzch, S, and Colombi, A: Intraocular pressure (IOP) in patients on long-term hemodialysis treatment, Kidney Int 7:365, 1975

72. Levy, NS, and Rawitscher, R: The effect of systemic hypotension during cardiopulmonary bypass on intraocular pressure and visual function in humans, Ann Ophthalmol 9:1547, 1977

73. Lieb, WA, Geeraets, WJ, and Guerry, D, III: Sickle-cell retinopathy: ocular and systemic manifestations of sickle-cell disease, Acta Ophthalmol Suppl 58:1, 1959

74. Lilleaasen, P, and Horven, I: Intra-ocular pressure levels during extracorporeal circulation in man, Scand J Thor Cardiovasc Surg 16:51, 1982

75. Linnér, E: The rate of aqueous flow and the adrenals, Trans Ophthalmol Soc UK 79:27, 1959

76. Luntz, MH, and Schenker, HI: Retinal vascular accidents in glaucoma and ocular hypertension, Surv Ophthalmol 25:163, 1980

77. Mapstone, R, and Clark, CV: The prevalence of autonomic neuropathy in glaucoma, Trans Ophthalmol Soc UK 104:265, 1985

78. Mapstone, R, and Clark, CV: Prevalence of diabetes in glaucoma, Br Med J 291:93, 1985

79. Matti Saari, K: Acute glaucoma in hemorrhagic fever with renal syndrome (nephropathia epidemica), Am J Ophthalmol 81:455, 1976

80. Matti Saari, K, Vänttinen, T, Pasternack, A, and Helin, H: Acute glaucoma in acute hemorrhagic tubulointerstitial nephritis, Glaucoma 3:269, 1981

81. Mendelsohn, AD, Jampol, LM, and Shoch, D: Secondary angle-closure glaucoma after central retinal vein occlusion, Am J Ophthalmol 100:581, 1985

82. Meretoja, J: Comparative histopathological and clinical findings in eyes with lattice corneal dystrophy of two different types, Ophthalmologica 165:15, 1972

83. Meretoja, J, and Tarkkanen, A: Occurrence of amyloid in eyes with pseudo-exfoliation, Ophthalmic Res 9:80, 1977

84. Neuner, HP, and Dardenne, U: Augenveränderungen bei Cushing-Syndrom, Klin Monatsbl Augenheilkd 152:570, 1968

85. Nielsen, NV: The prevalence of glaucoma and ocular hypertension in type 1 and 2 diabetes mellitus, an epidemiological study of diabetes mellitus on the island of Falster, Denmark, Acta Ophthalmol 61:662, 1983

86. Pantieleva, VM, Klyachko, VR, and Barkman, SM: Ocular hydrodynamics in primary hypothyroidism, Vestn Oftalmol 3:18, 1971

87. Paton, D, and Duke, JR: Primary familial amyloidosis (ocular manifestations with histopathologic observations), Am J Ophthalmol 61:736, 1966

88. Pohjanpelto, P: The thyroid gland and intraocular pressure (tonographic study of 187 patients with thyroid disease), Acta Ophthalmol Suppl 97:9, 1968

89. Polland, W, and Thorburn, W: Transient glaucoma as a manifestation of mumps, Acta Ophthalmol 54:779, 1976

90. Radius, RL, and Finkelstein, D: Central retinal artery occlusion (reversible) in sickle trait with glaucoma, Br J Ophthalmol 60:428, 1976

91. Raitta, C, Vannas, S, and Aurekoski, H: Aqueous humor dynamics after central retinal vein occlusion, Acta Ophthalmol 46:26, 1968

92. Ramsell, JT, Ellis, PP, and Paterson, CA: Intraocular pressure changes during hemodialysis, Am J Ophthalmol 72:926, 1971

93. Reese, AB, and McGavic, JS: Relation of field contraction to blood pressure in chronic primary glaucoma, Arch Ophthalmol 27:845, 1942

94. Safir, A, Paulsen, EP, Klayman, J, and Gerstenfeld, J: Ocular abnormalities in juvenile diabetics: frequent occurrence of abnormally high tensions. Arch Ophthalmol 76:557, 1966

95. Schmelzer, H: Hypophyse and Glaukomgenese, Klin Monatsbl Augenheilkd 129:114, 1956

96. Segawa, K: The fine structure of the iridocorneal angle tissue in glaucomatous eyes. V. Glaucoma secondary to primary familial amyloidosis, Jpn J Clin Ophthalmol 30:1375, 1976

97. Shapiro, AL, and Baum, JL: Acute open-angle glaucoma in a patient with sickle cell trait, Am J Ophthalmol 58:292, 1964

98. Shiose, Y, and Kawase, Y: A new approach to stratified normal intraocular pressure in a general population, Am J Ophthalmol 101:714, 1986

99. Sitprija, V, Holmes, JH, and Ellis, PP: Intraocular pressure changes during artificial kidney therapy, Arch Ophthalmol 72:626, 1964

100. Sjolie, AK: Ocular complications in insulin treated diabetes mellitus, an epidemiological study, Acta Ophthalmol Suppl 63:1, 1985

101. Sonty, S, and Schwartz, B: Vascular accidents in acute angle closure glaucoma, Ophthalmology 88:225, 1981

102. Sorokanich, S, Wand, M, and Nix, HR: Angle closure glaucoma and acute hyperglycemia, Arch Ophthalmol 104:1434, 1986

103. Steinmann, W, et al: A case-control study of the association of sickle cell trait and chronic open-angle glaucoma, Am J Epidemiol 118:288, 1983

104. Stellpflug, H, Busse, H, Niedermeier, M, and Dittrich, H: Augenveränderungen während extrakorporaler Zirkulation, Ophthalmologica 179:249, 1979

105. Stone, RA, and Scheie, HG: Periorbital scleroderma associated with heterochromia iridis, Am J Ophthalmol 90:858, 1980

106. Traisman, HS, Alfano, JE, Andrews, J, and Gatti, R: Intraocular pressure in juvenile diabetics, Am J Ophthalmol 64:1149, 1967

107. Tsukahara, SM, and Matsuo, T: Secondary glaucoma accompanied with primary familial amyloidosis, Ophthalmologica 175:250, 1977

108. Tuovinen, E, and Raudasoja, R: Poikilodermatomyositis with retinal hemorrhages and secondary glaucoma, Acta Ophthalmol 43:669, 1965

109. Ullman, S, Wilson, RP, and Schwartz, L: Bilateral angle-closure glaucoma in association with the acquired immune deficiency syndrome, Am J Ophthalmol 101:419, 1986

110. van Bijsterveld, OP, and Richards, RD: Pituitary tumors and intraocular pressure, Am J Ophthalmol 57:267, 1964

111. Vannas, S, and Tarkkanen, A: Retinal vein occlusion and glaucoma, tonographic study of the incidence of glaucoma and of its prognostic significance. Br J Ophthalmol 44:583, 1960

112. Waitzman, MB: Hypothalamus and ocular pressure, Surv Ophthalmol 16:1, 1971

113. Walker, SD, and Brubaker, RF: Aqueous humor dynamics in myotonic dystrophy, Invest Ophthalmol 19(suppl):140, 1980

114. Wan, WL, Minckler, DS, and Rao, NA: Pupillary-block glaucoma associated with childhood cystinosis, Am J Ophthalmol 101:700, 1986

115. Wax, MB, Ridley, ME, and Margargal, LE: Reversal of retinal and optic disc ischemia in a patient with sickle cell trait and glaucoma secondary to traumatic hyphema, Ophthalmology 89:845, 1982

116. Weekers, R, Prijot, E, and Laverne, G: Mesure de la pression oculaire, de la résistance à l'ecoulement de l'humeur aqueuse et de la rigidité dans les exophthalmies endocriniennes, Ophthalmologica 139:382, 1960

117. Weiss, DR: Glaucoma and systemic disease. In Duane, TD, editor: Clinical ophthalmology. vol 5, New York, 1979, Harper & Row, Publishers

118. Welch, RB, and Goldberg, MF: Sickle-cell hemoglobin and its relation to fundus abnormality, Arch Ophthalmol 75:353, 1966

119. Wilson, DM, and Martin, JHS: Raised intraocular tension in renal transplant recipients, Med J Aus 1:482, 1973

120. Winder, AF, Paterson, G, and Miller, SJH: Biochemical abnormalities associated with ocular hypertension and low-tension glaucoma, Trans Ophthalmol Soc UK 94:518, 1974

121. Womack, LW, and Liesegang, TJ: Complications of herpes zoster ophthalmicus, Arch Ophthalmol 101:42, 1983

122. Yanoff, M, and Fine, BS: Ocular pathology: a text and atlas, New York, 1975, Harper & Row, Publishers

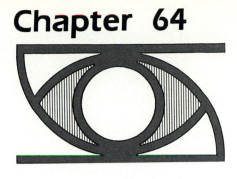

Chapter 64

Corticosteroid-induced Glaucoma

Michael A. Kass
Tim Johnson

HISTORICAL BACKGROUND

At one time it was postulated that adrenal extracts had a beneficial effect on glaucoma.[48] However, this idea soon proved to be false, and a number of reports indicated that systemically administered glucocorticoids elevated intraocular pressure in normal eyes[30,93] and eyes with uveitis.[34,62,66] François[34] and Goldmann[42] noted that individuals who received long-term treatment with corticosteroid eyedrops could develop findings that resembled open-angle glaucoma, including increased intraocular pressure, optic nerve head cupping and visual field loss. Over the subsequent years, there have been literally hundreds of reports linking topical, systemic and periocular corticosteroid administration with elevated intraocular pressure and secondary open-angle glaucoma.

During the 1960s and 1970s there was widespread interest in the association between the intraocular pressure response to topically administered glucocorticoids and the inheritance of primary open-angle glaucoma. Many different groups underwent topical corticosteroid testing, including normal volunteers,* senior citizens,[11] prisoners,[56] Africans,[33] American Indians,[81] glaucoma patients,[4,19,20,61,89] and glaucoma suspects.[61] Based on these studies it became clear that marked ocular hypertensive responses occurred less frequently in normal individuals than in patients with primary open-angle glaucoma[4,19,20] and their first-degree relatives[17,18,31,37,72] (Table 64-1). Armaly[7,8] and

*References 3, 4, 6-8, 15, 61, 89.

Becker[15] classified individuals according to their intraocular pressure responses to topical corticosteroid administration as low, intermediate, and high responders (Table 64-2). Despite the fact that they used different criteria for their classification systems, these two investigators concluded that the intraocular pressure response to corticosteroids was inherited and that the genes controlling this response were related to the inheritance of primary open-angle glaucoma.

The theories relating the intraocular pressure response to topical corticosteroids and primary open-angle glaucoma have lost favor over the past decade for a number of reasons. First, twin studies revealed a lower concordance of glucocorticoid testing results than would be expected from the Armaly and Becker theories.[84,85] Furthermore, the intraocular pressure response to topical dexamethasone was not very reproducible except in the high responder group.[71] Some authorities tried to explain this lack of reproducibility by invoking variable medication compliance among subjects.[69] Finally, glucocorticoid testing did not improve the accuracy of the predictions concerning the development of glaucomatous visual field loss in glaucoma suspects.[101]

Some investigators extended the Becker and Armaly hypotheses and proposed that individuals with primary open-angle glaucoma had a generalized sensitivity to the effects of corticosteroids. Evidence for this theory came from tests of dexamethasone suppression of plasma cortisol[22] and glucocorticoid inhibition of mitogen stimulated

Table 64-1 Topical corticosteroid testing in normal individuals and glaucoma patients

	Low responders (%)	Intermediate responders (%)	High responders (%)
Normal volunteers			
Armaly[3]	66	29	5
Becker[15]	58	36	6
Patients with primary open-angle glaucoma			
Armaly[4,7,8]	6	48	46
Becker[15,19,20]	0	8	92

Table 64-2 Intraocular pressure response to topical corticosteroid administration

	Becker[15]	Armaly[6-8]
Frequency of administration	4 times daily	3 times daily
Duration of administration	6 weeks	4 weeks
Parameter for classification	Final intraocular pressure	Change in intraocular pressure
Classification system		
Low responder	IOP* < 20 mm Hg	IOP† Δ < 6 mm Hg
Intermediate responder	IOP 20 to 31 mm Hg	IOP Δ 6 to 15 mm Hg
High responder	IOP > 31 mm Hg	IOP Δ > 15 mm Hg

*Based on final intraocular pressure.
†Based on change in intraocular pressure from baseline.

lymphocytic transformation.[25,26] However, these findings were not confirmed in subsequent studies.[23,65,78] A thorough discussion of corticosteroid responsiveness and glaucoma is beyond the scope of this chapter and readers wishing additional information are referred to several excellent reviews on the subject.*

Regardless of the heritability of the corticosteroid response or its relationship to primary open-angle glaucoma, three clinical points deserve emphasis. First, a substantial minority of the general population develops elevated intraocular pressure when treated with long-term topical, systemic, or periocular glucocorticoids (see Table 64-1). Second, certain individuals, particularly those with primary open-angle glaucoma,[4,19,20] their first-degree relatives,[15,18,31,72] diabetics,[16] and high myopes[76] are at greater risk of developing increased intraocular pressure when treated with corticosteroids. Third, physicians who prescribe corticosteroids are not sufficiently aware of this problem. Ophthalmologists must remind their colleagues of this potentially blinding side effect. Even though corticosteroid glaucoma has been well described for many years, it remains a common cause of visual loss.

CLASSIFICATION

It is possible to classify the cases of corticosteroid glaucoma by the source of the drug (see box

*References 8, 9, 18, 21, 68, 83.

CORTICOSTEROID-INDUCED GLAUCOMA

A. Exogenous corticosteroids
　1. Ocular
　　a. Eyedrops
　　b. Ocular ointments
　　c. Inadvertent administration to the eye from the lids or face
　2. Periocular injection
　3. Systemic
　　a. Oral
　　b. Topical (to the skin)
　　c. Injection
B. Endogenous corticosteroids
　1. Adrenal hyperplasia
　2. Adrenal adenoma or carcinoma
　3. Ectopic ACTH syndrome

---

above) even though this does not imply differences in the pathogenesis of the condition or its clinical presentation. Almost all cases of corticosteroid glaucoma are caused by exogenous glucocorticoids administered topically, periocularly, or systemically. It is important to emphasize that the category of topical glucocorticoids includes not only drops and ointments applied for therapeutic purposes to the eye but also creams, lotions, and ointments that inadvertently reach the eye from the face or eyelids.[95,104]

Systemic administration of glucocorticoids may

raise intraocular pressure after weeks to years of treatment.* Patients who require long-term corticosteroid treatment should be monitored periodically as long as they are receiving the medication. Many individuals receive both systemic and topical ocular glucocorticoids (e.g., patients with collagen vascular disease and uveitis), and it is important to remember that the ocular hypertensive effects of these administrations are additive.[41] Corticosteroids applied topically to the skin may be absorbed in sufficient quantity to act systemically and raise intraocular pressure.[90] This is most common when potent fluorinated glucocorticoids are applied with occlusive dressings to large areas of the body.

Periocular corticosteroid injections (subconjunctival, sub-Tenon's, or retrobulbar) have been reported to raise intraocular pressure.[39,46,49,70,74] The most persistent elevations of pressure have occurred after injection of repository or "depo" corticosteroid preparations.

Occasionally, corticosteroid glaucoma is caused by endogenous production of glucocorticoids (see box at left). Bayer and Neuner[13,14,79] reported a series of patients with adrenal hyperplasia and elevated intraocular pressure. After adrenal surgery, intraocular pressure fell 5 to 12 mm Hg in all cases. Haas and Nootens[43] described a patient with Cushing's syndrome who had elevated intraocular pressure and reduced tonographic facility of outflow. After surgery for an adrenal adenoma, the intraocular pressure and facility of outflow returned to normal. The patient and several of his relatives were high intraocular pressure responders upon topical corticosteroid testing. The authors concluded that the intraocular pressure response to high levels of endogenous glucocorticoids depended on the genetic predisposition of the individual.

CLINICAL PICTURE

A rise in intraocular pressure may be noted as early as 1 week after initiating glucocorticoid treatment, or it may not occur for months to years. The latent period before the intraocular pressure begins to rise and the magnitude of the pressure elevation are related to the potency of the drug, the dose administered, the frequency of administration, the route of administration, the presence of other ocular and systemic diseases, and most important, the responsiveness of the patient.

The clinical picture of corticosteroid glaucoma is affected by the age of the patient and the pres-

ence of other ocular diseases. Young children with corticosteroid glaucoma are often diagnosed as having primary infantile glaucoma on the basis of typical symptoms, such as tearing, photophobia, blepharospasm, and enlarged eyes, and typical physical findings, such as enlarged cloudy corneas, breaks in Descemet's membrane, elevated intraocular pressure, and glaucomatous cupping of the optic disc.[2,50,82,96] The anterior chamber angle of infants with corticosteroid glaucoma does not resemble that of infants with congenital glaucoma, but this can be a subtle distinction. The correct diagnosis is reached when the ophthalmologist elicits a history of glucocorticoid administration. Often these children were prescribed combined corticosteroid-antibiotic preparations by family physicians or pediatricians for presumed lacrimal obstruction.

In older children and adults, corticosteroid glaucoma usually resembles primary open-angle glaucoma in that the eyes are quiet with elevated intraocular pressure, open anterior chamber angles, cupped optic discs, and glaucomatous visual field loss. Most of these patients are asymptomatic, although occasionally intraocular pressure is elevated sufficiently to cause corneal edema with attendant halo vision, blurred vision, and discomfort. Uniocular topical corticosteroid administration elevates intraocular pressure in the treated eye. Binocular topical corticosteroid administration and systemic glucocorticoid administration elevate intraocular pressure in both eyes. It is ironic that many cases of corticosteroid glaucoma occur in patients who used glucocorticoids for minor conditions, such as contact lens discomfort, blepharitis, and conjunctival hyperemia.

Corticosteroid glaucoma can also resemble low-tension glaucoma.[94] Patients who were treated with glucocorticoids in the past may have optic disc cupping and glaucomatous visual field loss in the face of normal intraocular pressure and outflow facility. Once again, the key to the correct diagnosis is a careful history of past corticosteroid treatment.

The clinical picture of corticosteroid glaucoma may be confounded by the presence of other ocular diseases or conditions. For example, a patient with corticosteroid glaucoma and uveitis may appear to have elevated intraocular pressure from ocular inflammation. In contrast, a patient with corticosteroid glaucoma and a shallow anterior chamber may appear to have chronic angle-closure glaucoma.

Corticosteroid glaucoma may masquerade as uncontrolled open-angle glaucoma. Glaucoma patients who had been previously well controlled and who now take glucocorticoids may present with marked elevations of intraocular pressure that are poorly responsive to medical treatment. Unfortunately, some glaucoma patients administer topical glucocorticoids to relieve the irritation caused by their ocular hypotensive medications (e.g., conjunctival hyperemia from epinephrine).

Ophthalmologists may also note other sequelae of topical corticosteroid administration including posterior subcapsular cataract,[47,63,83] ptosis,[67] mydriasis,[5,67] skin atrophy of the eyelids,[95] ocular infection with herpes simplex or fungi,[95] delayed wound healing, corneal ulceration, and corticosteroid-induced uveitis.[58] Individuals treated with systemic glucocorticoids may appear cushingoid with moon facies, truncal obesity, hirsutism, plethora, buffalo hump, cutaneous striae, easy bruising, hypertension, diabetes, osteoporosis, infection, myopathy, renal calculi, fluid retention, and psychiatric disorders.

PATHOPHYSIOLOGY

Many of the physiologic and pharmacologic effects of the glucocorticoids are mediated by specific cytoplasmic receptors. After binding, the steroid-receptor complex passes into the cell nucleus where it alters chromatin structure and/or function and effects messenger RNA (mRNA) synthesis. The mRNA leaves the nucleus and modulates the synthesis of a variety of proteins including enzymes. Ocular tissues, including tissues of the outflow channels, contain specific steroid receptors and the necessary enzymes for the metabolism of circulating glucocorticoids.[45,87,88,98,100] It is unclear whether corticosteroid glaucoma is mediated by specific cytoplasmic steroid receptors and whether this entity involves a single metabolic pathway.

Corticosteroids raise intraocular pressure by lowering the facility of outflow.[3,59,67,97] Although a few investigators find that glucocorticoids increase aqueous humor production,[32,38,64] the balance of the evidence suggests that this effect has little importance in human eyes.[29]

A number of theories have been proposed to explain the diminished outflow facility noted in corticosteroid glaucoma. Perhaps the most widely discussed theory has been that glucocorticoids reduce outflow facility by effecting glycosaminoglycan (GAG) metabolism.* In a number of experiments, corticosteroids caused an accumulation of GAGs in the trabecular meshwork more likely by inhibiting catabolism rather than by stimulating

synthesis.* It has been further postulated that corticosteroids stabilize lysosomal membranes and thereby inhibit the release of enzymes that depolymerize GAGs. Although this theory has considerable appeal, it does not explain why some individuals are more susceptible than others to the ocular hypertensive effect of glucocorticoids. The varying response to glucocorticoids could be explained by differential metabolism or drug penetration, differential sensitivity of the outflow system, or a preexisting difference in the outflow pathways. However, there is no clear evidence to support any of these theories.

Other investigators have proposed alternative explanations for cortosteroid-induced elevations of intraocular pressure. Bill[27] has suggested that glucocorticoids inhibit the phagocytosis of foreign material by trabecular endothelial cells. This leads to an accumulation of debris that clogs the outflow channels. Weinreb et al.[99] have proposed that corticosteroids inhibit the synthesis of prostaglandins that modulate intraocular pressure. These investigators used radioimmunoassay to study prostaglandin synthesis by human trabecular endothelium in tissue culture. They found that dexamethasone inhibited the synthesis of prostaglandins E_2 and $F_{2\alpha}$ and suggested that these compounds regulate outflow facility. Southren et al.[87,88,100] have studied homogenates of trabecular meshwork taken from eyes with primary open-angle glaucoma and demonstrated changes in cortisol metabolism. These investigators found a 100-fold increase in the concentration of Δ^4-reductase and a four-fold decrease in the concentration of 3-oxidoreductase levels. These metabolic changes caused an accumulation of 5α (5β)-dihydrocortisol; 5β-dihydrocortisol potentiated the ocular hypertensive effect of dexamethasone in young rabbits.[88] Southren et al.[87,88,100] postulated that 5β-dihydrocortisol could also potentiate the effects of exogenous glucocorticoids in susceptible individuals.

Histopathologic studies of human eyes with corticosteroid glaucoma demonstrate increased density of the cribriform meshwork[80] and thinning of the endothelial lining of Schlemm's canal.[51] It is not clear whether these pathologic changes are primary or secondary.

DIAGNOSIS

To reach the proper diagnosis, clinicians must maintain a high index of suspicion and question patients specifically about their use of corticoste-

---

*References 10, 35, 51, 90, 92, 103.

*References 10, 35, 36, 44, 53, 54, 86, 103.

roid eyedrops, ointments, skin preparations, and pills. This is especially important when dealing with physicians and other health care professionals who have ready access to medication. Any unlabeled drug must be identified.

The key test for diagnosing corticosteroid glaucoma is to discontinue the medication and monitor the intraocular pressure response. Although most patients respond within a few days to several weeks after discontinuing the drug, there are a few reports of persistent elevations of intraocular pressure after glucocorticoid treatment.[37,90,91] In these cases, it is possible that the corticosteroid treatment unmasked underlying primary open-angle glaucoma or that prolonged elevation of intraocular pressure chronically damaged the outflow channels. It should be pointed out that there is a low order correlation between the length of glucocorticoid treatment and the time required for intraocular pressure to return to baseline after discontinuation of the drug.

It is more difficult to make the diagnosis of corticosteroid glaucoma when the drug is used to treat an eye disease that itself can be associated with elevated intraocular pressure (e.g., uveitis). If the clinician stops glucocorticoid treatment in a patient with uveitis and intraocular pressure falls, it may be impossible to distinguish the effect of the drug from the hypotony associated with increased inflammation. If the disease involves one eye, it may be helpful to determine the intraocular pressure response of the fellow eye to topical corticosteroid administration.

MANAGEMENT

Before initiating corticosteroid therapy it is important to obtain a baseline ocular examination. Although an occasional patient develops a marked ocular hypertensive response within several days of initiating treatment, it is reasonable to check the intraocular pressure after 2 to 3 weeks. If the intraocular pressure is still normal and if additional glucocorticoid therapy is needed, the ophthalmologist should reexamine the patient every 2 to 3 weeks for the first few months, and every 2 to 3 months thereafter. Unfortunately there is no time period beyond which a patient is incapable of developing corticosteroid glaucoma.

The key to managing corticosteroid glaucoma is stopping the drug. In almost all cases, the intraocular pressure returns to baseline over a few days to several weeks. During this period, treatment with standard antiglaucoma medications may be required to control the intraocular pressure. If glu-

cocorticoid treatment must continue despite elevated intraocular pressure, a weaker drug,[77] a lower concentration of the drug,[77] or a drug with less tendency to elevate intraocular pressure may be substituted.[28] Both medrysone and fluorometholone appear to cause less intraocular pressure elevation for a given antiinflammatory effect than some other corticosteroid preparations.[28] This conclusion is based on clinical impression and in vitro tests of lymphocyte transformation rather than direct measures of ocular antiinflammatory potency. It is important to realize that medrysone and fluorometholone can produce elevated intraocular pressure in susceptible individuals.

Elevated intraocular pressure associated with periocular corticosteroid injection is usually treated by standard medical means. However, in some patients intraocular pressure can remain elevated for 12 to 18 months or longer after repository glucocorticoid injection. If the intraocular pressure cannot be controlled and is threatening vision, the residual glucocorticoid material beneath the conjunctiva should be removed.[46]

A synthetic antiglucocorticoid compound, RU 486-6, has shown promise as a peripheral corticosteroid receptor antagonist. Phillips et al.[75] found that RU 486-6 lowered intraocular pressure in rabbits and speculated that the pressure reduction might be due to blockade of steroid receptor sites. Topical agents that block peripheral corticosteroid receptors may hold promise for the medical management of corticosteroid glaucoma.

Corticosteroid glaucoma that is resistant to medical management may require filtering surgery. It is possible to withhold surgery when the optic nerve is healthy, even if intraocular pressure cannot be controlled. However, such patients must be followed carefully. If progressive optic nerve and visual field damage occurs or seems very likely to occur, surgical intervention is indicated. Unfortunately laser trabeculoplasty seems to be of little help in the treatment of corticosteroid glaucoma.

After filtering surgery, the ophthalmologist can use topical, subconjunctival, and oral corticosteroids as needed to control inflammation and scarring. If systemic glucocorticoids are administered, the intraocular pressure of the fellow eye must be monitored carefully. There are a few reports of corticosteroid-induced intraocular pressure elevations occurring in eyes with functional filtering operations.[102] However, most authorities believe that a functional filtering operation precludes a corticosteroid-induced intraocular pressure elevation.[55,57]

REFERENCES

1. Alfano, JE: Changes in the intraocular pressure associated with systemic steroid therapy, Am J Ophthalmol 56:345, 1963
2. Alfano, JE, and Platt, D: Steroid (ACTH) induced glaucoma simulating congenital glaucoma, Am J Ophthalmol 61:911, 1966
3. Armaly, MF: Effects of corticosteroids on intraocular pressure and fluid dynamics. I. The effect of dexamethasone in the normal eye, Arch Ophthalmol 70:482, 1963
4. Armaly, MF: Effect of corticosteroids on intraocular pressure and fluid dynamics. II. The effect of dexamethasone in the glaucomatous eye, Arch Ophthalmol 70:492, 1963
5. Armaly, MF: Effect of corticosteroids on intraocular pressure and fluid dynamics. III. Changes in visual function and pupil size during topical dexamethasone application, Arch Ophthalmol 71:639, 1964
6. Armaly, MF: Statistical attributes of the steroid hypersensitive response in the clinically normal eye. I. The demonstration of three levels of response, Invest Ophthalmol Vis Sci 4:187, 1965
7. Armaly, MF: The heritable nature of dexamethasone-induced ocular hypertension, Arch Ophthalmol 75:32, 1966
8. Armaly, MF: Inheritance of dexamethasone hypertension and glaucoma, Arch Ophthalmol 77:747, 1967
9. Armaly, MF: Genetic factors related to glaucoma, Ann NY Acad Sci 151:861, 1968
10. Ashton, N: The role of the trabecular structure in the problem of simple glaucoma, particularly with regard to the significance of mucopolysaccharides. In Newell, FW, editor: Glaucoma: transactions of the 4th Conference, vol 4, New York, 1960, Josiah Macy, Jr., Foundation
11. Ballin, N, and Becker, B: Provocative testing for primary open-angle glaucoma in "senior citizens," Invest Ophthalmol Vis Sci 6:126, 1967
12. Barany, EH, and Southbrook, S: Influence of testicular hyaluronidase on the resistance to flow through the angle of the anterior chamber, Acta Physiol Scand 33:240, 1953
13. Bayer, JM: Ergebnisse und Beurteilung der subtotalen Adrenalektomie beim hyperfuncktions-Cushing, Langenbecks Arch Klin Chir 291:531, 1959
14. Bayer, JM, and Neuner, NP: Cushing-Syndrom und erhohter Augeninnendruck, Dtsch Med Wochenschr 92:1971, 1967
15. Becker, B: Intraocular pressure response to topical corticosteroids, Invest Ophthalmol Vis Sci 4:198, 1965
16. Becker, B: Diabetes mellitus and primary open-angle glaucoma: the XXVII Edward Jackson Memorial Lecture, Am J Ophthalmol 77:1, 1971
17. Becker, B, and Chevrette, L: Topical corticosteroid testing in glaucoma siblings, Arch Ophthalmol 76:484, 1986
18. Becker, B, and Hahn, KA: Topical corticosteroids and heredity in primary open-angle glaucoma, Am J Ophthalmol 57:543, 1964
19. Becker, B, and Mills, DW: Corticosteroids and intraocular pressure, Arch Ophthalmol 70:500, 1963
20. Becker, B, and Mills, DW: Elevated intraocular pressure following corticosteroid eye drops, JAMA 185:884, 1963
21. Becker, B, and Podos, SM: Hypersensitivity to glucocorticoids and primary open-angle glaucoma. In Etienne, R, and Patterson, GD, editors: International Glaucoma Symposium Albi, 1974, Lyon, France, 1975, Imprimerie
22. Becker, B, Podos, SM, Asseff, CF, and Cooper, DG: Plasma cortisol suppression in glaucoma, Am J Ophthalmol 75:73, 1973
23. Ben Ezra, D, Ticho, U, and Sachs, U: Lymphocyte sensitivity to glucocorticoids, Am J Ophthalmol 82:866, 1976
24. Bernstein, NH, and Schwartz, B: Effects of long-term systemic steroids on ocular pressure and tonographic values, Arch Ophthalmol 68:742, 1962
25. Bigger, JF, Palmberg, PF, and Becker, B: Increased cellular sensitivity to glucocorticoids in primary open-angle glaucoma, Invest Ophthalmol Vis Sci 11:832, 1972
26. Bigger, JF, Palmberg, PF, Zink, H, and Becker, B: Sensitivity to glucocorticoids in primary open-angle glaucoma, New Engl J Med 287:992, 1972
27. Bill, A: The drainage of aqueous humor, Invest Ophthalmol Vis Sci 14:1, 1975
28. Cantrill, HL, et al: Comparison of in vitro potency of corticosteroids with ability to raise intraocular pressure, Am J Ophthalmol 79:1012, 1975
29. Brubaker, RF: The physiology of aqueous humor formation. In Drance, SM, and Neufeld, AH, editors: Glaucoma: applied pharmacology in medical treatment, New York, 1984, Grune & Stratton
30. Covell, LL: Glaucoma induced by systemic steroid therapy, Am J Ophthalmol 45:108, 1954
31. Davies, TG: Tonographic survey of the close relatives of patients with chronic simple glaucoma, Br J Ophthalmol 52:32, 1968
32. Draeger, J: Der Einfluss lokaler Steroidgaven auf den Augeninnendruck, Klin Monats Augenheilkd 147:386, 1965
33. Easty, DL, and Luntz, MH: Influence of topical corticosteroids on intraocular pressure in Africans, Am J Ophthalmol 68:640, 1969
34. François, J: Cortisone et tension oculaire, Ann Ocul 187:805, 1954
35. François, J: The importance of the mucopolysaccharides in intraocular pressure regulation, Invest Ophthalmol Vis Sci 14:173, 1975
36. François, J, Benozzi, G, Victoria-Troncoso, V, and Bohgn, W: Ultrastructural and morphometric study of corticosteroid glaucoma in rabbits, Ophthalmic Res 16:168, 1984

37. François, J, Heintz-deBrée, CH, and Tripathi, RC: The cortisone test and the heredity of primary open-angle glaucoma, Am J Ophthalmol 62:844, 1966

38. Frandsen, E: Glaucoma and posterior subcapsular cataract following prednisolone (ultracorticol therapy), Acta Ophthalmol (Copenh) 42:108, 1964

39. Garber, MI: Methylprednisolone in the treatment of exophthalmos, Lancet 1:958, 1966

40. Godel, V, Feiler-Ofry, V, and Stein, R: Systemic steroids and ocular fluid dynamics. I. Analysis of the sample as a whole; influence of dosage and duration of therapy, Acta Ophthalmol (Copenh) 50:655, 1972

41. Godel, V, Feiler-Ofry, V, and Stein, R: Systemic steroids and ocular fluid dynamics. II. Systemic versus topical steroids, Acta Ophthalmol (Copenh) 50:664, 1972

42. Goldmann, H: Cortisone glaucoma, Arch Ophthalmol 68:621, 1962

43. Haas, JS, and Nootens, RH: Glaucoma secondary to benign adrenal adenoma, Am J Ophthalmol 78:497, 1974

44. Hernandez, MR, et al: The effect of dexamethasone on the in vitro incorporation of percursors of extracellular matrix components in the outflow pathway region of the rabbit eye, Invest Ophthalmol Vis Sci 24:704, 1983

45. Hernandez, MR, et al: Glucocorticoid target cells in human outflow pathway: autopsy and surgical specimens, Invest Ophthalmol Vis Sci 24:1612, 1983

46. Herschler, J: Intractable intraocular hypertension induced by repository triamcinolone acetonide, Am J Ophthalmol 74:501, 1972

47. Hovland, KR, and Ellis, PP: Ocular changes in renal transplant patients, Am J Ophthalmol 63:283, 1967

48. Josephson, EM: Effect of cortin on intraocular tension in glaucoma, Science 82:62, 1935

49. Kalina, RE: Increased intraocular pressure following subconjunctival corticosteroid administration, Arch Ophthalmol 81:788, 1969

50. Kass, MA, Kolker, AE, and Becker, B: Chronic topical corticosteroid use simulating congenital glaucoma, J Pediatr 81:1175, 1972

51. Kayes, J, and Becker, B: The human trabecular meshwork in corticosteroid-induced glaucoma, Trans Am Ophthalmol Soc 67:354, 1969

52. Kitazawa, Y: Acute glaucoma due to systemic corticosteroid administration, Acta Soc Ophthalmol Jpn 70:2179, 1966

53. Knepper, PA, Breen, M, Weinstein, HG, and Black, LJ: Intraocular pressure and glycosaminoglycan distribution in the rabbit eye: effect of age and dexamethasone, Exp Eye Res 27:567, 1978

54. Knepper, PA, Collins, JA, and Federick, R: Effect of dexamethasone, progesterone and testosterone on IOP and GAGs in the rabbit eye, Invest Ophthalmol Vis Sci 26:1093, 1985

55. Kolker, AE: Discussion of Wilensky, JT, Snyder, D, and Gieser, D: Steroid-induced ocular hypertension in patients with filtering blebs, Ophthalmology 87:243, 1980

56. Kolker, AE, Stewart, RM, Alton, E, and LeMon, L: Dexamethasone testing in prison inmates, Invest Ophthalmol Vis Sci 10:198, 1971

57. Kronfeld, PC: The effects of topical steroid administration on intraocular pressure and aqueous outflow after fistulizing operations, Trans Am Ophthalmol Soc 62:375, 1964

58. Krupin, T, et al: Uveitis in association with topically administered corticosteroids, Am J Ophthalmol 70:883, 1970

59. Kupfer, C: Pseudofacility in the human eye, Trans Am Ophthalmol Soc 69:383, 1971

60. Laval, J, and Collier, R, Jr: Elevation of intraocular pressure due to hormonal steroid therapy in uveitis, Am J Ophthalmol 39:175, 1955

61. Levene, R, et al: Topical corticosteroid in normal patients and glaucoma suspects, Arch Ophthalmol 77:593, 1967

62. Lijo-Pavia, J: Cortisona y tonus ocular, Rev Oto-neurophthalmol 27:14, 1952

63. Lindholm, B, Linnér, E, and Tengroth, B: Effects of long-term systemic steroids on cataract formation and aqueous humor dynamics, Acta Ophthalmol (Copenh) 43:120, 1965

64. Linnér, E: Adrenocorticol steroids and aqueous humor dynamics, Doc Ophthalmol 12:210, 1959

65. McCarty, G, Schwartz, B, and Miller, K: Absence of lymphocyte glucocorticoid hypersensitivity in primary open-angle glaucoma, Arch Ophthalmol 99:1258, 1981

66. McLean, JM: Discussion of Woods, AC: Clinical and experimental observation on the use of ACTH and cortisone in ocular inflammatory disease, Trans Am Ophthalmol Soc 48:293, 1959

67. Miller, D, Peczon, JD, and Whitworth, CG: Corticosteroids and functions in the anterior segment of the eye, Am J Ophthalmol 59:31, 1965

68. Miller, SJH: Genetic aspects of glaucoma, Trans Ophthalmol Soc UK 86:25, 1966

69. Mindel, JS, Goldberg, J, and Tavitian, HO: Similarity on the intraocular pressure response to different corticosteroid esters when compliance is controlled, Ophthalmology 86:99, 1979

70. Nozik, RA: Periocular injection of steroids, Trans Am Acad Ophthalmol Otolaryngol 76:695, 1972

71. Palmberg, PF, et al: The reproducibility of the intraocular pressure response to dexamethasone, Am J Ophthalmol 80:844, 1975

72. Paterson, G: Studies of the response to topical dexamethasone of glaucoma relatives, Trans Ophthalmol Soc UK 85:295, 1965

73. Paterson, GP, and Owen, R: Further studies on systemic steroids. In Patterson, G, Miller, SJH, and Paterson GD, editors: Drug mechanisms in glaucoma, Boston, 1966, Little Brown & Co

74. Perkins, ES: Steroid-induced glaucoma, Proc R Soc Med 58:531, 1965

75. Phillips, CI, et al: Eye drops of RU 486-6, a peripheral steroid blocker, lower intraocular pressure in rabbits, Lancet 1:767, 1984

76. Podos, SM, Becker, B, and Morton, WR: High myopia and primary open-angle glaucoma, Am J Ophthalmol 62:1039, 1966

77. Podos, SM, Krupin, T, Asseff, C, and Becker, B: Topically administered corticosteroid preparations, Arch Ophthalmol 86:251, 1971

78. Polansky, J, et al: Cellular sensitivity to glucocorticoids in patients with primary open-angle glaucoma: steroid receptors and responses in cultured skin fibroblasts, Invest Ophthalmol Vis Sci 26:805, 1985

79. Radnot, M: Der Augenbefund bei cushinger Krankheit, Ophthalmologica 104:301, 1942

80. Rohen, JW, Linner, E, and Witmer, R: Electron microscopic studies on the trabecular meshwork in two cases of corticosteroid glaucoma, Exp Eye Res 17:19, 1973

81. Rosenbaum, LJ, Alton, E, and Becker, B: Dexamethasone testing in Southwestern Indians, Invest Ophthalmol Vis Sci 9:325, 1970

82. Scheie, HG, Rubinstein, RA, and Albert, DM: Congenital glaucoma and other ocular abnormalities with idiopathic infantile hypoglycemia, J Pediatr Ophthalmol Strab 1:45, 1964

83. Schwartz, B: Corticosteroids and the eye, Int Ophthalmol Clin 6:753, 1966

84. Schwartz, JT, et al: Twin study on ocular pressure after topical dexamethasone. I. Frequency distribution of pressure response, Am J Ophthalmol 76:126, 1973

85. Schwartz, JT, et al: Twin study on ocular pressure following topically applied dexamethasone. II. Inheritance of variations in pressure responses, Arch Ophthalmol 90:281, 1973

86. Sossie, N, Hajek, A, and Palmberg, P: Dexamethasone phosphate causes increased accumulation of hyaluronic acid in the cell layer of cultured human trabecular endothelial cells, Invest Ophthalmol Vis Sci 22:192, 1982

87. Southren, AL, et al: Altered cortisol metabolism in cells cultured from trabecular meshwork specimens obtained from patients with primary open-angle glaucoma, Invest Ophthalmol Vis Sci 24:1413, 1983

88. Southren, AL, et al: 5-Beta-dihydrocortisol: possible mediator of the ocular hypertension in glaucoma, Invest Ophthalmol Vis Sci 26:393, 1985

89. Spaeth, GL: Effects of topical dexamethasone on intraocular pressure and the water drinking test, Arch Ophthalmol 76:772, 1966

90. Spaeth, GL, Rodrigues, MM, and Weinreb, S: Steroid-induced glaucoma: A. Persistent elevation of intraocular pressure. B. Histopathologic aspects, Trans Am Ophthalmol Soc 75:353, 1977

91. Spiers, F: A case of irreversible steroid-induced rise in intraocular pressure, Acta Ophthalmol (Copenh) 43:419, 1965

92. Starka, L, and Obenberger, J: Steroids and intraocular pressure, J Steroid Biochem J 7:979, 1976

93. Stern, JJ: Acute glaucoma during cortisone therapy, Am J Ophthalmol 36:389, 1953

94. Sugar, HS: Low-tension glaucoma: a practical approach, Ann Ophthalmol 11:1155, 1979

95. Tukey, RB: Glaucoma following the application of corticosteroid to the skin of the eyelid, Br J Dermatol 95:207, 1976

96. Turner, JB: A clinical review of congenital glaucoma, South Med J 64:1362, 1971

97. Weekers, R, Grieten, J, and Collignon-Brach, J: Contribution a l'étude de l'hypertension oculaire provoquée par la dexamethasone dans le glaucome à angle ouvert, Ophthalmologica 152:81, 1966

98. Weinreb, RN, et al: Detection of glucocorticoid receptors in cultured human trabecular cells, Invest Ophthalmol Vis Sci 21:403, 1981

99. Weinreb, RN, Mitchell, MD, and Polansky, JR: Prostaglandin production by human trabecular cells. In vitro inhibition by dexamethasone, Invest Ophthalmol Vis Sci 24:1541, 1983

100. Weinstein, BI, Munnangi, P, Gordon, GG, and Southren, AL: Defects in cortisol-metabolizing enzymes in primary open-angle glaucoma, Invest Ophthalmol Vis Sci 26:890, 1985

101. Wilensky, JT, Podos, SM, and Becker, B: Prognostic indicators in ocular hypertension, Arch Ophthalmol 91:200, 1974

102. Wilensky, JT, Snyder, D, and Gieser, D: Steroid-induced ocular hypertension in patients with filtering blebs, Ophthalmology 87:240, 1980

103. Zimmerman, L: Demonstration of hyaluronidase-sensitive acid mucopolysaccharide, Am J Ophthalmol 44:1, 1957

104. Zugerman, C, Saunders, D, and Levit, F: Glaucoma from topically applied steroids, Arch Dermatol 112:1326, 1976

Chapter 65

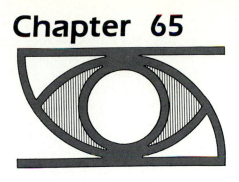

Effects of Nonsteroidal Drugs on Glaucoma

Robert M. Mandelkorn
Thom J. Zimmerman

The subject of this chapter is not true secondary glaucoma but drugs that can cause elevation of intraocular pressure in patients with open-angle glaucoma, precipitate angle-closure attacks, or worse, quietly promote the development of chronic angle-closure. The ophthalmologist and the non-ophthalmic physician should be aware that many commonly used drugs can secondarily cause or aggravate glaucoma. Drugs prescribed for such diverse conditions as depression, allergy, and hypertension can cause elevation of intraocular pressure, pupillary dilation, and lens swelling. The patient with narrow angles or previously undiagnosed angle-closure glaucoma is in particular danger. Since patients are not likely to bring the range of their complaints to the attention of a specialist, it is necessary that their physicians be alert to the dangers.

To the casual observer, the wide diversity of agents that are associated with glaucoma can present a bewildering morass of data. However, if one understands the basic mechanisms by which glaucoma can be precipitated, a clearer picture can be obtained. Cautions regarding specific drugs that have been associated with attacks of angle-closure glaucoma or aggravation of open-angle glaucoma are given in the *Physicians' Desk Reference (PDR)*. For a list of these drugs, refer to Tables 65-1 through 65-9. These drugs produce their unwanted effects through a variety of mechanisms, an understanding of which will help the physician anticipate problems. The contraindication to many of the drugs that cause pupillary dilation pertains not only to angle-closure glaucoma, but essentially to angle-closure eyes in which iridectomy has not been performed. At the present time, the majority of persons in this category probably consist of those in whom the diagnosis has not been made. Most of these drugs are safe to use in treated open-angle glaucoma. It is important for all physicians prescribing such medications, particularly those using psychotropic agents, to be aware of this and not to consider these drugs to be absolutely contraindicated in patients with "glaucoma." In addition, physicians should be aware of possible drug interactions in patients taking glaucoma medication and their possible adverse effects. These drugs include common agents such as aspirin, caffeine, and nicotine.

Through the mechanism of lens swelling (that is, the sulfa drugs), narrow angles can be further compromised and precipitate an episode of angle-closure glaucoma. Systemically used agents that can dilate the pupils (for example, psychotropics, antidepressants, antispasmolytics, antihistamines, monoamine oxidase inhibitors, antiparkinsonian agents, and the autonomic agents) may also precipitate acute angle-closure in susceptible patients. There are several classes of medication that may elevate intraocular pressure even in the controlled or not previously diagnosed open-angle glaucoma patient (Tables 65-1 through 65-9). The mechanism of this latter pressure elevation is poorly understood.

For the ophthalmologist, prevention of these problems lies in identifying patients at risk. Gonioscopy should be performed on all patients with glaucoma, shallow anterior chambers, or hyperopia. It is crucial that ophthalmologists be aware of the association between the glaucoma being treated and the patient's drug regimen. Patients with narrow angles that are judged occludable should be warned about the use of these medications. The ophthalmologist should routinely ask patients about every drug, prescribed or purchased over the counter, that they have taken in the recent past.

For the nonophthalmic physician the penlight or flashlight test is the simplest test available (see Fig. 46-5). Hold a penlight at the limbus of the eye. Note whether the light shines across the anterior chamber, fully illuminating the iris, or is partially blocked by forward bowing of the iris and therefore unable to illuminate the nasal side of the iris, as in patients with shallow anterior chambers. Also ask if the patient has seen colored halos around bright lights or has had blurred vision or eye pain. Any of these symptoms should raise suspicion of subacute attacks of angle-closure glaucoma.

Factors such as the small size of a hyperopic eye,[42,80] disproportion between the size of the lens and the size of the anterior segment of the eye,[28] and an abnormal insertion of the iris into the ciliary body[80] may predispose the patient to angle-closure glaucoma. The event itself is usually precipitated by placing the pupil in the middilated range. When the pupil is in the 3 to 5 mm range,[92] the possibility of angle-closure is greatest. Obviously, very little effect is required by either a weak mydriatic agent, such as dicyclomine (Bentyl), or a moderate miotic agent, such as a weak concentration of pilocarpine, to place the pupil, previously either constricted or dilated, in such a position. Dim light or darkness, emotional disturbance, shock, physical illness, and accident may lead to pupillary dilation.[4]

PSYCHOTROPICS

Phenothiazine Tranquilizers

The adverse ocular effects of phenothiazine compounds are well documented.[58] These agents exhibit both alpha-adrenergic and cholinergic blocking action, and either action may predominate in any one drug.[55] The former is seen with chlorpromazine, with which miosis occurs, and the latter occurs with most of the phenothia-

zines. However, the anticholinergic action of these agents is rather weak in comparison with that of atropine.[128] Indeed, only mepazine[116,127] has been shown to produce clinically observed mydriasis and cycloplegia, and only perphenazine and fluphenazine have been documented to precipitate angle-closure glaucoma (Table 65-1).

Although these agents generally have weak anticholinergic activity, when they are used together or in combination with other agents, especially the monoamine oxidase (MAO) inhibitors[56] and the tricyclic antidepressants,[55] their actions may be enhanced. In addition to their effects on the autonomic innervation of the eye, the phenothiazines (in particular, prochlorperazine [Compazine][153] and promethazine HCl [Phenergan][4]) may produce idiopathic lens swelling. Theoretically, this can precipitate angle-closure glaucoma in a susceptible patient. Although such attacks with the use of phenothiazines have not been documented, these problems are mentioned in the literature in connection with the use of sulfa compounds. This effect is probably attributable to a toxic reaction to the drug and has been reported only rarely (see section on sulfa drugs).

Table 65-1 Antipsychotic phenothiazine agents and their derivatives

Generic (brand)	PDR warning	Case reports of glaucoma
Phenothiazines		
Chlorpromazine HCl (Thorazine)	Yes	No
Triflupromazine HCl (Vesprin)	Yes	No
Thioridazine HCl (Mellaril)	No	No
Perphenazine (Trilafon)	Yes	Yes[37]
Prochlorperazine (Combid)	Yes	No
Prochlorperazine edisylate (Compazine)	No	No
Prochlorperazine (Pro-Iso capsules) maleate	No	No
Fluphenazine HCl (Permitil, Prolixin)	No	No
Fluphenazine decanoate (Prolixin)	Yes	Yes*
Acetophenazine maleate (Tindal)	No	No
Trifluoperazine HCl (Stelazine)	Yes	No
Promethazine HCl (Phenergan)	Yes	No
Thioxanthenes		
Chlorprothixene (Taractan)	Yes	No
Thiothixene HCl (Navane)	No	No
Butyrophenones		
Haloperidol (Haldol)	Yes	No
Dibenzoxepins		
Doxepin HCl (Sinequan)	Yes	No

*Personal observation of author (RMM)

Other Psychotropics

Two major classes of tranquilizers with anticholinergic action are represented by doxepin (Sinequan) and haloperidol (Haldol). Doxepin is a dibenzoxepin, a modification of the phenothiazine structure. Its anticholinergic effect is much stronger than that of the phenothiazines.[128] Haloperidol is a butyrophenone.[55] The use of both drug classes in patients with glaucoma is cautioned against in the PDR, but neither has actually been documented to exacerbate or precipitate glaucoma.

Table 65-2 Tricyclic antidepressants

Generic (brand)	PDR warning	Case reports of glaucoma
Amitriptyline (Elavil, Amitril)	Yes	Yes[88]
Imipramine (Tofranil)	Yes	No
Protriptyline (Vivactil)	Yes	No

Table 65-3 MAO inhibitors that may potentiate the adverse effects of drugs from Tables 65-1, 65-4, and 65-7

Generic (brand)	PDR warning	Case reports of glaucoma
Phenelzine sulfate (Nardil)	Yes	Yes[37]
Pargyline HCl (Eutonyl)	Yes	No
Tranylcypromine sulfate (Parnate)	Yes	Yes[37]

Table 65-4 Antihistamines

Generic (brand)	PDR warning	Case reports of glaucoma
Ethanolamines		
Diphenhydramine HCl (Benadryl)	Yes	No
Dimenhydrinate (Dramamine)	No	No
Orphenadrine citrate (Norgesic)	Yes	Yes[58]
Ethylenediamines		
Tripelennamine HCl (Pyribenzamine)	Yes	No
Antazoline phosphate (Vasocon-A)	Yes	No
Methapyrilene HCl (Histadyl)	No	No
Alkylamines		
Chlorpheniramine maleate (Chlor-Trimeton)	No	No
Brompheniramine (Dimetane)	Yes	No
Piperazine		
Cyclizine HCl (Marezine)	Yes	No
Phenothiazine		
Promethazine HCl (Phenergan)	Yes	No

ANTIDEPRESSANTS

Tricyclic Agents

The tricyclic antidepressants are a closely related group of agents that also have anticholinergic action.[55] However, their action is much stronger than that of the phenothiazines.[128] Indeed, amitriptyline (Elavil, Amitril), imipramine (Tofranil), and protriptyline (Vivactil) have all been shown to cause mydriasis in normal use.[44,139] When taken in overdoses,[132] amitriptyline, the strongest anticholinergic agent,[128] has been associated with attacks of angle-closure glaucoma.[88] All of these agents carry warnings about their use in patients with glaucoma (Table 65-2). It should also be noted that their actions may be augmented by the MAO inhibitors.[56]

Monoamine Oxidase Inhibitors

The MAO inhibitors are antidepressants with extremely weak anticholinergic action, comparable to that of the phenothiazines.[128] Although these agents have been reported to produce pupillary dilation in toxic dosages[87] and attacks of angle-closure glaucoma,[37] the major risk is that they may potentiate the effects of other drugs,[56] such as phenothiazines, tricyclic antidepressants, antiparkinsonian drugs, and sympathomimetic agents (amphetamines and ephedrine).

This drug interaction is mentioned in the PDR under the specific agent headings, and a warning is given cautioning against the use of these agents in patients with glaucoma (Table 65-3).

ANTIHISTAMINES

The antihistamines (Table 65-4) are a diverse group of drugs that have in common the ability to block the effect of histamine. The H_1 antihistamines[55] block the histamine effect on capillary permeability, and on vascular, bronchial, and other smooth muscles. H_1 antihistamines also have a sedative effect, an anticholinergic effect, and local anesthetic properties. The H_2 antihistamines[55] block the secretion of gastric acid, as well as blocking the histamine effect on smooth muscles of peripheral blood vessels.

H_1 Blocking Agents

The anticholinergic action is usually weak in H_1 blocking agents[55]; however, an acute overdose may precipitate an atropine-like toxic state[55,57] with fever, flushed face, and dilated pupils, which could exacerbate glaucoma. Only one case of precipitation of angle-closure glaucoma by one of these drugs, orphenadrine citrate (Norgesic), has been reported.[58] Another antihistamine, promethazine HCl, has been documented to cause an idiopathic swelling of the lens.[4] Even though glaucoma did not result in this case, similar incidents with other agents (sulfa)[90] have precipitated attacks of angle-closure glaucoma, so these agents should be carefully watched.

Krupin et al[83] found that when H_1 blocking agents were applied topically to male albino rabbits, various effects were observed. Doxylamine, (Bendectin, Nyquil), diphenhydramine (Benadryl), pyrilamine (Triaminic Tablets), tripelennamine (Pryibenzamine), chlorothen, brompheniramine (Dimetane), and pheniramine (Triaminic Tablets and Poly-Histine-D) had no effect on the intraocular pressure. Antazoline (Vasocon-A) was found to lower the intraocular pressure, and cyclizine HCl (Marezine) was observed to elevate the intraocular pressure significantly. This increase in intraocular pressure was thought to be related to prostaglandin production, as evidenced by the fact that this pressure elevation could be prevented by pretreatment with systemic indomethacin, an inhibitor of prostaglandin synthesis.

H_2 Blocking Agents

The H_2 blocking agents include burinamide, metiamide, cimetidine, and ranitidine. H_2 receptors are present in the brain in both the intracranial and extracranial blood vessels, on the external ocular surface, and in the stomach.[55] Their primary use today is the inhibition of gastric acid secretion in the treatment of peptic ulcer disease.

Reported effects of these agents on intraocular pressure have been variable. Dobrilla et al[40] reported that cimetidine and ranitidine caused an elevated intraocular pressure in a glaucoma patient being treated for a duodenal ulcer. Others were unable to duplicate this effect in both normal and glaucomatous patients when cimetidine was given intravenously and topically.[29,47,86]

Recently Trzeciakowski and Fry[141] produced elevated intraocular pressure in unanesthetized New Zealand white rabbits by injecting cimetidine and ranitidine into the cerebral ventricles. In contrast, histamine produced a biphasic effect on the intraocular pressure. The authors hypothesized that "central mechanisms may mediate the actions of some histamine receptor agonists and antagonists on intraocular pressure."

ANTIPARKINSONIAN DRUGS

The antiparkinsonian drugs can be divided into two groups: (1) agents that replenish the dimin-

Table 65-5 Antiparkinsonian agents

Generic (brand)	PDR warning	Case reports of glaucoma
Benztropine mesylate (Cogentin)	Yes	No
Trihexyphenidyl HCl (Artane)	Yes	Yes[49]
Biperiden HCl (Akineton)	Yes	No
Cycrimine HCl (Pagitane)	Yes	No
Procyclidine HCl (Kemadrin)	Yes	No

ished stores of dopamine in the corpus striatum (caudate nucleus and putamen) and (2) agents that improve clinical symptoms through a strong anticholinergic action. Of the first group of agents used, the classic drug today is levodopa. Because dopamine is the precursor of epinephrine and norepinephrine, the administration of dopamine[131] and levodopa[130] increases sympathetic tone and dilates the pupils. This action by itself is usually not enough to aggravate glaucoma. However, when used with MAO inhibitors,[56] the sympathomimetic action of levodopa may be increased, so that an eye with narrow angles is at greater risk.

The remaining agents act through strong anticholinergic action.[128] Trihexyphenidyl HCl (Artane)[49] has been reported to precipitate angle-closure glaucoma (Table 65-5). These agents should be used cautiously in all patients with glaucoma.

MOOD-ALTERING AGENTS

Minor Tranquilizers

The minor tranquilizers do not appear to have autonomic activity. However, there has been one report of an attack of angle-closure glaucoma in a patient taking diazepam (Valium).[74] The cause is not clear, as evidenced by the subsequent debate in the literature.[23]

Sedatives and Stimulants

The sedatives,[110] including barbiturates, paraldehyde, morphine, meperidine, reserpine, mephenesin, and phenytoin, may produce pupillary dilation when given in toxic dosages, but this appears to have no significant ill effects on the eye.[56,139] They may even lower the intraocular pressure in certain situations (see section on anesthetic agents).

The stimulants, including amphetamines, caffeine, and methylphenidate (Ritalin), do cause a transient rise in intraocular pressure in patients with glaucoma.[58] The significance of these findings is uncertain. In addition, MAO inhibitors will

Table 65-6 Antispasmolytic agents

Generic (brand)	PDR warning	Case reports of glaucoma
Methscopamine bromide (Pamine)	Yes	No
Propantheline bromide (Pro-Banthine)	Yes	Yes[99]
Oxyphenonium bromide (Antrenyl)	Yes	No
Tridihexethyl chloride (Pathilon)	Yes	No
Diphemanil methysulfate (Prantal)	Yes	No
Hexocyclium methysulfate (Tral)	Yes	No
Dicyclomaine HCl (Bentyl)	Yes	Yes[99]

potentiate the actions of amphetamines.[56] The amount of caffeine given orally or intravenously in the experiments was considerably more than the amount in a cup of coffee.

The amphetamines have also been documented to cause significant pupillary dilation when taken in toxic amounts.[119,145] Theoretically, this would place patients with narrow angles at increased risk. Although none of these agents have been documented to cause glaucoma, only phendime-trazine tartrate is mentioned in the PDR as contraindicated in patients with glaucoma.

The methylxanthines, including caffeine, theophylline, and theobromine methylxanthine, are known to block the enzyme phosphodiesterase and increase the levels of cyclic AMP. This action is in direct contrast to that of the beta-adrenergic blocking agent timolol, which blocks the formation of cyclic AMP. Weber and Opremcak[146] reported that pretreatment with oral caffeine may block the crossover response to topical timolol.

Lysergic acid diethylamide (LSD) may cause significant pupillary dilation.[118] This is thought to be caused by a sympathetic stimulation of the mesencephalon and medullary centers of the brain.[26] No cases of glaucoma have been reported.

ANTISPASMOLYTIC AGENTS

The ability of the antispasmolytic agents (Table 65-6) to reduce both gastric secretion and motility of the stomach is directly related to their anticholinergic actions. Herxheimer[70] compared these agents with atropine and showed their potency to range from oxyphenonium, which has 50% the potency of atropine, to propantheline, which has 22% the potency of atropine. Ironically, the weakest anticholinergic agents, dicyclomine and propantheline (Pro-Banthine),[70] which do not dilate the pupil, have actually been found to raise the intraocular pressure as high as 10 to 14 mm Hg when given to patients with open-angle glaucoma.[99] This transient pressure elevation is believed to be caused by their anticholinergic action. No cases of angle-closure glaucoma caused by these agents have yet been documented.

ANTIBIOTICS

Sulfa Drugs

The sulfa drugs, particularly acetazolamide (Diamox), lower intraocular pressure by reducing aqueous humor formation and are commonly used in the medical treatment of glaucoma.

In addition, an idiosyncratic response has been documented, consisting of acute myopia caused by swelling of the lens, associated with elevated intraocular pressure, retinal edema, and shallowing of the anterior chamber.[90] This phenomenon was believed to be caused by a toxic reaction of the ocular tissue, specifically lens and retina, to the chemical. Because these episodes do not respond to cycloplegic drugs and because the pupils are not affected in these cases, we believe that contraction of the iris and the ciliary body is not involved. This leads us to assume that this phenomenon is caused by an idiopathic swelling of the lens or by an alteration of the lens position.[58] Hook et al.[71] performed A-scan measurement and cycloplegic refraction of one such patient and confirmed that the transient myopia was caused by swelling and anterior movement of the lens. The authors thought the myopia was caused by ciliary body edema that resulted in an exaggerated relaxation of the lens zonules.

This phenomenon has been associated with sulfa drugs not only used as antibiotics, but also used in other forms. These include antihypertensive agents, hydrochlorothiazide (Hydrodiuril),[7] chlorthalidone (Hygroton),[45,98] and, most recently, trichlormethiazide (Methahydrin),[8] and antiglaucoma medications acetazolamide,[101] dichlorphenamide (Daranide, Oratrol),[102] and ethoxzolamide (Ethamide, Cardrase).[63]

Acute myopia also has been seen with tetracycline,[43] prochlorperazine,[153] promethazine,[4] hydralazine (Apresoline) and hexamethonium in combination,[62] spironolactone (Aldactone),[15] phenformin (DBI),[123] corticotropin,[8] and acetylsalicylic acid (Aspirin).[122] Obviously, those eyes with increased risk factors, such as those with shallow anterior chambers (for example, the hyperopic patient), are at greater risk of an attack of angle-closure glaucoma and should be carefully monitored for this development. Table 65-7 lists the drugs that can cause idiopathic lens swelling.

Table 65-7 Agents that cause idiopathic lens swelling

Generic (brand)	PDR warning	Case reports of glaucoma
Spironolactone (Aldactone)	No	No
Ethoxzolamide (Ethamide, Cardrase)*	No	No
Dichlorphenamide (Daranide, Oratrol)*	No	No
Phenformin (DBI)*	No	No
Hydrochlorothiazide (Hydrodiuril, Esidrix)*	No	No
Chlorothiazide (Diuril)*	No	No
Chlorthalidone (Hygroton)*	No	No
Polythiazide (Renese)*	No	No
Promethazine (Phenergan)	No	No
Sulfanilamide (AVC Cream, Vagitrol)*	No	Yes[90]
Tetracycline	No	No
Acetylsalicylic acid (Aspirin)	No	Yes[122]
Trichlormethiazide (Metahydrin)*	No	No
Acetazolamide (Diamox)*	No	No

*Sulfa agents.

Additional Antibiotics

Procaine penicillin has been found to produce dilated pupils in association with an acute psychotic reaction.[142] This was thought to be related to intravascular leakage of penicillin and was short lived in all cases. No incidence of glaucoma was observed.

Several agents, including neomycin sulfate, colistin, kanamycin sulfate, streptomycin sulfate, bacitracin, and polymixin B, have been shown to produce a myasthenic-like syndrome consisting of apnea and flaccid paralysis of skeletal and smooth muscles and are associated with hallucinations,[94] convulsions, and coma. The antibiotics colistin[111] and neomycin sulfate[93] have been observed to produce pupillary dilation during these episodes. These episodes are thought to be related to the neuromuscular blocking abilities of these agents in association with ether anesthesia, the use of other neuromuscular agents, hypocalcemia, and renal disease.[94]

Interestingly, in a review of ocular adverse effects of antibiotics, Davidson[37] stated that one third were attributed to the antibiotic nalidixic acid. These complaints were usually associated with visual disturbances involving the appearance of brightly colored objects. In addition, several cases of pupillary dilation were observed. No cases of glaucoma were mentioned.

CARDIAC AGENTS

Cardiac agents used to control dysrhythmias comprise a diverse group of drugs. Digitalis,

through the reduction of the Na-K ATPase activity in the ciliary processes, has been shown to reduce aqueous humor formation[16] and intraocular pressure[38] in humans and animals when given intravenously. Unfortunately, toxic side effects limit its use in glaucoma.[109] When digitalis is given in toxic dosages, scotomas and dilated pupils may be seen.[117] No effect on the intraocular pressure was noted by the authors.[117]

Quinidine also does not appear to have any effect on intraocular pressure. However, disopyramide phosphate (Norpace), a new agent used for cardiac dysrhythmias, does have some anticholinergic action (0.06% as strong as atropine)[105] and has been documented[140] to precipitate an attack of angle-closure glaucoma.

A new group of cardiac agents is the calcium channel blockers. Monica et al.[100] showed a mild drop in intraocular pressure when nitrendipine 20 mg was given orally to 10 patients with mild essential hypertension.

In contrast, Beatty et al.[9] produced an elevated intraocular pressure with the topical administration of the calcium channel blockers verapamil HCl, diltiazem HCl, and nifedipine in male albino rabbits. This effect was also observed in healthy human volunteers with topically applied verapamil. These researchers observed normal outflow facility and episcleral venous pressure; however, the aqueous humor flow and ocular blood volume was increased. They hypothesized that vascular changes might be responsible for the intraocular pressure elevation.

VASOACTIVE AGENTS

Vasodilator Agents

The vasodilator agents include the nitrates and tolazoline. Before the advent of gonioscopy, it was believed that acute glaucoma was caused by dilation of intraocular blood vessels, especially those of the ciliary body and the iris, and that the resultant swelling of the lens pushed the iris forward, obstructing the trabecular meshwork and aqueous humor outflow.[42] This led to the belief that these agents may precipitate angle-closure glaucoma in susceptible eyes. The nitrates, especially nitroglycerin (glyceryl trinitrate), have been shown to produce a transient partial blackout of vision. However, this is believed to be caused by a fall in blood pressure and the associated temporary loss of perfusion to the eye.[58]

The nitrates have also been shown to cause pupillary dilation.[58] However, when glaucoma patients with narrow angles took nitroglycerin[151] by mouth and inhaled amyl nitrate,[10] acute angle-clo-

Table 65-8 Sympathomimetic Agents

Generic (brand)	PDR warning	Case reports of glaucoma
Epinephrine (E-Carpine, E-Pilo, Mytrate, Epitrate, Epifrin, Glaucon, Epinal, Eppy N)*	Yes	Yes: a[75], b[68]
Ephedrine (Collyrium with Ephedrine)	No	Yes: b[53]
Norepinephrine	No	No
Dopamine	No	No
Metaraminol	No	No
Phenylephrine (Prefrin, Vasocidin, AK-Cide, Blephamide, Efricel, Murocoll, Neo-Synephrine, Vasosulf, Zincfrin, Vernacel Ophthalmic)	Yes	Yes: a[85], b[68]
Amphetamine (Delcobese, Obetrol)	Yes	Yes[58]
Naphazoline (AK-Con, Albalon, Clear Eyes, Degest-2, Naphcon, Vasoclear, Vasocon)	Yes	No
Tetrahydrozoline hydrochloride (Murine, Soothe, Tetracyn, Visine)	Yes	No
Pheniramine maleate (Naphcon-A, Vernacel)	Yes	No
Methoxamine (Vasoxyl)	No	No
Hydroxyamphetamine (Paredine)	Yes	Yes: b[53]

*This pupillary dilation may be exacerbated by timolol.[13]
a, Open-angle glaucoma; b, angle-closure glaucoma.

sure glaucoma could not be precipitated. Tolazoline (Priscoline), another vasodilator, was reported to have precipitated an attack of angle-closure glaucoma.[51]

The results are less clear regarding open-angle glaucoma. Oral nitroglycerin has been reported both to decrease[151] the intraocular pressure transiently in both normal and glaucomatous eyes and to increase[154] the intraocular pressure in glaucomatous eyes. The inhalation of amyl nitrate has also been reported to cause both a transient increase[79] and a decrease[33] of the intraocular pressure in glaucomatous individuals. In all cases the intraocular pressure change was not believed to be significant and did not last for more than several minutes.

Retrobulbar tolazoline has not been found to elevate intraocular pressure.[155] When given subconjunctivally as a provocative test for open-angle glaucoma, it has been found to cause a transient increase in intraocular pressure that is greater in patients with glaucoma than in normal patients.[133] This effect was not confirmed by Gandolfi[52] when he gave the drug topically. It has been claimed that tolazoline given subcutaneously lowers the in-

traocular pressure in normal and glaucomatous eyes.[154] However, further studies have questioned its ability to do so when given intravenously.[103]

Interestingly, additional studies done with dibenzylchlorethamine (Dibenamine), a weak vasoactive drug given intravenously, showed a transient lowering of the intraocular pressure.[103] However, because of its side effects, it was not studied further. The use of vasodilator agents appears to be safe for normal patients with narrow angles and open-angle glaucoma, with some exceptions. One reported case involved precipitation of angle-closure glaucoma with tolazoline[51] and in another patient with open-angle glaucoma the possible loss of medical control was noted after tolazoline was given subconjunctivally.[133]

Vasoconstricting Agents

The vasoconstricting agents are alpha-adrenergic agonists. Because the pupillary dilating fibers of the iris respond to these agents, pupillary dilation is possible. Table 65-8 summarizes the effects of these agents on intraocular pressure.

Becker and Christiansen[11] showed that the application of vasopressin (Beta-Hypophamine) reduced the intraocular pressure in both normal and glaucomatous patients. This effect was thought to be caused by a suppression of aqueous humor flow. Unfortunately, the effect was short term because of the rapid development of resistance in these eyes.

AUTONOMIC DRUGS
Sympathomimetic Agents

On the whole, the sympathomimetic agents (Table 65-8) lower the intraocular pressure. This effect has been well documented with epinephrine,[84] phenylephrine,[65,84] and ephedrine[65] in patients with open-angle glaucoma and with dopamine in rabbits.[125]

In spite of these results, it should be noted that a paradoxic elevation of intraocular pressure has been reported with use of these agents in patients with open-angle glaucoma.[85] Further study of these patients has documented that this effect is caused by an associated lowering of outflow facility.[85] The pupil dilation is also known to precipitate attacks of angle-closure glaucoma in predisposed patients with narrow anterior chamber angles.[53]

Sympathomimetic agents are used in inhalers for the treatment of bronchial asthma and nasal and respiratory congestion and as rectal suppositories for the treatment of hemorrhoids. Repeated use of these agents might possibly precipitate or aggravate glaucoma in the susceptible patient. Interestingly, the possible occurrence of eye pain and glaucoma is mentioned in the PDR only in the description of Wyanoid HC, used for the treatment of hemorrhoids.

Parasympathomimetic Agents

The parasympathomimetic agents, including pilocarpine and carbachol, although indicated in the treatment of open-angle glaucoma[28] and for breaking attacks of angle-closure glaucoma,[28] have to be used with caution in patients with narrow angles. These agents can cause congestion of the iris and ciliary body, relaxation of the zonules, and shallowing of the anterior chamber[80] (shown by ultrasound to be caused by an increase in the sagittal width of the lens and a net forward movement of the lens).[1]

Moderate concentrations of pilocarpine (2% and 4%) have been reported to precipitate rare attacks of angle-closure glaucoma.[28] Mapstone[92] believed this to be caused by several mechanisms in addition to those mentioned above. First, pilocarpine opens the anterior chamber angle[60] and increases trabecular meshwork outflow,[5] while at the same time reducing uveoscleral outflow.[19] The net result is an increase in the pressure differential from the posterior to the anterior chamber, allowing the iris to bow forward, further shallowing an already shallow anterior chamber. Second, pupils that were previously constricted will begin to redilate when pilocarpine begins to wear off, placing the pupil in the middilated position. According to Mapstone,[92] this is the critical pupillary position for precipitation of acute glaucoma. Therefore, eyes with narrow angles are theoretically at risk of an attack of angle-closure glaucoma when treated with miotic agents. In these patients a fine balance exists between the risk factors and the benefit of pulling the iris out of the anterior chamber angle, opening the trabecular meshwork, and reducing the intraocular pressure.

Obviously, the parasympathomimetic agents must be used carefully in the treatment of patients with narrow angles. Pilocarpine may exacerbate several other types of glaucoma. These situations include glaucoma caused by uveitis, malignant glaucoma, neovascular glaucoma, lens- and vitreous-induced pupillary-block glaucoma,[28] and recently a case of angle-recession glaucoma.[22]

In the treatment of glaucoma, the parasympathomimetic agents should not be used in conjunction with the anticholinesterase agents, such as echothiophate (Phospholine Iodide), eserine, and isoflurophate (Diisopropyl Flurophosphate,

DFP; or Floropryl). When used together, these different agents may actually cause the intraocular pressure to go up, rather than down.[21]

Swan et al[134] thought that those eyes treated with pilocarpine did not show a significant lowering of intraocular pressure after subsequent treatment with the anticholinesterase agents eserine and isoflurophate (Diisopropyl Fluorophosphate, DFP, Floropryl).

Bito and Merritt[21] observed that in monkey eyes treated for 16 days with the anticholinesterase agent echothiophate (Phospholine Iodide), subsequent treatment with pilocarpine caused the intraocular pressure to rise. This effect was observed to be dose related. The second eye in these monkeys, not pretreated with echothiophate, was observed to show a normal hypotensive response to pilocarpine. They hypothesized that pilocarpine acts upon two sites that have opposing action. Under normal conditions the predominant site would be the conventional outflow. Pretreatment with echothiophate might make this site subsensitive, allowing the nondominant site to become dominant. They hypothesized that this nondominant site was the uveoscleral outflow, shown by Bill and Walinder[19] to be reduced by pilocarpine.

Parasympatholytic Agents

The parasympatholytic agents appear to pose the same threats to the eye with either open-angle or angle-closure glaucoma as do the sympathomimetic agents. Indeed, atropine, homatropine, scopolamine, cyclopentolate, and tropicamide (Mydriacyl) all produce an elevated intraocular pressure in patients with open-angle glaucoma (23% versus 2% of normal patients).[66] Only eucatropine, a weak agent, showed no effect. These agents, as is the case with the sympathomimetic agents, have been well documented to precipitate angle-closure glaucoma in eyes anatomically predisposed (Table 65-9).

Table 65-9 Mydriatic agents

Generic (brand)	PDR warning	Case reports of glaucoma
Cyclopentolate HCl (Cyclogyl)	Yes	Yes:a[66], b[53]
Tropicamide (Mydriacyl)	Yes	Yes: a[66], b[58]
Hydroxyamphetamine (Paredrine)	Yes	Yes: b[53]
Atropine (Atropisol)	Yes	Yes: a[66], b[68]
Homatropine hydrobromide	Yes	Yes: a[66], b[68]
Scopolamine (Hyoscine)	Yes	Yes: a[66], b[68]

a, Open-angle glaucoma; *b*, angle-closure glaucoma.

Recently, CIBA has marketed scopolamine in a time-release contact disc for the treatment of motion sickness, under the label Transderm-Scop (originally Transderm-V) that releases 2.5 mg of scopolamine over 72 hours. Pupillary dilation has been documented following inadvertent contamination of the fingers after placement of the disc upon the body and subsequent contact with the eyes (in this case after a contact lens was removed from the eye).[27] In addition, supposedly through systemic absorption, an attack of angle-closure glaucoma was precipitated.[64] CIBA does warn of this pupillary dilation side effect and the risk of using this agent in patients with glaucoma. Unfortunately, those patients at greatest risk are those with undiagnosed angle-closure glaucoma. It is therefore recommended that all patients who use this disc be warned about the symptoms of an acute attack of glaucoma by their prescribing physician. It should be repeated that anticholinergic agents given systemically, including phenothiazines, tricyclic and MAO antidepressants, antispasmolytics and antiparkinsonian agents, either alone or in combination, may also be strong enough to move the pupil into the critical middilated position and precipitate an attack of angle-closure glaucoma.

ANESTHETIC AGENTS

General Anesthetic Agents

The general anesthetic agents, on the whole, are believed to lower the intraocular pressure. This has been confirmed with halothane[82] and methoxyflurane (Penthrane).[136] This drop in intraocular pressure has been hypothesized to be caused by depression of the diencephalic center, fall in arterial and venous pressure, relaxation of extraocular muscles, and changes in pupil size.[124]

The fall in intraocular pressure may also be related to the administration of oxygen.[50] In contrast, the retention of carbon dioxide has been reported to raise[77,112,121] the intraocular pressure.

Succinylcholine,[32] ketamine,[34] N_2O, and chloral hydrate,[115] in contrast, elevate intraocular pressure. This effect may be related to the increased tone of the extraocular and orbital muscles, seen when these agents are administered.[76] With ketamine,[34] these findings were not related to age, depth of anesthesia, arterial blood pressure, or amount of ketamine administered, whereas with succinylcholine[32] the deeper the anesthesia, the less the effect. The preanesthetic use of either a barbiturate or a narcotic (morphine sulfate or meperidine) lowered the intraocular pressure. Crossen and Hoy[34] attributed this to the patient's relaxed state and

reduced muscle tension. Pretreatment with Valium[35] also prevented the pressure rise with succinylcholine.

Other observers have noted that the intraocular pressure elevation seen in those patients given succinylcholine intravenously, in bolus or dilute drip form, wears off after 4 to 5 minutes.[76] Therefore, if succinylcholine is given intravenously in bolus or continuous drip form at least several minutes before intraocular surgery, the eye is at less risk than if the drug is given after the eye has been opened. Extreme care should be taken in selecting anesthesia for open or potentially open globes.

Any respiratory disturbance during the course of anesthesia, such as a cough, laryngospasm, or straining, which raises arterial and venous pressure, will result in an increase in intraocular pressure.[81] However, once general anesthesia has been induced, there tends to be an 8 to 10 mm Hg decrease of the intraocular pressure, associated with an increased coefficient of outflow. This is thought to be caused by both relaxation of the extraocular muscles and depression of the hypothalamus, where there may be a center for control of intraocular pressure.[41,81]

Fazio et al,[46] in a review of 750 charts, found 12 cases of acute angle-closure glaucoma precipitated by general anesthesia. Several of the cases were attributed to the use of mydriatic agents, including atropine, scopolomine, and ephedrine, used to induce anesthesia. In the remaining cases the authors thought other factors, such as stress, with resulting sympathetic discharge and pupillary dilation, may have precipitated these attacks. Pupillary dilation occurs in stage two of general anesthesia[41] and this may have precipitated some of the attacks.

Topical Anesthetic Agents

Most topical anesthetic agents have no effect on intraocular pressure.[91] One exception is cocaine, which can augment the response of sympathetically innervated organs to epinephrine, norepinephrine, and sympathetic nerve stimulations.[55] Thus, when cocaine is applied topically to the eye, there is increased sensitization of the adrenergic nerve terminals in the dilator muscle fibers of the iris to circulating catecholamines, resulting in mydriasis.[68] This same mydriasis may be observed when cocaine is given systemically or in cases of poisoning.[55]

The basis for this increased sympathetic tone is that cocaine acts by preventing the reuptake of norepinephrine at the adrenergic nerve terminals, thereby prolonging its action at the adrenergic receptor site. Cocaine apparently has no direct action on the adrenergic receptors. This fact is confirmed by the drug's lack of effect on sympathetically denervated eyes, as in Horner's syndrome.[144]

Because of the mydriasis that results from topical application of cocaine, it should be used with caution in patients with potential angle-closure glaucoma. Indeed, cases have been reported in the older literature in which cocaine precipitated angle-closure glaucoma in predisposed patients.[61] The initial reports of patients with open-angle glaucoma suggested that there was a lowering of the intraocular pressure.[61] However, subsequent reports on the use of cocaine in rabbits have shown no effect on intraocular pressure or outflow facility when the drug is given systemically.[108] This medication should be used with caution in all patients with glaucoma.

ANTIHYPERTENSIVE AGENTS

Antihypertensive agents usually have no effect on the eye, although clonidine (Catapres), an alpha-adrenergic sympathomimetic agent, increases the pupillary diameter when given systemically[135] and topically.[67] Even though clonidine lowers intraocular pressure when given topically to patients with open-angle glaucoma, one should be cautious about administering it to patients with narrow angles.

Several other agents (including chlorthiazide,[69] hydrochlorothiazide,[7] polythiazide,[54] chlorthalidone,[45,98] hydralazine and hexamethonium,[62] spironolactone,[15] and trichlormethiazide[8]) used to treat hypertension have been documented to cause idiopathic swelling of the lens, which might induce attacks of angle-closure glaucoma in those patients anatomically predisposed (Table 65-7).

HORMONAL AGENTS

Estrogen and Progesterone

The effect of hormonal agents is unclear. The intraocular pressure in women varies during the menstrual cycle.[120] Dalton[36] stated that the intraocular pressure was highest during the progestational phase of the menstrual period, including the 4 days preceding menstruation and the first 4 days of menstruation. However, Becker and Friedenwald[12] showed that during the progestational phase of the menstrual cycle and during pregnancy there are an increased facility of outflow and a lower intraocular pressure. In Becker and Friedenwald's study the intraocular pressure increased and the coefficient of outflow decreased

during the subsequent estrogenic postpartum and postmenopausal periods. They later confirmed their observations of the effects of progesterone on intraocular pressure by noting a reduction of intraocular pressure in several glaucoma patients treated with oral, intramuscular, and subconjunctival progesterone.

The role of estrogen is less clear. When given systemically, it has been found to increase intraocular pressure.[95] When given to rats in one study, an accumulation of glycosaminoglycans was found in the angle of the anterior chamber region.[114]

On the basis of Becker and Friedenwald's work, Meyer et al.[97] gave an estrogen-progesterone combination to patients with open-angle glaucoma and documented a fall in their intraocular pressure. However, Weinstein et al.[150] reported that three patients aged 26 to 36 years developed visual field and optic nerve changes while taking contraceptives. In all three patients these changes were associated with increased serum cortisol levels. One patient had a family history of glaucoma. A prospective study by Deufrains and Hempel[39] found a small increase in the intraocular pressure over the 2 years that their patients took contraceptive pills.

Several points can be raised regarding angle-closure glaucoma. Acute attacks of glaucoma occur more commonly in women during the menstrual period.[149] According to Duke-Elder,[42] this exacerbation of angle-closure glaucoma is caused by "fluid retention," which is often produced by estrogens. This property, in combination with the mydriasis seen with these hormones,[48] may be enough to precipitate an attack of angle-closure glaucoma, as documented recently in one patient taking oral contraceptives.[152]

ANTIPROSTAGLANDINS

The prostaglandins are among the most prevalent of autacoids in the body. Within the eye, prostaglandins have been isolated in the iris, ciliary body, cornea, retina, and trabecular meshwork.[80,147] The release of these agents within the eye has been observed to produce both an elevated[104,113] and a reduced intraocular pressure.[24,31] These agents may be involved in the elevated intraocular pressure observed after argon laser trabeculoplasty[148] and in several types of glaucoma, including trauma, uveitis, glaucomatocyclitic crisis, and primary open-angle glaucoma.[80] Unfortunately, topical prostaglandin synthetase inhibitors, including indomethacin and flurbiprofen, have not been able to prevent the pressure rise seen in the latter.[72,107,138]

Interestingly, Camras et al.[25] did show that the lowering of intraocular pressure by epinephrine may be reduced by systemic indomethacin, suggesting that the reduction in intraocular pressure seen with topical epinephrine may be medicated by the release of prostaglandins. Possibly we should review more carefully the use of indomethacin or other cyclooxygenase inhibitors, such as aspirin, in our glaucoma patients using epinephrine eye drops.

DRUGS USED AS ADJUVANTS TO SURGERY

Alpha-chymotrypsin

Alpha-chymotrypsin, commonly used in routine intracapsular cataract surgery to lyse zonules, causes a significant rise in intraocular pressure in the first week after surgery.[75,78] The lysed zonules are believed to obstruct the trabecular meshwork[2] (see Chapter 71).

Viscoelastic Substances

Hyaluronic acid (Healon)[59] and sodium chondroitin sulfate,[129] used to protect the corneal endothelium during lens implantation, have been associated with a significant intraocular pressure rise postoperatively.[20,89,106] Berson et al.[17] showed in the enucleated human eye that this is caused by a decrease in outflow facility. Pape[106] hypothesized that this pressure rise is viscosity dependent and has shown that with washout of hyaluronic acid from the eye the pressure rise is reduced.

Hultsch[73] in studying owl monkey eyes showed that the pressure rise may be prevented with the use of low-molecular-weight Healon. Barron et al[6] attempted to repeat these findings by comparing Healon (1% sodium hyaluronate) with Viscoat, a low molecular weight combination of chrondroitin sulfate and hyaluronic acid, which has a lower viscosity than Healon. Both substances produced a significant postoperative rise in intraocular pressure despite removal at the end of surgery (see Chapter 71).

ACETYLSALICYLIC ACID (ASPIRIN)

In cases of salicylate poisoning, the intraocular pressure may be lowered[143] because of a generalized acidosis.[55] Diminished pupillary reaction to light and edema of the optic nerve head and retina with diminished visual acuity, leading to optic atrophy, have also been observed.[58] Because of mydriasis, patients with narrow angles should be carefully observed. Patients with narrow angles are at risk also because of an idiopathic reaction that can

occur, producing lens swelling, myopia, shallowing of the anterior chamber, and intraocular pressure elevation.[122] One should be cautious with patients who complain of a sudden onset of blurred vision after ingesting aspirin, even in the prescribed fashion. This effect is not mentioned in the PDR.

TOBACCO

Surprisingly, few studies have been done on the effects of tobacco on the eye. Bellarminoff[14] and Bietti and Cima[18] showed a small increase in intraocular pressure after nicotine was applied topically to rabbit eyes. This effect was confirmed in rabbit eyes when nicotine was also given intravenously. Colle et al.[28] thought that this effect was caused by contraction of the extraocular muscles.

Attia et al.[3] observed 100 patients with primary open-angle glaucoma who smoked. They were able to convince 25 patients to stop smoking completely for 1 month. In this group 10 patients had a drop in intraocular pressure of 2 to 7 mm Hg. The 75 patients who did not stop smoking had no change in intraocular pressure.

EPIDEMIC DROPSY

Sanguinarine

Epidemic dropsy, an acute disorder occurring primarily in India, but also in Mauritius, Fiji, and South Africa, is another interesting condition related to drug-induced glaucoma. It results from ingestion of an alkaloid, sanguinarine, which is found in the seeds of the Mexican poppy *Argemona Mexicana*. These seeds outwardly resemble the seeds of the mustard plant and may be accidentally mixed in with them, producing mustard oil that is contaminated with sanguinarine and dihydrosanguinarine. Epidemics have occurred following consumption of other oils as well, and the possibility of intentional contamination exists.

Ocular features consist of glaucoma, retinal vascular dilation and tortuosity, venous congestion, retinal hemorrhages, and papillophlebitis.[99a,115a,119a,137]

The disease derives its name from a rapid onset of pitting edema of the legs and feet. The overlying skin is tender, warm, and erythematous. Other symptoms include diarrhea, hair loss, fever, malaise, exertional dyspnea, hepatomegaly, and hyperpigmentation. Sanguinarine may be found in the serum and urine early in the disease process.[126,137]

A chronic bilateral open-angle glaucoma occurs in approximately 10% of patients with epidemic dropsy. All ages may be affected, but young adults have been most commonly afflicted. Intraocular pressures are usually over 50 mm Hg. There is an elevation of protein in the aqueous humor and a marked dilation of the small vessels of the uveal tract without evidence of inflammation.[42] Aqueous humor levels of both prostaglandin E_2 and histaminelike activity are significantly elevated. Pilocarpine is ineffective in lowering intraocular pressure and a mechanism based on aqueous hypersecretion has been postulated.[119b]

Elevated concentrations of histamine in the plasma and erythrocytes of patients with open-angle glaucoma who had had epidemic dropsy 20 years previously have been reported.[96] The controls consisted of normal subjects rather than patients who had had epidemic dropsy without glaucoma.

REFERENCES

1. Abramson, DH, Coleman, DJ, Forbes, M, and Frazen, LA: Pilocarpine: effect on the anterior chamber and lens thickness, Arch Ophthalmol 87:615, 1972

2. Anderson, DR: Experimental alpha-chymotrypsin glaucoma studied by scanning electron microscopy, Am J Ophthalmol 71:470, 1971

3. Attia, H, Bakir, M, and Abdel-Rahman, H: Tobacco in relation to glaucoma, Bull Ophth Soc Egypt 71, 1978

4. Bard, LA: Transient myopia associated with promethazine (Phenergan) therapy: report of a case, Am J Ophthalmol 58:682, 1964

5. Bárány, EH: The mode of action of pilocarpine on outflow resistance in the eye of a primate (Circopithecus ethiops), Invest Ophthalmol 1:172, 1962

6. Barron, BA, Busin, M, Page, C, Bergsma, DR, and Kaufman, HE: Comparison of the effects of Viscoat and Healon on postoperative intraocular pressure, Am J Ophthalmol 100:377, 1985

7. Beasley, FJ: Transient myopia and retinal edema during hydrochlorothiazide (Hydrodiuril) therapy, Arch Ophthalmol 65:212, 1961

8. Beasley, FJ: Transient myopia during trichlormethiazide therapy, Ann Ophthalmol 12:705, 1980

9. Beatty, JF, Krupin, T, Nichols, PF, and Becker, B: Elevation of intraocular pressure by calcium channel blockers, Arch Ophthalmol 102:1072, 1984

10. Becker, B: In conference on glaucoma, Transactions of first conference, New York, 1955, Josiah Macy Jr Foundation

11. Becker, B, and Christensen, RE: Beta-Hypophamine (vasopressin): Its effect upon intraocular pressure and aqueous flow in normal and glaucomatous eye, Arch Ophthalmol 56:1, 1956

12. Becker, B, and Friedenwald, JS: Clinical aqueous out-flow, Arch Ophthalmol 50:557, 1963

13. Becker, B, et al: Timolol and epinephrine: a clinical study of ocular interactions, Arch Ophthalmol 98:484, 1980

14. Bellarminoff, L: Untersuchungen mit der quantitativen colorimetrischen Methode uber die Resorption in die vordere Augenkammer, v Graefe's Arch Ophthalmol 39:38, 1893

15. Belci, C: Miopia transitoria in corso di terapia con diuretici, Boll Ocul 47:24, 1968

16. Berggren, L: Effect of composition of media and of metabolic inhibitors on secretion in vitro by the ciliary processes of the rabbit eye, Invest Ophthalmol 4:83, 1965

17. Berson, FG, Epstein, DF, and Patterson, MM: Obstruction of outflow facility by sodium hyaluronate in post-mortem enucleated human eyes, Invest Ophthalmol Vis Sci (Suppl) 20:119, 1981

18. Bietti, GB, and Cima, V: Klin Monatsbl Augenheilkd 124:386, 1954

19. Bill, A, and Walinder, P: The effect of pilocarpine on the dynamics of aqueous humor in a primate (Macaca irus), Invest Ophthalmol 5:170, 1966

20. Binkhorst, CG: Inflammation and intraocular pressure after the use of Healon in intraocular lens surgery, Am Intraocular Implant Soc J 6:340, 1980

21. Bito, LT, and Merritt, SQ: Paradoxical ocular hypertensive effect of pilocarpine in echothiophate iodide treated primate eyes, Invest Ophthalmol Vis Sci 19:371, 1980

22. Bleiman, B, and Schwartz, AL: Paradoxical response to pilocarpine, Arch Ophthalmol 97:1305, 1979

23. Bowden, CL, and Giffen, MB: Psychotropics and glaucoma, Am J Psychiatry 134:1314, 1977

24. Camras, CB, Bito, LZ, and Eakens, KE: Reduction of intraocular pressure by prostaglandins applied to the eyes of conscious rabbits, Invest Ophthalmol Vis Sci 16:1125, 1977

25. Camras, CB, et al: Inhibition of the epinephrine-induced reduction of intraocular pressure by systemic indomethacin in humans, Am J Ophthalmol 100:169, 1985

26. Carlson, VR: Individual pupillary reactions to certain centrally acting drugs in man, J Pharmacol Exp Ther 121:501, 1957

27. Carlston, JA: Unilateral dilated pupil from scopolamine disc, JAMA 248:1, 1982

28. Chandler, PA, and Grant, WM: Glaucoma, ed 2, Philadelphia, 1979, Lea & Febiger

29. Cohen, MM, Feldman, F, Clark, L, and Hudy, D: Effect of cimetidine on intraocular pressure in patients with glaucoma, Can J Ophthalmol 19:212, 1984

30. Colle, J, Duke-Elder, LM, and Duke-Elder, WS: Studies on the intraocular pressure. I. The action of drugs on the vascular and muscular factors controlling the intraocular pressure, J Physiol London 71:1, 1931

31. Crawford, K and Kaufman, PL: Pilocarpine antagonizes prostaglandin, F_2 induced ocular hypotension in monkeys, Arch Ophthalmol 105:1112, 1987

32. Craythorne, NWB, Rothenstein, HS, and Dripps, RD: The effect of succinylcholine on intraocular pressure in adults, infants and children during general anesthesia, Anesthesiology 21:59, 1960

33. Cristini, G, and Pagliarani, N: Amyl nitrate test in primary glaucoma, Br J Ophthalmol 37:741, 1953

34. Crossen, G, and Hoy, JE: A new parenteral anesthetic—C1581: its effect on intraocular pressure, J Pediatr Ophthalmol 4:20, 1967

35. Cunningham, AT, Albert, O, Cameron, T and Watson, AG: The effect of intravenous diazepam on rise of intraocular pressure following succinylcholine, Can Anaesth Soc J 28:591, 1981

36. Dalton, K: Influence of menstruation on glaucoma, Br J Ophthalmol 50:557, 1963

37. Davidson, SJ: Reports of ocular adverse reactions, Trans Ophthalmol Soc UK 43:455, 1974

38. Desvignes, P, Amar, L, and Regnault, F: Étude des effects de la digoxine sur les hypertensions ocularies, Bull Soc Ophthalmol Fr 63:832, 1963

39. Deufrains, A, Hempel, E, and Klengic, G: Results of a prospective ophthalmologic study with reference to hormonal contraction, Dtsch Gesundhestsw 30:901, 1975

40. Dobrilla, G, Felder, M, Chilovi, F, and DePretis, G: Exacerbation of glaucoma associated with both cimetidine and ranitidine, Lancet 1:1078, 1982

41. Dripps, RD, Eckenoff, JE, Vandam, LD: Determination of the depth of anesthesia. In Introduction to anesthesia: the principles of safe practice, ed 4, Philadelphia, 1972, WB Saunders Co

42. Duke-Elder, S: System of ophthalmology, vol 11, Diseases of the lens and vitreous: glaucoma and hypotony, St Louis, 1969, The CV Mosby Co

43. Edwards, TS: Transient myopia due to tetracycline, JAMA 186:69, 1963

44. English, HL: An alarming side effect of Tofranil, Lancet 1:1231, 1959

45. Ericson, LA: Hygroton-induced myopia and retinal edema, Acta Ophthalmol 41:538, 1963

46. Fazio, DT, Bateman, JB and Christensen, RE: Acute angle-closure glaucoma induced by general anesthesia, Arch Ophthalmol 103:360, 1985

47. Feldman, F, and Cohen, MV: Effect of histamine-2 receptor blockade by cimetidine on intraocular pressure in humans, Am J Ophthalmol 93:351, 1982

48. Fraunfelder, FT: Drug-induced ocular side effects and drug interactions, Philadelphia, 1976, Lea & Febiger

49. Friedman, Z, and Neuman, E: Benzhexalol induced blindness in Parkinson's disease, Br Med J 1:605, 1972

50. Gallin-Cohen, PF, Podos, SM, and Yablonski, ME: Oxygen lowers intraocular pressure, Invest Ophthalmol Vis Sci 19, 43, 1980

51. Gallois, J: Glaucoma aigu après Priscol, Bull Soc Ophthalmol Fr 131, 1951

52. Gandolfi, C: L'azione del Priscol sulla pressione arteriosa retinica (P.A.R.), Ann Ottal 73:336, 1947

53. Gartner, S, and Billet, E: Mydriatic glaucoma, Am J Ophthalmol 43:975, 1957

54. Gastaldi, GM: Considerazioni sulla miopia transitoria dopo somministrazione di diuretici saluretici, Rass Ital Ottal 34:178, 1965-1966

55. Gilman, AG, Goodman, LS, Roll, TW, Murad, R: Goodman and Gillman: the pharmacological basis of therapeutics, ed 7, New York, 1985, MacMillan

56. Goldberg, LT: Monamine oxidase inhibitors: adverse reactions and possible mechanisms, JAMA 190:456, 1964

57. Gott, PH: Cyclizine toxicity-intentional drug abuse of a proprietary antihistamine, N Engl J Med 279:596, 1968

58. Grant, WM: Toxicology for the eye, ed 2, Springfield, Ill, 1974, Charles C Thomas, Publisher

59. Graue, EL, Polack, FM, Balazs, EA: The protective effect of Na-Hyaluronate to corneal endothelium, Exp Eye Res 31:119, 1980

60. Grierson, I, Lee, R, and Abraham, S: Effects of pilocarpine on the morphology of the human outflow apparatus, Br J Ophthalmol 62:302, 1978

61. Groenouw, A: Uber die Anwendung des Cocains bei glaucomatosen Zustanden, Ber. 25 vers, Ophthalmol Ges Heidelb, p. 198, 1896; Ber Ophthalmol 27:369, 1896

62. Grossman, EE, and Hanley, W: Transient myopia during treatment for hypertension with autonomic blocking agents, Arch Ophthalmol 63:853, 1960

63. Halpern, AE, and Kulvin, MM: Transient myopia during treatment with carbonic anhydrase inhibitors, Am J Ophthalmol 65:212, 1961

64. Hamill, MB, Sueflow, JA, and Smith, JA: Transdermal scopolamine delivery system (TRANSDERM-V) and acute angle-closure glaucoma, Ann Ophthalmol 15:1011, 1983

65. Hardesty, JF: Control of intraocular hypertension by systemic medication, Trans Am Ophthalmol Soc 32:497, 1934

66. Harris, LS: Cycloplegia-induced intraocular pressure elevations: a study of normal and open-angle glaucomatous eyes, Arch Ophthalmol 79:242, 1968

67. Harrison, R, and Kaufmann, CS: Clonidine effects of a topically administered solution on intraocular pressure and blood pressure in open-angle glaucoma, Arch Ophthalmol 95:1368, 1977

68. Havener, WH: Ocular pharmacology, ed 5, St. Louis, 1983, The CV Mosby Co

69. Hermann, MP: Myopia spasmodique au cours des traitements diuretique, Bull Soc Ophthalmol Fr 63:719, 1963

70. Herxheimer, A: A comparison of some atropine-like drugs in man, with particular reference to their end-organ specificity, Br J Pharmacol 13:184, 1958

71. Hook, SR, Holladay, JT, Prager, TC, and Goosey, JD: Transient myopia induced by sulfonamides, Am J Ophthalmol 101:495, 1986

72. Hotchkiss, ML, Robin, AL, Pollack, IR, and Quigley, HA: Nonsteroidal anti-inflammatory agents af-

ter argon laser trabeculoplasty: a trial with flurbiprofen and indomethacin, Am J Ophthalmol 91:969,
1984

73. Hultsch, E: Low molecular weight hyaluronic acid
in experimental anterior segment surgery: an alternative to Healon, Ophthalmol Aug Suppl 90:102,
1983

74. Hyams, SW, and Keroub, C: Glaucoma due to diazepam, Am J Psychiatry 134:447, 1977

75. Jaffe, NS: Cataract surgery and its complications,
ed 4, St Louis, 1984, The CV Mosby Co

76. Katz, RL, and Eakins, KB: Mode of action of succinylcholine on intraocular pressure, J Pharmacol
Exp Ther 162:1, 1968

77. Kielar, RA, Teraslinno, P, Kearney, ST and Barker,
D: Effect of changes in pCO$_2$ on intraocular tension,
Invest Ophthalmol 16:534, 1977

78. Kirsch, RE: Glaucoma following cataract extraction
associated with use of alpha-chymotrypsin, Arch
Opthalmol 72:612, 1964

79. Kochman, M, and Romer, P: Experimental investigation of pathologic fluid exchange in the eye,
Arch Opthalmol 8:528, 1914

80. Kolker, AE, and Hetherington, J, Jr: Becker-Schaf-
fer's diagnosis and therapy of the glaucomas, ed 4,
St Louis, 1976, The CV Mosby Co

81. Kornblueth, W, Aladjenoff, L, Magora, F and Gab-
bay, A: Influence of general anesthesia on intraocular pressure in man: the effect of diethyl ether,
cyclopropane, vinyl ether, and thiopental sodium,
Arch Ophthalmol 61:1884, 1959

82. Krupin, T, et al: Halothane anesthesia and aqueous
humor dynamics in rabbit eyes, Invest Ophthalmol
Vis Sci 19:518, 1980

83. Krupin, T, et al: The effect of H$_1$-blocking antihistamines on intraocular pressure in rabbits, Ophthalmology 87:1167, 1980

84. Langham, ME, Kitazawa, Y, and Hart, RW: Adrenergic responses in the human eye, J Pharmacol Exp
Ther 179:47, 1971

85. Lee, PF: The influence of epinephrine and phenylephrine on intraocular pressure, Arch Ophthalmol 50:863, 1958

86. Leon, T, et al: Cimetidine-gyrilamine eye drops: effect on intraocular pressure in human glaucoma,
Glaucoma 8:54, 1986

87. Lipkin, D and Kuschnick, T: Pargyline hydrochlo-
rine poisoning in a child, JAMA, 201:135, 1967

88. Lowe, RF: Amitryptyline and glaucoma, Med J Aust
2:509, 1969

89. MacRae, SM, et al: The effects of sodium hyaluronate, chondroitin sulfate, and methylcellulose
on the corneal endothelium and intraocular pressure, Am J Ophthalmol, 95:332, 1983

90. Maddalena, MD: Transient myopia associated with
acute glaucoma and retinal edema following vaginal
administration of sulfanilamide, Arch Ophthalmol
80:186, 1968

91. Mansour, AM, Goldberg, S, Marouf, L, and Bin-
stock, L: Topical anesthesia and intraocular pressure, Glaucoma, 8:13, 1986

92. Mapstone, R: Closed-angle glaucoma: theoretical
considerations, Br J Ophthalmol 58:46, 1974

93. McCorkle, RG: Neomycin toxicity: a case report,
Arch Pediatr 75:435, 1958

94. McQuillen, MP, Cantor, HE, and O'Rourke, JR: My-
asthenia syndrome associated with antibiotics,
Arch Neurol 18:402, 1968

95. Medgyaszay, A: Intraokularer Druck und Hormon-
benhandlung, Ophthalmogoca 114:168, 1947

96. Mehra, KS, et al: Histamine in relation to epidemic
dropsy glaucoma, Ann Ophthalmol 6:367, 1974

97. Meyer, EJ, Leibowitz, H, Christman, EH, and Nif-
fenegger, JA: Influence of norethynodrel with mes-
tranol on intraocular pressure in glaucoma. II. A
controlled double-blind study, Arch Ophthalmol
75:771, 1966

98. Michaelson, TT: Transient myopia due to Hygroton, Am J Ophthalmol 54:1146, 1962

99. Mody, MV, and Keeney, AH: Propantheline (Pro-
Banthine) bromide in relation to normal and glaucomatous eyes: effects on intraocular tension and
pupillary size, JAMA 159:1113, 1955

99a. Mohan, M, et al: Ocular and clinico-epidemiolog-
ical study of epidemic dropsy, Ind J Med Res
80:449, 1984.

100. Monica, ML, Hesse, RJ, and Messerli, FH: The effect of a calcium channel blocking agent on intraocular pressure, Am J Ophthalmol 96:814, 1983

101. Muirhead, JF, and Scheie, HG: Transient myopia
after acetazolamide, Arch Ophthalmol 63:315, 1960

102. Neuschler, R: Myopia transitoria in corso di terapia
con dichlorofenamide, Boll Ocul 43:507, 1964

103. Newell, FW, Ridgway, WL, and Zeller, RW: The
treatment of glaucoma with Dibenamine, Am J
Ophthalmol 34:527, 1951

104. Ober, M, and Scharrer, H: Entwicklung des Au-
geninnendruckes bei prostaglandin-induziertem
Schuangerschaftsabbruck (Changes in intraocular
pressure during prostaglandin-induced abortion),
Klin Mhl Augenheilk 180:230, 1982

105. Oradell, NJ: Physician's Desk Reference, ed 40, Lit-
ton, Indiana, 1986, Medical Economics Co

106. Pape, LG: Intracapsular and extracapsular techniques of lens implantation with Healon, Am Intraocular Implant Soc J 6:342, 1980

107. Pappas, HR, et al: The effect of topical indomethacin on the acute intraocular pressure rise of argon
laser trabeculoplasty, Invest Ophthalmol Vis Sci
25:194, 1984

108. Paterson, CA: The effect of sympathetic nerve stimulation on the aqueous humor dynamics of the cocaine pretreated rabbit, Exp Eye Res 5:37, 1966

109. Peczon, JD: Clinical evaluation of digitalization in
glaucoma, Arch Ophthalmol 71:504, 1964

110. Peczon, JD, and Grant, WM: Sedatives, stimulants,
and intraocular pressure in glaucoma, Arch
Ophthalmol 72:178, 1964

111. Perkin, RL: Apnea with intramuscular colistin therapy, JAMA, 190:421, 1964

112. Petoanis, AD, Chondrelli, S, and Vadaluka-Seikioti, A: Effect of hypercapnea and hyperventilation on human intraocular pressure during general anaesthesia following acetazolamide administration, Br J Ophthalmol 64:422, 1980

113. Podos, SM, Becker, B, and Kass, MA: Prostaglandin synthesis, inhibition, and intraocular pressure, Invest Ophthalmol 12:426, 1973

114. Polgar, J, Vass, Z, and Tiboldi, T: Histochemical changes in the rat's eye after prolonged administration of esterone, Szemeszet 106:178, 1969

115. Radtke, N, and Waldman, J: The influence of enflurane anesthesia on intraocular pressure in youths, Anesth Analg 54:212, 1975

115a. Rathore, MK: Ophthalmological study of epidemic dropsy, Br J Ophthalmol 66:573, 1982.

116. Reboton, J, Weedly, RD, Bylenga, ND, and May, RH: Pigmentary retinopathy and iridocycloplegia in psychiatric patients, J Neurosurg Psychiat 3:311, 1961-1962

117. Robertson, DM, Hollenhorst, RW, and Callahan, JA: Ocular manifestations of digitalis toxicity, Arch Ophthalmol 76:640, 1966

118. Rothlin, E: Lysergic acid diethylamide and related substances, Ann NY Acad Sci 66:668, 1956

119. Rubin, RF: Acute psychotic reaction following ingestion of phentermine, Am J Psychiatry 120:1124, 1964

119a. Sachdev, MS, et al: Optic disc vasculitis in epidemic dropsy, Jpn J Ophthalmol 31:467, 1987

119b. Sachdev, MS, et al: Pathogenesis of epidemic dropsy glaucoma, Arch Ophthalmol 106: 1221, 1988

120. Salvati, M: L'influence de la menstruation sur la tension oculaire, Ann Ocul 160:586, 1923

121. Samuel, TR and Beaugie, A: Effect of carbon dioxide on the intraocular pressure in man during general anaesthesia, Br J Ophthalmol 58:62, 1974

122. Sanford-Smith, JH: Transient myopia after aspirin, Br J Ophthalmol 58:698, 1974

123. Scialdone, D, and Artifoni, E: Miopia transitoria in corso di terapia con Debinyl, B Ital Oftal 16:92, 1963; Zentralbl Ges Ophthalmol 91:107, 1964

124. Self, WG and Ellis, PO: The effect of general anesthetic agents on intraocular pressure, Surv Ophthalmol 21:497, 1977

125. Shannon, RP, Mead, A, and Sears, ML: The effect of dopamine on the intraocular pressure and pupil of the rabbit eye, Invest Ophthalmol 15:371, 1976

126. Shenolikar, IS, Rukmini, C, Krishnamachari, KAVR, and Satyanarayana, K: Sanguinarine in the blood and urine of cases of epidemic dropsy, Food Cosmet Toxicol 12:699, 1974

127. Sigg, EB: Autonomic side effects induced by psychotherapeutic agents. In Etron, DN, editor: Psychopharmacology, a review of progress 1957-1967, proceedings of the Sixth Annual Meeting of the American College of Neuropsychopharmacology, San Juan, Puerto Rico, Dec. 12-15, 1967, Public Health Service Pub No 1836, Washington, DC, 1968, American College of Neuropsychopharmacology

128. Snyder, SH, and Yamamura, HI: Antidepressants and the muscarinic acetylcholine receptor, Arch Gen Psych 34:236, 1977

129. Soll, D, and Harrison, S: The use of chondroitin sulfate in protection of the corneal endothelium, Ophthalmology 88(suppl):51, 1981

130. Spiers, ASD: Mydratic responses to sympathomimetic amines in patients treated with L-DOPA, Lancet 2:1301, 1969

131. Spiers, ASD, and Calne, DB: Action of dopamine on the human iris, Br Med J 4:333, 1969

132. Steele, CM, O'Duffy, J, and Brown, SS: Clinical effects and treatment of imipramine and amitriptyline poisoning in children, Br Med J 3:663, 1967

133. Sugar, HS, and Santos, R: The priscoline provocative test, Am J Ophthalmol 40:510, 1955

134. Swan, KC, and Gehrsitz, L: Competitive action of miotics on the iris sphincter, Arch Ophthalmol 46:471, 1951

135. Tahnke, R, and Iham, HW: The effect of clonidine on intraocular pressure and pupillary diameter, Klin Monatsbl Augenheilkd 161:78, 1972

136. Tammisto, T, Hamalainen, L, and Tarkkanen, L: Halothane and methoxyflurane in ophthalmic anesthesia, Acta Anaesthesiol Scand 9:173, 1965

137. Tandon, RK, et al: Epidemic dropsy in New Delhi, Am J Clin Nutr 28:883, 1975

138. Taulonen, A: The effect of topical indomethacin on acute pressure elevations of laser trabeculoplasty on capsular glaucoma, Acta Ophthalmol 63:245, 1985

139. Tolle, R, and Porksen, N: Thymoleptic mydriasis in the course of treatment, Int Pharmacopsychiatry 2:86, 1969

140. Trope, GE, and Hind, VMD: Closed-angle glaucoma in patient on disopyramide, Lancet 1:329, 1978

141. Trzeciakowski, JP, and Fry, GD: Effects of intraventricular histamine and H_2 receptor antagonists on intraocular pressure, J Ocular Pharmacol 3:55, 1987

142. Utley, PL, Luca, JB, and Billings, TE: Acute psychotic reaction to aqueous procaine penicillin, South Med J 59:1271, 1966

143. Varady, J, and Jahn, F: Uber die Bulbushypotonie bei Vergiflurgen mit Salizylsaurepraparaten, Dtsch Med Wochenschr 66:322, 1940

144. Walsh, FB, and Hoyt, WF: Clinical neuro-ophthalmology, vol 1, ed 3, vol 3, ed 3, Baltimore, 1969, Williams & Wilkins

145. Waud, SP: The affects of toxic dosages of benzylmethylcarbinamine (Benzedrine) in man, JAMA, 110:206, 1938

146. Weber, PA, and Opremcak, EM: Clinical interaction of timolol and systemic caffeine on intraocular pressure, Third Annual Resident Research Symposium, Ohio State University, 1983

147. Weinreb, RN, Mitchell, MD, and Polansky, JR: Prostaglandin production by human trabecular cells: invitro inhibition by dexamethasone, Invest Ophthalmol Vis Sci 24:1541, 1983

148. Weinreb, RN, Ruderman, B, Juster, R, and Zweig, K: Immediate intraocular pressure response to argon laser trabeculoplasty, Am J Ophthalmol 95:279, 1983

149. Weinstein, P: Relation of glaucoma to blood pressure, Arch Ophthalmol 13:181, 1935

150. Weinstein, P, Ahi, D, and Anda, L: Oral contraceptives and glaucoma, Klin Monatsbl Augenheilkd 162:798, 1973

151. Whitworth, CG, and Grant, WM: Use of nitrate and nitrite vasodilators by glaucomatous patients, Arch Ophthalmol 71:492, 1964

152. Wood, R: Ocular complications of oral contraceptives, Ophthalmol Sem 2:371, 1977

153. Yasuna, E: Acute myopia associated with prochlorperazine (Compazine) therapy, Am J Ophthalmol 54:793, 1962

154. Zahn, K: The effect of vasoactive drugs on the retinal circulation, Trans Ophthalmol Soc UK 86:529, 1966

155. Zarrabi, M: Quelques observations sur le Priscol en ophthalmologie, Ophthalmologica 122:76, 1951

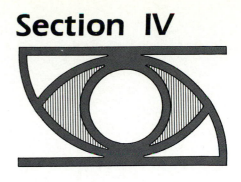

Section IV

Glaucomas Associated with Inflammation and Trauma

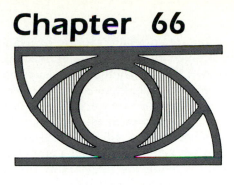

Chapter 66

Glaucoma Secondary to Keratitis, Episcleritis, and Scleritis

Peter G. Watson

Glaucoma associated with inflammation of the cornea, episclera, and sclera is sufficiently common that one should measure intraocular pressure in every patient with these inflammations and do so every time the patient is seen. It is a tragic experience for one to have spent weeks or months treating an inflamed eye, eventually obtaining an optically clear medium, only to find the disc cupped and pale and the patient without useful vision.

Many of the problems arise because of a reasonable reluctance to measure the intraocular pressure in a patient with active keratitis, either because of the possibility of damaging an already unhealthy epithelium or because of the very real danger of cross infection. Unfortunately, even the most elaborate apparatus for sterilizing Goldmann tonometer heads is ineffective against such viruses as the adenovirus group, and vigorous rubbing with a sterile swab is essential before each use. This problem can be avoided by the use of the American Optical or Keeler Air puff tonometers. If the cornea is irregular, however, these instruments may fail to give a reading. Digital tonometry can occasionally be an acceptable alternative and is better than nothing. If the pressure is very high, this assessment will be sufficient to determine that treatment needs to be given. The MacKay-Marg tonometer or pneumatonometer with disposable rubber covers are probably the best instruments to use, but the corneal epithelium can still be damaged with these instruments.

MECHANISMS OF ASSOCIATED GLAUCOMAS

There are as many causes of raised intraocular pressure in these conditions as there are causes for glaucoma. It is often assumed that the rise in pressure is directly related to the inflammatory condition of the eye, but this is often not the case. It is also often assumed that because the disc is pale and cupped, the rise in intraocular pressure is the sole reason for the change, yet many inflammatory diseases are accompanied by or associated with active vasculitis, and there may be other reasons for vascular insufficiency and capillary closure at the optic nerve head. The mechanism of the raised intraocular pressure in each patient must be considered. Is the angle closed? Is there a predisposition to angle-closure glaucoma, and does the fellow eye need treatment? Is the patient already suffering from primary open-angle glaucoma? Is the rise in pressure caused by an elevated episcleral venous pressure, edema of the meshwork, or obstruction by synechiae? Motzu, in the fourth century BC, said "The physician . . . has to know the course of the ailment before he can treat it." This is as true today as ever it was in the past.

Unfortunately, the investigation is hampered by the possibility of damaging an already diseased cornea or rupturing a thin sclera or cornea. Gonioscopy is often difficult or impossible in patients with severe keratitis, in which case one may attempt to assess the width of the angle by comparing one eye with the other and noting the position of the iris in relation to the cornea at the limbus. Although by no means foolproof, this method will often indicate whether the glaucoma is caused by a narrow angle. Gonioscopy in scleritis rarely presents a problem unless the sclera or limbus is very thin. It is, however, essential to use a three-mirror lens because, as will be seen later, a narrow angle may be the result of either a granuloma behind the iris overlying the ciliary body or a granuloma in the posterior sclera itself.

Visual field examination can be extremely confusing in patients with keratitis. It is valuable, however, if open-angle glaucoma is suspected, if there is segmental atrophy of the optic nerve head, or if a vascular occlusion is suspected. In patients with posterior scleritis with a localized lesion, optic nerve head edema, or exudative detachment, the visual field examination can be invaluable in assessing the progress of the disease and the effect of treatment.

Although almost any variety of glaucoma can occur in this group of conditions, some are much more common than others, and others are specific for one particular condition. It is useful, therefore, to consider these specific types under separate headings, the most common being mentioned first.

CLASSIFICATION OF GLAUCOMA MECHANISMS

I. Episcleritis
  A. Steroid-induced glaucoma
  B. Acute open-angle glaucoma associated with conjunctival chemosis and elevated episcleral venous pressure
  C. Acute angle-closure glaucoma
  D. Preexisting open-angle glaucoma
II. Anterior scleritis
  A. Open-angle glaucoma
    1. Secondary open-angle glaucoma
      a. Associated with uveitis
      b. Associated with active limbal scleritis resulting in trabecular destruction in severe cases
      c. As a result of vasculitis of the episcleral vessels
      d. Steroid-induced
    2. Preexisting primary open-angle glaucoma
  B. Angle-closure glaucoma
    1. Primary angle-closure glaucoma
      a. Induced by anterior segment edema; no peripheral anterior synechiae (PAS) formation
      b. Predisposition to angle-closure glaucoma precipitated by inflammation
    2. Secondary angle-closure glaucoma with uveitis and PAS formation
  C. Pupillary block glaucoma
  D. Neovascular glaucoma
III. Posterior scleritis
  A. Angle-closure glaucoma caused by forward movement of the lens-iris diaphragm
  B. Secondary angle-closure glaucoma with PAS formation
  C. Neovascular glaucoma
IV. Keratitis with little or no anterior uveitis
  A. Open-angle glaucoma
    1. Acute inflammatory change associated with bacterial, viral, or fungal keratitis
    2. Destructive changes in connective tissue and degenerative diseases
    3. Chronic degenerative changes associated with chronic keratitis
  B. Primary angle-closure glaucoma
    1. Associated with acute inflammation
    2. Chemical injury
  C. Secondary angle-closure: associated with acute and chronic inflammatory disease and PAS formation

EPISCLERITIS

Simple Episcleritis

Simple episcleritis is a benign, recurrent condition that, although uncomfortable, never causes permanent harm. The condition is twice as common in men as in women, has its peak incidence in the fourth decade of life, and may affect one eye or both simultaneously or at different times.

The clinical presentation is the same in all the various types. Without prior warning, the eye becomes prickly, red, and slightly tender. These symptoms increase in intensity over the next 24 hours, often accompanied by tearing but never discharge. The symptoms can range from a mild pricking and discomfort with slight redness of the eye to a very red, inflamed eye accompanied by intense conjunctival and episcleral chemosis, swelling of the lids, and a temporary miosis and myopia. Having reached a peak, the symptoms gradually decline again over the next several days, after which there is a short respite before the inflammation recurs either at the same or at another site. In 60% of patients, this pattern will persist for 3 to 5 years. The intervals between the attacks then increase until no further attacks occur. In a few patients the attacks may last up to 30 years.

The cause remains unknown. The initial attack frequently follows a viral infection, and many patients give a definite history of an exogenous antigen. Seven percent of the patients have clinical gout, but more often than not, no specific etiologic agent can be found. In many patients the disease behaves as a type I hypersensitivity reaction.

Nodular Episcleritis[36]

The symptoms, course, age, and sex distribution of nodular episcleritis are the same as for simple episcleritis, but this condition runs a much more protracted course, and the episcleral inflammation, instead of spreading throughout the tissue, localizes in one or several spots with the formation of a nodule within the episcleral tissue. This nodule can be moved under the conjunctiva, and the underlying sclera is not edematous. If the tissues are very inflamed, a drop of 1% epinephrine or 10% phenylephrine will blanch the tissues sufficiently to enable one to observe the underlying sclera.

Glaucoma Associated with Episcleritis

Steroid-induced glaucoma

Patients with episcleritis have been treated with topical steroids but such treatment is neither necessary or even desirable.[6,7] These patients develop recurrences and may be treated at intervals from as short a period as 2 weeks to as long as 30 years for a benign condition. Fifteen percent of patients treated this way develop posterior subcapsular cataracts,[35] and 16% develop a rise in intraocular pressure.[21] Considering the period of time over which they are liable to be given topical steroids, their chances of developing intractable glaucoma and cataracts are high indeed. A double-masked trial of placebo versus betamethasone versus oxyphenbutazone ointments in this condition showed that betamethasone gave symptomatic relief, oxyphenbutazone was equally effective, and neither shortened the course of the condition.[37] Similar results have been obtained in a recent trial using clobetasone butyrate drops and placebo drops.[18]

Occasionally, in a patient who has attacks that are incapacitating because of watering eyes, swollen lids, and conjunctiva, it is necessary to use intensive, strong topical steroids within minutes of the start of an attack. This will sometimes abort the attack. In all other situations, if the patient demands treatment, nonsteroidal antiinflammatory drops or lubricants should be used. If the attacks are severe, frequent, and incapacitating, systemic oxyphenbutazone or indomethacin will usually bring relief.

There is no hereditary tendency to develop episcleritis, but it has been suggested that the normal population can be divided into three groups regarding pressure response to topical steroids: (1) marked responders with rises in intraocular pressure above 30 mm Hg (homozygous [gg]), (2) responders with moderate rises in intraocular pressure to between 20 and 30 mm Hg (heterozygous [ng]), and (3) homozygous (nn) nonresponders who have no rise in intraocular pressure after 6 weeks of topical steroid application.[1,2] Four percent of the normal population are homozygous (gg), 32% heterozygous (ng), and 64% homozygous (nn) nonresponders.

Although 16% of the patients with episcleritis in one study showed transient rises in intraocular pressure of more than 20 mm Hg during the course of local steroid treatment, only 9 of 301 eyes (3%) developed glaucoma (i.e., permanent rises in intraocular pressure with disc and field changes, requiring medication or surgery for control).[35] During treatment of the episcleritis, four of these eyes were known to have open-angle glaucoma before treatment started, and one eye developed acute open-angle glaucoma (see below). The remaining four eyes could be regarded as having steroid-induced glaucoma (1.3%). It is probable that these patients were homozygous (gg) responders in whom the changes in the trabecular meshwork had become irreversible, but there was no evidence to show that the two conditions of episcleritis and glaucoma were otherwise linked.

Fortunately, the majority of patients who experience an intraocular pressure rise after using steroids recover completely once the steroids are withdrawn. Recurrent episcleritis may need to be controlled by systemic medication, or the glaucoma may recur. If antiglaucomatous medication fails, trabeculectomy must be performed.

Acute open-angle glaucoma

Acute open-angle glaucoma is an unusual but apparently specific entity that arises in those patients who develop markedly infiltrated, edematous episclera and swollen lids (Fig. 66-1). In addition to the signs of episcleritis, the patient has an extremely painful eye and deteriorating vision.[16,20] Because neither pain nor reduced vision are features of episcleritis, additional problems should be suspected. The intraocular pressure is markedly raised, the cornea moderately edematous, and the pupil miotic. The angle is open, but there is no reflux of blood into Schlemm's canal.

The cause seems to be edema of the trabecular meshwork. The episcleral venous pressure may also be somewhat raised, but the venous congestion usually associated with glaucoma of this cause is absent.

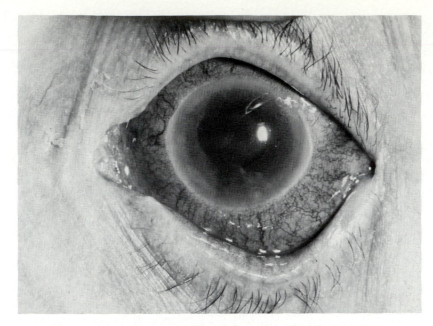

Fig. 66-1   Simple episcleritis and open-angle glaucoma in 60-year-old woman. Onset of pain, discomfort, and blurred vision was sudden. Episcleral and conjunctival tissue was edematous, and there was slight edema of cornea. Angle was wide open.

The two patients whom my colleagues and I have seen with this condition responded well to treatment with acetazolamide, dilation of the pupil with short-acting mydriatics, and intensive treatment of the episcleral inflammation with hourly application of 0.3% prednisolone drops, which was continued until the inflammation disappeared. Recurrent attacks have been controlled by starting the treatment as soon as the symptoms begin, and this has reduced the inflammatory response sufficiently to prevent the onset of the glaucoma.

Acute angle-closure glaucoma

We have seen two patients subject to attacks of episcleritis who also developed acute angle-closure glaucoma. Both patients responded to the standard therapy for acute angle-closure glaucoma, and peripheral iridectomies were performed through a corneal incision without complication.

Preexisting open-angle glaucoma

Since up to 80% of patients with open-angle glaucoma are (gg) or (ng) steroid responders, it is important to determine whether they have this condition or a family history of it before starting treatment. Beta blockers may result in underperfusion of the meshwork and further accumulation of abnormal substances and thus may fail to control the glaucoma. Trabeculectomy, if necessary, should be performed through an area of unaffected sclera.

SCLERITIS

In contradistinction to episcleritis, scleritis is a severe, painful, potentially destructive eye disease requiring vigorous therapy for its control, sometimes with extremely toxic and dangerous drugs. It is therefore important to distinguish between these two conditions, which can almost always be recognized when the patient is first seen. This is achieved by taking a careful history and by observing the depth of the inflammation.[35,36] In 1830 Mackenzie[19] gave this exact description:

The pain is at its onset of the stinging kind extending from the eyeball to the orbit and neighbouring parts of the head. These parts feel hot to the patient and even to the hand of the observer. The pain is strikingly augmented by warmth. It often extends to the forehead, cheekbone and the teeth; . . . pulsating . . . and particularly round the orbit, it consists rather in an agonizing kind of feeling which distresses and wearies out patience of the person affected. It never ceases entirely so long as the disease continues but it varies much in degree, coming on with severity about four or six or eight o'clock in the evening; continuing during the night becoming most severe about midnight and aborting towards five or six in the morning till then totally preventing sleep and occasioning great distress."

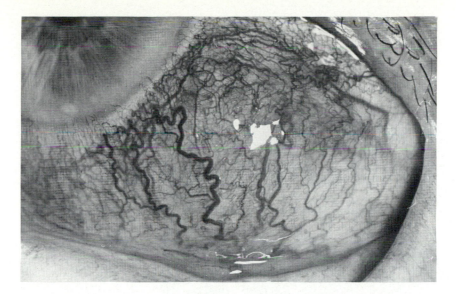

Fig. 66-2 Diffuse anterior scleritis. Intraocular pressure was raised in this patient. Angle was narrow and congested in area of scleral inflammation. There were some cells in anterior chamber. This is possibly clinical counterpart of Fig. 66-13.

With such severe pain, it is surprising that photophobia and tearing are not prominent features.[32,35] The pain is a consequence of swelling or destruction of the scleral tissue. Clinically this gives rise to scleral edema if the disease is anterior to the equator or to choroidal swelling and secondary retinal detachment if the disease is posterior to the equator. Destruction of the sclera (necrotizing scleritis) is a late feature and is almost always preventable if the disease is detected early enough.

Forty-six percent of patients with scleritis have some other systemic disease—usually connective tissue disease. The mortality is also high: between 30% and 45% of patients die within 5 years, primarily of cardiovascular disease related to the systemic cause of the scleritis[21,35] Several clinically distinct varieties of scleritis can be identified:
A. Anterior scleritis
   1. Diffuse
   2. Nodular
   3. Necrotizing
      a. With inflammation
      b. Without inflammation (scleromalacia perforans)
B. Posterior scleritis

Anterior Scleritis

Diffuse and nodular anterior scleritis[36]

The onset of diffuse scleritis and of nodular anterior scleritis is often insidious, pain being the prominent feature and the redness of the eye becoming completely ignored. Examination reveals edema of the deep scleral tissue and an overlying episcleral congestion (Figs. 66-2 and 66-3). In nodular scleritis, the scleral inflammation is localized to one or more nodules, which can become immense. Biopsy specimens should not be taken from these nodules, which are often full of pultaceous material and extremely tender, because they fail to heal. One feature that helps distinguish these varieties from the less important episcleritis is that the vascular plexuses lose their regular arrangement, and large bypass channels form. Treatment is with systemic antiinflammatory agents, such as flurbiprofen 100 mg three times a day or indomethacin 25 mg four times a day, until the inflammation disappears.

Necrotizing anterior scleritis[36]

Necrotizing anterior scleritis is always accompanied by severe inflammation (Fig. 66-4). Although only 10% of patients with scleral inflammation have necrotizing scleritis, the diagnosis must be considered at all times. Failure to treat it adequately leads to irreparable loss of tissue and the onset of glaucoma and uveitis, which may lead to loss of the eye.

Fortunately, it is almost always possible to detect the necrotizing type of scleritis at the outset; the patient has the condition initially rather than as a progression from the more benign scleritis. The pain is intense, and the eye is congested up to but usually not including the equator of the globe. In contrast to nodular scleritis, the conges-

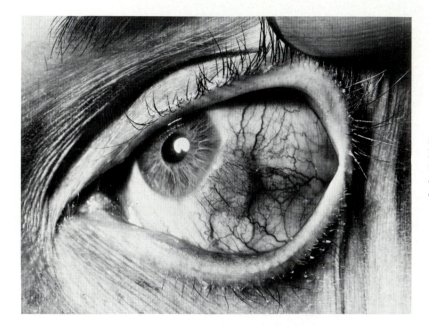

Fig. 66-3 Nodular anterior scleritis. Intraocular pressure was raised, angle wide open, and trabecular band was prominent. Outflow was reduced. Other eye was normal. This is possibly clinical counterpart of Fig. 66-6.

Fig. 66-4 Necrotizing anterior scleritis. Angle was open but narrow and congested in area adjacent to scleral inflammation. This probably is appearance of Fig. 66-8. (From Watson, P: Diseases of the sclera and episclera. In Duane, TD, editor: Clinical ophthalmology, vol 4, New York, 1980, Harper & Row Publishers, Inc)

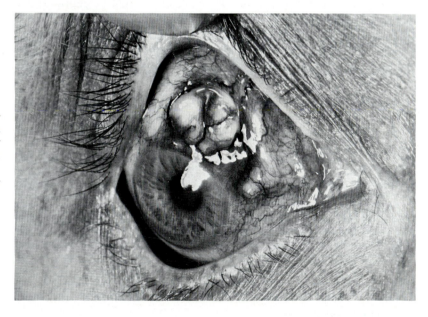

tion is more to the edges of the swollen area (representing the site of the active granuloma), and the episclera and sometimes the conjunctiva are hypoperfused on fluorescein angiography.[33] They may be avascular over the center of the lesion, which may break down, leading to loss of tissue. The course of the lesion is insidiously progressive and, if not stopped, will progress both around the globe and backward to involve the posterior segment. Treatment is with systemic steroids in high dosage.[22,35,36]

Necrotizing scleritis without inflammation (scleromalacia perforans)

The term scleromalacia perforans[30] is a specific disorder and should not be used indiscriminately. The patients are almost always female, with long-standing rheumatoid arthritis, who develop obliterative vasculitis of the episcleral vasculature. This inevitably leads to avascular necrosis and sequestration of the underlying sclera. The prominent feature is that there is little or no inflammation surrounding the necrotic tissue, and treatment is rarely indicated unless other complications supervene. Subconjunctival steroids are contraindicated in this disease, since they may induce necrosis leading to perforation of the globe.

Posterior Scleritis

Posterior scleritis is a much underdiagnosed condition and is present in three fourths of the eyes that require enucleation. Some 45% of these eyes have never had the diagnosis made before enucleation.[12] The site of the granuloma determines the symptoms and signs. Thus if the inflammation affects the area adjacent to the pars plana, cyclitis

and pars planitis will result (Fig. 66-5). If the inflammation overlies the midchoroid, an exudative retinal detachment will be produced; if the inflammation is at the disc, papilledema will result; and, if there is a large posterior granuloma, proptosis will result.[5] The diagnosis often depends on considering the possibility and, if necessary, giving a trial of steroid therapy. Ultrasonography and computed tomographic (CT) scanning can be helpful. Treatment is as for anterior scleritis. Nonsteroidal antiinflammatory agents work dramatically and should be tried first, but it is usually necessary to resort to the use of high-dose systemic steroids.

Glaucoma Associated with Anterior Scleritis

In 301 eyes of patients attending the scleritis clinic at Moorfields Eye Hospital, the intraocular pressure was found to be raised in 12% of the patients with scleritis, but only 3% required surgery for its control (Table 66-1). However, in a histopathologic study of 92 eyes removed because of scleral disease, 49% had glaucoma.[38] The most common reason for enucleation was intractable glaucoma and uveitis, so the presence of glaucoma must be regarded as having sinister import in patients with scleral inflammation.

Clinically, 90% of the patients with scleritis had inflammation anterior to the equator, and no inflammatory signs could be detected in the posterior segment, even on the closest examination. However, of the eyes that were removed and that also had glaucoma, inflammation was limited to the anterior segment in only 13 (26%) and to the posterior segment in only 6 (12%); the rest (62%) had a combination of both anterior and posterior disease. This underlines the importance of detecting and

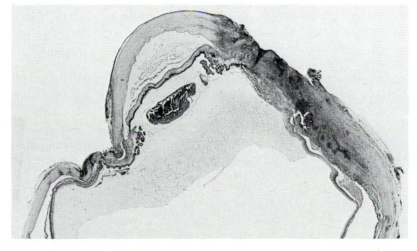

Fig. 66-5 Anterior necrotizing scleritis complicated by cataract, uveitis, and glaucoma. Eye was removed because of intractable pain and intolerance of steroid therapy. Inflammation has spread to involve posterior segment as well as angle structures. (From Watson, P: Diseases of the sclera and episclera. In Duane, TD, editor: Clinical ophthalmology, vol 4, New York, 1980, Harper & Row Publishers, Inc)

Table 66-1 Glaucoma in scleritis

Type of scleritis	Total eyes	Total with glaucoma	Primary open-angle glaucoma	Primary angle-closure glaucoma	Secondary glaucoma	Steroid-induced glaucoma
Diffuse anterior	119	12	6	0	6	0
Nodular anterior	134	11	6	0	5	0
Necrotizing	29	8	2	0	5	1
Scleromalacia perforans	13	4	0	0	4	0
Posterior	6	0	0	0	0	0
TOTAL	301	35	14	0	20	1

Of the patients with secondary glaucoma, nine had no abnormality other than scleritis, seven had keratitis, and six had uveitis. Sclerokeratitis coexisted in some patients. Five patients with episcleritis developed steroid-induced glaucoma.

treating the condition early if irreversible changes are not to supervene.

Further analysis of both the clinical and histopathologic data indicate that different mechanisms are at work in the production of the glaucoma.

Open-angle glaucoma

Primary open-angle glaucoma. Five percent of the patients with scleritis in the above clinical study were diagnosed as having primary open-angle glaucoma. The wide-open angle did not appear to be abnormal in any way. These patients had not been taking topical steroids, but most had had systemic steroids at some time or another. This incidence, which is twice what might be expected in the population as a whole, might be accounted for either by the presence of a mild degree of inflammation in a trabecular meshwork already compromised by glaucoma or perhaps by an abnormal steroid response. Treatment with miotics or trabeculectomy was successful. Again, trabeculectomy must be performed in an area where the conjunctiva and sclera appear normal.

Secondary open-angle glaucoma. Secondary open-angle glaucoma is an extremely difficult diagnosis to make clinically because the intraocular pressure sometimes rises to very high levels, but the angles appear normal and the disc and field changes are variable. Its presence, however, can be implied from a very rapid response to treatment of the scleritis and from the somewhat congested appearance of the trabecular band when viewed gonioscopically. This appearance is not a constant feature, but although it is independent of the presence of uveitis, it does seem to be related to an adjacent area of scleritis. In the histopathologic study, 80% of the glaucomatous eyes had a focus of scleritis overlying the angle structures as op-

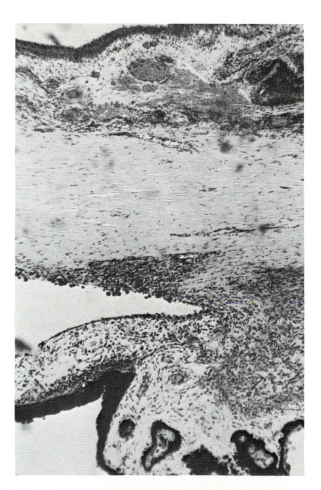

Fig. 66-6 Open angle with inflammatory cells concentrated within outflow system. Intense inflammatory reaction involves episcleral and conjunctival vessels. (From Wilhelmus, K, Grierson, I, and Watson, PG. Published with permission from the American Journal of Ophthalmology 91:697, 1981. Copyright by the Ophthalmic Publishing Co)

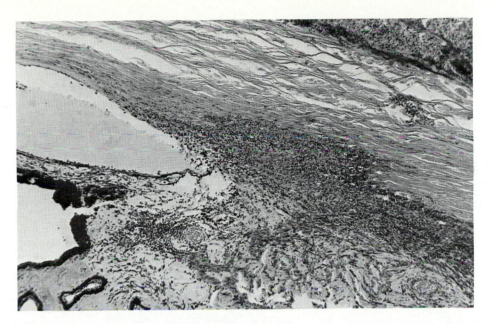

Fig. 66-7 Partially closed angle with intense inflammatory infiltrate within trabecular tissues. (From Wilhelmus, K, Grierson, I, and Waton, PG. Published with permission from the American Journal of Ophthalmology 91:697, 1981. Copyright by the Ophthalmic Publishing Co)

posed to 25% of the nonglaucomatous eyes (p < 0.005)[36] (Fig. 66-6).

GLAUCOMA ASSOCIATED WITH UVEITIS. Of the 14 eyes with open-angle glaucoma, 9 had severe anterior uveitis, and histologic examination showed that all of these patients had evidence of active trabecular inflammation without any evidence of peripheral anterior synechiae (PAS) formation[38] (Fig. 66-7). Uveitis is a common feature of eyes removed because of scleritis, being present in 84% of the glaucomatous ones, but it is not a common feature clinically. The combination of both uveitis and glaucoma must therefore be regarded with deep suspicion, and active measures taken to counteract it. Severe uveitis occurs only in the most severely affected eyes and seems to arise only when the inflammation has progressed circumferentially around the globe or has extended backward beyond the equator (Table 66-2). It is possible, therefore, that the glaucoma is a result of a combination of severe trabecular damage, damage to the episcleral outflow channels, anterior segment ischemia, and involvement of the uveal tract by the granulomatous reaction (Fig. 66-8).

Treatment is difficult, but it is essential to control both the glaucoma and the concomitant uveitis, Systemic medication with steroids or, in less severe cases, topical antiinflammatory agents, will usually control both the scleritis and the intraocular pressure. However, it may also be necessary to give

Table 66-2 Percentage of anterior uveitis in scleritis

Type of scleritis	Total eyes	Anterior uveitis (%)
Anterior		
Diffuse	119	35
Nodular	134	17
Necrotizing	29	37
Scleromalacia perforans	13	100
Posterior	6	66

Only two patients developed uveitis in the opposite, apparently unaffected eye.

mydriatic-cycloplegics and carbonic anhydrase inhibitors. Miotics are rarely effective in the presence of uveitis. Provided there is some relatively normal area of sclera and episcleral tissue, trabeculectomy undertaken at this site is almost always effective. If it fails, however, treatment becomes extremely difficult. Cyclocryotherapy is a poor procedure in an already inflamed eye. Setons need to be avoided if at all possible, because the presence of foreign material stimulates further inflammation.

GLAUCOMA IN THE PRESENCE OF ACTIVE LIMBAL SCLERITIS. Although scleritis involves the anterior segment, the inflammatory reaction is maximal about 3 to 5 mm from the limbus. If the inflammation does reach the limbus, it is rarely over more than an area of 45 degrees and, provided the tra-

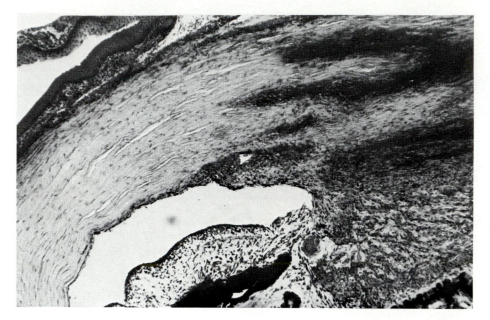

Fig. 66-8 Open angle with many inflammatory cells within outflow system. Deep scleral, interscleral, episcleral, and subconjunctival vessels are foci of inflammation. (From Wilhelmus, K, Grierson, I, and Watson, PG. Published with permission from the American Journal of Ophthalmology 91:697, 1981. Copyright by the Ophthalmic Publishing Co)

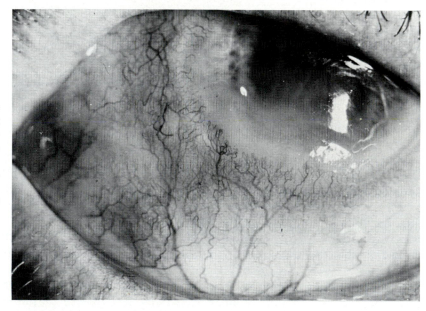

Fig. 66-9 Active limbitis in patient with severe anterior scleritis following herpes zoster and accompanied by keratitis and raised intraocular pressure. Angle was open. (From Wilhelmus, K, Grierson, I, and Watson, PG. Published with permission from the American Journal of Ophthalmology 91:697, 1981. Copyright by the Ophthalmic Publishing Co)

becular tissue is otherwise healthy, the remaining meshwork is sufficient to maintain the intraocular pressure at a normal level. However, particularly in patients with diffuse anterior scleritis, the whole circumference of the anterior segment can be involved, and very occasionally the scleritis is most active in the limbal area, in which case the intraocular pressure will rise (Fig. 66-9). In certain patients with long-standing circumferential necrotizing scleritis, the trabecular tissue becomes directly involved. In the histopathologic study, active limbal scleritis was more common in eyes with glaucoma than in those without glaucoma (p < 0.005)[36] (Fig. 66-10).

Because the inflammation causing the scleritis is the cause of this type of glaucoma, treatment of the scleral inflammation will reduce the intraocular

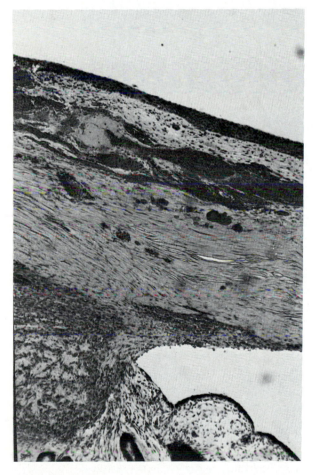

Fig. 66-10 Open-angle glaucoma with intense inflammatory infiltrate within outflow system. Inflammatory cuffing of limbal vessels is evident. (From Wilhelmus, K, Grierson, I, and Watson, PG. Published with permission from the American Journal of Ophthalmology 91:697, 1981. Copyright by the Ophthalmic Publishing Co)

pressure. In the acute phase of the inflammation, the intraocular pressure tends to rise to high levels. During this period, carbonic anhydrase inhibitors are usually necessary to control the pressure. There is, however, a long period of up to many weeks after the scleritis has disappeared clinically before the intraocular pressure normalizes. Carbonic anhydrase inhibitors can usually be discontinued when the inflammation subsides, but it may be necessary to continue treatment with pilocarpine or timolol during this period. Trabeculectomy is rarely necessary but is effective (Fig. 66-11). The delay in restoration of the intraocular pressure to normal is probably the result of damage to the proteoglycan matrix of the trabecular tissue, which requires time to return to normal.[34]

GLAUCOMA RESULTING FROM VASCULITIS OF THE EPISCLERAL VESSELS.[38] This is a condition that cannot be proved to exist except by anterior segment fluorescein angiography[33] or biopsy of episcleral tissue—a procedure not to be recommended unless it is part of a trabeculectomy procedure. It occurs in eyes with an open angle without anterior chamber inflammation or trabecular meshwork abnormality and where the scleritis is away from the limbus. On gonioscopy, the angle is wide open, but the response to miotics is poor. Tonography reveals a poor outflow.[14] Histologically the intrascleral outflow channels are surrounded by cuffs of lymphocytes, and there is often perivasculitis in the anterior uveal tissues (Figs. 66-8, 66-10, and 66-12). Vasculitis is a common feature of many of the connective tissue diseases associated with scleritis,[36] the generalized vasculitis and scleral necrosis often occurring simultaneously, and it is possible that the changes observed in the outflow channels are a manifestation of the systemic condition. The glaucoma usually resolves with the treatment of the scleritis or systemic disease.

STEROID-INDUCED GLAUCOMA. Since scleritis needs to be treated with systemic medication, steroid-induced glaucoma is much less of a problem in scleritis than in episcleritis. In a large series, only one case was definitely proved to be caused by steroids alone, although it is almost certain that some of the patients with open angles, many of whom must have been homozygous (gg) responders, had their glaucoma worsened by the use of steroids.[35] McGavin found raised intraocular pressure from this cause in 16% of the eyes that he treated for scleritis and rheumatoid arthritis, but many of these patients also had used local steroids

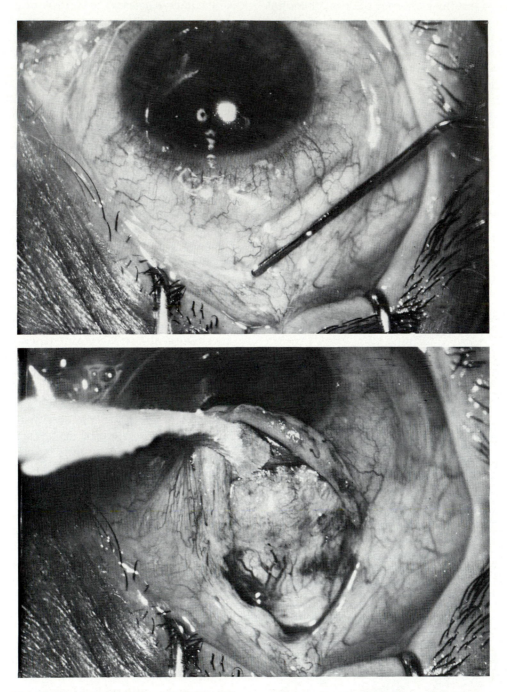

Fig. 66-11 Active limbitis and scleritis with open angle in patient in whom intraocular pressure could not be controlled. Trabeculectomy was successfully performed, and pressure has remained controlled for 5 years. Note gross episcleral and scleral edema.

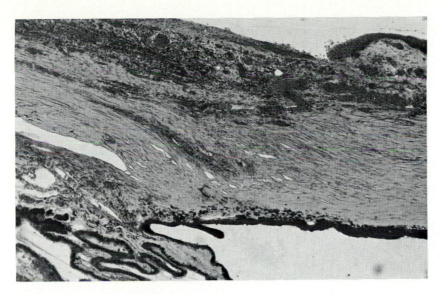

Fig. 66-12   Closed angle with atrophic thin iris and outflow system obliterated. Example shows clear evidence of scleritis and limbal vasculitis. (From Wilhelmus, K, Grierson, I, and Watson, PG. Published with permission from the American Journal of Ophthalmology 91:697, 1981. Copyright by the Ophthalmic Publishing Co)

as well.[21] Because of the possibility of steroid-induced glaucoma, we now rarely prescribe local steroids for patients with scleral disease and, if they are deemed essential, clobetasone butyrate, which has much less of a pressure-elevating effect, is used. Fortunately, most steroid-induced glaucomas resolve on withdrawal of the steroids, but again many patients must be given an antiglaucomatous medication for a prolonged period while the trabecular tissue returns to normal. Occasionally, however, the changes are irreversible, and trabeculectomy has to be undertaken.

GLAUCOMA FROM OTHER CAUSES.   If scleritis occurs in patients who already have the exfoliation syndrome, the scleritis does not appear to alter the course or treatment of the glaucoma. Histologically we have seen one example in which the exfoliation syndrome and scleritis occurred together. The angle of one eye, although wide open, was completely obstructed by a hyaline membrane. The cause of this is obscure but is probably a result of inflammation, fibrin exudation, and secondary hyaline formation from proliferation of the endothelium of the cornea.[9]

Angle-closure glaucoma

Primary angle-closure glaucoma.   Primary angle-closure glaucoma accompanying anterior scleritis is rare, but we have seen two patients whose attacks seemed to have been precipitated by the on-set of the scleral inflammation. Whether the combination of a narrow angle with simple dilation of the pupil, ciliary edema, partial obstruction of the outflow channels, or a combination of these factors caused the attack is uncertain. They responded well to antiglaucoma medication, systemic oxyphenbutazone, and peripheral iridectomy performed through the cornea. Two eyes in the histopathologic study, however, showed occluded angles without any evidence of synechiae formation or uveitis, and it is possible that the presence of the acute angle-closure glaucoma was not recognized, the pain being considered a concomitant part of the scleral inflammation (Fig. 66-13).

Secondary angle-closure glaucoma.   This is the least common type of glaucoma associated with scleral inflammation. The raised intraocular pressure invariably follows a prolonged uveitis that may or may not be severe. Fortunately, anterior uveitis occurs in less than a third of the patients with anterior scleritis. It is usually mild and can easily be controlled by dilation of the pupil and treatment of the scleritis. In some patients, particularly those with severe necrotizing disease, the uveitis is persistent and, although rarely acute, continues for months while the scleritis is poorly controlled. This gives rise to PAS formation and eventual occlusion of the angle (Fig. 66-14). In these patients it is most important to treat any acute attacks vigorously because severe "plastic" uveitis

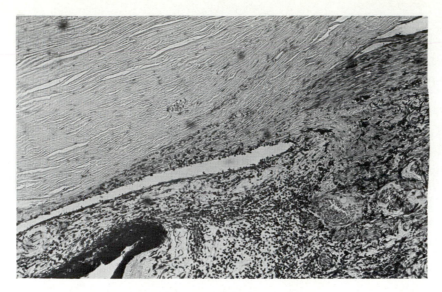

Fig. 66-13 Narrow angle with inflammatory reaction in anterior uvea. Schlemm's canal is closed; inflammatory cells are present within a hyalinized trabecular meshwork.

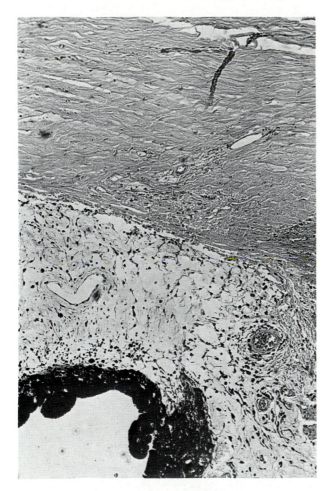

Fig. 66-14 Closed angle with thickened trabecular meshwork; inflammatory cells are present at site of iridotrabecular adhesion. (From Wilhelmus, K, Grierson, I, and Watson, PG. Published with permission from the American Journal of Ophthalmology 91:697, 1981. Copyright by the Ophthalmic Publishing Co)

inevitably leads to broad PAS formation and eventually to a false angle. Once this has occurred and the intraocular pressure becomes persistently raised, weak areas of sclera affected by the scleritis will start to bulge and staphyloma formation will result (Fig. 66-15). Staphyloma and spontaneous perforation is a rare event in scleritis and occurs (apart from accidental injury) only in eyes in which the intraocular pressure has been persistently raised.

Treatment is difficult. In the early stages, suppression of the uveitis and scleritis combined with antiglaucoma medication will prevent the continuation of the process, but once the angle has been occluded totally, it is difficult to control the intraocular pressure. Trabeculectomy is sometimes successful. This should be performed behind the scleral spur so that, after the scleral spur has been dissected from the underlying ciliary muscle, the synechiae can be dissected under direct vision. It is important to replace the superficial flap, since otherwise staphyloma formation can result if the pressure remains high. Success depends on a strict antiinflammatory postoperative regimen and a relatively normal area of episcleral and conjunctival tissue through which the aqueous can drain.

Pupillary block glaucoma

Although posterior synechiae are found in 70% of patients who develop uveitis with scleritis and in 40% of those who lose an eye from this disease, pupillary block glaucoma as the sole reason for the rise in intraocular pressure is rare. The one patient we have seen with this complication responded

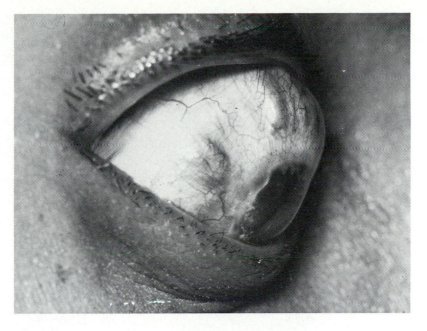

Fig. 66-15 Staphyloma formation in patient with anterior scleritis and persistently raised intraocular pressure. (From Watson, P: Diseases of the sclera and episclera. In Duane, TD, editor: Clinical ophthalmology, vol 4, New York, 1980, Harper & Row, Publishers)

well to a broad iridectomy with division of the synechiae followed by intensive anti-inflammatory therapy.

Neovascular glaucoma

Although we have seen this complication clinically only three times in over 1000 patients with scleral disease, it was found to be present in 31% of eyes removed presumably for the intractable pain often associated with this condition.[12] Scleritis was not even suspected as the diagnosis in 45% of these eyes, and it is possible, therefore, that neovascular glaucoma associated with anterior scleritis resulted from vaso-obliteration but was diagnosed as secondary glaucoma and uveitis. These patients all had deeply cupped discs, vascularization of the iris, and a neovascular membrane in the angle. Molteno[22] implants have been successful in secondary glaucoma following retinal venous occlusion. In the one patient who had a normal sclera where the plate was placed and was able to have the tube inserted, the pressure was reduced and the new vessels regressed. However, this did not, unfortunately, restore the vision.

Glaucoma Associated with Posterior Scleritis

Angle-closure glaucoma caused by choroidal effusion

Angle-closure glaucoma caused by choroidal effusion is a specific entity in posterior scleritis. If the cause is not recognized, the patient may be given inappropriate treatment and even submitted to unnecessary surgery.[25,27]

Scleral inflammation usually involves the anterior segment because the distribution of the anterior ciliary vessels is primarily affected, but because these vessels do supply the eye back to the equator, the granuloma can either start in this region or spread backward to it. If this happens, there is an inflammatory reaction in the region of the ciliary body and swelling of the adjacent tissue, which gives rise to an anterior choroidal effusion, which can be circumferential. This results in an anterior rotation of the ciliary body at the scleral spur and closure of the angle of the anterior chamber. A similar cause has been cited in other cases of anterior choroidal effusion[3,13,31,36] (Fig. 66-16).

The diagnosis is relatively simple if the patient has had anterior scleritis (usually of the diffuse type). Concomitant with the onset of the scleritis, the intraocular pressure rises and the anterior chamber shallows to the extent that it appears gonioscopically entirely occluded, whereas the opposite angle remains wide open. The diagnosis is much more difficult if the anterior scleritis is limited in extent or if the patient does not have a past history. Nevertheless, if a unilateral shallow anterior chamber is noted, this diagnosis should always be kept in mind.

Treatment with pilocarpine is contraindicated. Apart from not working, it actually will make the anterior chamber shallower,[26] thus making the condition worse. Treatment should be directed to the treatment of the scleritis with systemic nonsteroidal antiinflammatory agents (or systemic steroids) and dilation of the pupil with cycloplegics, together

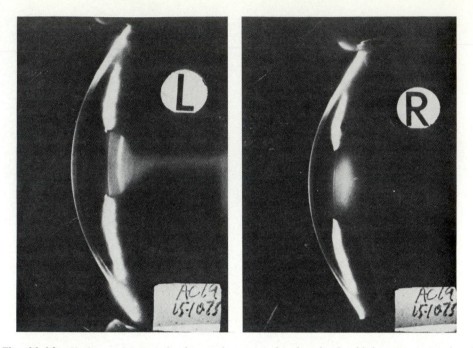

Fig. 66-16 Slit-lamp photograph of normal anterior chamber depth of left eye contrasted with very shallow anterior chamber of right eye in patient who had acute angle-closure attack in right eye. Angle-closure was found to be caused by anterior shift in lens-iris diaphragm resulting from posterior scleritis. (From Watson, PG, and Hazleman, BL: The sclera and systemic disorders, Longon, 1976, WB Saunders Co, Ltd; courtesy Nicholas P. Brown)

with carbonic anhydrase inhibitors if necessary. This course of treatment has so far been universally successful in resolving the acute attack and enables close observation of the posterior scleritis.

Secondary angle-closure glaucoma with PAS formation

Although we have not observed this situation clinically, in two of the eyes examined histologically, the scleritis was entirely posterior and the angle was occluded. It is probable that these patients had ciliary body effusions that were caused by the posterior scleritis but that were not recognized as such. Aided by concomitant mild uveitis, the angle became completely occluded, and intractable glaucoma resulted.

Neovascular glaucoma

Neovascular glaucoma has also not been observed clinically as a complication of posterior scleritis but has been observed in histologic specimens.[38] In the eyes studied, the granulomatous changes were all posterior to the equator and around the disc. Vasculitis was associated with the scleritis, so that it is reasonable to assume that this could have led to the vascular occlusion. There was no histologic evidence that the new vessel forma-

tion was caused by a generalized ischemia of the posterior segment.

Although glaucoma may manifest itself in many forms, it is almost always preventable and certainly treatable, provided care is taken in detection and the scleral inflammation treated early and energetically.

KERATITIS

Glaucoma induced by keratitis unaccompanied by uveitis is a rare event resulting from either direct involvement of the trabecular meshwork by the disease, which affects the cornea, or from the toxic results of the damage to the corneal stroma.

Chemical Burns to the Cornea

The most common corneal injury from chemicals is deliberate assault in which ammonia or lye is thrown at or squirted into the recipient's eyes and face. Caustic soda is widely used in industrial processes, and injuries still occur in spite of regulations requiring the use of protective goggles and clothing. Among other effects, these chemicals, together with chloroform, formalin mechlorethamine hydrochloride, and nitrogen mustards cause a marked rise in intraocular pressure.

The severity of the injury and type of response

depend on the concentration of the chemical and the length of time it is in contact with the cornea.[24] A patient who has been sprayed is immediately afflicted by intense pain, which subsides after 10 to 15 minutes only to be replaced within the hour by more severe pain and a clinical syndrome resembling acute angle-closure glaucoma.

This biphasic response has been thoroughly investigated in chemical burns in rabbits, and it has been shown that as soon as the alkali strikes the cornea, the epithelium is denatured and the collagen contracts, causing a rapid transient rise in intraocular pressure. As the chemical penetrates the cornea, there is an intense generalized ocular inflammatory response with miosis, ocular vasodilation, breakdown of the blood aqueous barrier, and a rise in intraocular pressure that reaches its maximum after 20 to 40 minutes. This pressure rise can be inhibited by polyphloretin phosphate and phenylephrine and has been shown to be a direct result of prostaglandin E and F release. The transient rise in intraocular pressure is also present to a lesser extent in the opposite, uninjured eye.

If the injury is severe, the uveitis and damage to the trabecular meshwork may lead to a late secondary open-angle glaucoma[10]; unfortunately, the ciliary processes are also frequently damaged, and as a result profound hypotension supervenes.

A similar type of secondary open-angle glaucoma has been observed in the few survivors of the mustard gas attacks of World War I. These have all been seen in those who have delayed mustard gas keratitis and peripheral corneal aneurysmal dilation of the vessels and corneal opacities. We have a trabeculectomy specimen from one of these patients in whom the trabecular tissue was well within the specimen, but its structure was almost indistinguishable because of excessive hyalinization.

Glaucoma Associated with Infections of the Cornea

The intraocular pressure will rise in any severe stromal infection whether it is caused by bacteria, virus, or fungus, and more so if the infection is accompanied by uveitis. If the infection is acute, it is possible that the rise in pressure is caused by prostaglandin release and the production of plasmoid aqueous. Generalized corneal and limbal edema will add to the problem through direct involvement of the trabecular meshwork, but it appears that the usual cause is obstruction of the meshwork by cellular exudate combined with some degree of local inflammation.[17]

The most common cause of keratitis with raised intraocular pressure is herpes simplex. Falcon and Williams[11] found that 28% of 183 patients with herpetic keratouveitis had an intraocular pressure of more than 25 mm Hg or a difference of 7 mm Hg in either eye (average 33; range 25 to 50). They found that the intraocular pressure never rose during the initial attack of herpes simplex; glaucoma was found exclusively in those with stromal disease, with 80% having either disciform keratouveitis or herpetic stromal keratouveitis. Five of their patients developed a glaucomatous field defect, and they concluded that the patients with limbitis were more likely to develop glaucoma than the others. They did not find an abnormal steroid response to be the cause of the raised intraocular pressure and as a consequence recommended that treatment with steroids and antiviral cover not be varied because of the glaucoma; rather, the glaucoma should be treated with the usual antiglaucomatous and antiinflammatory agents (such as oxyphenbutazone or indomethacin) as required.

Syphilitic interstitial keratitis has in the past been a potent cause of secondary glaucoma leading to buphthalmos in the infant, limbitis and scleritis in the juvenile, and secondary open- or closed-angle glaucoma as age advances.[8]

Glaucoma Caused by Systemic Syndromes with Corneal Manifestations

The trabecular meshwork occasionally becomes involved in syndromes that affect the cornea. The most common of these is Scheie's syndrome (mucopolysaccharidosis V),[28,29] in which the abnormal mucopolysaccharides have been shown to extend to the angle.

REFERENCES

1. Armaly, MF: Effect of corticosteroids on intraocular fluid dynamics. I. Effect of dexamethasone in the normal eye, Arch Ophthalmol 70:482, 1963
2. Becker, B, and Mills, BW: Corticosteroids and intraocular pressure. Arch Ophthalmol 70:500, 1965
3. Brockhurst, RJ, Schepens, CL, and Okamura, ID: Uveitis. II. Peripheral uveitis: clinical description, complications and differential diagnosis. Am J Ophthalmol 49:1257, 1960
4. Campbell, DM: Episcleritis, Ophthalmic Rec 12:517, 1903
5. Cleary, PE, Watson PG, McGill, JI, and Hamilton, AM: Visual loss due to posterior segment disease in scleritis, Trans Ophthalmol Soc UK 95:297, 1975
6. Duke-Elder, S: The clinical value of cortisone and ACTH in ocular disease, Br J Ophthalmol 35:637, 1951

7. Duke-Elder, S: A series of cases treated locally by cortisone (report to Medical Research Council), Br J Ophthalmol 35:672, 1951

8. Duke-Elder, S: System of ophthalmology, vol 11, Diseases of the lens and vitreous; glaucoma and hypotony, St. Louis, 1969, The CV Mosby Co

9. Duke-Elder, S, and Leigh, AG: Diseases of the outer eye, vol 8, part 2. In Duke-Elder, S: System of ophthalmology, St. Louis, 1965, The CV Mosby Co

10. Duke-Elder, S, and MacFaul, PA: Injuries, vol 14. In Duke-Elder, S: System of ophthalmology, St. Louis, 1972, The CV Mosby Co

11. Falcon, MG, and Williams, HP: Herpes simplex, kerato-uveitis and glaucoma, Trans Ophthalmol Soc UK 98:101, 1978

12. Fraunfelder, FT, and Watson PG: Evaluation of eyes enucleated for scleritis, Br J Ophthalmol 60:227, 1976

13. Gass, JDM: Retinal detachment and narrow angle glaucoma secondary to pseudo tumour of the uveal tract, Am J Ophthalmol 64:612, 1967

14. Givner, I: Uncommon complications of scleritis, Eye, Ear, Nose and Throat Mon 32;515, 1953

15. Grierson, I, Lee, WR, and Abraham, S: Effects of pilocarpine on the morphology of human outflow apparatus, Br J Ophthalmol 62:302, 1978

16. Harbin, T, and Pollack, J: Glaucoma in episcleritis, Arch Ophthalmol 93:948, 1975

17. Hogan, MJ, Kimura, ST, and Thygeson, P: Pathology of herpes simplex kerato-iritis. Am J Ophthalmol 57:551, 1964

18. Lloyd-Jones, D, Tokarewicz, A, and Watson, PG: Clinical evaluation of clobetasone butyrate eye drops in episcleritis, Br J Ophthalmol 65:641, 1981

19. Mackenzie, W: A practical treatise on the diseases of the eye, London, 1830, Longman

20. Mann, WA, and Markson, DE: A case of recurrent iritis and episcleritis on a rheumatic basis: treated with A.C.T.H., Am J Ophthalmol 33:459, 1950

21. McGavin, DD, et al. Episcleritis and scleritis: a study of the clinical manifestations and association with rheumatoid arthritis, Br J Ophthalmol 60:192, 1976

22. Meyer, PA, et al: Pulsed corneal and scleral disease, Eye 1:487, 1987

23. Molteno, ACB, Straughan, JL, and Ancker, E: Long tube implants in the management of glaucoma. South Afr Med J 50:1062, 1976

24. Paterson, CA, and Pfister, PR: Intraocular pressure changes after alkali burns, Arch Ophthalmol 91:211, 1974

25. Philips, CD: Angle closure glaucoma secondary to ciliary body swelling, Arch Ophthalmol 92:287, 1974

26. Poinooswamy, D, Nagasubramanian, S, and Brown, NAP: The effects of pilocarpine on the visual acuity and on the dimensions of the cornea and anterior chamber, Br J Ophthalmol 60:678, 1976

27. Quinlan, MP, and Hitchings, RA: Angle closure glaucoma secondary to posterior scleritis, Br J Ophthalmol 62:330, 1978

28. Rasteiro, A: Scheie's syndrome, Exp Ophthalmol Coimbra 3:62, 1977

29. Scheie, HG, Hambrick, GW, and Barness, LA: A newly recognized "forme fruste" of Hurler's disease (gargoylism), Am J Ophthalmol 53:753, 1962

30. van der Hoeve, J: Scleromalacia perforans, Ned Tijdschr Geneeskd 75:4733, 1931

31. Vogt, F: Scleritis in connection with choroidal detachment in rheumatic patients, Szemeszet 115:217, 1978

32. Wardrop, J: An account of the rheumatic inflammation of the eye with observation on the treatment of the disease, Medico Chir Trans 10:1, 1818

33. Watson, PG, and Bovey, E: Anterior segment fluorescein angiography in the diagnosis of scleral inflammation, Ophthalmology 92:1, 1985

34. Watson, PG, and Grierson, I: The place of trabeculectomy in the treatment of glaucoma, Ophthalmology 88:175, 1981

35. Watson, PG, and Hayreh, SS: Scleritis and episcleritis, Br J Ophthalmol 60:163, 1976

36. Watson, PG, and Hazleman, BL: The sclera and systemic disorders, London, 1976, WB Saunders Co, Ltd.

37. Watson, PG, et al: Treatment of episcleritis: a double blind trial comparing beta-methasone 0.1%, oxyphenbutazone 10% and placebo eye ointments, Br J Ophthalmol 57:866, 1973

38. Wilhelmus, K, Grierson, I, and Watson, PG: Histopathologic and clinical associations of scleritis and glaucoma, Am J Ophthalmol 91:697, 1981

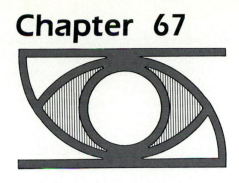

Chapter 67

Glaucoma Associated with Uveitis

Theodore Krupin
Marianne E. Feitl

Glaucoma secondary to uveitis presents a number of problems to the ophthalmologist. Although some forms of uveitis may be classified into clinical entities, most intraocular inflammations are nonspecific and can be broadly described only as anterior or posterior, granulomatous or nongranulomatous. Medical therapy is usually directed at relieving the resulting inflammation and elevated intraocular pressure and rarely at eliminating the underlying cause of the uveitis. The chronic and recurrent nature of the inflammation may produce permanent structural changes that in turn alter aqueous humor dynamics. It may be difficult to pinpoint the actual cause for the intraocular pressure elevation or to determine whether it results from active inflammation, insufficient antiinflammatory therapy, corticosteroid therapy, insufficient antiglaucoma therapy, or permanent changes in ocular structure. Secondary glaucoma can present as either open-angle or angle-closure glaucoma or as a combination of the two. To diagnose and manage the glaucoma properly, one must take into consideration all of these possibilities.

PATHOPHYSIOLOGY OF ELEVATED INTRAOCULAR PRESSURE

Inflammation

Trabecular block or dysfunction

Uveitis is usually associated with ciliary body inflammation and hyposecretion of aqueous humor. This may mask the effects of uveitis on the aqueous outflow channels, and intraocular pres-

sure may vary depending on whether outflow obstruction or aqueous humor hyposecretion predominates. The obstruction of outflow channels can be caused by swelling or dysfunction of trabecular sheets or endothelial cells or by the accumulation of inflammatory material in the outflow channels. Even though endothelial cells lining the trabeculum and juxtacanalicular tissue can be mobilized to remove inflammatory products from the outflow channels, they themselves can cause obstruction. Fibrin, white blood cell aggregates, and macrophages can also block outflow channels. In addition, normal serum components may become adsorbed or entrapped in the aqueous outflow system and cause obstruction.[19] There is limited capacity of the trabecular endothelial cells to regenerate, and each bout of recurrent inflammation may reduce the effectiveness of the trabecular meshwork as a biologic filter and produce additional permanent damage.

Prostaglandins

Prostaglandins, a group of naturally occurring lipid-soluble fatty acids with widespread distribution in mammalian tissues and diverse pharmacologic properties, can be involved in acute ocular inflammation. Prostaglandins can produce many of the signs of ocular inflammation, including vasodilation, miosis, and increased vascular permeability.[7] In addition, topical administration of prostaglandin E both elevates intraocular pressure and increases total outflow facility.[55] This suggests that

1205

an increase in aqueous humor production or a breakdown of the blood-aqueous barrier is responsible for the elevation of intraocular pressure. The suggestion is supported by the finding that topical administration of arachidonic acid, a precursor of prostaglandin E_2, also increases intraocular pressure, total outflow facility, and aqueous humor protein.[101] Inhibitors of prostaglandin synthesis, such as aspirin or indomethacin, block the responses after application of topical arachidonic acid. This may be of particular clinical interest, since prostaglandin-like activity may be present in the aqueous humor of patients with acute anterior uveitis.[17] Prostaglandins also may be an etiologic factor in glaucomatocyclitic crises.[79] If prostaglandins are partly responsible for many of the clinical signs in acute anterior uveitis, then substances that antagonize either their synthesis or action may be of value in controlling these diseases.

Altered vascular permeability

The structural changes that occur after ocular inflammatory disease may be permanent and could predispose the eye to subsequent recurrent inflammation. Altered vascular permeability may be present months after the cessation of active inflammation. The presence of aqueous protein in an apparently quiescent phase of chronic recurrent uveitis may be due to disruptions of the blood-aqueous barrier, including the ciliary epithelium.[39] This in turn may alter the normal mechanisms for transporting prostaglandins and other substances from the eye.[9]

Structural Changes

Uveitis, acute or chronic, can cause structural changes that lead to glaucoma. Clinical signs of acute iridocyclitis include perilimbal vascular injection, miosis, and photophobia. As stated, disruption of the blood-aqueous barrier results in cells and protein (flare) in the aqueous humor and anterior portion of the vitreous. Keratic precipitates are present. Corneal endothelial changes occur, including specular microscopic findings of intracellular and intercellularly located blackout areas, larger dark defects spanning several endothelial cells and bright, irregular patchy areas superimposed on the cell images.[1,92] The inflammation causes more than mere trabecular damage. The presence of albumin and fibrin in aqueous humor can result in posterior synechiae between the iris and lens or peripheral anterior synechiae in the iridocorneal angle.

Posterior synechiae

Adhesions of the iris to the lens occur at an early stage in the exudative types of iritis with a heavy aqueous flare, first by the formation of fibrinous adhesions and later by fibrovascular organization (see Plate IV, Fig. 5). The pupillary margin may be partially or completely involved. If the posterior synechiae are complete, they prevent aqueous humor from passing from the posterior to the anterior chamber through the pupil. This causes increased pressure in the posterior chamber and a forward ballooning of the iris periphery (iris bombé). Anterior chamber depth is normal at the pupil, but elsewhere it is shallowed by the iris bombé. Forward movement of the peripheral iris can produce acute angle-closure glaucoma.

Peripheral anterior synechiae

Peripheral anterior synechiae, adhesions between the iris and the trabecular meshwork or cornea, can form as a result of the inflammatory process. Synechia formation can be related to swelling of the iris periphery with the formation of adhesions, protein transudation and exudation in the angle (which pull the iris toward the cornea), or bridging of the angle by large keratic precipitates. Synechiae resulting from iritis are not uniform in shape or in the height of their trabecular attachment. They may be conical, cylindrical, or mound-like areas alternating with areas of completely open angle. The synechiae of intraocular inflammation differ from the synechiae of primary pupillary block, where iris segments are attached in a line parallel to Schwalbe's line. Although the iridocorneal angle can be closed by peripheral anterior synechiae, it is often difficult to estimate the extent to which the decrease in outflow facility is due to synechiae or to inflammatory damage to the trabecular meshwork.

MANAGEMENT

Medical treatment of glaucoma secondary to active anterior uveitis is directed toward controlling the inflammation and preventing its consequences, as well as lowering the elevated intraocular pressure. Efforts are made to dilate the pupil and decrease the inflammatory reaction so that damage, scarring, and visual loss are minimized. In all inflammatory processes, one hopes that the damaged outflow mechanism will restore itself to normal. As long as the outflow channels are impaired, one should attempt to maintain the intraocular pressure within normal limits through antiglaucoma therapy. If medical therapy fails to control the elevated intraocular pressure, surgery may become necessary.

Pupillary Dilation

Cycloplegic and sympathomimetic agents are used to break or prevent the formation of posterior synechiae and to prevent the development of a bound-down miotic pupil. They also reduce patient discomfort by decreasing spasms of the ciliary muscle and iris sphincter. Scopolamine, homatropine, and atropine are effective long-acting cycloplegic agents. If only a short duration of action is required, tropicamide or cyclopentolate can be used. Phenylephrine 2.5% or 10% may be added as a mydriatic to gain further effect of direct sympathetic stimulation on the iris dilator muscle.

Corticosteroids

The introduction of corticosteroids revolutionized the management of intraocular inflammation. Almost all inflammatory reactions, regardless of cause, can be inhibited nonselectively by steroids. Inhibition of the inflammatory response may improve outflow facility if the inflammation has caused trabecular swelling and increased outflow resistance. However, corticosteroids may not affect the underlying physiologic and biologic responses that caused the inflammation, and the eye often reverts to its original condition on their withdrawal.

The nonspecific antiinflammatory effect of corticosteroids on uveal inflammation has been ascribed to a decrease in capillary permeability,[18,71] to suppression of cellular exudates by interference with margination and "sticking" qualities of leukocytes,[18] and to an inhibition of the formation of granulation tissue.[70] Corticosteroids also exert a stabilizing effect on intracellular lysosomes associated with inflammatory responses.[126] This action may explain the inhibition of prostaglandin E release by antiinflammatory steroids.[21]

The antiinflammatory effect of corticosteroids on ocular structures can be obtained by topical, subconjunctival, or parenteral administration. Corticosteroids penetrate the cornea and sclera after topical administration. Penetration is increased in the inflamed eye. Experimental studies in rabbits suggest that phosphate derivatives may be less effective than acetate derivatives as topical antiinflammatory agents.[66] Most instances of anterior segment inflammation can be controlled with either topical dexamethasone 0.1% or prednisolone

1%. Tissue accumulation increases with the frequency of administration, and the drops should be instilled every 1 to 2 hours during the acute inflammatory process. When amelioration of the inflammation becomes evident, the time interval of administration may be lengthened. Frequently, the inflammatory reaction can be controlled by a minimum dose of 3 to 4 drops daily.

Although corticosteroids have been shown to be effective in relieving inflammation, their administration can result in other ocular complications, particularly increased intraocular pressure and cataract formation.[5,90] These complications can occur regardless of whether the corticosteroid is administered topically or systemically. Approximately 20% to 30% of the population may show an elevation of intraocular pressure after the topical administration of corticosteroids.[6] Steroid-induced elevation of intraocular pressure is extremely rare before 10 days of four-times-a-day topical dexamethasone administration. Certain corticosteroids (such as medrysone) show less tendency to elevate intraocular pressure but may not be as effective in reducing inflammation.[102] Fluoromethalone, either as a 0.1% or 0.25% suspension, is an effective antiinflammatory agent that is less likely to increase the intraocular pressure than is 0.1% dexamethasone.[54,121] It may be difficult to determine whether an elevated intraocular pressure is caused by the original disease process or by topical corticosteroids. If the inflammation occurs only in one eye, the corticosteroid can be tested on the noninvolved eye.

The increase in intraocular pressure during the steroid therapy may not necessarily be a side effect of corticosteroid administration but may in some cases be secondary to the elimination of inflammation-induced hyposecretion and a return of a normal rate of aqueous production by the ciliary body. Therefore, normal aqueous humor production in the face of a persistent inflammation-induced reduction in outflow facility results in an elevated intraocular pressure.

If the inflammation does not respond adequately to topical steroids, either subconjunctival or systemic corticosteroid therapy may be required. Subconjunctival or sub-Tenon's injection is effective in delivering high concentrations of steroids locally to the eye, resulting in a reduction of both systemic concentrations and potential systemic complications. The duration of the therapeutic effect may last for 1 to 6 weeks. Dexamethasone phosphate 4 mg (1 ml), prednisolone succinate 25 mg (1 ml), triamcinolone acetonide 4 mg (1 ml), and methylprednisolone acetate 20 mg (0.5 ml) are suitable steroid preparations. One should avoid using long-acting repository corticosteroids because they may produce a delayed rise in intraocular pressure.[33] Systemic corticosteroids should be reserved for special situations when the other routes of administration have been ineffective. The physician should use the oral preparation with which he has the most experience. We prefer prednisone, starting at 80 to 100 mg daily. This is maintained until evidence of clinical remission occurs, at which time the daily dosage is decreased by 10 to 20 mg every second or third day. The guiding principle for steroid therapy, either topical or systemic, is to use the minimum dose for the minimum time required to inhibit the inflammatory response.

The use of either systemic[90] or topical[5] corticosteroids for a prolonged period may induce posterior subcapsular cataracts. The systemic administration of corticosteroids may result in iatrogenic adrenal cortical insufficiency. Prolonged topical administration can cause considerable systemic absorption with resultant decreased plasma cortisol levels.[65] Titration of the corticosteroid is the most effective method of reducing steroid complications while controlling the inflammation. Not all inflammatory conditions respond to corticosteroids, (e.g., Fuchs' heterochromic cyclitis), and it is not unusual in other forms of uveitis to reach a state where there is a low-grade breakdown of the blood-aqueous barrier evidenced by flare, which does not respond to steroids. Excessive use of topical corticosteroids under these conditions increases the risk of steroid-induced cataract or elevated intraocular pressure without any benefit of the steroid for the uveitis. Also, corticosteroids themselves may induce anterior uveitis.[64] This is nongranulomatous and appears after termination of the steroid. If uveitis recurs on withdrawal of topical corticosteroids, the possibility of iatrogenic inflammation indistinguishable from that of the original ailment must be considered.

Nonsteroidal Antiinflammatory Therapy

Systemic nonsteroidal antiinflammatory agents are useful in the treatment of a number of inflammatory disorders. These agents may be effective in controlling anterior and posterior uveitis and can either reduce the dose or replace the need for corticosteroid therapy.[78] These agents produce their effects by inhibiting the prostaglandin cascade.

Immunosuppressive Therapy

Unfortunately, corticosteroid side effects may preclude prolonged use. Also, steroid therapy may fail to control the inflammatory process and prevent progressive ocular damage. In this event, the ophthalmologist may wish to consider, under appropriate medical direction, immunosuppressive therapy. Immunologic mechanisms are involved in the pathogenesis of endogenous uveitis.[99] Immunogenetic factors may influence either the susceptibility or expression of inflammatory eye diseases.[114,134] Immunosuppressive therapy has been employed with some success in a variety of eyes with chronic uveitis either intolerant or unresponsive to corticosteroids. Methotrexate[141] and combined low-dose prednisone with azathioprine or chlorambucil[4] result in a response rate of 60% to 70%. Cyclosporine A, an anti-T-cell immunosuppressive agent, may be effective in reducing severe intraocular inflammatory disease which is unresponsive to steroid or conventional immunosuppressive therapy.[88] Renal dysfunction is the most frequent side effect associated with cyclosporine.[133]

Antiglaucoma Therapy

Medical therapy

Topical mydriatics (phenylephrine), cycloplegics (atropine, scopolamine, cyclopentolate, or tropicamide), and corticosteroids are used in the treatment of the uveitis. The cycloplegics reduce the pain characteristic of iridocyclitis caused by relaxation of the inflamed ciliary body and iris muscles. These drugs may also help to stabilize a disrupted blood-aqueous barrier, thus reducing the outpouring of protein and inflammatory cells into the aqueous. Furthermore, atropine is useful in lowering intraocular pressure by increasing the rate of pressure-independent or uveoscleral outflow.[8] Movement of the pupil reduces formation of posterior synechiae, which could result in pupillary block; and pupillary dilation reduces the likelihood of a bound-down miotic pupil if synechiae do occur.

Therapy to lower intraocular pressure is primarily aimed at reducing aqueous humor formation and may include a topical beta-adrenergic antagonist, as well as a systemic carbonic anhydrase inhibitor. Occasionally, hyperosmotic agents may be necessary. Miotics are generally to be avoided because they may cause discomfort by aggravating ciliary spasm, may allow formation of posterior synechiae or an inflammatory membrane, and may even increase inflammation by accelerating the release of enzymes from polymorphonuclear leukocytes.[44] In addition, miotics are usually ineffective in improving reduced outflow facility when this results from inflammation. If the iridocorneal angle is open, epinephrine may be included in an effort to further facilitate aqueous humor outflow. In addition, it is possible that epinephrine may contribute to the reduction of aqueous humor secretion.[116]

Surgical therapy

Medical therapy may fail to control the secondary glaucoma, in which case surgery may become necessary. Iridectomy is the procedure of choice if pupillary block is a contributing factor. Rarely will maximum mydriasis or miosis terminate the pupillary block by mechanical lysis of posterior synechiae. Although iridectomy may not succeed in all such cases, it does not alter the prognosis if a subsequent filtering procedure becomes necessary. Iridectomy is a much safer and simpler procedure than filtration surgery, especially in inflamed eyes. A laser iridectomy, either with the argon or Nd:YAG, can be difficult to perform secondary to uveitis-induced iris congestion and edema. Also, the inflammatory process may become more active after laser surgery with an increased tendency for the iridectomy to close. Close follow-up is mandatory and repeated laser treatment may be necessary to maintain patency of the iridectomy. Surgical iridectomy should be reserved for cases of failure to achieve laser iris penetration or if the laser iridectomy does not remain patent.

Filtration surgery is less successful in eyes with preexisting uveitis, in which an increased postoperative inflammatory reaction and prolonged hypotony may increase the rate of failure. Filtration surgery is indicated when the intraocular pressure cannot be controlled medically at a level sufficient to prevent damage to the optic nerve or visual field. Standard filtration surgery (thermal sclerostomy or sclerectomy) has been reported to be more successful than filtering surgery under a scleral flap (trabeculectomy).[37] A modified goniotomy (trabeculodialysis) has been successful in approximately 60% of eyes with glaucoma secondary to uveitis.[38,52] In this technique, an irrigating goniotomy needle is introduced into the anterior chamber. Under direct visualization with a surgical goniotomy contact lens, the needle is passed across the chamber into the inferior iridocorneal angle. Peripheral anterior synechiae are retracted by depressing the base of the iris, and an incision is made just posterior to Schwalbe's line and the trabeculum retracted. The

use of seton devices at the time of surgery has been reported to be successful in secondary uveitic glaucoma.[63,84] The postoperative use of antimetabolites (e.g., subconjunctivally injected 5-fluorouracil) may improve filtration success in eyes with uveitic glaucoma (see Chapter 31). Postoperative high-dose corticosteroids (topical and subconjunctival or systemic) are often necessary.

SPECIFIC INFLAMMATORY CONDITIONS

Anterior segment inflammation accounts for a large percentage of secondary glaucomas. Most conditions are nonspecific and have intervals of exacerbation and remission. Intraocular pressure may be acutely elevated, depending on the balance of trabecular impairment and ciliary body hyposecretion. In addition, pupillary block with obstruction of aqueous flow from the posterior to the anterior chamber may result in secondary acute closed-angle glaucoma. If the inflammatory process is chronic, it may result in damage to the trabecular meshwork and in secondary glaucoma. Although most inflammatory conditions are purely ocular, some are associated with systemic disease.

Glaucoma in Fuchs' Syndrome of Heterochromic Cyclitis

Fuchs' syndrome, a mild, chronic form of cyclitis associated with heterochromia iridis, often with cataracts and sometimes with glaucoma, was first recognized by Lawrence[68] in 1853 but was described by Fuchs[25] in 1906. It comprises approximately 2% of all cases of uveitis.[60] Fuchs' heterochromic cyclitis appears most frequently in the third and fourth decades of life. Men and women are equally affected.[22] The onset is insidious, and the clinical course is chronic but usually mild. Pain, irritation, photophobia, and redness of the affected eye are absent; and the disease is usually present for a long time before it is discovered. More observant patients may note the heterochromia, which develops gradually.

Signs

The fully developed syndrome presents with the triad of heterochromia, cyclitis, and cataract. **Heterochromia.** Heterochromia, which increases slowly over the years, is more noticeable when the irides are brown. Typically, the hypochromic eye is the affected eye. However, occasionally the involved eye may be darker (heterochromia inversa) because of iris stromal atrophy exposing the pigment epithelium. Stromal iris atrophy begins at the pupillary margin and spreads to the sphincter and iris periphery. This results in the characteristic moth-eaten appearance of the pupillary region and the lacunae-like holes of the iris by retroillumination. Atrophy leads to exposure of the iris radial vessels. In one third of the cases characteristic, translucent, grayish-white nodules are present on the anterior surface of the iris, especially in the sphincter area. Although most cases are unilateral, from 3.5%[23] to 13%[22] may be bilateral. It is almost always possible to recognize Fuchs' syndrome without considering the heterochromia if a careful ophthalmologic examination is made.

Cyclitis. The one constant feature of this syndrome is very mild, chronic cyclitis. Aqueous flare and cells are always minimal in the face of an abnormally permeable blood-aqueous barrier.[50] Posterior synechiae never occur except after intraocular surgery. Keratic precipitates, seen typically in the pupillary area and in the lower portion of the cornea, are a constant finding and are characteristically small or medium, round or star-shaped, sharply circumscribed, never confluent, and white. Fine filaments may be present between the precipitates. Of diagnostic value is the presence of anterior vitreous opacities, which appear biomicroscopically as white dots rather than as the brownish ones seen in other types of uveitis.[132]

Cataract. Cataract represents a frequent but late complication of Fuchs' syndrome, which limits its value as a diagnostic sign. The cataract is a complicated type that starts in the posterior cortex beneath the capsule. It forms as a result of the long-standing cyclitis. Rapid progression can occur many years after the first cataract symptoms. In the hypermature stage, glaucomatous complications (phacolytic glaucoma) may be observed. Cataract surgery in patients with Fuchs' syndrome appears to be only slightly more complicated than routine surgery for senile cataracts. Elective removal of cataractous lenses in patients with this disease should not be delayed because of fear of a poor prognosis.[118]

Secondary glaucoma

The only serious late complication in Fuchs' syndrome is secondary glaucoma, with an incidence of 5% to 13% in unilateral cases and 25% to 33% in bilateral cases.[40] It usually resembles chronic open-angle glaucoma, with reduced outflow facility and normal episcleral venous pressure. The contralateral uninvolved eye may have abnormal tonometric or tonographic findings.[32]

Gonioscopic examination of the chamber angle may reveal the presence of multiple fine blood vessels, both radially and concentrically arranged, in the region of the trabecular meshwork. This may account for the apparently pathognomonic phenomenon in heterochromic cyclitis of a filiform hemorrhage in the angle after puncture of the anterior chamber. This usually occurs in the angle 180 degrees away from the site of puncture.[3]

In most instances, the glaucoma secondary to Fuchs' heterochromic cyclitis is a complication of the chronic inflammation. However, rubeosis iridis with secondary neovascular (hemorrhagic) glaucoma can occur in this disease.[72] Despite the favorable results of cataract removal, glaucoma may be a frequent postoperative complication.[32] However, it is difficult to assess the relation of glaucoma to cataract surgery because glaucoma is frequently encountered as a late complication in the natural course of this disease.

Diagnosis

Like other syndromes, Fuchs' heterochromic cyclitis can be diagnosed when some of its characteristic manifestations are missing. Heterochromia is not a constant sign, and the disease can be identified in its absence. The character and course of the cyclitis identifies the disease (i.e., the quiet, white eye with mild iridocyclitis, minimal aqueous flare and cells, vitreous opacities, small white discrete keratic precipitates, and total absence of synechia). Gonioscopic findings of vessels and the occurrence of an angle hemorrhage after anterior chamber puncture may be helpful in substantiating the diagnosis.

Fuchs' syndrome must be differentiated from the heterochromia secondary to uveitis of other causes in which there may be patchy iris stromal atrophy and posterior synechiae. None of the tests made in the usually exhaustive workup of a patient with uveitis are of any value in the diagnosis or management of heterochromic cyclitis. Therefore, prompt recognition saves both the examiner and the patient much time and expense.

Glaucomatocyclitic crisis must be considered in the differential diagnosis of Fuchs' syndrome. Three of nine patients in the original report by Posner and Schlossman[105] had definite heterochromia. Essential iris atrophy also must be considered in the differential diagnosis (see Chapter 54). An eccentric pupil, ectropion uveae, and progressive formation of peripheral anterior synechia should eliminate any diagnostic confusion.

Etiology

The cause of heterochromic cyclitis is unknown. The association with status dysraphicus or syringomyelia lends support to the theory of a degenerative or abiotrophic lesion.[98] Pharmacologic studies have demonstrated a sympathetic denervation of the iris.[24,49] This sympathetic disturbance, whatever it may be, leads to changes in the blood vessels and atrophy of the iris stroma and chromatophores. Heterochromic cyclitis has been observed in families and in identical twins.[77]

Pathology

Alterations of the iris are predominantly degenerative. There is a decrease in the number of stromal melanocytes; degeneration of the iris pigment epithelium, especially the posterior layer; and thickening and hyalinization of the iris blood vessels with narrowing of their lumens.[26] Electron microscopy and computerized image analysis of iris biopsies demonstrate that the depigmentation is secondary to a reduction in the number of deep stromal melanocytes, as well as a decrease in melanosomal size.[81] Chronic, nongranulomatous iridocyclitis is present with active trabeculitis characterized by the presence of lymphocytes and plasma cells in the trabecular meshwork and an inflammatory membrane over the meshwork. Rubeosis of the iridocorneal angle is patchy and discontinuous.[100]

Management

Corticosteroids, whether administered topically or parenterally, are of no value in the treatment of heterochromic cyclitis. Indeed, long-term corticosteroid therapy may hasten cataract development and/or result in steroid-induced glaucoma. As stated, cataract surgery in patients with Fuchs' syndrome is only slightly more complicated than routine surgery for senile cataracts. The secondary glaucoma may be difficult to control medically. If medical therapy is ineffective in maintaining the intraocular pressure at a level that prevents optic nerve or visual field damage, then filtration surgery becomes necessary. Patients with Fuchs' syndrome and neovascular glaucoma are managed as outlined in Chapter 60.

Glaucomatocyclitic Crises (Posner-Schlossman Syndrome)

The syndrome of glaucomatocyclitic crises occupies a unique and important position among the many and heterogeneous types of glaucoma associated with uveitis. The syndrome was first fully described by Posner and Schlossman in 1948.[105] The condition typically affects individuals 20 to 50 years old and is seldom seen after the age of 60. The patient generally gives a history of recurrent attacks of unilateral blurred vision and halos caused by corneal edema. Symptoms are remarkably few and slight in relation to the height of the intraocular pressure. Some episodes may be asymptomatic. There seems to be an association of glaucomatocyclitic crises with primary open-angle glaucoma.[53]

Signs

The features of glaucomatocyclitic crises as described by Posner and Schlossman are listed here.[105-106] A number of cases have since been reported that deviate from this description.

1. Unilateral involvement
2. Recurrent attacks of mild cyclitis
3. Findings of a slight decrease in vision, elevated intraocular pressure, open angles, and a few keratic precipitates; corneal edema, heterochromia, and a larger pupil on the affected side in some patients
4. Duration of crises from a few hours to a few weeks
5. Normal visual fields and optic discs
6. Between attacks all tests within normal limits, including intraocular pressure, outflow facility, and all provocative tests

Unilateral involvement. The process is usually unilateral with recurrent involvement of the same eye. Occasionally, bilateral cases are seen, with both eyes involved at the same time or on different occasions.[53,74]

Recurrent mild cyclitis. A history of recurrent attacks of variable frequency is common. Inflammatory signs are minimal, with occasional mild conjunctival injection. The signs of cyclitis do not precede glaucoma. Posterior synechiae are never found.

Attack. The most common presenting symptom is slight discomfort, but as a rule the patient does not complain of pain even at the height of the attack. Blurring of vision and halos may occur if the intraocular pressure is high and corneal edema is present. The affected eye has a larger pupil during an attack. The most frequently observed initial intraocular pressures are between 40 and 60 mm Hg, and the iridocorneal angle is open. There is only a trace of aqueous flare and a slight increase in the number of aqueous cells. Clearing of the corneal edema with topical glycerin may be necessary to observe these anterior chamber findings. Keratic precipitates are generally noted within 3 days of the onset of the attack and begin to disappear soon after they are formed. They are small, discrete, well defined, nonpigmented, flat, and round. There are seldom more than 25 precipitates, which tend to accumulate in the lower third of the cornea. Fresh precipitates may appear, however, with each exacerbation of the hypertension. Heterochromia, which was observed in three of the original nine cases studied by Posner and Schlossman,[105] is not characteristic of the syndrome. The duration of the elevated intraocular pressure can last from a few hours to several weeks.

Aqueous humor dynamics. Tonographic studies indicate a significant reduction in outflow facility during the attack.[28] The hypertension is also associated with a significant increase in the rate of aqueous humor formation.[120] The transfer coefficient of fluorescein in the anterior chamber by flow (volume of aqueous flowing into and out of the anterior chamber per unit time) and by diffusion (diffusional exchange between the anterior chamber and blood) are increased during attacks of glaucomatocyclitic crises.[85] During remission, both coefficients return to normal.

Relationship to primary open-angle glaucoma. Between attacks, the affected eye has normal intraocular pressure and outflow facility. However, in some patients there may be an association of glaucomatocyclitic crises with primary open-angle glaucoma. Patients with this syndrome have a higher than normal incidence of high-corticosteroid responsiveness to topical steroids, similar to patients with primary open-angle glaucoma.[53,107] A number of patients deviate from the original clinical description. These patients show, between crises, an elevated intraocular pressure, decreased outflow facility, cupping of the optic nerve head, and visual field loss in the nonaffected, as well as in the involved eye.[53,97,108] Careful follow-up of both eyes in patients with glaucomatocyclitic crises for evidence of primary open-angle glaucoma is important.

Diagnosis

The Posner-Schlossman syndrome represents a clinical entity that must be differentiated from other forms of glaucoma. Gonioscopy demonstrates an open iridocorneal angle in contrast to acute angle-closure glaucoma. In this syndrome, the glaucoma does not appear to be a result or complication of the uveitis, but both manifestations are concomitant expressions of a single disease entity. Absent are signs of glaucoma secondary to uveitis, such as posterior synechiae, ciliary injection, small and irregular pupils, numerous aqueous cells and distinct aqueous flare, pigmented keratic precipitates, and peripheral anterior synechiae. The glaucoma may be secondary to a direct inflammatory effect on the trabecular meshwork—a trabeculitis. Differentiation from heterochromic cyclitis is discussed earlier in the chapter.

Etiology

The mechanism responsible for the production of glaucomatocyclitic crises is obscure. A possible allergic factor has been entertained.[125] Recently, prostaglandins, particularly prostaglandin E, have been found in high concentrations in aqueous humor during the attack and within normal limits during the remission.[79] In rabbit eyes, prostaglandin E increases blood-aqueous barrier permeability and ultrafiltration in association with the elevation of intraocular pressure.[86] The increase in flow and diffusion coefficients for fluorescein in human eyes with glaucomatocyclitic crises is consistent with the observation of the response of animal eyes to prostaglandin E. The findings by angiography of iris congestion and fluorescein leakage at the pupillary border are also consistent with a prostaglandin-mediated response.[108] However, elevated prostaglandins, which in rabbits increase outflow facility, do not account for the reduced outflow facility in glaucomatocyclitic crises.

Management

A glaucomatocyclitic crisis is a self-limited glaucoma that usually subsides spontaneously regardless of treatment. Since the duration of the attack varies, it is difficult to provide well-matched control cases for drug effect studies. Topical corticosteroids may be effective in controlling the inflammatory process[125] but may elevate the intraocular pressure further. In the phase of high intraocular pressure, the use of systemic carbonic anhydrase inhibitors or topical therapy with epinephrine or beta blockers usually reduces the intraocular pressure to normal.

Antiglaucoma therapy does not prevent recurrences and is not necessary between attacks. Prolonged treatment with corticosteroids should be avoided because it may elicit a hypertensive ocular response in high-corticosteroid responders and complicate the condition.

Indomethacin, which inhibits the synthesis of prostaglandin E_2 from arachidonic acid, may be an effective treatment. Oral indomethacin, 75 to 150 mg/day, has been reported by Masuda et al.[79] to decrease intraocular pressure faster than the combination of acetazolamide and topical epinephrine and/or dexamethasone. These same authors have reported that a subconjunctival injection of polyphloretin phosphate, an inhibitor of prostaglandin E_2 effects, reduces intraocular pressure within a few hours. The effectiveness of prophylactic administration of prostaglandin synthesis inhibitors (indomethacin or aspirin) in preventing recurrent attacks is unknown. Glaucoma surgical procedures are not effective in preventing recurrences.

Glaucoma Associated with Syphilis

Ocular involvement may result from congenital syphilis (infection of the fetus in utero) or from acquired adult disease. The association between secondary glaucoma and congenital syphilitic interstitial keratitis was first made by Hutchinson.[42] Glaucoma can occur with the early iritis or during the acute phase of interstitial keratitis and uveitis. After healing of the cornea, intraocular pressure elevation may not become a problem until years later.

Congenital syphilis

Congenital syphilis is caused by the transplacental transmission of the *Treponema pallidum* organism from the mother to the fetus. It usually occurs after the fourth gestational month, and approximately 70% of infants exposed to the organism who are born alive will develop the disease. Early congenital syphilis can cause a variety of systemic signs and symptoms, including maculopapular rash, mucopurulent discharge from the nose (snuffles), osteochrondritis and multiple fractures, meningitis, fever, anemia, hepatosplenomegaly with jaundice, nephritis, and pneumonitis. Ocular findings include acute and chronic iritis, interstitial keratitis, chorioretinitis ("salt and pepper retinopathy"), retinal periphlebitis, optic neuritis, and secondary cataracts. Pupillary abnormalities and optic atrophy may occur if neurosyphilis results. Acute iritis may be present at birth but more commonly begins when the infant is about 6 months of age.

The most characteristic ocular lesion of congenital syphilis is interstitial keratitis. This abnormality, together with peg teeth (Hutchinson's incisors, adult teeth) and labyrinthine deafness, form Hutchinson's triad. The keratitis, however, may be the only physical sign of the syphilitic condition.

Interstitial keratitis, which occurs in about 15% of cases, forms one of the late manifestations of congenital syphilis. It commonly appears between the sixth and twelfth years. While it may at first be unilateral, the condition becomes bilateral in at least 90% of patients. Its onset is heralded by lacrimation and photophobia. Corneal edema, infiltrates, and vascularization of the deep corneal layers are characteristic. Vessel formation may be so marked as to give the cornea a pink or "salmon patch" appearance. Anterior uveitis is almost invariable. The process may remain active from 1 week to several months. In healed lesions, the vascular channels at the level of Descemet's membrane persist even though they may be devoid of circulating blood ("ghost vessels"). Local injury and nonspecific inflammation may cause a reopening of these vascular channels, leading to an apparent late relapse, which may in fact be only a nonspecific local vasomotor reaction.

Acquired syphilis

Acquired syphilis, with an incubation period of 2 to 4 weeks, is divided into primary, secondary, and tertiary stages. The initial lesion is a chancre from which *T. pallidum* may be demonstrated on darkfield microscopic examination. During the secondary stage, 4 to 6 months after the appearance of the chancre, iridocyclitis may occur in association with the syphilitic skin rash. Meningitis with optic nerve and chiasmatic arachnoiditis can occur during the secondary stage, along with ocular findings of chorioretinitis followed by pigment proliferation and retrobulbar neuritis. The tertiary stage occurs 10 years or more after the chancre and is characterized by gumma formation. Central nervous system disease may develop as tabes dorsalis (degenerative involvement of the posterior columns) or paresis (inflammatory central involvement with organic psychosis). Optic atrophy, Argyll Robertson pupils, and iridocyclitis are other ocular signs of tertiary syphilis.

Acquired syphilis may cause interstitial keratitis in approximately 3% of patients. Corneal disease can occur soon after the acquisition of the infection, but as a rule it is a late manifestation occurring, on the average, 10 years later. Interstitial keratitis in acquired syphilis resembles the congenital variety but is usually uniocular, frequently milder, and limited to a sector-shaped area of the cornea.

Diagnosis of syphilis

Diagnosis is based on the eye findings and other stigmata of congenital or acquired syphilis, together with positive serologic tests. Interstitial keratitis can occur as a complication of tuberculosis, leprosy, mumps, lymphogranuloma venereum, trypanosomiasis, onchocerciasis, and in association with Cogan's syndrome. The rapid plasma reagin (RPR) test may be used as a screening test for the disease. It must be noted that this test may be negative in very early syphilis. The RPR test is useful in ascertaining adequate treatment, since it will revert to negative after a patient has been treated. The serum fluorescent treponemal antibody-absorption (FTA-ABS) test has become the definitive serologic test for syphilis, approaching 94% to 97% accuracy.[130] The FTA-ABS will remain positive in syphilis patients even after therapy. However, permanent false positive FTA-ABS test results can occur in leprosy, Hashimoto's thyroiditis, and systemic lupus erythematosus. A false positive result can also be seen in malaria, infectious mononucleosis, tuberculosis, and brucellosis; however, this result is transient, appearing only during the first 6 months of these diseases.

Secondary glaucoma

Active uveitis. Secondary glaucoma developing after systemic spirochetal infections may have multiple causes. Iridocyclitis, with acutely elevated intraocular pressure, can occur in all stages and during the active phase of interstitial keratitis. In addition, anterior uveitis with secondary glaucoma can occur in late adult life in eyes that had interstitial keratitis in youth.[29] The relationship of this inflammatory type of glaucoma to the original keratitis is unknown.

Late glaucoma after congenital syphilis with interstitial keratitis. The association of interstitial keratitis in young age with adult secondary glaucoma has been well documented. This glaucoma occurs in 15% to 20% of patients years after the original inflammation has become inactive. The series by Tsukahara[129] indicates an average age of 16 years for the onset of interstitial syphilitic keratitis, with secondary glaucoma occurring an average of 27 years later. The clinical course suggests two main types of late glaucoma involvement: the predominantly open-angle type described by Knox[61] and the closed-angle type reported by Sugar,[123] which occur with equal frequency.

Open-angle type. The onset is insidious, and the disease course resembles that of chronic simple glaucoma. Gonioscopy shows open angles. Evidence of the initial inflammatory condition may persist as old peripheral anterior synechiae, and trabecular pigmentation. The open portions of the angle have a "dirty" appearance.[29] Similar gonioscopic findings are present in eyes with congenital syphilitic interstitial keratitis but without glaucoma. The degree of synechial closure may not accurately indicate the amount of outflow obstruction. One half of patients with open-angle glaucoma secondary to syphilis show involvement of both eyes. Although the glaucoma damage may be progressive, there are no observations demonstrating an increase in the angle abnormalities with time.

These eyes show pathologic changes of congenital syphilis, such as interstitial keratitis and extensive atrophy of the choroid and retina. In addition to the peripheral anterior synechiae, there is extensive endothelialization and glass membrane formation in the anterior chamber overlying all angle structures and the iris.[61] These membranes cover the trabecular meshwork and extend along newly formed endothelium.[131]

In general, this type of glaucoma is reported to respond poorly to antiglaucoma medications, with control achieved in only 25% to 50% of cases.[29,129] Miotics are tolerated and used in combination with carbonic anhydrase inhibitors, epinephrine, or beta blockers. Routine filtration surgery is successful only in about 50% of cases. While surgery does not activate the old intraocular inflammation, these eyes are prone to more postoperative inflammation and external bleb scarring.

Closed-angle type. The closed-angle type of secondary glaucoma may have an acute onset with pain and high intraocular pressure, or it may present as chronic angle-closure. The eyes characteristically have small anterior segments and shallow anterior chambers.[123] In addition to the angle closure, old inflammatory peripheral anterior synechia and pigment residues are present in the angle. Interstitial keratitis in infancy may predispose these eyes to angle-closure by resulting in abnormally small anterior segments[76] and vertically oval corneas.[34] Lichter and Shaffer[75] have described gonioscopic findings resembling cases of intraepithelial cysts of the iris and ciliary body, which may be an additional mode of angle-closure in this disease.

Iridectomy is often successful in the closed-angle type of glaucoma. Approximately 60% to 70% of eyes are controlled after iridectomy and 80% to 90% of eyes with iridectomy and medical therapy.[29,129] The remaining eyes require filtration surgery. Prophylactic iridectomy is indicated in contralateral eyes with extremely narrow angles in which closure appears to be imminent.

Glaucoma in Sarcoid Uveitis

Sarcoidosis is a systemic noncaseating granulomatous disease of undetermined cause. Although the first description of sarcoidosis is attributed to Hutchinson,[43] its ocular features received little attention until 1936, when Herrfordt's syndrome of uveitis, salivary gland enlargement, and cranial nerve palsies was recognized as a sign of sarcoidosis.[12] Subsequently, sarcoidosis has been recognized as commonly having ocular involvement and as being a foremost cause of uveitis.

Systemic findings

Sarcoidosis is a multisystem disorder most commonly affecting young adults. The disease shows a number of immunologic changes, including depression of delayed-type hypersensitivity, hyperactive circulating antibody responses, and the Kveim skin test phenomenon.[48] The condition occurs more frequently in blacks than in whites. The most common systemic changes are diffuse fibrosis of the hili of the lungs and lymph nodes and cutaneous involvement, with soft, brown or red papules, nodules, and plaques. In addition there can be systemic involvement of the lung parenchyma (53%), liver (22%), spleen (13%), musculoskeletal system (7%), and central nervous system (9%).[89]

Ocular findings

Ocular manifestations are a prominent feature of this condition, occurring in 10% to 38% of patients with systemic sarcoidosis[36,47,89,117] and most commonly in blacks.

Approximately 20% of patients seek medical attention because of eye-related complaints, which are second only to pulmonary symptoms in frequency. Ocular abnormalities can be classified into three categories: (1) anterior segment disease, (2) posterior segment disease, and (3) orbital and other disease.

Anterior segment disease. Anterior segment structures are involved more frequently than other parts of the eye. Sarcoid anterior uveitis is a common and important ocular sign, occurring in 25% to 53% of patients.[47,89] The characteristic picture is nodular iritis that may be painless. Iris nodules are multiple small white superficial lesions in the crypts (Busacca nodules) and on the pupillary border (Koeppe nodules). Sarcoid nodules frequently involve the iris root and the iridocorneal angle.[83] In the acute stage, ocular inflammation can be unilateral. As the disease becomes chronic, bilateral involvement usually develops. Chronic granulomatous uveitis is exemplified by mutton fat keratic percipitates, iris nodules, and synechiae. Iris inflammatory changes often result in the formation of a pupillary membrane. Cataracts can be caused by chronic inflammation or treatment with corticosteroids. Conjunctival follicles or nodules and band keratopathy also occur.

Posterior segment disease. Involvement of the posterior segment occurs in approximately one fourth of patients with ocular sarcoidosis.[89] While retinopathy may be the sole ophthalmic expression of the ailment,[73] posterior segment disease usually accompanies anterior involvement. Predominant posterior manifestations are chorioretinitis and retinal periphlebitis. The chorioretinitis is clinically indistinguishable from that caused by other factors. Retinal periphlebitis, producing the ophthalmoscopic appearance of "candle wax drippings" in the more severe cases, is a hallmark of the disease.[27] Characteristic grayish white inferior vitreous opacities, occurring in chains like a "string of pearls," are frequently found.[67]

Orbital and other disease. Lacrimal gland involvement in sarcoidosis is well established. Bilateral lacrimal enlargement may be the sole ophthalmic manifestation.[89] Orbital involvement is a rare cause of unilateral proptosis and problems with motility. Posterior segment sarcoidosis is accompanied by involvement of the central nervous system in 20% to 35% of cases.[27,89] This emphasizes the need for a thorough neurologic examination in patients with this form of ocular sarcoidosis. Optic nerve involvement is manifested by papilledema, papillitis, optic neuritis, and rarely by granulomas of the optic disc. When sarcoidosis affects the brain, the intracranial portion of the optic nerve may be involved by the inflammatory reaction.

Secondary glaucoma

Glaucoma is observed in approximately 12% of patients with ocular sarcoidosis at some time during the course of the disease.[46] A higher incidence of secondary glaucoma, blindness, and subsequent enucleation occurs in blacks.[89] Mechanisms for impairment of aqueous humor outflow can include nodular infiltration of the trabeculum, peripheral anterior synechiae, or obstruction of the trabecular meshwork by particulate matter.[45] Secondary angle-closure glaucoma can result from dense posterior synechia formation or occlusion of the pupil by a connective tissue pupillary membrane.

Diagnosis

Chest x-ray examination is the most important screening test and is abnormal in more than 90% of patients with ocular sarcoidosis.[89] A biopsy of accessible tissue, such as skin or lymph nodes, is essential for diagnosis. A conjunctival biopsy can confirm a histologic diagnosis if follicles are observed.[10] Because conjunctival biopsy is a safe and simple procedure, it has been advocated for the diagnosis of sarcoidosis even in the absence of clinically apparent conjunctival lesions. Positive conjunctival biopsy results are obtained in approximately one third of patients with histologically confirmed sarcoidosis, irrespective of the presence or absence of visible ocular lesions.[58]

Although the Kveim skin test is positive in 75% of patients with sarcoidosis, it may also be positive in other granulomatous conditions.[41] Also, although serum lysozyme is elevated in patients with sarcoidosis and active uveitis,[93,135] elevated serum lysozyme levels are not specific for sarcoidosis. They have also been correlated with disease activity in tuberculosis, uremia, Crohn's disease, megaloblastic anemia, myelomonocytic leukemia, rheumatoid arthritis, and osteoarthritis.[135] Serum angiotensin-converting enzyme (ACE) has proven useful for diagnosing sarcoidosis and monitoring the effectiveness of steroid therapy.[112,136] ACE reflects the total amount of granulomas found throughout the body and is most commonly increased when the disease is widespread and involves the lungs.[87] Therefore, ACE activity can be within normal levels in patients with localized ocular sarcoid. Aqueous humor ACE levels may be increased in these patients with localized disease.[137]

Pathology

In sarcoidosis, one sees the typical nonnecrotic epitheloid tubercle. The tubercles are all the same size, although they may coalesce to form conglomerate masses that typically involve the iris and ciliary body. The tubercles are surrounded by a small zone of inflammatory cells, mainly lymphocytes.

Management

Corticosteroids are usually effective in the treatment of systemic and ocular sarcoidosis. Patients with acute iritis, erythema nodosum, and hilar lymphadenopathy tend to have a benign, self-limiting course, whereas those individuals with chronic uveitis, skin plaques, pulmonary fibrosis, and bone cysts respond poorly to treatment with corticosteroids and almost invariably have a prolonged, complicated course.[47] Topical corticosteroids are effective in suppressing anterior segment inflammation, whereas periocular or systemic therapy is usually required for posterior involvement. Parenteral corticosteroids or other forms of immunosuppression are necessary for treating systemic sarcoidosis including central nervous system involvement. Steroid side effects can frequently occur during therapy for this chronic condition.

Secondary glaucoma should be treated medically, with avoidance of the use of miotic therapy. Filtration surgery may become necessary in patients who are not medically controlled. Postoperative steroid therapy is necessary because of the chronically persistent inflammation of the iris and ciliary body. Iridectomy is the treatment of choice if the disease is complicated by secondary pupillary block glaucoma.

Glaucoma and Anterior Uveitis Associated with Arthritis

Anterior uveitis can be associated with various types of arthritis: ankylosing spondylitis, adult rheumatoid arthritis, juvenile rheumatoid arthritis, and Reiter's syndrome. The incidence of uveitis and associated complications, as well as systemic manifestations, differ for each of these conditions.

Ankylosing spondylitis (Marie-Strümpell disease)

Fifteen percent to 25% of patients with ankylosing spondylitis develop intermittent nongranulomatous anterior uveitis.[11] Cervical vertebra involvement often makes it difficult for the patient to place his head at the slit-lamp. The lumbosacral spine is involved as frequently as the cervical spine and easily escapes diagnosis. Recurrent attacks of uveitis may precede the onset of symptoms of ankylosing spondylitis. The severity of the joint disease does not seem to be related to that of the eye disease. The HLA-B27 antigen, present in 5% of the white population, is found in 96% of patients with ankylosing spondylitis and in 58% of the patients with uveitis.[11] Abnormal technetium bone scans of the sacroiliac joints have been reported in 60% of patients with HLA-B27 antigen, acute nongranulomatous anterior uveitis and normal lumbosacral spine x-ray films.[113] This suggests that acute anterior uveitis may represent a manifestation of spondylitic diathesis even in the complete absence of any suggestive symptomatic or radiologic joint change.

The uveitis is an acute nongranulomatous condition that responds to corticosteroid drops and pupillary dilation. Posterior synechia, peripheral anterior synechia, and trabecular damage can occur, leading to secondary glaucoma.

Adult rheumatoid arthritis

Adult rheumatoid arthritis, a chronic systemic disease of unknown cause, has an insidious onset in people between the ages of 25 and 50 and causes pain and swelling in one or more joints. Women are affected more often than men (75% vs 25%). The disease may become chronic and involve all joints with contraction and deformity. Ocular manifestations are caused by inflammatory and/or exudative alterations of connective tissue elements. About 5% of adults with rheumatoid arthritis develop iritis.[119]

Juvenile rheumatoid arthritis

The term juvenile rheumatoid arthritis covers a range of clinical syndromes. The spectrum can be divided into three major types based on the degree of articular and systemic involvement at the time of onset.[13]

Acute systemic juvenile rheumatoid arthritis (Still's disease). This accounts for 20% of cases and occurs principally in young boys. The disease begins with a high fever, rash, anemia, lympadenopathy, hepatosplenomegaly, and pericarditis. Most patients subsequently develop chronic polyarthritis. Still's original description[122] included this type of arthritis. Uveitis has not been reported in patients with this disease.

Polyarticular-onset juvenile rheumatoid arthritis. This accounts for 50% of cases and occurs principally in girls. The polyarticular onset simultaneously involves five or more joints. There is a low incidence of systemic features, but the children appear ill. This variant has been called adult-type-onset juvenile rheumatoid arthritis, but serum rheumatoid factor and subcutaneous nodules are rarely found. Uveitis occurs in a small percentage of patients.[115]

Monoarticular-onset juvenile rheumatoid arthritis. This accounts for 30% of cases and is more common in girls than in boys (3:1 ratio). Characteristically, there is insidious swelling, pain, and stiffness in a large joint, most frequently the knee. Occasionally, a small joint in the foot, hand, or elsewhere is affected. These children are apparently healthy, and their arthritis responds well to treatment. In most cases, the disease remains monoarticular or pauciarticular, involving four or fewer joints. Antibody and rheumatoid factor are absent. Systemic signs are rare. However, iridocyclitis is common, occurring in approximately 30% of patients.[115]

Uveitis in juvenile rheumatoid arthritis. In most children the iridocyclitis is a mild, insidious, chronic anterior segment inflammation that produces few symptoms. However, up to 45% of patients may have symptoms of severe pain, redness, and photophobia.[14,16] The iritis is nongranulomatous, with fine- or medium-keratic precipitates, cells, and flare, and in a few cases cells in the anterior vitreous. Posterior synechiae and pigment deposition on the anterior lens capsule are frequent. Arthritis precedes the uveitis in approximately 90% of patients, with the iridocyclitis developing 2 months to 12 years later. There is no parallel between the activity of the iridocyclitis and the joint disease. Whereas the arthritis tends to disappear in adult life, the iridocyclitis persists.[57] There can be extended periods of quiescence; however, these rarely last longer than 4 years. Eventually most patients have persistent aqueous flare, which probably indicates altered vascular permeability.

Chronic iridocyclitis can result in complications of band keratopathy (4% to 49%), posterior synechiae (38% to 61%), and rarely macular edema and papillitis.[16,51,57] Cataracts are common, occurring in up to 50% of children. These cataracts can be related to chronic inflammation or to chronic corticosteroid therapy.

Secondary glaucoma

Glaucoma is a relatively common complication. The occurrence increases with the duration of the disease, approaching an incidence of 20%. Glaucoma may be secondary to posterior synechiae and iris bombé resulting in angle closure, to peripheral anterior synechiae, or to trabecular obstruction by particulate matter.

Management

Arthritis. Systemic long-term corticosteroids are frequently necessary for treatment of the systemic manifestations. This therapy can be a causative factor in the development of posterior subcapsular cataracts. Both the dose and duration of systemic steroid therapy are important. A high frequency of posterior subcapsular cataracts is observed in patients receiving more than 20 mg/day of prednisone (0.5 mg/kg/day). Cataracts do not occur in patients receiving corticosteroid therapy for less than 6 months. These cataracts may be reversible on withdrawal of the steroid.[91] This highlights the necessity of a team approach to meet the medical, orthopedic, and ophthalmologic needs of these patients.

Uveitis. Approximately 50% of patients respond to topical corticosteroids and pupillary dilation. It is important to keep the pupil mobile to prevent the formation of posterior synechiae. In many eyes topical corticosteroids have no effect on anterior chamber cells and flare. Only about one third of patients respond to treatment with systemic corticosteroids.[51] The results of immunosuppressive therapy (chlorambucil, cyclophosphamide, or azathioprine) have been disappointing.

Cataracts. Surgical treatment of cataracts formerly was discouraging.[16] More favorable results were reported by Key and Kimura[57] with the use of periocular and systemic corticosteroids both preoperatively and postoperatively to quell the surgical inflammatory response. They reported improved vision in 12 of 20 eyes after extracapsular procedures.

Glaucoma. The possibility of a steroid-induced glaucoma should be kept in mind. Medical therapy avoids the use of miotics. Iridectomy is indicated if a pupillary block mechanism exists. There is no best method to achieve external filtration if it becomes necessary. A modified goniotomy technique described by Haas[31] was reported to have been successful in 7 of 15 eyes for up to 2 years. However, these results are similar to goniotomy, thermosclerostomy, or trabeculectomy in this condition.[57] The advent of 5-fluorouracil and other antifibrotic agents offers great promise in improving success rates of filtration surgery.

Reiter's syndrome

Reiter's syndrome is a complex of signs and symptoms characterized by conjunctivitis, urethritis, arthritis, and, frequently, mucocutaneous lesions.[109] It most commonly affects young men and is sometimes associated with venereal disease or dysentery. The cause of Reiter's syndrome is unknown; however, the high frequency of occurrence of the HLA-B27 genotype may be an indication that an unusual host response to an infectious agent or some unknown antigen occurs.[69]

Nonophthalmic manifestations include rheumatologic findings in 98% of patients, urethritis in 74%, mucocutaneous lesions in 42%, and nonspecific electrocardiologic changes in 27% of patients.[2]

The frequency of venereal disease may be as high as 25%, with gonorrhea the most common.

Ophthalmic manifestations are common, with conjunctivitis (58%) the most frequent eye finding.[2] Nongranulomatous iridocyclitis (13%), keratitis (14%), and episcleritis (1%) also occur in Reiter's syndrome. In a recent series of 113 patients with Reiter's syndrome, only one patient developed glaucoma secondary to the ocular inflammation.[2]

The conjunctivitis and keratitis in patients with this syndrome are usually self-limited and require no special therapy. Iridocyclitis usually responds to standard therapy with topically applied corticosteroids and cycloplegics.

Viral Uveitis and Secondary Glaucoma

Various types of viral infections can cause uveitis and secondary glaucoma. The elevated intraocular pressure is related to the intraocular inflammation and can be secondary to pupillary block or to outflow damage as a result of peripheral anterior synechiae, trabecular inflammatory damage, or trabecular obstruction by inflammatory debris.

Herpesvirus

This group of viruses contains three members pathogenic for humans: (1) herpesvirus hominis, the virus of herpes simplex; (2) herpesvirus varicellae, which causes chickenpox and herpes zoster; and (3) herpesvirus simiae, which causes a subclinical infection in monkeys but a fatal central nervous system disease when transmitted to humans.

Herpes simplex. This endemic virus infection occurs in nonimmune individuals and usually results in a subclinical and self-limited disease. Type 1 virus causes herpetic infections of the eye, whereas type 2 virus is associated with genital infections. Up to 90% of adults have circulating antibodies to the type 1 virus and carry the virus in an inactive state. Secondary or recurrent ocular herpes simplex develops in patients with neutralizing antibodies and can result in conjunctivitis, keratitis (superficial or deep), uveitis (with or without keratitis), or trophic (postherpetic) keratitis.

Herpes simplex keratouveitis may be associated with an increased intraocular pressure. In a study by Falcon and Williams,[20] the associated herpetic ocular signs in 50 patients with secondary glaucoma included the following: disciform keratouveitis (44%), stromal keratouveitis (36%), disciform keratitis (10%), stromal keratitis (4%), scleral keratitis (2%), and metaherpetic ulcer (4%). These cases represent 28% of patients with herpes keratouveitis seen by Falcon and Williams. In this series, active corneal ulcers were not present at the time of raised intraocular pressure. Herpetic ocular hypertension is characterized by intermittent attacks, with a mean duration of 8 weeks of raised intraocular pressure. The frequency of ocular hypertensive attacks is greater in patients with irregular stromal keratitis than in patients with disciform keratitis.

Herpesvirus has been described as the causal agent in anterior uveitis.[59] Viral particles have been identified in the human iris,[138] and fluorescent antibody techniques provide a clinical method for establishing the diagnosis.[56,95] Elevated intraocular pressure is related to trabecular blockade or trabeculitis.[20,35,128] Angle-closure is not implicated.[20]

The management of herpes simplex keratouveitis and glaucoma is directed initially toward halting or preventing activation of the viral disease. Two different antiviral drugs are currently available for treatment of herpetic keratitis: idoxuridine (IDU) and vidarabine (Ara-A). Neither of these drugs achieves therapeutic levels in the deep corneal stroma, anterior chamber, or iris. However, two antiviral agents, trifluridine[96,124] and acyclovir,[103] have been demonstrated to penetrate through the cornea into the anterior chamber after topical application. These are the antiviral agents of choice for herpetic keratouveitis.[80,82,103] Corticosteroids are effective in suppressing the associated intraocular inflammation. However, steroids can reactivate epithelial herpes simplex. Antiviral coverage must be given concurrently with topical corticosteroids to reduce reactivating epithelial herpes.[94] Supplementary hypotensive treatment with systemic carbonic anhydrase inhibitors and topical epinephrine or timolol may be required. Although elevated intraocular pressure occurs before corticosteroid therapy, the possibility of corticosteroid-induced increases should be kept in mind.[127] The intraocular pressure usually returns to normal as the inflammation subsides. Approximately 12% of patients will develop a persistent secondary glaucoma requiring continued therapy after the uveitis has cleared. Filtration surgery may occasionally be required.[20]

Herpes zoster. Herpes zoster ophthalmicus results from invasion or reactivation of the virus in the Gasserian ganglion and the first (ophthalmic) branch of the trigeminal nerve. A vesicular rash on an erythematous base occurs along this division of the fifth nerve but does not cross the midline. Lancinating pain precedes the rash by 24 to 48 hours.

The skin over the tip of the nose is supplied by the nasociliary branch of the fifth nerve, and lesions in this area frequently are followed by keratitis and uveitis. The iridocyclitis is associated with mutton fat keratic precipitates, posterior synechiae, and sector iris atrophy. Hypopyon may be present. Corneal sensation is lost and is never fully recovered.

Secondary glaucoma is said to occur commonly in association with keratitis and uveitis from herpes zoster but perhaps not so frequently as herpes simplex.[15] Glaucoma results from intraocular inflammation and its consequences as previously described. The true incidence of glaucoma in herpes zoster ophthalmicus is not as well defined as in herpes simplex keratouveitis. However, as many as 25% of affected eyes may be found to have intraocular pressure elevation.[62]

Steroids are effective for the uveitic manifestation of herpes zoster. Topical steroids usually control the acute, as well as the chronic, form of uveitis. Occasionally, subconjunctival or systemic corticosteroids are necessary. When maintaining patients with this disease on a regimen of long-term steroids, one must consider the possibility of steroid-induced glaucoma. Topical trifluridine or acyclovir may be effective in the therapy of this infection.[82]

Rubella

The importance to the developing fetus of prenatal infection with rubella virus was first recognized by Gregg in 1941.[30] A large variety of congenital defects can occur in infants whose mothers contract the disease during the first trimester of pregnancy. The incidence of embryopathy varies and is more severe the earlier in pregnancy the disease occurs. Associated ocular disorders in decreasing rank of incidence include retinopathy, strabismus, cataracts, nystagmus, microphthalmus and microcornea, optic atrophy, corneal haze and leukomas, glaucoma, lid defects, and iris atrophy.[139] Besides ocular manifestations, other defects include congenital heart disease, deafness, mental retardation, and microcephaly.

The reported incidence of glaucoma in congenital rubella varies. Glaucoma seems to be associated with more advanced cases of the disease. A summary of retrospective studies up to 1969 reveals that of 730 patients with congenital rubella, 22 had glaucoma and 230 had cataracts.[139] Rubella keratitis, which results in corneal clouding, can present a problem in differential diagnosis with corneal edema of congenital glaucoma. Corneal haze, which is usually permanent, is deep, is diffuse or disciform, and resists attempts at clearing by removal of the epithelium. It can cause difficulty in measuring intraocular pressure. The MacKay-Marg tonometer or the pneumatonometer may be the most accurate method.

Glaucoma can be transient or permanent. An inflammatory reaction is probably responsible for the transient condition. The iritis is nongranulomatous with diffuse and focal infiltration of the anterior uvea by lymphocytes, plasma cells, and histiocytes.[142] The iritis may become chronic.[140] This type of glaucoma is best managed medically with the combined use of corticosteroids and antiglaucoma therapy. The permanent type of glaucoma is related to the developmental defects of the iridocorneal angle that occur in some rubella patients. Gonioscopically and pathologically the anterior chamber angle appears not unlike that of typical congenital glaucoma (see Chapter 37).

Mumps

Mumps is an acute contagious systemic disease characterized by painful enlargement of the salivary glands (most commonly the parotid gland) and, after puberty, by orchitis. Lymphocytic meningitis, pancreatitis, and involvement of other organs occur rarely. Ocular manifestations of mumps include dacryoadenitis, optic neuritis, keratitis, conjunctivitis, scleritis, and iritis.[111] Secondary glaucoma can occur in conjunction with the iritis.[110] One case of transient bilateral glaucoma was reported in a man during convalescence from mumps in which there were no signs of scleritis or iritis.[104] In this patient, with open angles and reduced outflow facility, the glaucoma is reported to have responded to treatment with acetazolamide and topical corticosteroids.

REFERENCES

1. Alanko, HI, Vuorre, I, and Saari, KM: Characteristics of corneal endothelial cells in Fuchs heterochromic cyclitis, Acta Ophthalmol 64:623, 1986
2. Amett, FG, McClusky, OE, Schacter, BZ, and Lordon, RE: Incomplete Reiter's syndrome: discriminating features and HL-A W27 in diagnosis, Ann Intern Med 84:8, 1976
3. Amsler, M, and Verrey, F: Hétérochromie de Fuchs et fragilité vasculaire, Ophthalmologica 3:117, 1946
4. Andrasch, RH, Pirofsky, B, and Burns, RP: Immunosuppressive therapy for severe chronic uveitis, Arch Ophthalmol 96:247, 1978
5. Becker, B: Cataracts and topical corticosteroids, Am J Ophthalmol 58:872, 1964
6. Becker, B: Intraocular pressure response to topical corticosteroids, Invest Ophthalmol 4:198, 1965
7. Beitch, BR, and Eakins, KE: The effects of prostaglandins on the intraocular pressure of the rabbit, Brit J Pharmacol 37:158, 1969
8. Bill, A: Conventional and uveo-scleral drainage of aqueous humor in the cynomolgus monkey (Macaca iras) at normal and high intraocular pressures, Exp Eye Res 5:45, 1975
9. Bito, LZ: The effects of experimental uveitis on anterior uveal prostaglandin transport and aqueous humor composition, Invest Ophthalmol 13:959, 1974
10. Bornstein, JS, Frank, MI, and Radner, DB: Conjunctival biopsy in the diagnosis of sarcoidosis, N Engl J Med 267:60, 1962
11. Brewerton, DA, et al: Ankylosing spondylitis and HLA-B27, Lancet 1:904, 1973
12. Bruins Slot, WJ: Zeikle van Besnier-Boeck en Febris uveoparotidea (Herrfordt), Ned Tijdschr Geneesk 80:2859, 1936
13. Calabro, JJ, and Mareschano, JM: The early natural history of juvenile rheumatoid arthritis, Med Clin North Am 52:567, 1968
14. Calabro, JJ, et al: Chronic iridocyclitis in juvenile rheumatoid arthritis, Arthritis Rheum 13:406, 1970
15. Chandler, PA, and Grant, WM: Glaucoma, Philadelphia, 1965, Lea & Febiger
16. Chylack, LT, Bierfang, DC, Bellows, HR, and Stillman, JS: Ocular manifestations of juvenile rheumatoid arthritis, Am J Ophthalmol 79:1026, 1975
17. Eakins, KE, Whitelock, RAF, Bennett, A, and Martenet, AC: Prostaglandin-like activity in ocular inflammation, Br Med J 3:452, 1972
18. Ebert, RH, and Barclay, WR: Changes in connective tissue reaction induced by cortisone, Ann Intern Med 37:506, 1952
19. Epstein, DL, Hashimoto, JM, and Grant, WM: Serum obstruction of aqueous outflow in enucleated eyes, Am J Ophthalmol 86:101, 1978
20. Falcon, MG, and Williams, HP: Herpes simplex kerato-uveitis and glaucoma, Trans Ophthalmol Soc UK 98:101, 1978
21. Floman, Y, Floman, N, and Zor, U: Inhibition of prostaglandin E release by anti-inflammatory steroids, Prostaglandins 2:592, 1976
22. Franceschetti, A: Heterochromic cyclitis: Fuchs' syndrome, Am J Ophthalmol 39:50, 1955
23. François, J: L'hétérochromie iriènne de Fuchs, Ann Ocul 179:559, 1946
24. François, J: Contribution a l'étude de l'hétérochromie de Fuchs et de ses troubles pupillaires (pathogénie sympathique), Ann Ocul 182:585, 1949
25. Fuchs, E: Uber Komplikationen der Heterochromie, Z Augenheilkd 15:191, 1906
26. Goldberg, MF, Erozan, YS, Duke, JR, and Frost, JK: Cytopathologic and histopathologic aspects of Fuchs' heterochromic iridocyclitis, Arch Ophthalmol 74:604, 1965
27. Gould, H, and Kaufman, HE: Sarcoid of the fundus, Arch Ophthalmol 65:453, 1961

28. Grant, WM: Clinical measurements of aqueous outflow, Arch Ophthalmol 46:113, 1951
29. Grant, WM: Late glaucoma after interstitial keratitis, Am J Ophthalmol 79:87, 1975
30. Gregg, NMA: Congenital cataract following German measles in the mother, Trans Ophthalmol Soc Aust 3:35, 1941
31. Haas, JS: Surgical treatment of open-angle glaucoma. In Transactions of the New Orleans Academy of Ophthalmology: Symposium on glaucoma, St Louis, 1967, The CV Mosby Co
32. Hart, CT, and Ward, DM: Intra-ocular pressure in Fuchs' heterochromic uveitis, Br J Ophthalmol 52:739, 1967
33. Herschler, J: Intractable intraocular hypertension induced by repository triamcinolone acetonide, Am J Ophthalmol 74:501, 1972
34. Hoehne, H: Ueber Keratitis parenchymatosa, Klin Monatsbl Augenheilkd 105:656, 1940
35. Hogan, MJ, Kimura, SJ, and Thygeson, P: Pathology of herpes simplex keratitis, Trans Am Ophthalmol Soc 61:75, 1963
36. Hoover, DL, Khan, JA, and Giangiacomo, J: Pediatric ocular sarcoid, Surv Ophthalmol 30:215, 1986
37. Hoskins, HD: Secondary glaucomas. In Heilmann, K, and Richardson, KT, editors: Glaucoma: concepts of a disease, Stuttgart, Germany, 1978, Georg Thieme
38. Hoskins, HD, Jr, Hetherington, J, Jr, and Shaffer, RN: Surgical management of the inflammatory glaucomas, Perspect Ophthalmol 1:173, 1977
39. Howes, EL, Jr, and Cruse, VK: The structural basis of altered vascular permeability following intraocular inflammation, Arch Ophthalmol 96:1668, 1978
40. Huber, A: Glaucoma as a complication in heterochromia of Fuchs, Ophthalmologica 142:66, 1961
41. Hurley, TH, Sullivan, JR, and Hurley, JV: Reaction of Kveim test material in sarcoidosis and other diseases, Lancet 1:494, 1975
42. Hutchinson, J: Diseases of the eye and ear consequent on inherited syphilis, London, 1863, Churchill Livingstone
43. Hutchinson, J: Anomalous disease of skin of fingers, etc. (papillary psoriasis?). In Illustrations of clinical surgery, vol 1, London, 1878, Churchill Livingstone
44. Ignarro, LJ, and Columbo, C: Enzyme release from polymorphonuclear leukocyte lysosomes: regulation by autonomic drugs and cyclic nucleotides, Science 4:1801, 1973
45. Iwata, K, Nanba, K, Sobue, K, and Abe, H: Ocular sarcoidosis: evaluation of intraocular findings, Ann NY Acad Sci 278:445, 1976
46. Jabs, DA, and Johns, CJ: Ocular involvement in chronic sarcoidosis, Am J Ophthalmol 102:297, 1986
47. James, DG, Anderson, R, Langely, D, and Ainslie, D: Ocular sarcoidosis, Br J Ophthalmol 48:461, 1964
48. James, DG, Neville, E, and Walker, A: Immunology of sarcoidosis, Am J Med 59:388, 1975
49. James, JL, and Nigam, MP: Pupillary autonomic functions in heterochromia iridis, Arch Ophthalmol 89:291, 1973
50. Johnson, D, Leisegang, TJ, and Brubaker, RF: Aqueous humor dynamics in Fuchs' uveitis syndrome, Am J Ophthalmol 95:783, 1983
51. Kanski, JJ: Anterior uveitis in juvenile rheumatoid arthritis, Arch Ophthalmol 95:1974, 1977
52. Kanski, JJ, and McAllister, JA: Trabeculodialysis for inflammatory glaucoma in children and young adults, Ophthalmology 92:927, 1985
53. Kass, MA, Becker, B, and Kolker, AE: Glaucomatocyclitic crisis and primary open-angle glaucoma, Am J Ophthalmol 75:668, 1973
54. Kass, MA, Cheetham, J, Duzman, E, and Burke, PJ: The ocular hypertensive effect of 0.25% fluorometholone in corticosteroid responders, Am J Ophthalmol 102:159, 1986
55. Kass, MA, Podos, SM, Moses, RA, and Becker, B: Prostaglandin E_1 and aqueous humor dynamics, Invest Ophthalmol 11:1022, 1972
56. Kaufman, HE, Kanai, A, and Ellison, ED: Herpetic iritis: demonstration of virus in the anterior chamber by fluorescent antibody techniques and electron microscopy, Am J Ophthalmol 71:465, 1971
57. Key, SN, III, and Kimura, SJ: Iridocyclitis associated with juvenile rheumatoid arthritis, Am J Ophthalmol 80:425, 1975
58. Khan, F, Wessely, Z, Chazin, SR, and Seriff, NS: Conjunctival biopsy in sarcoidosis: a simple, safe and specific diagnostic procedure, Ann Ophthalmol 9:671, 1977
59. Kimura, SJ: Herpes simplex uveitis: a clinical and experimental study, Trans Am Ophthalmol Soc 60:440, 1962
60. Kimura, SJ, Hogan, MJ, and Thygeson, P: Fuchs' syndrome of heterochromic cyclitis, AMA Arch Ophthalmol 54:179, 1955
61. Knox, DL: Glaucoma following syphilitic interstitial keratitis, Arch Ophthalmol 64:44, 1961
62. Kolker, AE, and Hetherington, J, Jr: Becker-Shaffer's diagnosis and therapy of the glaucomas, ed 4, St Louis, 1976, The CV Mosby Co
63. Krupin, T: Surgical treatment of glaucoma with the Krupin-Denver Valve. In Cairns, JE, editor: Glaucoma, London, 1986, Grune & Stratton, Inc
64. Krupin, T, et al: Uveitis in association with topically administered corticosteroid, Am J Ophthalmol 70:883, 1970
65. Krupin, T, Mandell, AI, Podos, SM, and Becker, B: Topical corticosteroid therapy and pituitary-adrenal function, Arch Ophthalmol 94:919, 1976
66. Kupferman, A, and Leibowitz, HM: Anti-inflammatory effectiveness of topically administered corticosteroids in the cornea without epithelium, Invest Ophthalmol 14:252, 1975
67. Landers, PH: Vitreous lesion observed in Boeck's sarcoid, Am J Ophthalmol 32:1740, 1949
68. Lawrence, W: Treatise on diseases of the eye, ed 3, Philadelphia, 1853, Isaac Hays

69. Lee, DA, et al: The clinical diagnosis of Reiter's syndrome: ophthalmic and nonophthalmic aspects, Ophthalmology 93:350, 1986

70. Leopold, IH: Treatment of eye disorders with antiinflammatory steroids, Ann NY Acad Sci 82:939, 1959

71. Leopold, IH, et al: Local and systemic cortisone in ocular disease, Am J Ophthalmol 34:361, 1951

72. Lerman, S, and Levy, C: Heterochromic iritis and secondary neovascular glaucoma, Am J Ophthalmol 57:479, 1964

73. Letocha, CE, Shields, JA, and Goldberg, RE: Retinal changes in sarcoidosis, Can J Ophthalmol 10:184, 1975

74. Levatin, P: Glaucomatocyclitic crises occurring in both eyes, Am J Ophthalmol 41:1056, 1956

75. Lichter, PR, and Shaffer, RN: Interstitial keratitis and glaucoma, Am J Ophthalmol 68:241, 1969

76. Luyckx-Bacus, J, and Delmarcelle, Y: Récherches biometriques sur des yeux présentant une microcornée ou une megalocornée, Bull Soc Belge Ophthalmol 149:433, 1968

77. Makley, TA, Jr: Heterochromic cyclitis in identical twins, Am J Ophthalmol 41:768, 1956

78. March, WF, and Coniglione, TC: Ibuprofen in the treatment of uveitis, Ann Ophthalmol 17:103, 1985

79. Masuda, K, Izawa, Y, and Mishima, S: Prostaglandins and glaucomato-cyclitic crisis, Jpn J Ophthalmol 19:368, 1975

80. Maudgal, PC, Vrijghem, JC, Molemans, M, and Missotten, L: Effect of topical acyclovir therapy on experimental herpes simplex keratouveitis, Arch Ophthalmol 103:1389, 1985

81. McCartney, ACE, Bull, TB, and Spalton, DJ: Fuchs' heterochromic cyclitis: an electron microscopy study, Trans Ophthalmol Soc UK 105:324, 1986

82. McGill, J, Tormey, P, and Walker, C: The clinical use of acylovir in the treatment of herpes simplex corneal ulceration. In Sundmacher, R, editor: Herpetic eye diseases, West Germany, 1981, JF Bergmann Verlag

83. Mizuno, K, and Watanabe, T: Sarcoid granulomatous cyclitis, Am J Ophthalmol 81:82, 1974

84. Molteno, ACB: Implants for draining neovascular glaucoma, Br J Ophthalmol 61:120, 1977

85. Nagataki, S, and Mishima, J: Aqueous humor dynamics in glaucomato-cyclitic crisis, Invest Ophthalmol 15:365, 1976

86. Neufeld, AH, and Sears, ML: Prostaglandin and eye, Prostaglandins 4:157, 1973

87. Nosal, A, et al: Antigiotensin converting enzyme and gallium scan in noninvasive evaluation of sarcoidosis, Ann Intern Med 90:328, 1979

88. Nussenblatt, RB, Palestine, AG, and Chan, CC: Cyclosporin: A therapy in the treatment of intraocular inflammatory disease resistant to systemic corticosteroids and cytotoxic agents, Am J Ophthalmol 96:275, 1983

89. Obenauf, CD, Shaw, HE, Sydnor, CF, and Klintworth, GK: Sarcoidosis and its ophthalmic manifestations, Am J Ophthalmol 86:648, 1978

90. Oglesby, RB, Black, RL, von Sallmann, L, and Bunim, JL: Cataracts in patients with rheumatic diseases treated with corticosteroids, Arch Ophthalmol 66:625, 1961

91. Ohguchi, M, et al: Posterior subcapsular cataracts in children on long-term corticosteroid therapy, Jpn J Ophthalmol 19:254, 1975

92. Olsen, T: Transient changes in specular appearance of the corneal endothelium and in corneal thickness during anterior uveitis, Acta Ophthalmol 59:100, 1981

93. Pascual, RS, Gee, BL, and Finch, SC: Serum lysozyme analysis and diagnosis and evaluation of sarcoidosis, N Engl J Med 289:1074, 1973

94. Patterson, A: Management of ocular herpes simplex, Br J Ophthalmol 51:494, 1967

95. Patterson, A, Sommerville, RG, and Jones, BR: Symposium of kerato-uveitis, Trans Ophthalmol Soc UK 88:243, 1968

96. Pavan-Langston, D, and Nelson, DJ: Intraocular penetration of trifluridine, Am J Ophthalmol 87:814, 1979

97. Perdviel, G, Raynaud, G, and Gayard, M: Syndrome de Posner-Schlossman et glaucome, Bull Soc Ophthalmol Fr 62:611, 1962

98. Perkins, ES: Heterochromic uveitis, Trans Ophthalmol Soc UK 81:53, 1962

99. Perkins, ES: Recent advances in the study of uveitis, Br J Ophthalmol 58:432, 1974

100. Perry, HD, Yanoff, M, and Scheie, HG: Rubeosis in Fuch's heterochromic iridocyclitis, Arch Ophthalmol 93::337, 1975

101. Podos, SM, Becker, B, and Kass, MA: Prostaglandin synthesis, inhibition, and intraocular pressure, Invest Ophthalmol 12:426, 1973

102. Podos, SM, Krupin, T, Assef, C, and Becker, B: Topically administered corticosteroid preparations: comparison of intraocular pressure effects, Arch Ophthalmol 86:251, 1971

103. Poirier, RH, et al: Intraocular antiviral penetration, Arch Ophthalmol 100:1964, 1982

104. Polland, W, and Thorburn, W: Transient glaucoma as a manifestation of mumps: a case report, Acta Ophthalmol 54:779, 1976

105. Posner, A, and Schlossman, A: Syndrome of unilateral recurrent attacks of glaucoma with cyclitic symptoms, Arch Ophthalmol 39:517, 1948

106. Posner, A, and Schlossman, A: Further observations on the syndrome of glaucomatocyclitic crises, Trans Am Acad Ophthalmol Otolaryngol 57:531, 1953

107. Raitta, C, and Klemetti, A: Steroidbelastung bei Posner-Schlossmanschem Syndrom, v Graefes Arch Klin Exp Ophthalmol 174:66, 1967

108. Riatta, C, and Vannas, A: Glaucomatocyclic crisis, Arch Ophthalmol 95:608, 1977

109. Reiter, H: Ueber eine bisher unerkannte Spirachäteninfektion (Spirochaetosis arthritica), Dtch Med Wochenschr 42:1535, 1916

110. Riffenburgh, RS: Iritis and glaucoma associated with mumps, Arch Ophthalmol 51:702, 1954

111. Riffenburgh, RS: Ocular manifestations of mumps, Arch Ophthalmol 66:739, 1961

112. Romer, RK, Schmidt, T, and Geday, H: Angiotensin-converting enzyme in uveitis and sarcoidosis, Acta Ophthalmol 58:243, 1980

113. Russell, AS, Lentle, BC, Percy, JC, and Jackson, FI: Scintigraphy of sacroiliac joints in acute anterior uveitis, Ann Intern Med 85:606, 1976

114. Saari, KM, et al: Genetic background of acute anterior uveitis, Am J Ophthalmol 91:711, 1981

115. Schaller, J, Kupfer, C, and Wedgewood, RJ: Iridocyclitis in juvenile rheumatoid arthritis, Pediatrics 44:92, 1969

116. Schenker, HI, et al: Fluorophotometric study of epinephrine and timolol in human subjects, Arch Ophthalmol 99:1212, 1981

117. Siltzbach, LE, et al: Course and prognosis of sarcoidosis around the world, Am J Med 57:847, 1974

118. Smith, RE, and O'Connor, R: Cataract extraction in Fuch's syndrome, Arch Ophthalmol 91:39, 1974

119. Sorsby, A, and Gormaz, A: Iritis in rheumatic affections, Br Med J 1:597, 1946

120. Spivey, BE, and Armaly, MF: Tonographic findings in glaucomatocyclitic crises, Am J Ophthalmol 55:47, 1963

121. Stewart, RH, and Kimbrough, RL: Intraocular pressure response to topically administered fluorometholone, Arch Ophthalmol 97:2137, 1979

122. Still, GF: On a form of chronic disease in children, Med Chir Trans 80:47, 1897

123. Sugar, HS: Late glaucoma associated with inactive syphilitic interstitial keratitis, Am J Ophthalmol 53:602, 1962

124. Sugar, J, Varnell, E, Centafanto, Y, and Kaufman, HE: Trifluorothymidine treatment of herpetic iritis in rabbits in intraocular penetration, Invest Ophthalmol 12:532, 1973

125. Theodore, FH: Observations of glaucomatocyclitic crises: Posner-Schlossman syndrome, Br J Ophthalmol 36:207, 1952

126. Thomas, L: The role of lysosomes in tissue injury. In Zeifach, BW, Grant, L, and McCluskey, RT, editors: The inflammatory process, New York, 1965, Academic Press, Inc

127. Thygeson, P: Chronic herpetic kerato-uveitis, Trans Am Ophthalmol Soc 65:211, 1967

128. Townsend, WM, and Kaufman, HE: Pathogenesis of glaucoma and endothelial changes in herpetic kerato uveitis in rabbits, Am J Ophthalmol 71:904, 1971

129. Tsukahara, S: Secondary glaucoma due to inactive congenital syphilitic interstitial keratitis, Ophthalmologica 174:188, 1977

130. Tuffanelli, DL, Wuepper, KD, Bradford, LL, and Wood, RM: Fluorescent treponemal-antibody absorption tests: studies of false-positive reactions to tests for syphilis, N Engl J Med 276:258, 1967

131. Van Horn, DI, and Schultz, RE: Electronmicroscopy of syphilitic interstitial keratitis, Invest Ophthalmol 10:469, 1971

132. Vogt, A: Lehrbuch und Atlas der Spaltlampenmikroskopie des lebenden Auges, vol 1, Berlin, 1930, Springer-Verlag

133. Von Graffenried, B, and Harrison, WB: Renal function in patients with autoimmune diseases treated with cyclosporine, Transplant Proc 17(suppl 1):215, 1985

134. Wakefield, D, Breit, SN, Clark, P, and Penny, R: Immunogenetic factors in inflammatory eye disease: influence of HLA-B27 and α_1-antitrypsin phenotypes on disease expression, Arthritis Rheum 25:1431, 1982

135. Weinberg, RS, and Tessler, HH: Serum lysozyme in sarcoid uveitis, Am J Ophthalmol 82:105, 1976

136. Weinreb, RN, and Kimura, SJ: Uveitis associated with sarcoidosis and angiotensin converting enzyme, Trans Am Ophthalmol Soc 77:280, 1979

137. Weinreb, RN, Sandman, R, Ryder, MI, and Friberg, TR: Angiotensin-converting enzyme activity in human aqueous humor, Arch Ophthalmol 103:34, 1985

138. Witmer, RS, and Iwamoto, J: Electron microscope observation of herpes-like particles in the iris, Arch Ophthalmol 79:331, 1968

139. Wolff, SM: The ocular manifestations of congenital rubella, Trans Am Ophthalmol Soc 70:577, 1972

140. Wolter, JR, Insel, PA, Willey, EN, and Brittain, HP: Eye pathology following maternal rubella: a study of four children, J Pediatr Ophthalmol 3(2):29, 1966

141. Wong, VG, and Hersch, EM: Methotrexate in the therapy of cyclitis, Trans Am Acad Ophthalmol Otolaryngol 69:279, 1965

142. Zimmerman, LE, and Font, RL: Congenital malformations of the eye: some recent advances in the knowledge of the pathogenesis and histopathological characteristics, JAMA 196:684, 1966

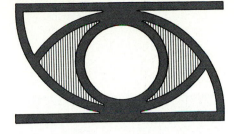

Chapter 68

Trauma and Elevated Intraocular Pressure

Jonathan Herschler
Michael Cobo

Trauma to the globe, both directly to the eye and indirectly to the orbit or head, is a frequent occurrence in everyday life. In the case of blunt trauma, the severity of the injury to the ocular structures depends on several factors, including the size, weight, and speed of the injuring object and its direction and point of impact. In addition, ocular injury may occur secondary to other forms of trauma, such as chemical burns, therapeutic irradiation, and electrical injury. In many situations, trauma to the eye may result in elevated intraocular pressure. In each instance, knowledge of the mechanism of increased intraocular pressure is essential for proper choice of effective treatment.

BLUNT TRAUMA

Blunt trauma can be associated with anterior segment injuries, including hyphema, iris sphincter tear, iridodialysis, cyclodialysis, trabecular tear, inflammation, and zonular rupture with lens subluxation. A posttraumatic elevation in intraocular pressure may occur in association with any of these findings.

Hyphema

Clinical findings

The most common presenting symptom after blunt trauma is reduction of visual acuity, which is usually because of a hyphema. If the intraocular pressure is measured shortly after injury accompanied by a hyphema, it may be elevated in comparison with the fellow eye. Soon thereafter, however, the intraocular pressure falls to a mildly sub-

normal level for approximately 5 days.[25] If a different pattern of intraocular pressure fluctuation occurs, more than just a simple hyphema should be suspected. For example, if hypotony is severe or persistent, then a cyclodialysis, uveitis, or a rupture of the globe should be strongly suspected.

The usual source of bleeding is a tear into the face of the ciliary body between the longitudinal and circular fibers (Fig. 68-1). Small branches of the major arterial circle are torn and then bleed into the anterior chamber.[25] As the intraocular pressure rises, bleeding diminishes and a clot forms. Clot lysis and retraction occur 2 to 4 days after the injury and the maximal incidence of rebleeding from the injured vessels occurs at this time.[49] The rebleed is often more severe than the initial episode and can lead to a total hyphema, also known as a "black-ball" or "eight-ball" hyphema. Unlike the typical initial bleeding episode, total hyphema is usually associated with extreme pain, nausea, and other symptoms related to acute glaucoma.

The mechanism for the increase in intraocular pressure is mechanical obstruction of the trabecular meshwork by red blood cells and blood products (Fig. 68-2) and sometimes pupillary block from a clot.[18] The typical black appearance of the anterior chamber fluid is probably caused by deoxygenated hemoglobin.

Medical management

Many treatments have been advocated to lessen the incidence of rebleeding. One difficulty in evaluating these reports is the wide variation in

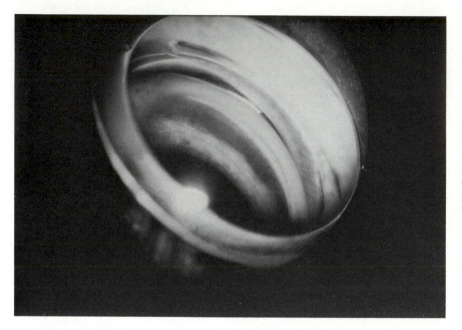

Fig. 68-1 Goniophotograph through Koeppe lens of human eye 2 days after blunt anterior segment trauma with mild hyphema. Large tear into face of ciliary body can be seen with raw, exposed longitudinal fibers remaining attached to scleral spur.

Fig. 68-2 Histologic section through trabecular meshwork and ciliary body of monkey eye after blunt anterior segment trauma. Note torn trabecular meshwork with large adherent blood clot blocking access of aqueous humor into that portion of Schlemm's canal.

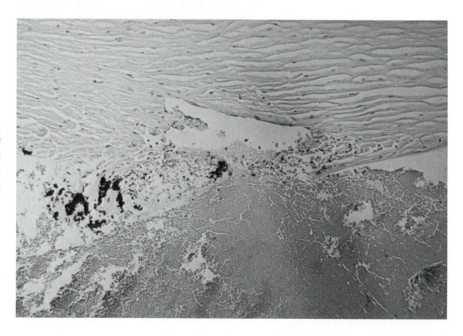

the incidence of rebleeding in the "control" populations studied. As low as 4% rebleeding without any special management to as high as 33% has been reported.[33,53] Randomized studies using oral ε-aminocaproic acid indicate a significant reduction in rebleeding rates in the treated group.[27,33] The use of ε-aminocaproic acid (a fibrinolysin inhibitor) is based on the belief that blocking lysis of the clot that formed after the initial bleeding episode will reduce the incidence of rebleeding. However, the rebleed rates in the control populations (23% to 33%[27,33]) were unusually high. In addition, the high complication rate, including gastrointestinal distress, and the increased cost associated with the ε-aminocaproic acid makes us reluctant to recommend this as a routine approach.

A recent study suggested that the same efficacy but a reduced incidence of side effects could be achieved with ε-aminocaproic acid by halving the recommended dose to 50 mg/kg every 4 hours.[38] Because epsilon aminocaproic acid can only be administered on an inpatient basis, the perceived benefits of this treatment must be weighed against the cost and morbidity. At present, home care or hospitalization, with limited activity, and the use of a protective shield for the injured eye would appear prudent.[18] A decision for or against the use of ε-aminocaproic acid should be made on the basis of the perceived risk of rebleed and the ocular and medical status of the individual. A patient with a hyphema in an only seeing eye, with sickle cell trait, or who has already had a rebleed is a candidate for hospitalization and the use of ε-aminocaproic acid.

If a total hyphema occurs, conservative treatment of elevated intraocular pressure with drugs that reduce aqueous formation (beta blockers and carbonic anhydrase inhibitors) and hyperosmotic agents frequently results in sufficient pressure lowering to allow gradual resorption of the hyphema. Improvement is signaled by the appearance of a mixture of brighter blood and aqueous near the upper limbus. If no further rebleeding occurs, total resorption of the residual blood usually occurs within 7 to 10 days.[44]

The occurrence of a hyphema in a patient with sickle cell disease or trait may require earlier and more aggressive management. Because of sludging and sickling, sickled red blood cells have more difficulty in traversing the trabecular meshwork than do normal red blood cells.[34] In addition, the risk of occlusion of the central retinal artery is greatly increased in patients with sickling.[19]

Surgical management

The optimal time and method of surgical intervention for medically unresponsive cases of total hyphema from blunt trauma is an often-debated subject. Early intervention should be avoided because it often results in rebleeding. Furthermore, if intervention is delayed 3 to 5 days, a significant number of cases will resolve spontaneously. Severe, unremitting pain and early blood staining of the cornea argue for surgical intervention.

Experimental work by Sears[49] on clot retraction suggested the optimum time for surgical intervention to be 4 days. At this point the clot is freest of adherence to adjacent structures. Total removal of the clot is unnecessary for resolution of the glaucoma and also exposes the patient to an increased risk of rehemorrhage and loss of uveal tissue that may adhere to the clot.

Suggested surgical approaches include paracentesis[37] and irrigation with balanced salt solution or fibrinolytic agents[42,43,47] or aspiration with an emulsification or vitrectomy type of instrument.[24,32] We favor draining the anterior chamber via a trabeculectomy approach. A fornix-based conjunctival approach is combined with a half-thickness equilateral 4 mm triangular scleral flap. A 1×3 mm segment of the deeper limbal tissues is removed anterior to the scleral spur. Before removal of this window of tissue, a paracentesis tract is made in the temporal cornea. Twisting the blade in the tract allows a small amount of fluid to escape and serves to reduce the pressure in a slow and controlled manner. The tract also provides a second entry site for the later irrigation of the clot. The injection of a viscoelastic agent through this paracentesis tract often facilitates extrusion of a resistant clot. The relatively large trabeculectomy window allows free exit of the clot, but removal should be slow and controlled, with careful visual inspection of all contents before removal from the anterior chamber. The clot may be adherent to iris and can be gently separated by irrigation with balanced salt solution. Patience and care will help avoid the inadvertent removal of iris. In no instance is it advisable or necessary to reach into the anterior chamber to remove clot. Instrumentation within the anterior chamber can cause traction on the uvea with resultant new hemorrhage or lens injury.

In our experience, the trabeculectomy approach has accomplished the goal of immediate reduction of intraocular pressure and clot removal, with no recurrence of hemorrhage. Usually a permanent filtration bleb is not established, but during the first few weeks postoperatively, external filtration occurs while the traumatized trabecular meshwork has a chance to recover.

Lens Subluxation

Pupillary block can occur after blunt trauma with subluxation of the lens. Rupture of a portion of the zonules may allow formed vitreous to herniate around the tilted lens equator, or the lens itself may become incarcerated in the pupil, thereby increasing the normal physiologic obstruction to aqueous flow through the pupil. This may cause increased bulging of the peripheral iris, leading to angle-closure glaucoma.

Miosis usually aggravates the problem. Dilation may allow vitreous to come through the pupil and fill the anterior chamber, and angle-closure attacks may be alleviated in this manner. Unfortunately, the eye may be at risk for repeated attacks of pupillary block and angle closure, depending on the relationship between the pupil, lens, and vitreous. Iridectomy or lens extraction may be necessary. Treatment should be vigorous and timely to prevent the formation of peripheral anterior synechiae.

A dislocated lens may fall into the vitreous cavity. This is usually not a problem unless the lens becomes hypermature and causes phacolytic glaucoma (see Chapter 58). A totally dislocated lens may also fall forward into the anterior chamber and cause pupillary block and angle-closure glaucoma. This is an emergency because of early corneal decompensation from lens-endothelial touch.

Forward Movement of the Lens-iris Diaphragm

Angle closure resulting from forward displacement of the lens-iris diaphragm can occur after trauma. It can be difficult to distinguish from pupillary block with lens subluxation, although the former may have more shallowing of the central anterior chamber. The mechanism appears to be ciliary block, and although the exact cause is unknown, severe edema of the choroid, retina, and ciliary body secondary to the acute trauma could be initiating factors. The condition is best treated with cycloplegics and corticosteroids and is usually self-limited, resolving in 3 to 5 days. Iridectomy is not necessary as a rule.

Inflammation

Inflammation from trauma may compromise the outflow structures due to obstruction by inflammatory cells, debris, or protein. Inflammatory cells may be difficult to distinguish from red blood cells. Inflammatory cells should be suspected if the intraocular pressure is elevated with a cell count in the anterior chamber that does not appear to be proportional to the height of the pressure because similar quantities of fresh red blood cells do not elevate the intraocular pressure in eyes with normal outflow facility.

Treatment with topical corticosteroids usually helps to resolve the inflammation and decrease the intraocular pressure. Chronic use of corticosteroids should be avoided, however, because pressure elevations may occur. If systemic corticosteroids are employed, their possible adverse side effects must be borne in mind.

Occasionally, as an anterior chamber hemorrhage resolves, the fresh red blood cells are gradually replaced with fine tan-colored cells. The intraocular pressure, which may have declined toward normal, may now start to rise. Rather than uveitis, ghost cell glaucoma should be suspected. This is caused by degenerated red blood cell ghosts coming forward into the anterior chamber from a vitreous hemorrhage secondary to the original trauma[10] (see Chapter 69).

A rare cause of glaucoma several months after trauma is a retinal detachment related to traumatic retinal dialysis.[48] Inflammatory changes in the anterior segment and major swings in intraocular pressure are typically seen. Although rare, it is an important consideration in the differential diagnosis because surgical reattachment cures this type of glaucoma (see Chapter 59).

Trabecular Injury

Clinical findings

The most common cause of elevated intraocular pressure in the early postinjury period is mechanical damage to the trabecular meshwork. Tears in the trabecular meshwork (Fig. 68-3) occur frequently after blunt trauma but are often overlooked.[4] One study reported evidence of trabecular injury in 13 of 17 patients with mild hyphemas examined gonioscopically within 48 hours of the injury.[21]

The actual trabecular tear does not decrease outflow facility; however, the resultant scarring of the trabecular meshwork can lead to severe outflow obstruction (Fig. 68-4).

Increased intraocular pressure due to trabecular scarring usually does not respond well to medical therapy. However, if treated conservatively, this problem is usually self-limited, probably because of regeneration or repair of the damaged tra-

Fig. 68-3 Artist's conception of tear in trabecular meshwork after acute blunt anterior segment trauma. Note clot adhering to trabecular flap created by anterior segment trauma. Also note large tear into face of ciliary body with raw appearance of torn ciliary muscle.

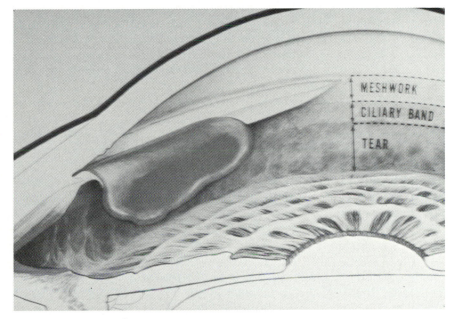

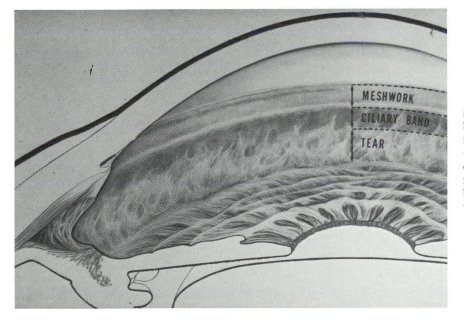

Fig. 68-4 Artist's conception of trabecular and ciliary body tear 9 days after injury. Trabecular tear is sealed, since trabecular flap has rotated back to its original position and scar tissue is forming. Note scar tissue formation in ciliary body tear with resultant narrowing of visible angle recession.

becular meshwork. Filtration surgery in the early posttraumatic period, therefore, should be avoided if at all possible.

Mechanisms of glaucoma

Tears in the ciliary body after trauma were first demonstrated experimentally in 1942.[25] However, the association of blunt ocular trauma and the later development of glaucoma was not noted clinically until 1945[13] and was not correlated pathologically until 1962.[54] The ciliary body tears noted histopathologically (clinically called angle recession) originally were thought to be evidence of past trauma but not the cause of the increased intraocular pressure.

Attempts have been made to correlate the later development of glaucoma with the extent of angle recession visible years after the initial injury.[8] Glaucoma is more frequent in angle recession involving 270 degrees or more.[23] Prospective studies suggest that the incidence of later developing glaucoma after angle recession is from 2% to 10%.[23,52]

The fresh tear into the ciliary body, which splits the longitudinal and circular fibers, begins to scar soon after injury.[21] The depth and extent of the visible cleft changes markedly in the first weeks and months after injury because of synechia formation (Fig. 68-5). Some eyes show obliteration of the angle recess and even peripheral anterior synechiae, which obscure the angle recession.

Rather than looking solely for angle recession, one can frequently recognize past trauma to the anterior segment by absent or torn iris processes,

a localized depression or tear in the trabecular meshwork, and increased whitening and visibility of the scleral spur (Figs. 68-6 and 68-7).

Although asymmetric cupping and visual field loss are common in primary open-angle glaucoma, asymmetry of pressure is not. When it is encountered, a secondary cause (e.g., exfoliation syndrome or trauma) should be considered. In our experience, careful gonioscopic examination of referred patients requiring surgery for primary open-angle glaucoma shows that prior trauma has occurred more often than previously thought.

It is rare to find a truly unilateral glaucoma years after a blunt anterior segment injury. Decrease in outflow facility from trauma probably occurs soon after the initial injury. The further loss in outflow facility is due to an underlying predisposition to the development of open-angle glaucoma. In a series of 18 patients suffering from glaucoma associated with previous trauma, an average of 16.5 years elapsed between injury and discovery of increased intraocular pressure. Of interest was the finding that the fellow, uninjured eye had an average intraocular pressure of 23.5 mm Hg.[21] An underlying predisposition to glaucoma in eyes with an intraocular pressure rise after trauma is further supported by the work of Armaly[2] indicating that the uninvolved eye of patients with traumatic glaucoma responded to steroid-provocative testing, as would the eye of a patient with primary open-angle glaucoma.

How does anterior segment trauma affect patients who already have established primary open-

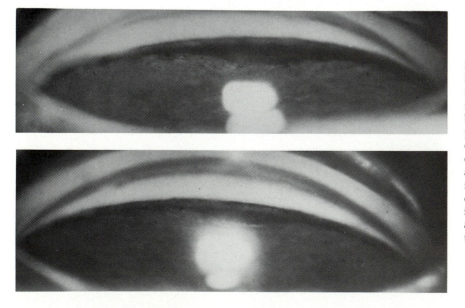

Fig. 68-5 Goniophotograph of monkey eye after blunt anterior segment trauma. Upper portion of figure is photographed 1 week after experimental blunt anterior segment injury with hyphema. Note both depth and horizontal extent of ciliary body tear. Lower portion of figure shows same area pictured above 3 months after injury. Note narrowing of angle recession in areas beside deepest portion of ciliary body tear. This is caused by scar contraction. Peripheral anterior synechiae actually occlude portions of trabecular meshwork.

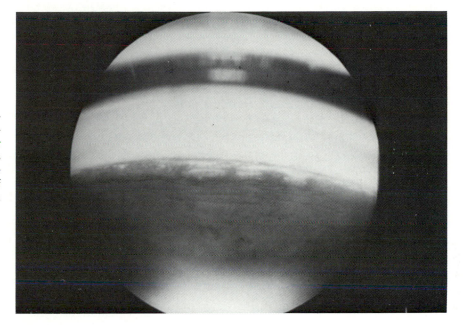

Fig. 68-6 Goniophotograph of human eye in patient with traumatic glaucoma 10 years after blunt anterior segment injury. Note area of torn iris processes with gray appearance of face of ciliary body. Also note whitening of trabecular meshwork and scleral spur in injured area.

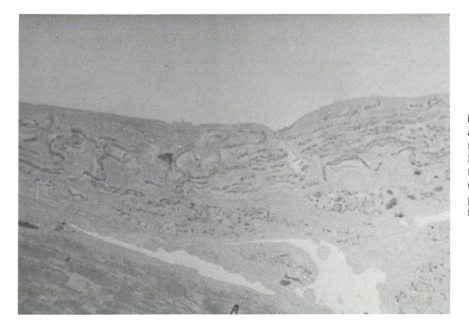

Fig. 68-7 Histologic section obtained at time of filtration surgery from area of filtration angle pictured in Fig. 68-6. Note collapse and scarring of adjacent trabecular sheets. Schlemm's canal is patent, but trabecular meshwork itself appears impermeable to aqueous humor flow.

angle glaucoma? Initially, it may be more difficult to clear the anterior chamber of red blood cells with a resultant increase in intraocular pressure. However, if an extensive trabecular tear has occurred (in effect, a traumatic trabeculotomy), outflow facility may increase. Sometimes this increase in facility is only temporary, but occasionally a long-lasting improvement in intraocular pressure regulation may occur.

Cuticular membranes have been seen histopathologically in eyes enucleated for glaucoma resulting from trauma.[28] It is difficult to know if the membrane was the initial factor in decreasing the outflow because eyes enucleated with traumatic glaucoma are usually blind and painful with long-standing glaucoma. The pain is often due to bullous keratopathy and intraocular inflammation. Many eyes with chronic inflammation from causes other than trauma also develop cuticular membranes over the filtration meshwork.

PENETRATING INJURIES

Injury Without a Retained Foreign Body

The most significant glaucoma problem associated with a perforating injury to the globe is prolonged flattening of the chamber in an inflamed eye with the formation of permanent peripheral anterior snyechiae. The best treatment for this problem is prophylaxis. Adequate wound closure with fine, permanent suture material, postoperative mydriasis, and the use of topical corticosteroids, lessens the incidence of this complication.

A related cause for PAS formation is pupillary block. If the iris is not adequately dilated after injury and inflammation causes seclusion of the pupil, iris bombé with secondary angle-closure will result. Again, prophylaxis is the most effective way to avoid this problem. However, if seclusion occurs, a prompt laser iridectomy is imperative to avoid chronic angle-closure glaucoma.

A perforating injury that breaks the lens capsule can result in swelling of the lens, with a relative pupillary block and angle-closure glaucoma or phacolytic glaucoma. Aspiration of the swollen lens material is the definitive therapy.

As in blunt trauma, bleeding can occur from a perforating injury, and total hyphema with glaucoma and ghost cell glaucoma can occur.

Epithelial ingrowth (see Chapter 73), causing mechanical obstruction of the trabecular meshwork, is a rare complication of a perforating injury. It should be suspected as the cause of glaucoma if the eye remains chronically irritated after a perfo-

rating injury. A gray membrane is seen on the posterior surface of the cornea and/or the anterior surface of the iris.

Another rare cause for glaucoma after perforating trauma associated with a chronically inflamed eye is sympathetic ophthalmia. Usually the condition is bilateral, but one eye may be more affected than the other. Glaucoma results from inflammatory obstruction of the trabecular meshwork. The advent of vitrectomy to rehabilitate severely traumatized eyes may be associated with an increased incidence of sympathetic ophthalmia.[30]

Injury with a Retained Foreign Body

A patient sustaining an intraocular foreign body may have early elevation in intraocular pressure, either as a consequence of direct trauma to ocular structures or secondary to the effects of blunt trauma on the trabecular meshwork, as previously discussed. In addition, glaucoma may develop as a late sequela of a retained, often unsuspected, metallic foreign body.

A rupture of the lens capsule is present in about 50% of eyes injured by a metallic intraocular foreign body[40] and may result in a concurrent phacogenic glaucoma at the time of presentation. On occasion, this may be the presenting sign of an occult intraocular foreign body. The correct diagnosis may be suggested by a sealed corneal perforation site, a hole or transillumination defect in the iris, or direct visualization of the foreign body after pupillary dilation.[11] Appropriate x-ray studies, ultrasonography, and computerized axial tomography may confirm the clinical suspicion. On occasion, it may not be possible to detect a minute foreign body in the anterior segment by these techniques in spite of strong clinical signs. In this situation, an alternate approach is the use of a pediatric dental x-ray cassette, lodged lengthwise in the medial canthal region after the instillation of a topical anesthetic. On occasion, this may accurately localize an otherwise undetectable foreign body in the anterior segment. Such documentation is important, since appropriate therapy includes removal of the metallic foreign body to prevent the late complications of siderosis or chalcosis.

Intraocular foreign bodies may cause the onset of late elevation in intraocular pressure by several mechanisms. As in nonpenetrating injuries, the blunt trauma associated with the injury itself may damage the angle or trabecular meshwork. Flattening of the anterior chamber and concurrent inflammation may produce peripheral anterior syn-

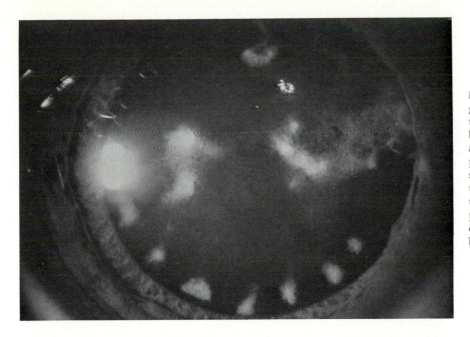

Fig. 68-8 Anterior segment photograph of siderotic cataract in construction worker with occult retained foreign body. Multiple small rust-colored spots are seen to lie subcapsularly, and nonpharmacologic mydriasis secondary to siderosis can be appreciated. Other features present but not demonstrated photographically include rusty staining of posterior corneal surface, heterochromia, and retained magnetic foreign body lodged in retina.

echiae.[46] Finally, iron deposition in the trabecular meshwork of eyes with siderosis from a retained magnetic foreign body may explain the reduced aqueous outflow and secondary glaucoma.[15,16] This process, however, develops over months to years. In this era of vitreous surgery and increasingly sophisticated intraocular instrumentation, such complications are not common. Nevertheless, patients may have unsuspected intraocular foreign bodies and unilateral glaucoma.[35] Heterochromia, mydriasis, a rust-colored stain to the posterior corneal surface, and multiple rust-colored anterior subcapsular lens deposits (Fig. 68-8) are the classic clinical signs of siderosis and should lead the clinician to the appropriate diagnosis.

CHEMICAL INJURIES

Alkali burns (and, to a lesser extent, acid burns) of the eye carry a poor prognosis, in part because the early florid external manifestations of the injury may mask the internal damage from uncontrolled elevations of intraocular pressure. Recognition and treatment of glaucoma through all phases of the injury are extremely important in the management of these patients.

Various pathogenic mechanisms responsible for an elevation in intraocular pressure may become manifest at different times after the injury, thus posing a constant threat to the visual potential of the chemically injured eye. To manage glaucoma secondary to a chemical injury, one must understand its pathogenesis, the difficulties in accurately measuring the intraocular pressure and documenting optic nerve damage, and, finally, the therapeutic modalities available.

Glaucoma secondary to a chemical burn can occur in three phases of the injury. The early phase (first hours to few days) is characterized by acute tissue destruction and the release of inflammatory mediators. It is followed by an intermediate phase (weeks to months) of repair, scarring, and ongoing inflammation. As inflammatory signs abate, the transition is made to a late phase characterized by extraocular and intraocular cicatrization and consequent functional disturbances.

Early Phase of Damage

Structural damage to the anterior segment occurs within minutes after contact with the offending chemical and may be associated with an early rise in intraocular pressure. Although early copious irrigation and removal of particulate matter is recommended, animal studies indicate that saponified alkaline chemicals are detected in the anterior chamber within seconds of the injury.[22,29] The severity of the injury is a function of the rapidity of ocular penetration, chemical concentration, and duration of exposure.

Alkaline substances generally cause more profound damage through destruction of the lipid barriers of the anterior segment. This results in ischemia of the anterior circulation, reflected in a

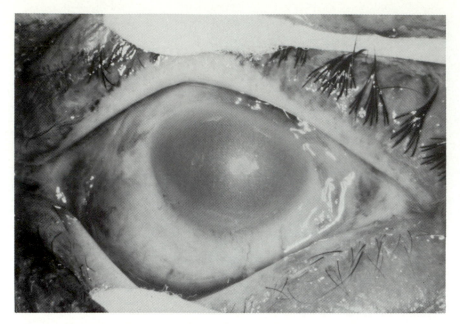

Fig. 68-9 External photograph of human eye 6 hours after chemical injury with potassium hydroxide. Whitening of inferior perilimbal sclera and conjunctiva can be seen, indicating ischemia. Cornea demonstrates typical beaten silver appearance seen after severe alkali chemical injury.

whitened sclera and in death of the cellular elements of the anterior segment (Fig. 68-9). Acids, on the other hand, cause coagulation of tissue proteins and generally result in a more superficial, corrosive injury.[17,29] However, if the eye is exposed to high concentrations of acid for prolonged periods of time, deeper tissue destruction can occur, producing a clinical picture not unlike the more rapidly destructive alkali burn.

Early elevations of intraocular pressure may result from scleral shrinkage secondary to the caustic injury, possibly coupled with the release of intraocular prostaglandins.[39] Conversely, in the most severely injured eyes, damage to the ciliary body may result in hypotony.[41]

Accurate documentation of the intraocular pressure may be difficult in this early period as a result of periorbital swelling and a thickened or irregular corneal surface. Conventional Schiøtz or applanation tonometry may be difficult in this setting, and the presence of corneal edema may result in underestimation of the intraocular pressure with these instruments. In the presence of corneal edema, measurements are more easily and accurately obtained with a pneumatometer.[45]

Treatment of early elevation of intraocular pressure is limited to agents that decrease aqueous production, such as beta blockers and carbonic anhydrase inhibitors, and to epinephrine compounds. Miotics are relatively contraindicated, since they augment the inflammatory response and may contribute to pupillary block if synechiae are formed between pupil and lens. If it is not possible to measure the intraocular pressure because of alterations of the anterior segment, prophylactic use of a carbonic anhydrase inhibitor may be reasonable until one can obtain accurate measurements.

Intermediate Phase of Damage

During the intermediate or reparative phase, lid and conjunctival changes evolve while the cornea attempts to reepithelialize areas of potential stromal breakdown and concurrent endothelial damage. The trabecular meshwork may have been structurally damaged by the initial direct, toxic injury or by synechia formation as a result of inflammation and tissue necrosis. More inflamed eyes, in particular those with hypopyon, are prone to develop glaucoma in this phase.[9] Medical reduction of aqueous production remains the cornerstone of antiglaucoma therapy, coupled with antiinflammatory medications. However, topical corticosteroids may be contraindicated in the first few weeks if corneal stromal lysis is present.[14] Oral corticosteroids may be administered to reduce anterior chamber inflammation if topical corticosteroids are contraindicated because of stromal lysis.

Trabecular meshwork damage is the principal but not sole cause of elevation of intraocular pressure during the intermediate phase. The pupillary portion of the iris, which frequently becomes unresponsive after a chemical injury, may become adherent to the lens, resulting in pupillary block glaucoma. This condition should be anticipated and mydriatic treatment initiated early with the effect on pupil size noted. If pupillary block develops, intensive therapy with topical steroids and mydriatics should be undertaken. If this fails and if the cornea is sufficiently clear, laser iridectomy may be sufficient to reverse the pupillary block. As a last resort, one may be required to undertake a conventional surgical iridectomy.

Progressive cataract formation may occur and can contribute to increased intraocular pressure, either on the basis of pupillary block from a swollen lens or from the release of lens material.[9] Medical therapy may allow surgery to be deferred. However, lens extraction may be required, in which case lens aspiration through a small wound is recommended, if possible.

Late Phase of Damage

After the anterior segment has stabilized relative to lid deformities and corneal resurfacing, it may become necessary to manage more chronic elevations of intraocular pressure. This is required not only to prevent optic nerve damage, but also to improve the prognosis of a rehabilitative procedure, such as a penetrating keratoplasty or keratoprosthesis.

If corneal surface irregularities or corneal edema exist, the pneumatometer should be used to obtain more accurate intraocular pressure measurements. This instrument may be used with a (bandage) soft contact lens in situ without markedly altering accuracy. Scarred, opaque media make visual field and optic nerve head evaluation more difficult and less accurate for follow-up. However, other less precise parameters may be helpful. If the injury is monocular, the consensual response of the normal pupil may demonstrate an afferent pupillary defect, indicating significant optic nerve damage or coexisting retinal disease. Using a Goldmann perimeter with larger peripheral targets may provide reproducible parameters that can be followed. If perimetry is not possible, confrontation fields with a bright light should discriminate between a residual temporal island or remaining central field. Ultrasound examination may detect advanced "beanpot" glaucomatous cupping, although a normal examination does not rule out advanced glaucomatous damage.

In the chronic, noninflammatory phase of pressure elevation, miotics may be effective in increasing outflow facility. Topical corticosteroids are ineffective during this stage and may have undesirable side effects of retarding corneal reepi-

thelization, augmenting corneal stromal lysis, and causing secondary elevation of intraocular pressure. It has been proposed that an acquired (non-genetic) form of corticosteroid-induced ocular hypertension exists, with susceptibility in part resulting from trabecular meshwork damage, suggesting that eyes with chemical injuries affecting the trabecular meshwork may be more prone to this complication.[1]

An additional consideration in antiglaucoma therapy of eyes with chemical injuries is related to the potential deleterious effect of topical beta-blocking agents, which may retard reepithelization. Presumably, this is a consequence of a beta-adrenergic antagonist effect on the corneal epithelium with lower cyclic adenosine monophosphate levels and retardation of corneal epithelial wound healing.[36] Persistent epithelial defects secondary to chemical burns are notoriously problematic, and it may be necessary to limit potentially toxic drugs, such as the beta-adrenergic antagonists. Promising adjuncts in these difficult surgical cases include conjunctival transplantation.[20,51]

Antiglaucoma surgery, which one would be hesitant to undertake in the acute or intermediate stages, may now be considered if the intraocular pressure is not adequately controlled medically. Because widespread conjunctival necrosis and subsequent scarring and symblepharon frequently occur, there is often no suitable site for a filtration operation. However, if damage is limited to the exposed interpalpebral fissure, there may be a reasonable site for filtration in an undamaged area. If not, the only alternative is cyclodestructive surgery, most commonly cyclocryotherapy.[50] However, because of ciliary body necrosis, aqueous production may already be reduced. Consequently, cyclocryotherapy should be limited to treatment of no more than 90 to 180 degrees at one time. A freeze-thaw rather than a freeze-thaw-refreeze technique may lessen the likelihood of hypotony and phthisis.

RADIATION THERAPY

Radiation therapy for periocular and intracranial neoplasia may result in elevations of intraocular pressure from heterogeneous causes.[3] A secondary open-angle glaucoma, often associated with generalized conjunctival telangiectasis, can occur and may respond to conventional antiglaucoma treatment.[5] More intractable elevations in pressure may result from rubeosis iridis or intraocular hemorrhage, presumably related to coexisting retinal radiation damage.[31] Generally, this occurs in the presence of widespread ocular damage, and the prognosis for these eyes is poor.

More recently, radiation has been used in the treatment of uveal melanoma. Neovascular glaucoma develops in approximately 10% of these eyes, most commonly in association with the presence of a large tumor.[26]

ELECTRICAL INJURY

Although no conclusive data establish glaucoma as a complication of electrical injury, abnormalities of the iris pigment, resulting from accidental and therapeutic (e.g., cardioversion, electroconvulsive therapy) electrical trauma, have been reported.[6,7] In these patients, there may be mild to extensive loss of the iris pigment epithelium, which is best demonstrated by slit-lamp retroillumination. A concurrent dispersion of pigment onto the anterior lens capsule, anterior iris surface, and corneal endothelium is also seen. Although a transient elevation of intraocular pressure is noted in some patients who have had previous electroconvulsive therapy, a direct connection between electrical injury, dispersion of iris pigment, and glaucoma remains to be established.

REFERENCES

1. Akingbehin, AO: Corticosteroid-induced ocular hypertension. II. An acquired form, Br J Ophthalmol 66:541, 1982

2. Armaly, ME: Steroids and glaucoma. In Transactions of the New Orleans Academy of Ophthalmology: Symposium on glaucoma, St Louis, 1967, The CV Mosby Co

3. Barron, A, McDonald, JE, and Hughes, WF: Long-term complications of beta radiation therapy in ophthalmology, Trans Am Ophthalmol Soc 68:112, 1970

4. Bechetoille, A: Aspects gonioscopiques des lesions traumatiques de l'angle, Clin Ophthalmol 3:17, 1971

5. Bedford, MA: Corneal and conjunctival complications following radiotherapy, Proc R Soc Med 59:529, 1966

6. Berger, RO: Ocular complications of cardioversion, Ann Ophthalmol 10:161, 1978

7. Berger, RO: Ocular complications of electroconvulsive therapy, Ann Ophthalmol 10:737, 1978

8. Blanton, FM: Anterior chamber angle recession and secondary glaucoma: a study of the after effects of traumatic hyphemas, Arch Ophthalmol 72:39, 1964

9. Brown, SI, Tragakis, MP, and Pearce, DB: Treatment of the alkali burned cornea, Am J Ophthalmol 74:316, 1972

10. Campbell, DG, Simmons, RJ, and Grant, WM: Ghost cells as a cause of glaucoma, Am J Ophthalmol 75:205, 1973

11. Crouch, ER, and Frenkel, M: Aminocaproic acid in the treatment of traumatic hyphema, Am J Ophthalmol 81:355, 1976

12. Davidson, SI: Intraocular foreign bodies: clinical recognition, Int Ophthalmol Clin 8:171, 1968

13. D'Ombrain, A: Traumatic monocular chronic glaucoma, Trans Ophthalmol Soc Aust 5:116, 1945

14. Donshik, PC, et al: The effect of topical corticosteroids on ulceration in alkali-burned corneas, Arch Ophthalmol 96:2117, 1970

15. Duke-Elder, S: System of ophthalmology: diseases of the lens and vitreous; glaucoma and hypotony, vol 11, St Louis, 1969, The CV Mosby Co

16. Duke-Elder, S, and MacFaul, P: Injuries. I. Mechanical injuries, vol 14. In Duke-Elder, S, editor: System of ophthalmology, St Louis, 1972, The CV Mosby Co

17. Duke-Elder, S, and MacFaul, P: Injuries. II. Non-mechanical injuries, vol 14. In Duke-Elder, S, editor: System of ophthalmology, St Louis, 1972, The CV Mosby Co

18. Edwards, WC, and Layden, WE: Traumatic hyphema: a report of 184 consecutive cases, Am J Ophthalmol 75:110, 1973

19. Goldberg, MF: The diagnosis and treatment of sickled erythrocytes in human hyphemas, Trans Am Ophthalmol Soc 76:481, 1978

20. Herman, WK, Doughman, DJ, and Lindstrom, RL: Conjunctival autograft transplantation for unilateral ocular surface disease, Ophthalmology 90:1121, 1983

21. Herschler, J: Trabecular damage due to blunt anterior segment injury and its relationship to traumatic glaucoma, Trans Am Acad Ophthalmol Otolaryngol 83:239, 1977

22. Hughes, WF: Alkali burns of the eye. I. Review of the literature and summary of the present knowledge, Arch Ophthalmol 35:423, 1946

23. Kaufman, JH, and Tolpin, DW: Glaucoma after traumatic angle recession: a ten-year prospective study, Am J Ophthalmol 78:648, 1974

24. Kelman, CD, and Brooks, DL: Ultrasonic emulsification and aspiration of traumatic hyphema: a preliminary report, Am J Ophthalmol 71:1289, 1971

25. Kilgore, GL: An experimental study of iridodialysis, Trans Am Ophthalmol Soc 40:516, 1942

26. Kim, MK, et al: Neovascular glaucoma after helium ion irradiation for uveal melanoma, Ophthalmology 93:189, 1986

27. Kutner, B, et al: Aminocaproic acid reduces the risk of secondary hemorrhage in patients with traumatic hyphema, Arch Ophthalmol 105:206, 1987

28. Lauring, L: Anterior chamber glass membranes, Am J Ophthalmol 68:308, 1969

29. Lemp, MA: Cornea and sclera, Arch Ophthalmol 92:158, 1974

30. Lewis, ML, Gass, JDM, and Spencer, WH: Sympathetic uveitis after trauma and vitrectomy, Arch Ophthalmol 96:263, 1978

31. Macfaul, PA, and Bedford, MA: Ocular complications after therapeutic irradiation, Br J Ophthalmol 54:237, 1970

32. McCuen, BW, and Fung, WE: The role of vitrectomy instrumentation in the treatment of severe traumatic hyphema, Am J Ophthalmol 88:930, 1979

33. McGetrick, JJ, et al: Aminocaproic acid decreases secondary hemorrhage after traumatic hyphema, Arch Ophthalmol 101:1031, 1983

34. Michelson, PE, and Pfaffenbach, D: Retinal arterial occlusion following ocular trauma in youths with sickle-trait hemoglobinopathy, Am J Ophthalmol 74:494, 1972

35. Miles, DR, and Boniuk, M: Pathogenesis of unilateral glaucoma, Am J Ophthalmol 62:493, 1966

36. Nork, TM, et al: Timolol inhibits corneal epithelial wound healing in rabbits and monkeys, Arch Ophthalmol 103:1224, 1984

37. Oksala, A: Treatment of traumatic hyphema, Br J Ophthalmol 51:315, 1967

38. Palmer, DJ, et al: A comparison of two dose regimens of epsilon amino caproic acid in the prevention and management of secondary traumatic hyphemas, Ophthalmology 93:102, 1986

39. Paterson, CA, and Pfister, RR: Intraocular pressure changes after alkali burns, Arch Ophthalmol 91:211, 1974

40. Percival, SPB: Late complications from posterior segment intraocular foreign bodies, Br J Ophthalmol 56:462, 1972

41. Pfister, RR, Friend, J, and Dohlman, CH: The anterior segments of rabbits after alkali burns, Arch Ophthalmol 86:189, 1971

42. Polychronakos, D, and Razoglou, C: Treatment of total hyphema with fibrinolysin, Ophthalmologica 154:31, 1967

43. Rakusin, W: Urokinase in the management of traumatic hyphema, Br J Ophthalmol 55:826, 1971

44. Read, J, and Goldberg, MF: Comparison of medical treatment of traumatic hyphema, Trans Am Acad Ophthalmol Otolaryngol 78:799, 1974

45. Richter, RC, Stark, WJ, Cowan, C, and Pollack, IP: Tonometry on eyes with abnormal corneas, Glaucoma 2:508, 1980

46. Roper-Hall, MJ: Intraocular foreign bodies: prognosis, Int Ophthalmol Clin 8:257, 1968

47. Scheie, HG, Ashley, BJ, and Burns, DT: Treatment of total hyphema with fibrinolysin, Arch Ophthalmol 69:147, 1963

48. Schwartz, A: Chronic open-angle glaucoma secondary to rhegmatogenous retinal detachment, Am J Ophthalmol 75:205, 1973

49. Sears, ML: Surgical management of black ball hyphema, Trans Am Ophthalmol Otolaryngol 74:820, 1970

50. Shields, MB: Cyclodestructive surgery for glaucoma: past, present, and future, Trans Am Ophthalmol Soc 83:285, 1985

51. Thoft, RA: Conjunctival transplantation, Arch Ophthalmol 95:1425, 1977

52. Tonjun, AM: Intraocular pressure and facility of outflow late after ocular contusion, Acta Ophthalmol (Copenh) 46:886, 1968

53. Witteman, GJ: Traumatic hyphema, letter to the editor, Arch Ophthalmol 102:356, 1984

54. Wolff, SM, and Zimmerman, LE: Chronic secondary glaucoma associated with retrodisplacement of iris root and deepening of the anterior chamber angle secondary to contusion, Am J Ophthalmol 54:547, 1962

Chapter 69

Ghost Cell Glaucoma

David G. Campbell
M. Bruce Shields
Jeffrey M. Liebmann

In the previous chapter, fresh red blood cells in the anterior chamber (hyphema) was considered as one mechanism of blood-induced glaucoma. There are other situations in which degenerated erythrocytes or blood products, usually derived from a vitreous hemorrhage, may also lead to secondary glaucoma.

HISTORY AND TERMINOLOGY

In 1960, Vannas[25] discussed the role of hemosiderin in eyes with intraocular hemorrhage as a mechanism of intraocular pressure elevation, often occurring years after the initial bleed. While hemosiderin-filled macrophages were found during the first few months after a hemorrhage, it appeared that iron-containing substance in the tissues of the aqueous outflow system, possibly promoting degenerative-inflammatory changes in these structures, was responsible for the secondary glaucoma. This form of late-onset glaucoma following intraocular hemorrhage has been called "hemosiderotic glaucoma" and is apparently rare.

In 1963, Fenton and Zimmerman[12] emphasized the role of macrophages as a mechanism of blood-induced glaucoma. They noted that degenerated blood products originated in the vitreous and passed forward into the anterior chamber to obstruct the trabecular meshwork. Their light microscopic findings led them to believe that the associated glaucoma was due to red blood cell debris and macrophages. Noting the similarity to phacolytic glaucoma, they introduced the term "hemolytic glaucoma." Although follow-up reports seemed to confirm these findings,* continued study of the association between degenerated blood and elevated intraocular pressure suggested that macrophages rarely, if ever, are the main cause of this form of secondary glaucoma.

In 1975, Campbell and Grant[8] and, in 1976, Campbell, Simmons, and Grant[9] described a secondary glaucoma associated with vitreous hemorrhage that they thought was caused primarily by degenerated red blood (ghost cells, erythrocyte ghosts). Their light and electron microscopic studies of anterior chamber aspirates showed little or no debris and few to no macrophages. They named this condition "ghost cell glaucoma" and defined it as a transient, secondary glaucoma resulting from obstruction of the trabecular meshwork by degenerated erythrocytes. The ghost cells develop within the vitreous cavity after several types of hemorrhage. They then enter the anterior chamber through a disruption in the anterior hyaloid face.

PATHOGENESIS

Red Blood Cell Degeneration within the Vitreous Cavity

An understanding of ghost cell glaucoma requires knowledge of the fate of blood within the vitreous cavity after vitreous hemorrhage. Morphologic, colorimetric, and rheologic changes occur in the erythrocyte after it arrives in the vitreous cavity.[1,7] The normal erythrocytes degenerate from

---

*References 2, 11, 13, 14, 17, 24.

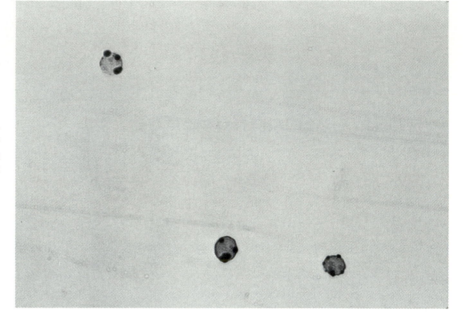

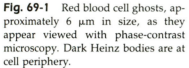

Fig. 69-1   Red blood cell ghosts, approximately 6 μm in size, as they appear viewed with phase-contrast microscopy. Dark Heinz bodies are at cell periphery.

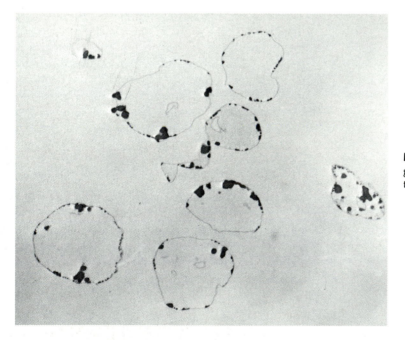

Fig. 69-2   Transmission electron micrograph of ghost cells withdrawn from anterior chamber of patient with traumatic ghost cell glaucoma.

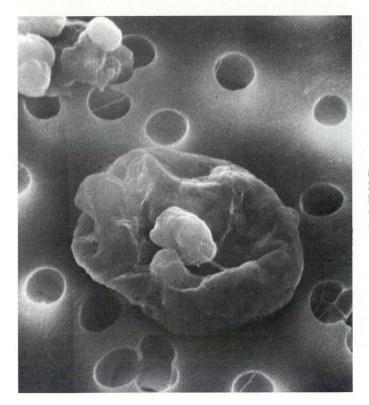

Fig. 69-3   Scanning electron micrograph of ghost cells collected on Nucleopore filter, showing protruding Heinz bodies. Specimen was taken from anterior chamber of patient with ghost cell glaucoma developing after cataract extraction.

red, biconcave, pliable cells to tan or khaki-colored, spherical and hollow, less pliable ghost cells (Figs. 69-1 to 69-3). The conversion begins within days and is generally almost complete within 1 to 3 weeks. After the ghost cells have formed, they do not rapidly degenerate further and can remain in this form within the vitreous cavity for many months. During the conversion to the ghost cell form, intracellular hemoglobin is lost, presumably through leaky membranes, into the extracellular vitreous space (Fig. 69-4). The hemoglobin that remains within the cell denatures and forms clumps called Heinz bodies, which adhere to the inner surface of the plasma membrane. The extracellular hemoglobin also becomes denatured and clumped, often forming small to large accumulations that tend to adhere to vitreous strands. The adherence to and the entrapment within vitreous strands (Fig. 69-5) prevents these extracellular clumps of hemoglobin from moving freely and from passing into the anterior chamber. In contrast, the red blood cell ghosts do not adhere to each other or to the vitreous strands and are free to move anteriorly. Erythrocyte ghosts are generally 4 to 7 μm in size, and the extracellular hemoglobin clumps are generally 2 to 20 μm in size. Studies of the vitreous show that macrophages are common and ingest

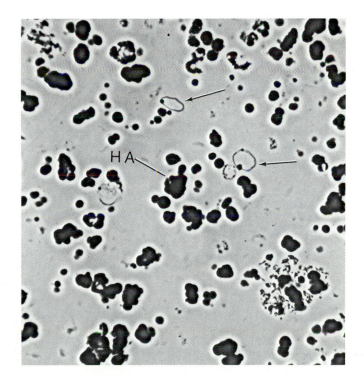

Fig. 69-4   Phase-contrast micrograph of vitreous hemorrhage specimen showing ghost cells *(arrows)*, much extracellular hemoglobin *(HA)*, and macrophage *(lower right)*. (From Campbell, DG, and Esigmann, EM: Arch Ophthalmol 97:2141, copyright 1979, American Medical Association)

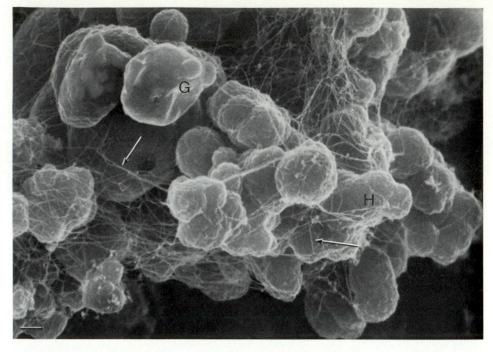

Fig. 69-5 Scanning electron micrograph of vitreous with hemorrhage showing free ghost cells *(G),* enmeshed extracellular hemoglobin clumps *(H),* and vitreous strands *(arrows).* (From Campbell, DG, and Esigmann, EM: Arch Ophthalmol 97:2141, copyright 1979, American Medical Association)

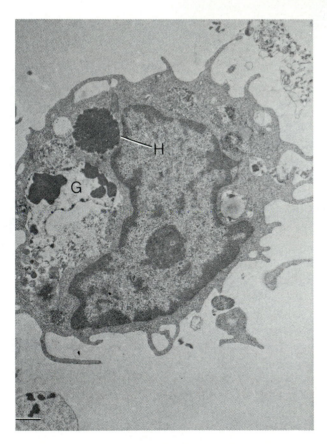

Fig. 69-6 Macrophage removed from vitreous cavity of patient with vitreous hemorrhage. Cell has ingested both extracellular hemoglobin clump *(H)* and ghost cell *(G).* (From Campbell, DG, and Esigmann, EM: Arch Ophthalmol 97:2141, copyright 1979, American Medical Association)

both the extracellular clumps and the ghost cells (Fig. 69-6).

The anterior hyaloid face serves as a natural boundary for the products of vitreous hemorrhage. Laboratory studies show that neither fresh erythrocytes nor ghost cells are able to pass across the intact anterior hyaloid face. Clinical observations show further that if the anterior hyaloid face is intact after a vitreous hemorrhage, fresh or degenerated products of the hemorrhage are not seen in the anterior chamber. If, however, there has been a disruption of the anterior hyaloid face, caused by either trauma, surgery, or perhaps a rare spontaneous disruption, the cells pass forward in large numbers. Once in the anterior chamber, the ghost cells obstruct the trabecular meshwork and cause glaucoma.

Rheologic Characteristics of the Ghost Cell

Ghost cells are less pliable than fresh red blood cells.[9] They cannot pass through a 5-μm Millipore filter and cannot pass through the human trabecular meshwork with ease, whereas fresh red blood cells do both. Ghost cells cause approximately three times more obstruction to outflow than an equal number of fresh erythrocytes. Lambrou et al.[15] demonstrated that injection of erythrocyte ghosts into the anterior chamber of cat and monkey eyes produced a significantly greater rise in intraocular pressure than an even larger injection of viable red blood cells. Histologic studies have shown that the

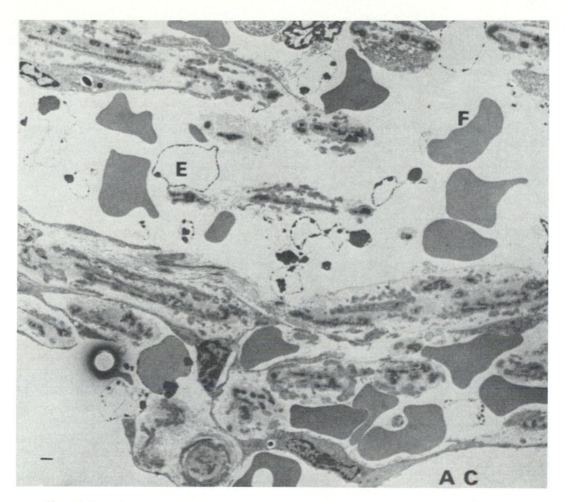

Fig. 69-7 Electron micrograph of outer one third of trabecular meshwork, adjacent to anterior chamber *(AC),* in human autopsy eye perfused with fresh red blood cells *(F)* and ghost cells *(E),* showing both cell types in intertrabecular spaces. Ghost cells do not pass easily beyond this level of meshwork. Bar gauge = 1 μ (×3,125). (From Campbell, DG, Simmons, RJ, and Grant, WM: Am J Ophthalmol 81:441, 1979. Published with permission, copyright by The Ophthalmic Publishing Co)

ghost cells tend to lodge in the outer and midportion of the trabecular meshwork, whereas fresh red blood cells pass to the inner meshwork and to Schlemm's canal with relative ease (Fig. 69-7). Fixed ghost cells can be used to induce glaucoma in primates,[18] a finding that provides laboratory confirmation of previously reported clinical and laboratory observations.

CLINICAL FORMS

The clinical history of a patient with ghost cell glaucoma invariably includes a history of vitreous hemorrhage, usually resulting from trauma, surgery, or primary retinal disease, such as diabetic retinopathy. The clinical history usually includes an event likely to have disrupted the anterior hyaloid face, such as cataract extraction, vitrectomy, or trauma. A number of different clinical presentations of ghost cell glaucoma have been found; the majority of cases have followed vitrectomy, cataract extraction, or trauma.

Ghost Cell Glaucoma after Vitrectomy

After closed pars plana vitrectomy for vitreous hemorrhage, ghost cell glaucoma often occurs.[10] The surgical procedure generally disrupts the anterior hyaloid face, and ghost cells left behind at surgery pass into the anterior chamber and cause glaucoma within days to weeks after the procedure. The glaucoma generally lasts weeks to months. This glaucoma was relatively common when vitrectomy was first introduced because in some cases the initial procedure cleared away only a central corridor of hemorrhagic material, leaving much peripheral material, including ghost cells, behind. Later, as vitreous surgeons began removing more of the hemorrhagic content, the incidence of this entity after vitrectomy decreased considerably. This glaucoma occurred after vitrectomy with or without lensectomy but seemed slightly more common after lensectomy and the creation of a larger opening in the anterior hyaloid face.

Ghost Cell Glaucoma after Cataract Extraction: Three Presentations

Early postoperative bleed

The most common way that ghost cell glaucoma occurs after cataract extraction involves the following sequence of events: A patient undergoes an uneventful intracapsular or extracapsular cataract extraction, after which a large hyphema develops with extension into the vitreous cavity within the first few days after the surgical procedure.[7] Usually, the anterior chamber hemorrhage clears at least partially, permitting a view of the vitreous hemorrhage. The elevation of intraocular pressure associated with the initial hemorrhage usually resolves within 1 or 2 weeks, but this is followed within 2 to 6 weeks postoperatively by an intraocular pressure elevation in association with the appearance of a multitude of tiny ghost cells in the anterior chamber. The pressure rise is due to obstruction of the trabecular meshwork by ghost cells that have reentered the anterior chamber. The original hyphema, which began in the anterior chamber, presumably extended back into the vitreous cavity through a disruption in the anterior hyaloid face created at the time of cataract removal. This same opening then allowed ghost cells to enter the anterior chamber at a later time. Ghost cell glaucoma has also been observed after cataract extraction and intraocular lens (IOL) implantation, in which cases, it was speculated that the IOL might have been a factor in recurrent bleeding.[20,23]

Preoperative bleed

The second presentation may occur after cataract extraction when a patient has a vitreous hemorrhage, usually from a retinal source existing before the cataract extraction. Large numbers of ghost cells existing within the vitreous cavity migrate into the anterior chamber immediately after the cataract extraction, which has disrupted the anterior hyaloid face, causing a marked elevation of intraocular pressure within days.

Late postoperative bleed

The third and least common presentation after cataract extraction occurs when a patient has a cataract extraction with disruption of the anterior hy-

aloid face and then develops a vitreous hemorrhage as a result of retinal disease at a later date. The red blood cells degenerate in the vitreous and then slowly pass forward into the anterior chamber. In this case, the contents of the anterior chamber are mixed with fresher red blood cells as well.

Ghost Cell Glaucoma after Trauma

Trauma to the eye, either blunt or penetrating, may result in the formation of a hyphema with hemorrhage into the vitreous cavity.[5] In some cases, the hyphema clears, allowing a view of the vitreous cavity filled with blood. Ghost cells form in the vitreous cavity and begin to pass forward into the anterior chamber weeks to months after the original injury. Characteristically, the anterior chamber hyphema has cleared or almost cleared when the infusion of tan-colored ghost cells becomes apparent. The intraocular pressure, which may have been high after the hyphema, has spontaneously decreased, when the infusion of ghost cells causes it once more to rise.

Occasionally an eight-ball hyphema is complicated by ghost cell glaucoma in association with a vitreous hemorrhage.[6] A high pressure rise occurs in the immediate days after the injury, but this generally begins to ameliorate 1 to 2 weeks after the injury. The anterior chamber is typically still obscured by dark purple material when a second elevation of intraocular pressure occurs. Anterior chamber aspirate studies at this time have shown large numbers of ghost cells that presumably passed forward from the vitreous cavity, in addition to the contents of the eight-ball hyphema, consisting of fresher red blood cells, white blood cells, macrophages, and fibrin.

Ghost Cell Glaucoma with No Prior Trauma or Surgery

Ghost cell glaucoma has been observed in phakic eyes with long-standing, spontaneous vitreous hemorrhage, usually from diabetic retinopathy or central retinal vein occlusion.[2,16] The glaucoma may appear years after the vitreous hemorrhage. In these cases, it is presumed that a defect in the anterior hyaloid face develops spontaneously, possibly as the vitreous liquefies and degenerates.

CLINICAL FEATURES

Intraocular Pressure

When a large number of erythrocyte ghosts exists within the anterior chamber, the patient may either by asymptomatic or complain of ocular pain caused by high intraocular pressure. If large numbers of ghost cells have entered the chamber, the pressure rises quickly over a period of days to a level as high as 60 to 70 mm Hg. The elevated intraocular pressure may persist for several months. However, ghost cells do not always cause a pressure rise, especially if there is only a small number of them circulating in the anterior chamber.

Conjunctiva

The conjunctiva is generally white unless it has been inflamed by extreme elevation of intraocular pressure or previous surgery. The presence of ghost cells alone in the anterior chamber does not incite an inflammatory response, which explains the relatively normal conjunctiva in the company of a markedly cellular anterior chamber.

Cornea

The cornea is typically normal but may be edematous with extreme elevation of intraocular pressure. If the cornea is edematous, topical glycerin is very useful in clearing it to allow examination of the contents of the anterior chamber. The corneal endothelium is either normal or has collections or layers of fine khaki-colored cells scattered on the surface. Keratic precipitates, characteristic of inflammation, do not form in association with ghost cells and when seen should lead the observer away from the diagnosis of ghost cell glaucoma toward an inflammatory cause.

Anterior Chamber

The aqueous humor is typically filled with a multitude of tiny tan-colored cells, often circulating slowly. The characteristic red color of fresh erythrocytes is absent. The tan-colored cells may be mistaken for white blood cells, resulting in the misdiagnosis of uveitis or endophthalmitis. The cells are tiny, generally 4 to 7 μm in size, and may be overlooked unless high-power examination of the anterior chamber contents (generally 25× magnification) is used. If the cells exist in large quantities, a pseudohypopyon, consisting of a layer of khaki-colored cells precipitated inferiorly, is often mistaken for a true hypopyon. However, true hypopyons, which are collections of white blood cells, are white; and the khaki color of a layer of red blood cell ghosts is easily distinguished and pathognomonic for ghost cells. If fresher red blood cells exist, two or more different layers are often seen, with the lighter khaki-colored layer of ghost appearing on top of a heavier, redder cell layer, imparting a candy-striped appearance (Fig. 69-8).

Gonioscopy

Gonioscopic examination generally reveals either a normal-appearing open angle; an open angle covered by a fine layer of khaki-colored cells, which have slightly to moderately discolored the trabecular meshwork; or a heavy layer filling the angle, generally inferiorly, with cells composing an early pseudohypopyon.

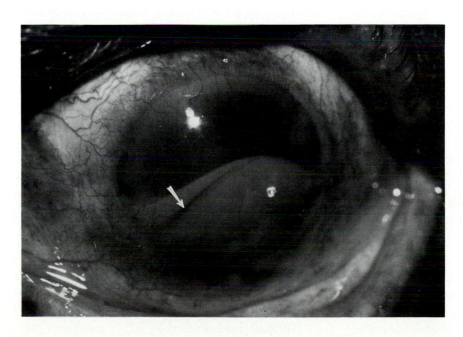

Fig. 69-8 Slit lamp view of eye with ghost cell glaucoma showing layer of fresher red blood cells *(arrow)* between two layers of khaki-colored ghost cells (candy-stripe appearance). (From Shields, MB, Textbook of Glaucoma, ed 2, Baltimore, Williams & Wilkins, 1987, p. 324; Courtesy David G. Campbell, M.D.)

Vitreous

Examination of the vitreous cavity reveals the characteristic khaki color typical of degenerated hemorrhage. Often, many fine ghost cells, along with extracellular hemoglobin clumps, frequently in sheets within the vitreous, can be seen. When the lens is absent, ghost cells can occasionally be seen streaming forward through a disruption in the anterior hyaloid face into the anterior chamber.

Anterior Chamber Aspiration Studies

The diagnosis can often be confirmed by examination of an anterior chamber aspiration specimen, usually obtained in conjunction with a therapeutic irrigation of the anterior chamber.[4,7,9,21] The diagnosis is made most easily by immediate examination of an unstained drop of aqueous humor placed on a slide, covered by a slightly elevated cover slip, and examined with phase-contrast microscopy[7,9,21] (see Fig. 69-1). This generally reveals a multitude of ghost cells with characteristic Heinz bodies. Some specimens contain occasional macrophages. Noncellular debris is typically absent, but 1 μm Heinz bodies may occasionally be seen. Polymorphonuclear leukocytes and lymphocytes are not found. Large extracellular clumps of hemoglobin commonly found within the vitreous cavity are also not found within the aqueous humor specimens, presumably because they remain entrapped and attached to vitreous strands (see Fig. 69-5). The diagnosis can also be made if the aspirate is filtered through a 1 μm Millipore filter and the surface is stained and examined by light microscopy. This is especially useful when phase contrast microscopy is not available and has the added advantage of providing a permanent specimen.[4] Characteristic ghost cells can be seen, but if, as is often the case, multitudes of cells are piled on each other, the cells appear to be amorphous debris. Scanning and transmission electron microscopic examination of the aspirates has confirmed the phase-contrast microscopic findings (see Figs. 69-2 and 69-3).

Often, while collecting the aspirate, the surgeon may note that a volume greater than 0.2 ml, the normal volume of the anterior chamber, can be aspirated without causing collapse of the chamber. This indicates that free communication exists with the fluid within the vitreous cavity and that this fluid is free to pass forward.[22]

DIFFERENTIAL DIAGNOSIS

Ghost cell glaucoma must be differentiated from other glaucomas that occur in association with vitreous hemorrhage, including neovascular, hemosiderotic, inflammatory, and hemolytic glaucomas.

Neovascular glaucoma, which is frequently associated with vitreous hemorrhage, can also be associated with extreme elevation of intraocular pressure. Neovascular glaucoma is differentiated from ghost cell glaucoma by the absence of ghost cells within the anterior chamber and the presence of neovascularization at the pupillary margin and in the angle.

Hemosiderosis, as previously discussed, causes a chronic open-angle glaucoma presumably caused by iron deposition in and damage to the trabecular meshwork.[25] This extremely rare glaucoma is more chronic, does not have ghost cells in the anterior chamber, and is characteristically associated with a slight discoloration of the meshwork. It occurs many years after the original injury, in contrast to ghost cell glaucoma, which occurs within weeks to months after the original injury.

Glaucoma secondary to uveitis has to be distinguished from ghost cell glaucoma. The tiny ghost cells may be misinterpreted as white blood cells, and the misdiagnoses of endophthalmitis and uveitis are not uncommon. The history of vitreous hemorrhage, disruption of the hyaloid face, a multitude of tiny khaki-colored cells, a relatively non-inflamed conjunctiva, and an absence of keratic precipitates differentiates this condition from uveitis and endophthalmitis. The white hypopyon of uveitis or endophthalmitis is easily distinguished from the khaki-colored pseudohypopyon associated with ghost cell glaucoma.

In regard to hemolytic glaucoma, the major question has been whether a glaucoma, separate and distinguishable from the one resulting from ghost cells, exists. We have not seen a patient or found an anterior chamber aspirate compatible with hemolytic glaucoma as originally described. It is possible that such a glaucoma exists, but if so, it is much rarer than ghost cell glaucoma. The diagnosis would be established by finding an aqueous humor specimen devoid of ghost cells but filled with macrophages and debris.

MANAGEMENT

The initial treatment of ghost cell glaucoma consists of standard medical therapy, including beta-adrenergic blocking agents, adrenergic agonists, parasympathomimetics, and carbonic anhydrase inhibitors. These may suffice to lower the intraocular pressure to a safe level until the supply of ghost cells within the vitreous cavity becomes exhausted and the glaucoma resolves.

Surgical intervention is often necessary because of a persistently elevated intraocular pressure despite maximum medical therapy. Thorough anterior chamber irrigation, repeated if necessary, is usually successful in removing sufficient numbers of ghost cells to lower the intraocular pressure. Irrigation with 10 to 20 ml of fluid, directed toward the angle so that the fluid will circulate and help clear angle debris, is often effective. The initial paracentesis wound should be large enough to allow the aqueous humor and ghost cells to egress easily around the needle. If anterior chamber washout lowers the intraocular pressure successfully but the pressure rises again because of the further entrance of ghost cells from the vitreous, a washout of the anterior chamber can be repeated. If this relatively simple and safe procedure is unsuccessful, vitrectomy to remove the contents of the vitreous cavity may be required.[3,19]

Because ghost cell glaucoma is not inflammatory, topical steroids are ineffective. If the patient is a steroid responder, long-term topical steroid use will cause further elevation of pressure. Steroids should be omitted or used in low doses only if concomitant inflammation is thought to exist.

PROGNOSIS

Ghost cell glaucoma is typically transient, although it may last many months. Eventually, the supply of erythrocyte ghosts in the vitreous cavity becomes exhausted and cells stop passing forward into the anterior chamber. No permanent damage to the trabecular meshwork has been noted to date.

REFERENCES

1. Benson, WE, and Spalter, HF: Vitreous hemorrhage, Surv Ophthalmol 15:297, 1971
2. Brooks, AMN, and Gillies, WE: Haemolytic glaucoma occurring in phakic eyes, Br J Ophthalmol 70:603, 1986
3. Brucker, AJ, Michels, RG, and Green, WR: Pars plana vitrectomy in the management of blood-induced glaucoma with vitreous hemorrhage, Ann Ophthalmol 10:1427, 1978
4. Cameron, JD, and Havener, VR: Histologic confirmation of ghost cell glaucoma by routine light microscopy, Am J Ophthalmol 96:251, 1983
5. Campbell, DG: Ghost cell glaucoma following trauma, Ophthalmology 88:1151, 1981
6. Campbell, DG, and Bellows, AR: Erythrocyte ghost cells in eight-ball hyphemas, Invest Ophthalmol Vis Sci (Suppl) 1977
7. Campbell, DG, and Essigmann, EM: Hemolytic ghost cell glaucoma, further studies, Arch Ophthalmol 97:2141, 1979
8. Campbell, DG, and Grant, WM: Alterations in red blood cells that prevent passage through the trabecular meshwork in human eyes, Invest Ophthalmol Vis Sci (Suppl) 1977
9. Campbell, DG, Simmons, RJ, and Grant, WM: Ghost cells as a cause of glaucoma, Am J Ophthalmol 81:441, 1976
10. Campbell, DG, Simmons, RJ, Tolentino, FI, and McMeel, JW: Glaucoma occurring after closed vitrectomy, Am J Ophthalmol 83:63, 1977
11. Fenton, RH, and Hunter, WS: Hemolytic glaucoma in CPC, Surv Ophthalmol 10:355, 1965
12. Fenton, RH, and Zimmerman, LE: Hemolytic glaucoma, an unusual cause of acute open angle secondary glaucoma, Arch Ophthalmol 70:236, 1963
13. Hunter, WS: Hemolytic glaucoma, Trans Am Acad Ophthalmcl Otolaryngol 73:95, 1969
14. Kiess, JD, Burnes, KC, and Cohen, MM: Hemolytic glaucoma: a difficult clinical diagnosis, EENT Monthly 48:49, 1969
15. Lambrou, FH, Aiken, DG, Woods, WD, and Campbell, DG: The production and mechanism of ghost cell glaucoma in the cat and primate, Invest Ophthalmol Vis Sci 26:893, 1985
16. Mansour, AM, Chess, J, and Starita, R: Nontraumatic ghost cell glaucoma: a case report, Ophthalmol Surg 17:34, 1986
17. Phelps, CD, and Watzke, RC: Hemolytic glaucoma, Am J Ophthalmol 80:690, 1975
18. Quigley, HA, and Addicks, EM: Chronic experimental glaucoma in primates, Invest Ophthalmol Vis Sci 19:126, 1980
19. Singh, H, and Grand, MG: Treatment of blood-induced glaucoma by trans pars plana vitrectomy, Retina 1:255, 1981
20. Summers, CG, and Lindstrom, RL: Ghost cell glaucoma following lens implantation, Am Intra-Ocular Implant Soc J 9:429, 1983
21. Summers, CG, Lindstrom, RL, and Cameron, JD: Phase contrast microscopy: diagnosis of ghost cell glaucoma following cataract extraction, Surv Ophthalmol 28:342, 1984
22. Thomas, R, Alexander, TA, and Joseph, P: Ghost cell glaucoma, Ind J Ophthalmol 33:53, 1985
23. van Oye, R, and Gelisken, O: Pseudophakic glaucoma, Int Ophthalmol 8:138, 1985
24. Wollensak, J: Phakolytisches und hämolytisches Glaucom, Klin Monatsbl Augenheilkd 168:447, 1976
25. Vannas, S: Hemosiderosis in eyes with secondary glaucoma after delayed intraocular hemorrhages, Acta Ophthalmol 38:254, 1960

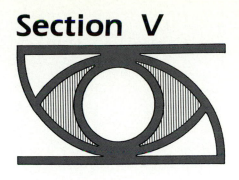

Section V

Glaucomas Associated with Ocular Surgery

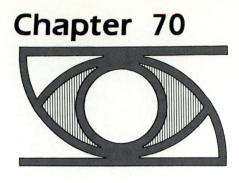

Chapter 70

Malignant Glaucoma

Richard J. Simmons
John V. Thomas
Moustafa K. Yaqub

Malignant glaucoma, first described by von Graefe[25] in 1869, is a rare but extremely serious form of glaucoma that has been responsible for the loss of one or frequently both eyes of many patients. It has been reported to occur in 2% to 4% of patients operated on for angle-closure glaucoma,[11,24] and occurs regardless of the type of conventional (not laser) operation performed. The fact that it may occur in both phakic and aphakic eyes with potentially devastating consequences makes it an important form of glaucoma.

The following characteristics have played an important role in its unusual destructiveness:

1. It is difficult to recognize early stages
2. Optimal medical therapy for the involved eye is often not instituted early enough or is ineffective
3. Prophylactic therapy for the fellow eye may be delayed
4. It is difficult to manage surgically

Knowledge of the unique characteristics of this form of glaucoma can help avoid many of these difficulties and ensure optimal success. Marked improvement in the management of malignant glaucoma has occurred over the past three decades and is largely because of the contributions of Chandler, Grant, and Shaffer.

DEFINITION

The term *malignant glaucoma* is used here as von Graefe used it to identify a specific type of glaucoma that occurs in several settings, most commonly as a complication after surgery for angle-closure glaucoma. In the classic sense, malignant glaucoma is a certain type of postoperative shallowing or flattening of the anterior chamber with an accompanying rise in intraocular pressure. It is referred to as "malignant" glaucoma because of the difficulty with which it responds to conventional treatment. The name does not imply malignancy in the sense of neoplastic disease. Weiss and Shaffer[27] have suggested the term *ciliary block glaucoma* as a substitute for malignant glaucoma, because it directs the attention of the clinician to the region of the ciliary body where, as is discussed below, some type of aqueous block appears to be present and because they find their term less alarming to the patient. However, thorough understanding of malignant glaucoma lies in the future, and many aspects of the presumed pathogenetic mechanism of malignant glaucoma remain unresolved or as yet unknown. In addition, malignant glaucoma is a term widely accepted by ophthalmologists. Therefore, we continue to retain it.

PATHOPHYSIOLOGY

Although many details of the mechanism of malignant glaucoma are unknown, most investigators accept the hypothesis originally proposed by Shaffer.[19] According to this hypothesis, aqueous humor is diverted posteriorly into, behind, or beside the vitreous cavity (Figs. 70-1, 70-2, and 70-3). Details of the specific mechanism that causes the posterior diversion of aqueous humor have not yet been identified. Relative block to the anterior movement of aqueous humor near the junction of the ciliary processes, lens equator, and anterior vitreous face, which causes aqueous to be diverted

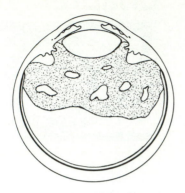

Fig. 70-1 Working hypothesis of fluid trapped in or behind vitreous body in phakic eye with malignant glaucoma.

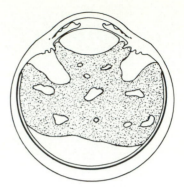

Fig. 70-2 Variation of Fig. 70-1, showing that fluid may, according to working hypothesis, occur at various sites in posterior segment.

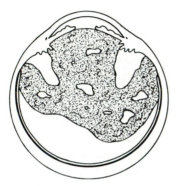

Fig. 70-3 Variation of Figs. 70-1 and 70-2, in an aphakic eye.

posteriorly, is a mechanism consistent with clinical observations. Shaffer's hypothesis is supported by the success of Chandler's vitreous surgery, which is designed to remove aqueous humor trapped in the vitreous cavity and restore the posteriorly diverted aqueous flow from the ciliary body to the anterior chamber.

Certain distinctive anatomic features have been regularly observed in the region of the ciliary processes, lens equator, and anterior vitreous face in eyes with malignant glaucoma. The tips of the ciliary processes may touch the lens when viewed through a peripheral iridectomy. The ciliary processes are frequently rotated anteriorly, their tips sometimes flattened against the lens. In one case, Grant observed ciliary processes firmly adherent to the lens by synechiae after an attack of malignant glaucoma had subsided. The spaces between the ciliary processes, however, are open, and through these spaces the posterior vitreous can be seen. In phakic eyes with malignant glaucoma, the anterior vitreous face may be abnormally forward behind

the ciliary processes, and in aphakic eyes it may touch and/or adhere to the ciliary processes.

Slit-lamp examination of the vitreous of certain eyes, both phakic and aphakic, with malignant glaucoma has revealed optically clear areas within the vitreous cavity, which have been interpreted as pockets of fluid. In a few cases in which the eye was unusually clear, a smooth vitreous face has been seen anterior to the middle of the vitreous cavity. We have interpreted this as the posterior hyaloid. The vitreous face in some eyes is smooth and seemingly bowed forward, with an optically clear space behind it.

Epstein et al.,[6] in experimental perfusion studies of normal, enucleated human and calf eyes, have provided support for Grant's speculation that in malignant glaucoma there may be a decrease in the permeability of the vitreous body or of the anterior hyaloid membrane to the anterior flow of aqueous humor, and that increased pressure in the space behind a posteriorly detached vitreous leads to a decrease in fluid movement through the vitreous gel. Epstein et al.[6] have also suggested that this resistance to the forward flow of aqueous humor could be further increased by apposition of the peripheral anterior hyaloid to the ciliary body and the peripheral lens, since there would be a decrease in available hyaloid surface area for fluid flow.

Fatt[8] measured the hydraulic flow conductivity of vitreous in vitro and noted that as pressure increased on the vitreous gel, the vitreous became dehydrated and fluid conductivity through the dehydrated vitreous decreased.

Quigley[15] postulated that malignant glaucoma may be initiated by the following sequence of events: (1) an event occurs that increases the posterior force applied to the vitreous gel (for example, increased fluid pressure in the cavity posterior to the detached vitreous); (2) fluid flows through the vitreous toward the anterior chamber at an increased rate, but some compaction (in effect, dehydration) of the gel occurs; (3) because of the dehydration, the fluid conductivity of the vitreous gel decreases, and with continued high pressure posteriorly, the gel undergoes a further decrease in conductivity, setting up a vicious cycle; and (4) the compressed vitreous gel is moved forward physically by the posterior-to-anterior pressure difference, leading to shallowing of the anterior chamber.

According to this explanation, osmotic agents are effective in malignant glaucoma, since they decrease the fluid content of the vitreous cavity, thereby lowering pressure behind the vitreous. The decrease in pressure would produce a decrease in compaction or dehydration of the vitreous, thereby allowing improved fluid conductivity, and possibly restoring normal tissue relationships and intraocular pressure. Surgical disruption of the vitreous gel structure would prevent the recurrence of the cycle, since there would be no intact vitreous gel to act as a diaphragm across the entire globe. An important detail that remains unexplained is how the initial increased pressure behind the vitreous body occurs.

Although much basic information on the mechanism of malignant glaucoma awaits firm documentation, much practical progress has been made in the recognition, medical management, and surgical therapy of this once hopeless situation.

Attention to the phenomena associated with malignant glaucoma has led a number of ophthalmologists to recognize forms of glaucoma identical to, very similar to, or related to classic malignant glaucoma. Although most commonly seen after surgery on phakic eyes with primary angle-closure glaucoma, the condition can persist after lens extraction on eyes afflicted with malignant glaucoma. Conditions similar to classic malignant glaucoma have been identified after cataract extraction alone on eyes without preexisting glaucoma, in eyes operated on for open-angle glaucoma, in eyes receiving miotic therapy,[17] in eyes being treated with miotics after surgery for open-angle glaucoma,[12] in eyes with spasm and swelling of the ciliary body,[14] in cases where inflammation and trauma have been prominent predecessors,[10] and in eyes without previous surgery or miotic therapy.[10,18]

Whether any of these conditions should be classified as forms of malignant glaucoma or as conditions that have similarity to classic malignant glaucoma will be definitively answered only as new knowledge becomes available.

DEVELOPMENT OF MALIGNANT GLAUCOMA

The chance of developing malignant glaucoma after surgery for angle-closure glaucoma is greatest in eyes in which some of the angle is closed at the time of operation.[21] In our experience, if the angle is open or has been opened by medical therapy at the time of operation, malignant glaucoma usually does not occur; however, when some of the angle remains closed, the danger of development of malignant glaucoma after surgery is still present. Its development as a consequence of surgery seems to have little relationship to the type of procedure performed, since it occurs after iridectomy, cyclodialysis, and filtration surgery of the conventional type with a full-thickness sclerostomy, as well as with a scleral flap, such as trabeculectomy.

The level of tension at the time of surgery for angle-closure glaucoma is not a reliable indicator of the possible occurrence of malignant glaucoma. Although frequently elevated at the time of surgery, the tension may be normal or low in some cases. In some eyes, the tension has become normal because of a low rate of aqueous humor formation, which may be a spontaneous reaction to a previous acute attack of angle-closure glaucoma, or it may be caused by use of medications.

Malignant glaucoma may be detected during surgery or at any time following surgery. Some cases develop months after the initial operation, perhaps as a result of the discontinuance of cycloplegic drops. Once the medication is stopped, the anterior chamber shallows or flattens and tension rises. In other instances, the development of malignant glaucoma is noticed when a regimen of miotic drops is begun long after surgery.

DIFFERENTIAL DIAGNOSIS

The three most important entities that may be confused with malignant glaucoma in an eye with elevated or normal tension and a flat or shallow anterior chamber are choroidal separation, pupillary block, and suprachoroidal hemorrhage. An accurate diagnosis may depend on consideration of a combination of (1) the characteristics of each condition, (2) the response of the eye to medical therapy, and (3) the use of a surgical confirmation procedure (see below) to gain the most precise and certain differentiation possible by performing several specific steps before vitreous surgery for the malignant glaucoma itself.

Choroidal Separation

Choroidal separation is common after filtration surgery and is usually found in a hypotonous eye.

When ophthalmoscopy is performed, elevations of the choroid in the peripheral fundus are visible, although in some cases the choroidal separation is shallow or low and cannot be easily discerned. At surgery, choroidal separation may be distinguished from malignant glaucoma by the presence of a characteristic straw-colored fluid of variable viscosity in the suprachoroidal space. In malignant glaucoma, such suprachoroidal fluid is almost never present.

In the combined experience of Chandler and Grant,[5] only one case of malignant glaucoma showed any fluid in the suprachoroidal space, and in this case the quantity of fluid was very small. When a shallow anterior chamber with hypotony and choroidal separation persist, it should be treated by drainage of the suprachoroidal fluid through one or more sclerotomies and reformation of the anterior chamber through a paracentesis incision.

Pupillary Block

Compared with choroidal separation, pupillary block is more difficult to distinguish from malignant glaucoma because it characteristically occurs as a flat or shallow anterior chamber with normal or elevated pressure.[24] It is essential to rule out pupillary block, which is more common, before accepting the diagnosis of malignant glaucoma. If there is no patent iridectomy, it is impossible with currently available means to reliably distinguish between pupillary block and malignant glaucoma. Pupillary block is relieved by a patent iridectomy, and malignant glaucoma is not; therefore, the coloboma in the iris should be inspected carefully for its presence and patency. If there is any doubt about the presence of a patent iridectomy, another should be created.

Although the creation of a patent iridectomy usually is intended at the time of glaucoma surgery, such as trabeculectomy or other filtration procedures, in a few instances, the attempt at iridectomy during surgery results only in removal of the anterior stroma of the iris, and the posterior pigment epithelium is left intact. When this is the case, blockage will persist until the posterior pigment epithelium is disrupted by laser treatment to the site of the imperforate iridectomy. In some cases the surgical wound is too far posterior for the creation of a patent iridectomy, and uveal tissue from the ciliary body is inadvertently excised at the time of intended iridectomy. This may result in hemorrhage into the anterior or posterior chambers or vitreous cavity and the absence of a patent coloboma in the peripheral iris. This can be avoided by carefully identifying anatomic landmarks during glaucoma surgery to ensure that the intended incision into the anterior chamber is not posterior to the scleral spur. In other cases, the iris may become incarcerated in the wound, or the iridectomy may be obstructed by intraocular tissue, such as Descemet's membrane, anterior hyaloid surface, or ciliary processes. The lack of functional patency can usually be identified by careful biomicroscopy with the slit-lamp and by gonioscopy.

In phakic, aphakic, and pseudophakic eyes, if pupillary block is present, the anterior chamber will readily deepen after iridectomy is performed. This deepening is usually associated with the sudden escape of aqueous humor through the iridectomy and confirms the diagnosis of pupillary block.

In pseudophakic eyes, however, a variant of pupillary block may be seen in which iris bombé develops despite the presence of a full-thickness surgical iridectomy. In some of these cases, the block may be relieved transiently by argon laser iridectomy, but will often require Nd:YAG laser photodisruption of the vitreous face for permanent relief.

Shrader et al.[20] felt that these cases demonstrate *iridovitreal block,* a variant of pupillary block. Iridovitreal block has been described in aphakic eyes, especially after intracapsular cataract surgery without lens implantation. Its cause appears to be the lack of free access of aqueous humor from the posterior to the anterior chamber because the anterior hyaloid face is apposed or adherent to the posterior iris surface. This concept of the mechanism is supported by the fact that both laser iridectomy and Nd:YAG photodisruption of the vitreous face were necessary to relieve the block. Before the availability of the Nd:YAG laser, some such cases were termed malignant glaucoma in aphakia, but we prefer Shaffer's term, iridovitreal block.

The pathophysiologic mechanism involved is distinctly different from malignant glaucoma, in which communication from the posterior to the anterior chamber is present, posterior diversion to and entrapment of aqueous humor in the vitreous cavity is present, and simple iridectomy with incision of the hyaloid face does not relieve the condition.

The initial step in recognizing pupillary and iridovitreal block in pseudophakic eyes is to perform a careful slit-lamp evaluation. Since the majority of these patients are asymptomatic and have normal intraocular pressures, the clinical condition may be missed in the early stages. If examination reveals even the slightest suggestion of an iris bombé configuration, the integrity of the cataract incision should be assessed, the intraocular pressure measured, the presence or absence of full-thickness surgical iridectomies determined, and in the case of an anterior chamber lens, the location of the haptics of the intraocular lens in relation to the iridectomy sites should be noted. If the intraocular pressure is greater than 10 mm Hg and if the possibility of a wound leak and choroidal detachment have been excluded, the diagnoses of pupillary block, iridovitreal block, and true aphakic malignant glaucoma must be considered.

Iridovitreal block is caused by anterior movement of the hyaloid face, causing apposition and sometimes, in the presence of postoperative inflammation, adherence to the posterior surface of the iris and the iridectomy. The diagnosis of iridovitreal block may be made by careful evaluation of the iridectomy site with high-power slit-lamp magnification, giving particular attention to the position of the anterior hyaloid. Vitrectomy for the relief of pupillary block in aphakia and pseudophakia appears to be unnecessary, since laser iridectomy relieves the block in nearly all such cases.[20]

Suprachoroidal Hemorrhage

Hemorrhage into the suprachoroidal space, like malignant glaucoma, may be characterized by a flat or shallow anterior chamber in the presence of a normal or elevated pressure. Hemorrhage into the suprachoroidal space can occur at the time of surgery or in the early hours or days after surgery, especially glaucoma surgery. It is sometimes associated with pain. Eyes with suprachoroidal hemorrhage may have the sudden onset of a flat anterior chamber on the first, second, or third postoperative day, and are usually quite injected. Ophthalmoscopy or ultrasonography may reveal the presence of single or multiple elevations of the choroid in the periphery of the fundus. The choroidal elevations may be similar in size and distribution to those in simple choroidal separation. Ophthalmoscopically, however, they are frequently dark reddish brown in color, as opposed to the lighter brown color of ordinary choroidal separations. The presence of these features should make one suspect suprachoroidal hemorrhage.

Suprachoroidal hemorrhage and choroidal separation can sometimes be differentiated by ultrasonography. However, this is usually unnecessary, since the treatment will be the same as outlined below, regardless of the results of ultrasonography.

If suprachoroidal hemorrhage is present, sclerotomy into the suprachoroidal space reveals liquified or partially liquified blood, which is usually dark red or black. Occasionally the fluid obtained is a mixture of clear, straw-colored fluid and reddish to black liquified blood. All the fluid obtained from the suprachoroidal space should be drained from two sclerotomies, and the anterior chamber should be formed with saline.

In rare cases intrachoroidal hemorrhage occurs without major penetration of the hemorrhage into the suprachoroidal space itself. In such cases all clinical features are identical to those associated with suprachoroidal hemorrhage except that little or no free blood is found in the suprachoroidal space, and drainage of the blood is not possible. Spontaneous absorption will occur slowly.

Table 70-1 summarizes the differential features of the clinical entities mentioned above.

Table 70-1 *Differential diagnosis*

	Malignant glaucoma	Choroidal separation	Pupillary block	Suprachoroidal hemorrhage
Anterior chamber	Flat or shallow	Flat or shallow	Flat or shallow	Flat or shallow
Intraocular pressure	Normal or elevated	Subnormal	Normal or elevated	Normal or elevated
Fundus appearance	No choroidal elevation	Large, smooth, light brown choroidal elevations	Normal	Dark brown or dark red choroidal elevations
Suprachoroidal fluid	Absent	Straw-colored fluid present	Absent	Light red or dark red blood present
Relief by drainage of suprachoroidal fluid	No	Yes	No	Yes
Relief by iridectomy	No	No	Yes	No
Patent iridectomy	Yes	Yes	No	Yes
Onset	At surgery or first 5 days postoperatively, but sometimes weeks to months postoperatively	First 5 days postoperatively, occasionally later	Early or late postoperatively	At surgery or first 5 days postoperatively, rarely later

MANAGEMENT

Medical therapy for malignant glaucoma should be employed once malignant glaucoma is suspected in an eye with a shallow or flat anterior chamber and a normal or elevated intraocular pressure. Also, all precautions must be taken to protect the fellow eye, since a patient who has malignant glaucoma in one eye is more likely to develop the same condition in the other eye.

Medical Therapy

Miotic therapy was used for many years with uniformly unsuccessful results in malignant glaucoma, suggesting to Chandler and Grant that miotics might in fact precipitate or aggravate malignant glaucoma. In the 1950s, carbonic anhydrase inhibitors were tried in combination with miotics, but this combination was also disappointingly ineffective.

The first major success in medical therapy for malignant glaucoma came in 1962 with the report of the successful relief of this condition with mydriatic-cycloplegic drops.[4] Mydriatic-cycloplegic treatment is beneficial in malignant glaucoma presumably because it tightens the zonules, pulling the lens back into the plane of the ciliary body against the force of the vitreous, which tends to push it forward. In cases of aphakic malignant glaucoma, mydriatic-cycloplegic drops are of little benefit. However, it is reasonable to use them for their effect on relaxation of the ciliary body muscle.

The inital treatment consisted of 4% atropine and 10% phenylephrine drops, each four or five times a day.[4] This treatment was uniformly successful in the first eight cases in which it was tried. It soon became apparent that continuation of cycloplegia for an indefinite period of time was important. Generally, when atropine was continued, the anterior chamber retained normal depth and the tension was lowered. However, when atropine was discontinued, the chamber became shallow or flat and tension rose. In most cases, but not all, this process was reversed by reestablishing the use of atropine. Our experience with these cases has emphasized the importance of continuing atropine or scopolamine indefinitely, since it cannot be certain that a recurrence of malignant glaucoma can be relieved by resumption of the drops.

If mydriatic-cycloplegic drops alone do not relieve the malignant glaucoma, the addition of a carbonic anhydrase inhibitor will be effective in some patients. Hyperosmotic agents relieve an additional number of patients. More recently we have added beta-adrenegic blocking agents in the expectation that it will decrease aqueous humor production, lower the pressure, and help relieve the malignant glaucoma.

From this experience, we believe that the optimal regimen of medical therapy for malignant glaucoma consists of the concurrent use of mydriatic-cycloplegic drops, beta-adrenergic blocking agents, carbonic anhydrase inhibitors, and hyperosmotic solutions in full dosage from the very beginning of treatment. Our preferred initial dosages consist of atropine 1%, 1 drop four times daily; phenylephrine 10%, 1 drop four times daily; timolol 0.5%, 1 drop two times daily; acetazolamide, 250 mg orally four times daily; and hyperosmotic solutions in maximal dosage. Undiluted 50% oral glycerol (1 ml per pound of body weight) or oral isosorbide 45% solution (1.5 ml per pound of body weight or 1.5 g per kg) should be given cold for palatability over a period of no more than 5 minutes. Mannitol 20%, 2 g (10 ml) per kg may be administered intravenously over a 45-minute period. The patient is not given any oral food or fluids for 2 hours before and after the administration of the hyperosmotic agent, to ensure that its osmotic effect is not altered. The hyperosmotic agents are given every 12 hours.

The dosage of any of the above medications should be reduced if the patient is intolerant of it. Where no contraindications exist, the entire regimen is surprisingly well tolerated by the average patient for 4 to 5 days. For patients who complain of nausea when oral glycerol is administered, the use of antiemetics 1 hour before administration can reduce this unpleasant side effect. This regimen should be continued until the anterior chamber forms and the pressure improves, or until it has been tried for 4 to 5 days. If the condition is relieved, the regimen is gradually tapered and discontinued over several days. Hyperosmotic agents are discontinued first, and then carbonic anhydrase inhibitors. Mydriatic (phenylephrine) drops are stopped, but the cycloplegic (atropine) drops are continued indefinitely. If the anterior chamber does not deepen and tension does not improve with the medical treatment outlined above, the treatment must not be considered a failure until it has been tried for 4 or 5 days. We have seen cases in which the condition was relieved after 2 or 3 or even 5 days of treatment. With the use of this regimen for 4 to 5 days, about 50% of cases of malignant glaucoma are relieved.

Laser Therapy

If medical therapy is unsuccessful, and if the ocular media are clear and the iridectomy visible, it may be reasonable to use the argon laser to shrink the ciliary processes. Herschler[9] reported success with this technique in five of six cases of malignant glaucoma unresponsive to medical therapy.

If the ciliary processes are visible through the peripheral iridectomy without the aid of a gonioscopy lens, the laser beam may be applied directly through the cornea. Before the ciliary processes are treated with the laser beam, topical glycerin may be required to clear corneal edema. The power used varies from 100 mW to 300 mW. The duration of treatment is 0.1 to 0.2 seconds, and the spot size varies from 100 to 200 μm. In successfully treated cases, the laser produced shrinkage of two to four ciliary processes. Immediately after treatment, slight deepening of the anterior chamber occurred, and medical therapy was continued. Full restoration of the depth of the anterior chamber, however, occurred after 3 to 5 days of continued medical therapy.

Herschler[9] has suggested that the efficacy of laser shrinkage of the ciliary processes in treating malignant glaucoma may be caused by relief of relative ciliolenticular block to the anterior flow of aqueous humor. However, many unanswered questions remain.[23] For example, does laser therapy contract the adjacent hyaloid membrane, which is in apposition to the ciliary processes? Does the heat of the laser on the ciliary processes rupture the hyaloid membrane itself or alter the permeability of the adjacent vitreous? Does it rupture adhesions of the hyaloid to the ciliary processes or lyse lens zonules in this region? Because medical therapy was given for a few days both before and after laser therapy, it is possible that medical therapy itself was responsible for relief of the malignant glaucoma. However, despite the hypothetical issues regarding the mechanism of malignant glaucoma, laser therapy to the ciliary processes involves little risks in such cases, and we believe it should be tried in eyes in which medical therapy has failed and in which the ciliary processes are visible in the coloboma.

Of particular interest to the treatment of malignant glaucoma is the current research being undertaken with the Nd:YAG laser. Recently Epstein[7] had suggested the use of Nd:YAG laser hyaloidotomy to disrupt the anterior vitreous face in cases of malignant glaucoma in aphakia. In four cases immediate deepening of the anterior chamber was obtained and sustained, and in one case pars plana vitrectomy was needed.

We believe that in such cases where there is no clear distinction between iridovitreal block and true malignant glaucoma, the relief of the condition may likely be caused by establishment of communication between the anterior and posterior chambers, indicating that these were cases of iridovitreal block rather than true malignant glaucoma. As pointed out previously, the success of Chandler's vitreous aspiration surgical technique for relief of malignant glaucoma is based on disruption of both the anterior and posterior hyaloid membranes, which relieves entrapment of aqueous humor within or behind the vitreous.

Surgical Therapy

If medical and laser therapy fail to relieve the condition, we recommend the use of what we call the "surgical confirmation procedure." This procedure will eliminate with certainty at surgery the other diagnostic possibilities in the differential diagnosis of malignant glaucoma (i.e., choroidal separation, pupillary block, and suprachoroidal hemorrhage), and allow the immediate performance of surgery for malignant glaucoma in cases where the diagnosis is confirmed. If, however, one of the other diagnostic possibilities is present, it can be treated surgically at that time and the procedure terminated.

Many surgical procedures have been employed for malignant glaucoma since its description in 1869. A simple posterior sclerotomy 8 to 10 mm from the limbus was recommended in 1877 by Weber,[26] who employed this procedure successfully in one case in which he applied pressure on the cornea for 2 minutes after making the posterior sclerotomy, presumably with the loss of vitreous through the wound site. This procedure was repeated by other surgeons, but it proved unreliable.

Lens extraction was first recommended by Pagenstecher[13] (1877) and first used by Rheindorf[16] (1887), possibly after a decade of cautious contemplation. Many eyes have been saved from malignant glaucoma by lens extraction. In Chandler's series, when vitreous was lost anteriorly, the malignant glaucoma was relieved. However, when vitreous was not lost anteriorly, the glaucoma usually continued.

In 1954 Shaffer[19] called attention to the importance of the role of the vitreous in phakic and aphakic eyes affected by malignant glaucoma. He noted that when lens extraction was performed without vitreous loss, the malignant course persisted, but it would respond to subsequent deep incision into the vitreous. This incision presumably disrupted the anterior and posterior hyaloid membranes. He postulated that aqueous humor was trapped in or behind the detached vitreous body.

In 1964 Chandler[3] devised a surgical technique

involving puncture and aspiration of the vitreous without removal of the lens. Since the primary disorder appeared to be one involving the relationship of aqueous humor and the vitreous, removal of the lens seemed superfluous. He postulated that the disturbance of the vitreous associated with vitreous loss at the time of cataract extraction for malignant glaucoma produced the beneficial effect and reported six cases in which a needle was passed into the vitreous around the lens and vitreous and/or fluid was aspirated. He postulated that the needle puncture would pierce the anterior and posterior hyaloid and that the vitreous would be decompressed by aspiration. This procedure was successful in relieving malignant glaucoma, but because of a high incidence of postoperative cataract formation, he abandoned it. However, Balakrishnan and Abraham[1] successfully employed this operation without complications.

In an effort to avoid damage to the lens, Chandler devised the procedure currently recommended, and in 1968, Chandler et al.[5] reported uniform success in a series of cases in which medical therapy had failed to relieve malignant glaucoma. The initial steps consist of the sequence of surgical diagnostic maneuvers referred to above as the surgical confirmation procedure. The combined experience of Chandler, Grant, and us now includes over 70 patients in whom some form of malignant glaucoma has played a role in one or both eyes. In over 30 of these eyes, Chandler's procedure has been used. In the vast majority of cases it has been successful in relieving the malignant glaucoma without complication, but it must be performed precisely according to the protocol and steps must not be altered or eliminated if its safety and efficacy are to be preserved.

Confirmation of communication between the posterior and anterior chamber

Before the patient enters the operating room, the anterior segment of the eye is studied carefully for the presence or absence of a patent iridectomy, since it is imperative that there be communication between the posterior and anterior chambers. If any question exists, an additional iridectomy is performed. A laser iridectomy may be attempted initially. If that is unsuccessful, a surgical peripheral iridectomy should be done to rule out pupillary block, since there is no currently reliable way to distinguish between pupillary block and malignant glaucoma in the absence of a patent iridectomy.

At the time of surgical iridectomy, if pupillary block is present, aqueous humor will be released

from the posterior chamber and the anterior chamber will deepen. The procedure can then be terminated. If the anterior chamber remains flat, the surgeon must proceed with other steps described below.

Sclerotomy to confirm the absence of suprachoroidal fluid or blood

A beveled incision is made in the peripheral cornea with a Wheeler knife or a similar instrument to allow access to the anterior chamber for later injection of fluid and air. The incision is made in the periphery of the cornea roughly parallel to the limbus. This incision should be tested to ensure that easy access with a syringe can be obtained. Later, access to the anterior chamber through this wound will be more difficult, when the eye is hypotonous.

At the sites chosen for sclerotomies, conjunctiva and Tenon's capsule should be incised with a radial incision (a radial incision is least traumatic and most convenient). Usually a site away from the area of previous ocular surgery is chosen (i.e., both lower quadrants are most commonly used when a filtration procedure or iridectomy has been previously performed above). A radial incision through the sclera to the suprachoroidal space, about 3 mm in length with its center a carefully measured distance of 3.5 mm behind the external limbus, is then made in both quadrants (Figs. 70-4 and 70-5). The incision should not be placed more posteriorly for reasons to be given later.

When sclerotomies are made in a case of malignant glaucoma, no fluid will be present in the suprachoroidal space. However, if straw-colored fluid is encountered in the suprachoroidal space, the diagnosis is choroidal separation, and the fluid should be drained completely from the suprachoroidal space through both sclerotomies. The anterior chamber is deepened through the previously placed beveled incision in the cornea with saline and in some cases, air. The diagnosis of choroidal separation is confirmed, and the case is terminated after closure of the conjunctival incision. The sclerotomy wounds themselves are left open without suturing in the hope that any future reaccumulation of fluid in the suprachoroidal space will be encouraged to drain spontaneously from the eye.

If suprachoroidal hemorrhage is present, blood or a mixture of old blood and suprachoroidal fluid will be found in the suprachoroidal space. This old blood should then be drained from the suprachoroidal space, the anterior chamber reformed with

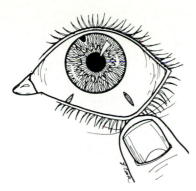

Fig. 70-4 Sclerotomy incisions. Note their relationship to limbus, as well as their circumferential positions.

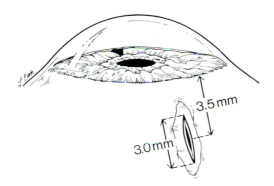

Fig. 70-5 Size of sclerotomy incision and its distance from limbus.

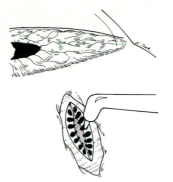

Fig. 70-6 Sclerotomy technique: Diathermy is placed at inner edges of scleral wound to cauterize inner scleral layers, as well as vessels in adjacent choroid. Diathermy should not be applied directly to choroid, since it may cause and stimulate bleeding.

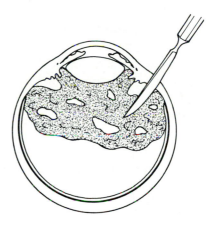

Fig. 70-7 Sclerotomy technique: Wheeler knife is used to pierce uvea and enter vitreous cavity. Knife should be kept away from lens by aiming it toward optic nerve head.

saline, and the conjunctival incision closed. As with choroidal separation, the sclerotomy wounds should not be sutured. The diagnosis of suprachoroidal hemorrhage is thus confirmed, and the operation is terminated.

If no fluid flows from the sclerotomies, a smooth spatula, such as a standard cyclodialysis spatula, should be passed circumferentially through the lips of the sclerotomy into the suprachoroidal space parallel to the limbus. Occasionally fluid or blood can be present in the suprachoroidal space, but is loculated and does not flow freely from the sclerotomy until this maneuver is performed. If iridectomy has been done and yet the anterior chamber remains shallow or flat, and if sclerotomies into the suprachoroidal space have been made and fluid or blood are not found, the diagnosis of malignant glaucoma is established.

Using the sclerostomies made for tapping of the suprachoroidal space, deep vitreous surgery for malignant glaucoma should be then carried out. The operation of choice is Chandler's deep vitreous surgery as described below. This can be performed by using the paracentesis entry into the anterior chamber and the sclerotomies made for the suprachoroidal drainage, without making additional incisions into the globe.

Vitreous surgery for malignant glaucoma

The vitreous surgery is performed through one of the sclerotomies. The lower temporal sclerotomy is convenient and has been successfully used in most of our cases. A ring of surface diathermy is placed around the inner layers of the scleral wound, using a strong RF diathermy current with a conical electrode and sufficient power to produce brown discoloration of the sclera and slight coagulation of the vessels in the underlying choroid (Fig. 70-6). Diathermy is used to try to avoid bleeding from the uvea when the uvea is later pierced. Next, a Wheeler knife is plunged into the vitreous cavity to a depth of about 10 mm through the ciliary body (Fig. 70-7), the knife being aimed toward the

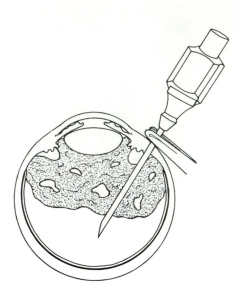

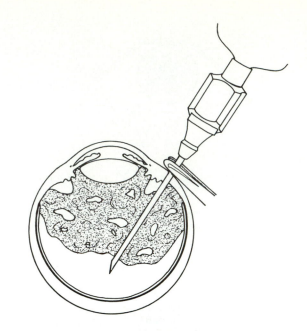

Fig. 70-8 Sclerotomy technique: 18 gauge needle is inserted 12 mm from the needle point. Hemostat guard to control depth of needle is shown.

Fig. 70-9 Sclerotomy technique: Syringe is attached to 18 gauge needle, and 1.0 to 1.5 ml of vitreous is aspirated.

optic nerve to avoid contact with the lens. The wound in the uvea is enlarged slightly anteriorly and posteriorly to a length, in radial direction, of about 3 mm with its center 3.5 mm behind the external limbus.

A hemostat is placed around the shaft of an 18-gauge needle a measured distance of 12 mm behind its tip to prevent excessively deep penetration into the globe. The needle is then passed through the wound into the vitreous cavity toward the optic nerve (Fig. 70-8). When the needle is fully inserted to the measured depth, its tip is moved back and forth about 4 mm in an arc of about 4 mm to allow slight separation of the vitreous membranes in its path. A syringe, such as a 5 ml Luer-Lok syringe, is then attached to the base of the needle by the assistant. The surgeon must use both hands to carefully control the position of the needle within the eye. After the syringe is attached to the needle, the surgeon continues to maintain the position of the needle with one hand and with the other hand aspirates 1 to 1.5 ml; if necessary, the assistant may aspirate while the surgeon holds the needle in place with both hands. The material thus obtained may be waterlike fluid, fluid vitreous, or vitreous (Fig. 70-9).

Before the needle is withdrawn from the eye, 0.25 ml of aspirated fluid is reinjected into the eye to clear the tip of the needle of any vitreous strands engaged within its lumen. The needle is then carefully withdrawn from the eye exactly along its path of entry. The eye at this point will be markedly hypotonous, with folds in the cornea and sclera. A small amount of saline is then injected into the anterior chamber through the previously placed beveled incision to partially restore the shape and configuration of the globe. It is important that the eye not be filled completely with saline, because in some cases saline will flow back into and behind the vitreous cavity and recreate the original malignant glaucoma. The quantity of saline injected should be just enough to partially restore the globe. A very large air bubble is then placed in the anterior chamber to fill the anterior chamber completely and force the iris and lens posteriorly (Figs. 70-10, and 70-11). The air bubble should be large enough to deepen the chamber to a depth greater than that usually encountered in the normal myopic eye. After injection of the air, the eye should still be hypotonous, since it is important not to fill out the eye completely to a normal contour and tension. A sterile Schiøtz tonometer can be placed on the eye at the end of the procedure, or a muscle hook can be used to test the pressure in the eye. If there is measurable pressure within the eye, too much saline has been injected.

The procedure is the same in aphakic eyes except that the wound of entry into the vitreous can

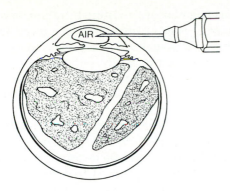

Fig. 70-10 Sclerotomy technique: Air bubble is placed in anterior chamber to deepen it.

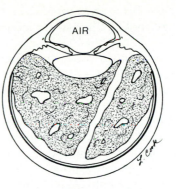

Fig. 70-11 Sclerotomy technique: Size of air bubble should be large enough to deepen chamber to a depth greater than usually encountered in a normal myopic eye.

be made at the limbus through a newly formed iridectomy or an existing iridectomy, since there is no lens to be injured by the anterior placement of the vitreous puncture. The needle is passed into the eye for a distance of 15 mm instead of 12 mm, since the wound of entry is at the limbus rather than 3.5 mm behind the limbus.

The scleral wounds are each closed with a single interrupted suture, and the conjunctival wounds are then closed with simple running or interrupted sutures.

Postoperative care

Atropine is instilled at the end of the operation and is continued postoperatively for weeks or months. We do not know with certainty whether cycloplegics can later be discontinued in all cases, but it has been our experience that after the eye has been stable for several weeks following surgery, the cycloplegics can be tapered and stopped with careful observation. Should reshallowing of the anterior chamber occur, of course, one would immediately restart cycloplegics. Miotics, including phospholine iodide, can also be used after the eye has stabilized without recurrence of malignant glaucoma. Topical steroids to suppress inflammation not only improve comfort postoperatively, but also may encourage significant beneficial filtration from the sclerostomy sites.

Result of Therapy

The operation is predictable and reliable as long as exacting attention is given to details.[22] Complications or lack of efficacy of the procedure can almost always be traced to a lack of diligent attention to the details of the procedure. For example,

if diathermy is not applied around the wound, hemorrhage into the suprachoroidal space and vitreous may occur. If the air bubble used at the end of the procedure is too small to force the lens, iris, and vitreous posteriorly, the procedure may not be successful. If the initial incision in the sclera is too far posterior, the procedure may become less effective or ineffective because the anterior vitreous is not affected adequately. The anterior placement of the wound for vitreous puncture in this procedure may be essential, since it is calculated to be anterior to the anterior portion of the anterior hyaloid membrane as the instrument is placed into the vitreous cavity. If the scleral incision is too anterior (i.e., if it is centered less than 3 mm from the limbus), injury to the lens with cataract formation may result.

It is obviously important to control the tip of the needle within the eye carefully and skillfully. The hemostatic guard must be placed precisely 12 mm from the needle tip and the surgeon must not move his eyes from the needle, nor lose hand control of the needle, nor lose concentration while the needle is within the eye.

At surgery, or postoperatively in some cases, the anterior chamber will appear to have flattened, but careful inspection will show that the air bubble instilled during surgery has slipped behind the iris. This is in no way an indication that the malignant glaucoma has recurred. Manipulation of the patient's head or eye or prolonged dilation of the pupil will often shift the air bubble back into the anterior chamber. Otherwise, it will gradually reabsorb, and the anterior chamber will gradually reform.

A few small, transient punctate fundus hemorrhages have been encountered in a few cases, but these have not resulted in any permanent damage.

Transient postoperative choroidal separation has occurred in about a third of our cases. It is important to distinguish choroidal separation after the procedure from recurrence of malignant glaucoma. If choroidal separation follows this procedure, the eye is soft; and although the anterior chamber is shallow or flat, suprachoroidal elevation in the peripheral fundus is present, and the condition will gradually clear spontaneously with improvement in the anterior chamber depth.

In several cases, malignant glaucoma has not responded to the first performance of Chandler's procedure, but we have merely resumed medical therapy for 2 to 3 days and then repeated the procedure. Following the second operation, these eyes have responded. In three cases, when we were attempting aspiration through a disposable 18-gauge needle, no fluid or vitreous entered the needle and syringe. We withdrew the needle from the vitreous and attempted to instill as much air as possible into the flat anterior chamber. We then resumed atropine therapy and the full medical regimen for malignant glaucoma, and in each case the eye responded to medical therapy, whereas it had not before the procedure. In one case, we were able to resume miotic therapy some months after the proecedure.

In our hands, Chandler's procedure has been considerably simpler, safer, and more effective than lens extraction. In many of these cases, a phakic eye with a clear lens resulted following relief of the malignant glaucoma. Even in cases where a cataract is present, we believe it is safer to carry out Chandler's procedure to relieve the malignant glaucoma and then some months later, when the eye is stabilized, to remove the cataract as a separate surgical procedure. We have some years later removed cataracts that have been present before surgery and have found a normal response of these eyes to lens extraction.

Role of standard pars plana vitrectomy with automated infusion-suction instrumentation

At the time that Chandler's procedure was devised, sophisticated instruments for vitrectomy were not available. Since their advent, many colleagues have mentioned to us the thought that vitrectomy might now be the treatment of choice for malignant glaucoma. At the present time, we feel that vitrectomy is not necessary to relieve malignant glaucoma and can be more traumatic to the external ocular tissues, existing filtration blebs, and conjunctiva. These eyes often have hazy anterior segments and visualization for vitrectomy in the usual manner is frequently impossible. We have had no case in which the malignant glaucoma could not be relieved by a combination of medical therapy followed when necessary by Chandler's procedure, with postoperative cycloplegic therapy in all cases, and one repetition of Chandler's procedure if needed. Should a case be encountered in which a trial of medical therapy and Chandler's procedure fails, we recommend that one repeat the medical therapy for an additional 3 days and then repeat Chandler's procedure. If the malignant glaucoma still does not respond after these two trials of medical therapy and two trials of Chandler's procedure, the use of pars plana vitrectomy should be strongly considered.

THE FELLOW EYE

All precautions must be taken to protect the fellow eye, since a patient who has malignant glaucoma in one eye is likely to develop the same condition in the other eye. To provide a greater margin of safety, it is reasonable to create a laser iridectomy in the fellow eye before surgical intervention on the involved eye. One or two iridectomy sites can be created, but our preference is to perform two, because if a single iridectomy closes, a serious attack of glaucoma can occur. Miotics may precipitate angle-closure and malignant glaucoma in a predisposed eye. Therefore "prophylactic" miotic drops, used in the belief that they will protect the fellow eye are contraindicated. This practice is unwise in ordinary primary angle-closure glaucoma and is particularly dangerous and proscribed in malignant glaucoma.

We have never known malignant glaucoma to occur in the fellow eye when iridectomy was performed with an entirely open angle and normal intraocular pressure. If angle-closure glaucoma is allowed to develop in the fellow eye, the treatment becomes much more difficult and the results far more uncertain. Laser iridectomy should be performed immediately. This should be attempted first without the customary pretreatment with miotics, but if full-thickness iridectomy cannot be achieved after attempts by both the argon and Nd:YAG lasers, weak miotics such as pilocarpine 1% should be employed to induce miosis to facilitate performance of the laser iridectomy. Following the successful creation of the laser iridectomy, mydriatic-cycloplegic therapy should be immediately employed and the patient should be closely observed to make sure that malignant glaucoma does not follow. If, for any reason, laser iridectomy cannot be performed, surgical peripheral iridectomy is indicated. Medical therapy to open the angle and lower intraocular pressure should be given before surgery, but miotics should be avoided.

If glaucoma is present in the fellow eye and the angle does not open on medical treatment, malignant glaucoma can be anticipated after surgery, whether or not the tension has been brought to normal. In such cases, an iridectomy is done, atropine is instilled at the conclusion of the operation, and the full optimal medical regimen for malignant glaucoma is begun at the end of surgery. This regimen is continued in the hope of aborting the expected malignant course. If the malignant course is successfully aborted, the intensive medical regimen is tapered. If malignant glaucoma occurs and persists despite the full medical regimen for 4 to 5 days, one must resort to laser or surgical therapy for the malignant glaucoma.

It is most important that the best opportunity for effective treatment of the fellow eye be seized promptly and that the opportunity not be lost because of preoccupation with the involved eye or procrastination. When an eye is badly involved with malignant glaucoma, there is a tendency to wait and do nothing to the second eye until we are sure of the outcome of the first, for fear of encountering unavoidable risk. This tendency must be strongly resisted, since it leads to the erroneous course of inaction; instead, the opposite course of prompt therapy for the fellow eye is the most conservative, prudent, and risk free. The absence of prompt appropriate therapy for the fellow eye has resulted in bilateral blindness in many patients.

REFERENCES

1. Balakrishnan, E, and Abraham, JE: Chandler's operation for malignant glaucoma, Arch Ophthalmol 82:723, 1969
2. Chandler, PA: Malignant glaucoma, Am J Ophthalmol 34:993, 1951
3. Chandler, PA: A new operation for malignant glaucoma: a preliminary report, Trans Am Ophthalmol Soc 62:408, 1964
4. Chandler, PA, and Grant, WM: Mydriatic-cycloplegic treatment in malignant glaucoma, Arch Ophthalmol 68:353, 1962
5. Chandler, PA, Simmons, RJ, and Grant, WM: Malignant glaucoma: medical and surgical treatment, Am J Ophthalmol 66:496, 1968
6. Epstein, DL, Hashimoto, JM, Anderson, PJ, and Grant, WM: Experimental perfusions through the anterior and vitreous chambers with possible relationships to malignant glaucoma, Am J Ophthalmol 88:1078, 1979
7. Epstein, DL, Steinert, RF, Puliafito, CA: Neodymium-YAG laser therapy to the anterior hyaloid in aphakic malignant (cilio-vitreal block) glaucoma, Am J Ophthalmol 98:137-143, 1984
8. Fatt, I: Hydraulic flow conductivity of the vitreous gel, Invest Ophthalmol Vis Sci 16:565, 1977
9. Herschler, J: Laser shrinkage of the ciliary processes—a treatment for malignant (ciliary block) glaucoma, Ophthalmology 87:1155, 1980.
10. Levene, R: A new concept of malignant glaucoma, Arch Ophthalmol 87:497, 1972
11. Mehner, A: Beitrag zu den Komplikationen bei Glaucomooperationen Speziell bei der Iridectomie, Klin Monatsbl Augenheilkd 70:491, 1923
12. Merrit, JC: Malignant glaucoma induced by miotics postoperatively in open-angle glaucoma, Arch Ophthalmol 95:1988, 1977
13. Pagenstecher, H: Uber Glaukoms, Arch Ophthalmol 10:7, 1877
14. Phelps, CD: Angle-closure glaucoma secondary to ciliary body swelling, Arch Ophthalmol 92:287, 1974
15. Quigley, HA: Malignant glaucoma and fluid flow rate (editorial), Am J Ophthalmol 89:879, 1980
16. Rheindorf, O: Uber Glaukom, Klin Monatsbl Augenheilkd 25:148, 1887
17. Rieser, JC, and Schwartz, B: Miotic induced malignant glaucoma, Arch Ophthalmol 87:706, 1972
18. Schwartz, AL, and Anderson, DR: "Malignant glaucoma" in an eye with no antecedent operation or miotics, Arch Ophthalmol 93:379, 1975
19. Shaffer, RN: Role of vitreous detachment in aphakic and malignant glaucoma, Trans Am Acad Ophthalmol Otolaryngol 58:217, 1954
20. Shrader, CE, et al: Pupillary and iridovitreal block in pseudophakic eyes, Ophthalmol 91:831, 1984
21. Simmons, RJ: Malignant glaucoma. In Epstein, D, editor: Chandler and Grant's glaucoma, ed 3, Philadelphia, 1986, Lea and Febiger
22. Simmons, RJ: Malignant glaucoma, Br J Ophthalmol 56:263, 1972
23. Simmons, RJ: Discussion of Herschler, J: Laser shrinkage of the ciliary processes—a treatment for malignant (ciliary block) glaucoma, Ophthalmology 87:1158, 1980
24. Simmons, RJ, and Dallow, RL: Primary angle-closure glaucoma. In Duane, TD, editor: Clinical ophthalmology, vol 3, New York, 1976, Harper & Row, Publishers
25. von Graefe, A: Beitrage zur Pathologie und Therapie des Glaucoms, Arch Ophthalmol 15:108, 1869
26. Weber, A: Die Ursache des Glaukoms, Arch Ophthalmol 23:1, 1877
27. Weiss, DI, and Shaffer, RN: Ciliary block (malignant) glaucoma, Trans Am Acad Ophthalmol Otolaryngol 76:450, 1972

Chapter 71

Secondary Glaucoma in Aphakia

Morris M. Podolsky
Robert Ritch

Temporary or permanent elevations of intraocular pressure frequently develop after cataract extraction by a variety of mechanisms that are emphasized in this chapter. We avoid the term *aphakic glaucoma*, which is misleading, because it implies that aphakia itself causes elevated intraocular pressure.

Routine cataract surgery has changed significantly in the past few years. The movement from predominantly intracapsular cataract extraction (ICCE) to extracapsular cataract extraction (ECCE) has led to the virtual disappearance of some previously common causes of secondary glaucoma, such as that induced by alpha-chymotrypsin. At the same time, such advances in technology as the use of viscoelastic substances and Nd:YAG posterior capsulotomy have been complicated by new types of secondary glaucomas. Rapid developments in laser and surgical therapy have led to a wide variety of potentially valuable improvements in the treatment of glaucoma in aphakia. These include the use of adjunctive 5-fluorouracil therapy in filtration surgery, transscleral cyclophotocoagulation, and trabeculectomy ab interno.

As is the case with the primary glaucomas, secondary glaucoma in aphakic eyes can be broadly categorized as open- or closed-angle. It is also possible for both mechanisms to occur coincidentally. Glaucoma may develop immediately after cataract extraction or weeks to months later (see box at right). The onset may be acute or insidious. Careful examination and analysis are imperative so that the

CAUSES OF GLAUCOMA IN APHAKIA

A. Open-angle glaucoma
  1. Early onset
     a. Preexisting open-angle glaucoma
     b. Early postoperative intraocular pressure rise
     c. Alpha-chymotrypsin–induced glaucoma
     d. Hyphema
     e. Viscoelastic-induced
  2. Intermediate onset
     a. Vitreous filling anterior chamber
     b. Hyphema
     c. Inflammation
     d. Lens particle glaucoma
     e. Steroid-induced glaucoma
     f. Ghost cell glaucoma
  3. Late onset
     a. Primary open-angle glaucoma
     b. Ghost cell glaucoma
     c. Epithelial ingrowth
     d. Fibrous proliferation
     e. Nd:YAG laser
     f. Failed bleb
B. Angle-closure glaucoma
  1. Early onset
     a. Preexisting peripheral anterior synechiae
     b. Air block
     c. Pupillary block
     d. Vitreociliary block (malignant glaucoma)
  2. Intermediate and late onset
     a. Pupillary block
     b. Neovascular glaucoma
     c. Nd:YAG posterior capsulotomy

optimal method of treatment may be instituted. Our approach in complicated cases is to enumerate the underlying mechanisms for the glaucoma and to then eliminate each one with as precise treatment as possible. The forms of glaucoma discussed in this chapter are those related to cataract extraction and aphakia. The approach to cataract extraction in patients with glaucoma is covered in Chapter 36 and glaucomas related to various types of intraocular lenses in Chapter 72.

OPEN-ANGLE GLAUCOMA ASSOCIATED WITH APHAKIA

Preexisting Open-angle Glaucoma

Primary open-angle glaucoma may be present before cataract extraction or may develop later, in which case the diagnosis is essentially one of exclusion.

Glaucoma present before cataract extraction should be carefully evaluated with tonometry, gonioscopy, perimetry, and tonography when applicable. This baseline information is important for preoperative preparation, intraoperative care, and evaluation of any postoperative changes in intraocular pressure. Precautions may be taken to minimize factors that increase the likelihood of a secondary glaucoma in the postoperative period, such as avoiding the use of sodium hyaluronate or alpha-chymotrypsin in an eye with advanced glaucomatous visual field loss.

The effect of cataract extraction per se on intraocular pressure has been controversial. In the immediate postoperative period there is often a self-limited episode of elevated intraocular pressure (see below). This is more common in eyes with preexisting open-angle glaucoma, even when the intraocular pressure is controlled preoperatively with medications and/or laser trabeculoplasty.

There is less consensus regarding long-term effects. Some studies have suggested that intraocular pressure may be reduced after ICCE or ECCE for a few weeks to several months.* In one study, intraocular pressure was reduced for up to 6 years postoperatively in patients in whom it had been controlled preoperatively with low dosages of miotics.[94] Handa et al[51] found a significant decrease in intraocular pressure and number of antiglaucoma medications administered following ECCE with posterior chamber lens implantation with a mean follow-up of 2 years. Other studies, however, have indicated that neither ICCE[41,66] nor

_____

*References 10, 45, 51, 56, 81, 90.

ECCE[86,118] leads to lower intraocular pressure. McGuigan et al[86] found no significant change in glaucoma control in medically treated eyes after 18 months follow-up of ECCE with posterior lens implantation.

Inadvertent filtration, formerly a major cause of lowered intraocular pressure postoperatively,[40,41] is much less common with the watertight closure of the cataract incision now commonly obtained with fine, nonabsorbable sutures placed with microsurgical techniques.[41,63,77]

The beneficial effect of argon laser trabeculoplasty persists after ECCE with or without intraocular lens implantation.[14,141] Since laser trabeculoplasty appears to be more successful when performed before cataract extraction, particularly if a posterior chamber lens is not implanted, one should consider carefully whether trabeculoplasty is indicated before cataract extraction.

Cataract extraction may adversely affect functioning filtering blebs. Overall experience suggests a 50% loss or reduction of functioning blebs. Suggested techniques for cataract extraction in the presence of a bleb have included incision through the bleb, corneal incision anterior to the bleb, and limbal incision in an area opposite the bleb.[33,106,131] Postoperative hypotony may lead to collapse of the bleb, and concomitant inflammation may lead to scarring of the walls of the bleb to the underlying episclera. After ICCE, the composition of the aqueous humor may predispose to stimulate fibroblast proliferation, leading to bleb failure.[57] Vitreous herniation into and occlusion of the pupil are less common in eyes with an intact posterior capsule.

Transient Postoperative Rise in Intraocular Pressure

A transient, early intraocular pressure rise may occur after uncomplicated ICCE[107,109] or ECCE.[59,60,115] Rich et al[109] demonstrated elevated intraocular pressure within several hours after surgery in all of 20 eyes undergoing ICCE without the use of alpha-chymotrypsin. The intraocular pressure rose to 26 to 50 mm Hg at a mean of 6.8 hours after surgery. In one series of nonglaucomatous eyes undergoing ECCE, 7 of 34 eyes developed an intraocular pressure of at least 40 mm Hg within 2 to 3 hours after surgery.[47a] The use of hyaluronate did not appear to influence this. Glaucomatous eyes appear to be at increased risk for an early postoperative pressure rise.[86,118] The incidence after phacoemulsification with a 3 mm incision needs further clarification.

One mechanism for this rise appears to be watertight closure of the corneoscleral wound. Exact reapproximation of the incision eliminates the "safety valve" of aqueous leakage allowed by earlier techniques of wound closure.

"Plasmoid aqueous," formed in the first hours after surgery, may contribute to the intraocular pressure elevation by obstructing the trabecular meshwork.[45] This may be mediated to some extent by prostaglandins. Aspirin and indomethacin have been found to blunt the postoperative intraocular pressure rise,[108] although this has been disputed.[41]

Third, edema in the region of the corneoscleral incision creates a deformational effect on the aqueous outflow structures.[70,71] A white ridge resembling an inverted snowbank with the incision at its crest protrudes into the anterior chamber (Fig. 71-1). This ridge usually recedes within 2 weeks. Tight corneoscleral sutures themselves may deform the outflow structures enough to raise the intraocular pressure.[15] After clear corneal incision, which should minimize trabecular damage, elevated intraocular pressure may[107] or may not[113] result.

Patients experiencing a significant rise in in-

traocular pressure immediately after cataract extraction often have ocular pain. Postoperative pain caused by operative trauma or inflammation usually responds to mild analgesics. Severe pain should arouse suspicion of corneal edema caused by elevated intraocular pressure or, less commonly, a postoperative suprachoroidal hemorrhage. Patients with severe pain should not be given routine narcotics but should be examined at the slit-lamp and treated appropriately. The incidence of wound complications, such as iris prolapse and wound leak, may be increased.[68]

One may wish to avoid watertight closure in a patient with extensive glaucomatous damage, since even a transient postoperative pressure rise may obliterate the remaining field.[72] However, even trabeculectomy combined with cataract extraction does not guarantee against the possibility of a significant early pressure rise. Postoperative intraocular pressures as much as 15 mm Hg higher than baseline have been documented in eyes undergoing trabeculectomy combined with cataract extraction and implantation of a posterior chamber lens.[128]

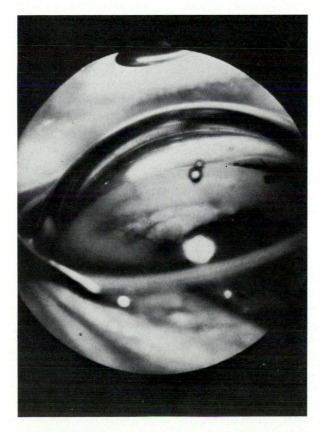

Fig. 71-1   "White ridge" after cataract extraction. In this gonioscopic view, ridge is present at right of photograph and represents edema of inner lips of cataract incision. Suture is visible through the trabecular meshwork as a dark mass in the angle recess. (Courtesy Ralph E. Kirsch, MD)

A transient postoperative rise in intraocular pressure is the most likely diagnosis when the intraocular pressure is elevated several hours after surgery and should be suspected when the angle is open and the anterior chamber is unremarkable. The diagnosis is most certain in retrospect, when the intraocular pressure soon returns to normal. Since this pressure rise usually resolves spontaneously within 36 hours, no treatment is necessary in the absence of preexisting glaucomatous damage unless the level of intraocular pressure is high enough to threaten the integrity of the incision or cause pain.

Intracameral acetylcholine[59] or carbachol[60] at the time of surgery decreases the intraocular pressure rise. The surgeon should institute prophylactic treatment with a beta-blocking agent or carbonic anhydrase inhibitor to blunt the rise and also measure intraocular pressure a few hours after cataract extraction. Beta-blockade has not been consistently reported effective either prophylactically or in blunting an existing intraocular pressure spike.[49] Pilocarpine gel applied postoperatively has been reported more effective than timolol in blunting the rise and without complications.[115] Hyperosmotic agents may be useful on a short-term basis.

Alpha-Chymotrypsin–induced Glaucoma (Zonulytic Glaucoma)

Alpha-chymotrypsin is commonly used for zonulysis during ICCE. Intraocular pressure elevations of 20 to 30 mm Hg, usually occurring from 2 to 5 days after cataract extraction, have been observed in up to 27% of patients in whom it has been used.[61,67,69,77,85]

Ultrastructural observations of particulate material in the trabecular meshwork of owl monkeys[2] and enucleated human eyes[147] after injection of alpha-chymotrypsin have been interpreted as suggestive of obstruction of the outflow pathway by zonular fragments. Other proposed mechanisms include direct toxic effects on the trabecular meshwork, damage to the meshwork from contaminants in the enzyme preparation, and alpha-chymotrypsin–induced inflammation. Damage to the meshwork and ciliary body after injection of alpha-chymotrypsin into the anterior chamber has been demonstrated experimentally,[34,79] as opposed to negative findings in earlier studies.[52,80] Running the preparation through a Millipore filter before intraocular instillation or instillation of the diluent alone does not result in elevated intraocular pressure.[67] Normal amounts of anti-alpha-chymo-

trypsin are present in the aqueous of responders to alpha-chymotrypsin,[39] and negative skin tests indicate lack of hypersensitivity to the enzyme.[68] Topical corticosteroids have no ameliorating effect.[68]

Patients with preexisting glaucoma have either no[43] or only a slightly increased[72] incidence of zonulytic glaucoma. No long-term effects on aqueous humor dynamics have been demonstrated in eyes that have had zonulytic glaucoma.[65]

Intraocular acetylcholine, preoperative acetazolamide or mannitol and postoperative acetazolamide, pilocarpine, or topical corticosteroids do not prevent zonulytic glaucoma.[11,39] Acetazolamide given after the onset of the intraocular pressure rise failed to shorten its duration in comparison with that of untreated eyes.[6] However, Packer et al[93] found prophylactic treatment with timolol and acetazolamide to blunt the rise in intraocular pressure.

Prevention is the most effective treatment. Alpha-chymotrypsin should be used judiciously and only when indicated by the patient's age or the maturity of the cataract. The use of minimum volumes and a 1:10,000 solution instead of a 1:5000 solution decreases the incidence of intraocular pressure elevation.[70] Irrigation of the anterior chamber before lens extraction may remove zonular fragments, but does not diminish the incidence of zonulytic glaucoma by removing the enzyme itself, since anti-alpha-chymotrypsin in the anterior chamber inactivates the enzyme within minutes after instillation.

When zonulytic glaucoma develops, temporizing measures are indicated, since it usually abates within 48 to 72 hours. Medical therapy with beta-blockers and/or carbonic anhydrase inhibitors usually suffices.

Glaucoma Caused by Viscoelastic Agents

Sodium hyaluronate (Healon) is commonly used as an adjunct in ECCE both with and without intraocular lens implantation to maintain the anterior chamber during the anterior capsulotomy and to deepen the anterior and posterior chambers before intraocular lens insertion. Its use has been associated with a significant postoperative rise in intraocular pressure,[9,22,42,95] which may occur more often and more severely in eyes with preexisting outflow impairment.

The elevation characteristically begins within the first postoperative day and abates spontaneously within 48 to 72 hours.[22,95] Intraocular pressure rises to as high as 60 mm Hg have been reported.[50] Similar effects have been reported with a combination of chondroitin sulfate and hyaluronic acid (Viscoat).[5] Pretreatment with carbonic anhydrase inhibitors or beta-adrenergic blocking agents has been reported to be variably efficacious in blunting a pressure rise.[91]

The amount of sodium hyaluronate instilled into the anterior chamber as well as the amount remaining at the end of the procedure may be important. Consequently, one should aspirate any residual material from the anterior chamber at the conclusion of surgery,[91] although a pressure rise may still occur.[9] One should consider avoiding its use in eyes with severe glaucomatous damage.

The mechanism of the pressure elevation most likely results from mechanical block of the trabecular meshwork.[95] Outflow facility was reduced in enucleated eyes in which sodium hyaluronate was instilled into the anterior chamber.[9] Hyaluronidase caused an increase in outflow facility in rabbits when instilled alone and blocked a hyaluronate-induced decrease in outflow facility when instilled with it.[51]

Intraocular pressure should be closely monitored in the immediate postoperative period when hyaluronate has been used. Prophylactic treatment with carbonic anhydrase inhibitors and/or beta-adrenergic blocking agents may be advisable in eyes with preexisting glaucoma. Miotics may prove useful.

Vitreous in the Anterior Chamber

Free vitreous in the anterior chamber usually results from spontaneous rupture of the anterior hyaloid face and has been associated with open-angle glaucoma.[46,116,127] It is rarely seen after ECCE unless the posterior capsule is inadvertently opened or a posterior capsulotomy is performed. Intraoperative vitreous loss may also lead to free vitreous in the anterior chamber when an anterior vitrectomy is not performed. Vitreous is often present in the anterior chamber without causing glaucoma, and this diagnosis is difficult to substantiate, remaining one of exclusion.

Glaucoma usually begins within weeks to months postoperatively. The mechanism appears to be direct obstruction of the trabecular meshwork by vitreous, which produces significant outflow obstruction when introduced into the anterior chambers of enucleated eyes.[46] When vitreous in the anterior chamber results from intraoperative loss of vitreous, concomitant inflammation may also

predispose the eye to pupillary block and formation of peripheral anterior synechiae.[84,127] The glaucoma may thus be complicated by more than one mechanism.

On slit-lamp examination, the anterior chamber is filled with vitreous. The angle is open, and vitreous appears to extend into the meshwork, but this is difficult to confirm by direct visualization.

The usual agents for control of open-angle glaucoma in the aphakic eye may be used. Mydriatics, by allowing withdrawal of the vitreous from the anterior chamber, may also be effective, as may hyperosmotic agents. Miotics, by causing the iris to draw the vitreous away from the meshwork, may occasionally be efficacious, but their effect is often unpredictable. When recondensation of the vitreous face occurs, the vitreous will spontaneously retract from the angle with subsequent resolution of the glaucoma. If the glaucoma is not controlled medically, anterior vitrectomy is indicated. Despite a complete anterior vitrectomy, a residual open-angle glaucoma may require medical therapy.

Hyphema

A hyphema most commonly occurs in the first week after surgery. The source of the hemorrhage is usually the site of the iridectomy or, less commonly, the cataract incision. A hyphema may also occur spontaneously or in association with minor trauma or heavy physical exercise months after surgery.[98,130,137] The source of this late hyphema is fine neovascularization of the inner aspect of the cataract incision. Fine, lacy, new vessels cross the site of the incision and may occasionally bleed if light pressure is applied with a gonioscopy lens.

Most postoperative hyphemas are limited in extent, are asymptomatic beyond blurring of vision, and are not associated with elevated intraocular pressure. More extensive hyphemas may cause a rise in pressure, and the patient may experience severe pain. Gonioscopy typically reveals an open angle. A cellular response of variable severity may occur in response to the blood in the anterior chamber, and the mechanism of the intraocular pressure rise is believed to be obstruction of the trabecular meshwork by hemosiderin-laden macrophages. The meshwork may also be obstructed by clotted blood. Chronic intermittent hyphemas may lead to secondary angle-closure caused by formation of peripheral anterior synechiae in the inferior angle where the blood settles. If the anterior hyaloid face is ruptured, the vitreous may fill with blood, which may cause delayed restoration of vision, as well as ghost cell glaucoma.

The hyphema and the associated secondary glaucoma are usually self-limited. Medical treatment is preferred, beta-blockers and carbonic anhydrase inhibitors being the agents of first choice. Pilocarpine probably should not be used, since this exacerbates inflammation. Hyperosmotic agents may be used to blunt an acute rise in intraocular pressure. Since clearance of the hyphema may depend on a sufficient rate of aqueous flow, medical therapy should be reserved for patients in whom the intraocular pressure level threatens corneal blood staining, the integrity of the wound, or visual field loss.

Surgical intervention should be reserved for those patients in whom medical therapy fails to control the intraocular pressure. Aspiration of the hyphema is less risky than in the phakic patient. If the hyphema is caused by wound neovascularization, the vessels may be photocoagulated with the argon laser.[98,125,139]

Uveitis

Intraocular inflammation may cause elevated intraocular pressure in the aphakic eye by obstruction of the meshwork by inflammatory cells and fibrinous aqueous, peripheral anterior synechiae, and pupillary block. The inflammation may be part of the postoperative course or may represent an exacerbation of preexisting uveitis and usually must be severe in order to result in a significant elevation of pressure. Sometimes a cause-and-effect relationship must remain presumptive. A detailed discussion of glaucoma caused by uveitis is given in Chapter 67.

Corticosteroid-induced Glaucoma

Topical corticosteroid treatment causes an elevation of intraocular pressure in susceptible patients, particularly those with primary open-angle glaucoma (see Chapter 64). Postoperative effects of corticosteroids on aqueous outflow may sometimes be masked by concomitant secretory hypotony and not be revealed until aqueous production is restored.

Increased penetration of topical corticosteroids in an inflamed eye may make the eye more susceptible to their hypertensive effects. Partial blockage of the trabecular meshwork by inflammatory debris may result in a higher intraocular pressure elevation than would otherwise occur. Cycloplegics, which may induce intraocular pressure elevations in glaucomatous patients, may also be an aggravating factor. Corticosteroids should be used judiciously in the postoperative period.

Ocular examination does not reveal an obvious cause of the pressure elevation, and the examiner must therefore always keep the possibility of this diagnosis in mind. A decrease in intraocular pressure after discontinuation of corticosteroids provides confirmatory evidence. The use of preparations that have less of an effect than dexamethasone on intraocular pressure, such as fluorometholone, should be considered. If necessary, concomitant use of antiglaucoma agents, especially beta-blockers, may be employed.

Lens Particle Glaucoma

A secondary glaucoma may develop after either planned or unplanned ECCE because of lens cortex remnants in the anterior chamber (see Chapter 57). This does not occur in all eyes with retained cortical material after cataract extraction. A variety of mechanisms may account for this rise, including obstruction of the meshwork by free lens particles, obstruction by macrophages swollen with lens material, and plugging of the meshwork by inflammatory debris. Angle-closure glaucoma may result from the development of a pupillary membrane, causing pupillary block, or from peripheral anterior synechiae formation.

The anterior chamber is filled with retained cortical material. There is usually a marked inflammatory response, and prominent white keratic precipitates are present on the corneal endothelium and vitreous face. Medical therapy usually suffices to control the intraocular pressure. Topical corticosteroids are indicated if inflammation is prominent. The glaucoma resolves as the retained cortical material resorbs. When medical therapy fails, surgical removal of the residual cortex is indicated.

Ghost Cell Glaucoma

Ghost cell glaucoma is caused by physical blockage of the outflow channels of the trabecular meshwork by the plasma membranes of degenerated erythrocytes (erythrocyte ghosts). These result from bleeding into the vitreous, either from a vitreous hemorrhage or from an anterior chamber hemorrhage that gains access to the vitreous. Blood in the vitreous may be present before the cataract extraction or may occur at the time of surgery or long afterward. The onset of ghost cell glaucoma depends on the presence of defects in the anterior hyaloid face, which allow the ghost cells to gain access to the anterior chamber. This topic is discussed fully in Chapter 69.

Epithelial Ingrowth and Fibrous Ingrowth

The onset of glaucoma in the late postoperative period should alert the examiner to rule out fibrous ingrowth and epithelial ingrowth. These late complications of cataract extraction are discussed in Chapter 73.

Pseudophakia

Glaucoma in the presence of an intraocular lens may occur at any time and may or may not be related to the lens. Secondary glaucomas may be associated with specific types of implants used over the years. This topic is covered in Chapter 72.

Neodymium-YAG Laser Capsulotomy

Nd:YAG capsulotomy has become the procedure of choice in managing opacification of the posterior capsule, which occurs in 25% to 50% of eyes in the months to years after ECCE.

Elevated intraocular pressure occurs in 39%[133] to 95%[21] of eyes undergoing Nd:YAG capsulotomy. There is a higher incidence in eyes with preexisting glaucoma.[35] The rise in pressure is usually modest, but can be significant and vision-threatening. It usually occurs 1 to 2 hours after treatment, but may develop later, and is generally self-limited. In one series, it had resolved in 60% of eyes in 24 hours and 90% of eyes by 1 week. Persistent elevations of intraocular pressure have been noted.[30] In one large series of 2110 cases, 1% had persistent intraocular pressure elevation.[133]

The mechanism of the pressure rise is unclear and may include iritis, trabecular blockage by debris, prostaglandin release,[75] and the shock wave effect of the laser on the ciliary epithelium.[21] The total amount of laser energy used and the size of the capsulotomy have also been proposed as factors, but pressure elevation may occur even with low energy levels. Outflow facility is reduced after capsulotomy.[110,129]

Patients undergoing capsulotomy should be monitored carefully and treated or pretreated as necessary. The reported efficacy of prophylactic treatment has been variable.[89] Brown et al[13] noted a 67% incidence of postlaser intraocular pressure elevation >10 mm Hg in untreated controls compared to 6% in eyes treated with 4% pilocarpine. Timolol may be effective in decreasing the elevation,[111] which may reappear even several weeks postlaser when glaucoma medications are withdrawn.[20] Recently, topical apraclonidine has been shown to be highly effective in preventing the postlaser rise in pressure.[100a] This topic is further covered in Chapter 57.

ANGLE-CLOSURE GLAUCOMA ASSOCIATED WITH APHAKIA

Preexisting Angle-closure Glaucoma

Cataract extraction is definitive therapy for eyes with angle-closure glaucoma caused by relative or absolute pupillary block which, for whatever reasons, have not previously undergone iridectomy. An eye with previous angle-closure may develop secondary open-angle glaucoma after cataract extraction and is more prone to do so if there has been previous damage to the trabecular meshwork.

Prevention of further compromise of trabecular function is accomplished by intensive control of postoperative inflammation and precautionary measures to avoid a postoperative flat anterior chamber and subsequent extension of peripheral anterior synechiae. Surgical intervention for a flat anterior chamber should be considered early in a patient with preexisting extensive peripheral anterior synechiae.

Pupillary Block

Pupillary block is defined as the failure of aqueous to pass from the posterior to the anterior chamber because of blockage of the pupil and iridectomy. The block is usually functional in phakic eyes, but in aphakic eyes is usually accompanied by the formation of adhesions between the hyaloid face, lens capsule, or lens optic and the iris.

Pupillary block is the most common cause of angle-closure after cataract extraction.[37] Its incidence has been reported as being between 1% and 7% after ICCE.[119] It is most common in the immediate postoperative period but may occur at any time. Cotlier[27] found 76% of cases occur within 2 weeks of surgery. Chances of pupillary block are enhanced when the iridectomy is incomplete (Fig. 71-2), too anterior, or included in an iris prolapse (Fig. 71-3). Pupillary block is most likely to occur if the iridectomy does not extend to within 1 mm of the iris root.[136] Even a sector iridectomy does not ensure against pupillary block if it is not truly basal (Fig. 71-4).

A number of conditions may predispose an eye to aphakic pupillary block (see box on p. 1274). After ICCE a wound leak is probably the most frequent early cause, since it permits the anterior hyaloid to adhere to the posterior iris. A flat anterior chamber with hypotony and choroidal detachment is often followed by pupillary block. Conversely, elevated intraocular pressure caused by pupillary block may cause a wound leak and flat anterior chamber.

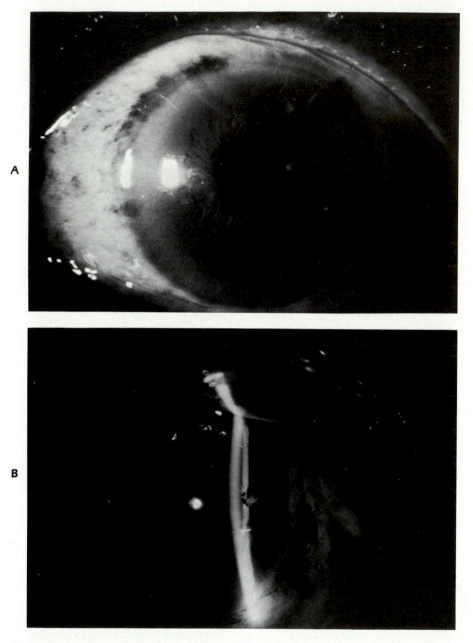

Fig. 71-2 Partial-thickness sector iridectomy, **A**, before and, **B**, after laser iridectomy. (From Ritch, R, and Podos, SM: Perspect Ophthalmol 4:129, 1980)

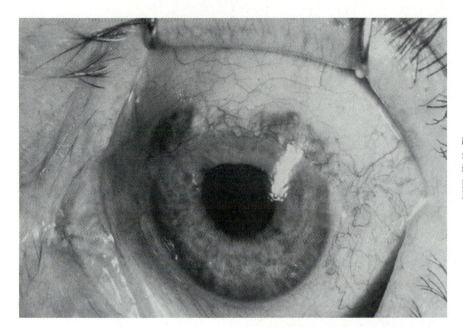

Fig. 71-3 Two peripheral iridecto-mies (10 o'clock and 2 o'clock position) incarcerated in wound with resultant pupillary block glaucoma. (Courtesy Max Forbes, MD)

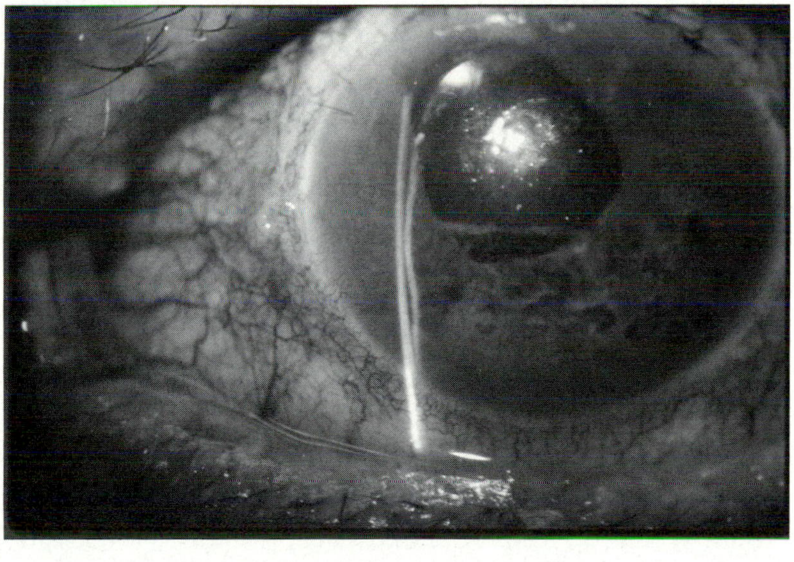

Fig. 71-4 Pupillary block in patient with a sector iridectomy and posterior chamber intraocular lens.

CAUSES OF PUPILLARY BLOCK

1. Wound leak
2. Postoperative inflammation
3. Pupillary occlusion
4. Posterior vitreous detachment
5. Air
6. Incomplete iridectomy
7. Iris prolapse
8. Iridectomy too anterior
9. Lens remnants

Some surgeons have argued against the necessity for routine peripheral iridectomy in ECCE.[31,97,121] However, pupillary block may occur after planned ECCE with or without an intact posterior capsule and even with an iridectomy* (Fig. 71-4).

Air in the anterior and/or posterior chambers may cause pupillary block within 24 to 48 hours of surgery.[4,64,120,124,148] Retained lens material may obstruct the iridectomy and induce greater inflammation, leading to adhesions.[62] Pupillary occlusion by a dense membrane may occur from such causes as marked inflammation or hyphema. Persistent postoperative inflammation is a frequent cause of later pupillary block. The anterior hyaloid may adhere to the iris at the pupillary border or may adhere to the posterior iris surface.

Pupillary Block by Air

Air may be placed into the anterior chamber at the end of the procedure. An eye in which the vitreous volume has been decreased by massage and hyperosmotics may be soft at the end of the procedure, even with a large air bubble. However, when the vitreous volume reconstitutes itself, the aqueous can pass out of the trabecular meshwork but the air cannot, and it becomes confined to a relatively smaller volume. Since the air is not compressible, the intraocular pressure may rise. A bubble filling the anterior chamber will block the flow of aqueous through the pupil, much as a lens does in the anterior chamber (Fig. 71-5). Aqueous behind the iris causes peripheral bombé and angle-closure. If some or all of the air is in the posterior chamber, the air itself may cause the iris to flatten against the trabecular meshwork (Fig. 71-6).

It may not be immediately apparent that the cause of intraocular pressure elevation is blockage of the trabecular meshwork, since the anterior

*References 8, 24, 36, 117, 142, 143, 145.

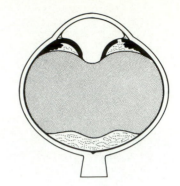

Fig. 71-5 Artist's conception of air bubble in anterior chamber causing pupillary block. Posterior aspect of bubble occludes both pupil and iridectomy.

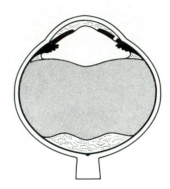

Fig. 71-6 Pupillary block caused by air in posterior chamber.

chamber depth is maintained centrally. Slit-lamp examination and gonioscopy will reveal peripheral iris bombé and angle-closure.

Intensive mydriasis may relieve the pupillary block until the air has been resorbed. Air in the posterior chamber may be released into the anterior chamber. If this is insufficient, the air may be removed by paracentesis with a 30-gauge needle. If too much air is removed, the anterior chamber may be reconstituted with balanced salt solution if necessary. Most air bubbles will resorb spontaneously in 24 to 48 hours.

Pupillary Block by Vitreous

This form of pupillary block is most common after ICCE, but may occur after ECCE if the posterior capsule is opened, either intentionally or unintentionally. When the pupil and iridectomy are obstructed by vitreous, the anterior vitreous face is almost invariably intact. A formed anterior hyaloid acts as a relatively impermeable barrier to the

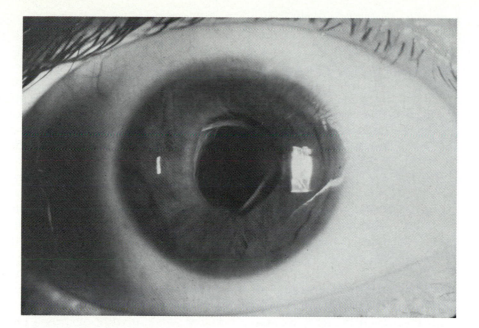

Fig. 71-7   Lens remnants after congenital cataract extraction. No iridectomy was performed. Patient developed pupillary block several years after surgery. (Courtesy Max Forbes, MD)

forward flow of aqueous. A broken vitreous face is only rarely associated with pupillary block.[96] Eyes with preexisting uveitis or iris neovascularization are especially susceptible to pupillary block from posterior synechiae caused by more severe postoperative inflammation.

A rent in the posterior capsule may allow vitreous to herniate anteriorly, predisposing to pupillary block. A posterior vitreous detachment may be associated with pooling of aqueous behind the vitreous, which forces the vitreous more anteriorly, making pupillary block more likely.

Clinical Characteristics

Pupillary block may be diagnosed at various stages in its progression. The patient may experience a decrease in vision and pain in the involved eye or may be asymptomatic. Commonly a shallow or flat anterior chamber with an elevated intraocular pressure and a middilated, nonreactive pupil is present. However, this presentation is by no means the rule, and one must be able to recognize the various earlier stages in order to minimize consequences to the eye.

The intraocular pressure is usually high in the absence of a leak and low if there is a wound leak or marked secretory hypotony. Pressure may be normal early in the course of pupillary block.

The anterior chamber may be flat, shallow, or deep. When the anterior chamber is shallow or flat,

pupillary block must be distinguished from a wound leak, choroidal effusion, or hemorrhage. A wound leak is suggested by the presence of a filtering bleb, a positive Seidel test, or visualization of a wound gape on gonioscopy. However, the Seidel test will be negative in some instances when there is insufficient aqueous to create a visible rivulet in the fluorescein-stained tear film. Fundoscopy and ultrasonography aid in evaluation of the posterior segment.

The anterior chamber may be deep early in the development of pupillary block, and the examiner is easily misled at this time. If the trabecular meshwork is blocked by the iris, restricted aqueous outflow may result in temporary maintenance of the chamber. However the chamber will shallow and flatten as aqueous exists by uveoscleral outflow or a wound leak even if the meshwork is completely blocked. If broad adhesions between the hyaloid face and posterior iris are present in some areas but not in others, the depth of the anterior chamber may be irregular.

The cornea may be clear or edematous, or it may exhibit folds in Descemet's membrane, depending on the intraocular pressure and the state of corneal compensation. The pupil and iridectomy may be occluded with vitreous, inflammatory membranes, or retained lens remnants (Fig. 71-7), although occasionally the pupillary margin may not appear to be secluded. In such situations posterior synechiae to the vitreous originate from the posterior surface of the iris rather than from the pupillary margin. The vitreous face is characteristically intact, and posterior synechiae or a pupillary membrane may be visible.

On gonioscopy, the angle is usually closed, but it may be open if the block is diagnosed at an early stage. The choroid may be intact or detached. If the anterior chamber is shallow or flat with separation of the choroid or ciliary body, the intraocular pressure is usually low.

If the diagnosis is in doubt, an intravenous injection of fluorescein can be given.[103] Fluorescein will appear in the anterior chamber of a normal aphakic eye in about 20 seconds, whereas in pupillary block, it may be absent entirely or trickle in slowly.

The incidence of a flat anterior chamber caused by a wound leak after cataract extraction has been greatly reduced with the advent of tight wound closure, and nonabsorbable sutures. The wound leak may result from faulty closure, premature dissolution of absorbable sutures, pressure on the globe, Valsalva maneuver, or an elevated intraocular pressure postoperatively.

A chain of events may ensue whereby transient pupillary block leads to an elevated intraocular pressure, which causes a wound leak. It is often difficult to decide whether the flat anterior chamber or the pupillary block was the primary cause when both are present. If the intraocular pressure is low, one should think of a wound leak. However, a secondary wound leak may also lead to a low intraocular pressure, and a prolonged flat chamber predisposes the eye to pupillary block. This blockage may remain even after the chamber is spontaneously or surgically reformed and may initiate the cycle again.

Choroidal detachments may also cause shallowing of the anterior chamber, initiating the chain of events cited above. In some instances the low intraocular pressure caused by a wound leak allows transudation of fluid into the suprachoroidal space by reversing the pressure gradient between the choroidal vasculature and the surrounding tissue. The detachment may develop at the time of surgery by the same mechanism. The choroidal detachment then produces forward pressure on the iris, causing shallowing of the anterior chamber.[18,26] Production of aqueous is diminished because of ciliary detachment, further shallowing the chamber.[19]

Prophylactic measures to guard against pupillary block include routine iridectomy in both ICCE and ECCE, and making sure that the iridectomy is basal if ICCE is performed. Wound closure should be adequate, and not too much air should be allowed to remain in the anterior chamber. Postoperative inflammation should be treated appropriately, as should wound leaks. Tonometry should be routinely performed postoperatively, as should gonioscopy as soon as is feasible, particularly if the intraocular pressure is elevated.

Medical therapy is the first line of treatment. Intensive mydriasis will often break the block if adhesions between the anterior hyaloid or posterior capsule and posterior iris are not too extensive.* Mydriasis may have only a temporary effect, since iridovitreal adhesions can still form, and topical corticosteroids should be used to reduce inflammation. Movement of the pupil by alternating mydriatics and miotics may be more effective than mydriatics alone. Miotics alone may be effective in breaking a pupillary block if the pupil is moderately dilated to begin with, or if the iridectomy is functionally blocked or caught up in an iris prolapse. Short-acting mydriatics are easier to reverse than long-acting ones, which should not be used routinely. Hyperosmotic agents may dehydrate the vitreous sufficiently to retract the anterior hyaloid and break adhesions. If the anterior chamber is flat, hyperosmotics may convert it to a shallow one, permitting pupillary movement or allowing laser treatment.

If a wound leak is a factor, pressure patching the eye may aid in breaking the cycle of the wound leak and pupillary block. The use of strong miotics and patching to deepen a shallow or flat anterior chamber has been reported to be successful often.[19,25,44,76,104] Surgical repair of the wound leak should be performed if it is not successful.

If medical treatment is unsuccessful, laser treatment should be attempted. Hyperosmotics are often valuable before treatment to deepen the anterior chamber by contracting the vitreous before either iridectomy or anterior hyaloidectomy. These procedures may also help clear the cornea, as may topical glycerine. Laser pupilloplasty,[23,96,139] and iridectomy[3,100,112,122,123] have been advocated for breaking pupillary block. If the cornea is edematous, one may attempt to break the block by peaking the pupil. If the pupil is clear, one should go directly to creating a new iridectomy with either the argon or the Nd:YAG laser.[123] In a few cases in which the cornea was edematous and pupilloplasty was unsuccessful, we have been able to lower the pressure with peripheral iridoplasty long enough

---

*References 16, 17, 19, 105, 134, 144.

for the cornea to clear sufficiently to perform an iridectomy. The technique is basically that used for creating an iridectomy in a phakic eye, with a few additional considerations.

The site chosen for the iridectomy should be opposite the site of the previous iridectomy. If only point adhesions are present at the pupillary margin (Fig. 71-8), then penetration of the iris at any point should result in release of aqueous and breakage of the block. However, penetration of the iris over an area of broad adhesions will open a path only to the anterior hyaloid face, and the block will remain (Fig. 71-9). If the first iridectomy is unsuccessful in releasing trapped aqueous, we create a second one at another site.

Laser iridectomy can be difficult to perform when the pupil is middilated or wider, since the iris stroma is correspondingly thicker. If miotics do not succeed in constricting the pupil, the iris stroma may be compacted with contraction burns and the iridectomy then performed either between or through them if an argon laser is used. The Nd:YAG laser may be more convenient in this situation.

Vitreociliary Block (Malignant Glaucoma)

Until recently, if two or three laser iridectomies did not succeed in breaking the block, surgical iridectomy was indicated. Sector iridectomy was felt to offer the greatest chance of finding smaller pockets of aqueous. If that failed, a diagnosis of vitreociliary block (aphakic malignant glaucoma, aqueous misdirection) was made and an incision of the anterior hyaloid face[1,28,127,135,138] or a partial anterior vitrectomy[29] was indicated to allow aqueous trapped behind the vitreous to reach the anterior chamber.

At the present time, we feel that it is safer to proceed with Nd:YAG posterior capsulotomy and/or anterior hyaloidectomy[12,32] before surgical intervention if laser iridectomies are unsuccessful. Hyperosmotics are often valuable before treatment, are often effective, and are a key component of treatment. Surgical treatment may be necessary if the condition does not respond to laser therapy. Infusion-suction cutters can also be used to remove membranes occluding the pupil.[62] This is fully discussed in Chapter 70.

Peripheral Anterior Synechiae

Peripheral anterior synechiae are seen most often in aphakic eyes when a flat anterior chamber from any cause has complicated the postoperative period. The incidence of synechia formation is re-

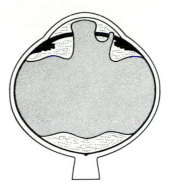

Fig. 71-8 Pupillary block caused by vitreous occlusion of pupil and iridectomy. Point adhesions are present between anterior hyaloid face and iris at pupillary margin.

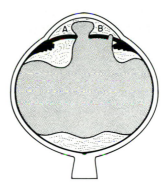

Fig. 71-9 Pupillary block with broad adhesions between anterior hyaloid face and iris in one area and point adhesions in another. Laser iridectomy will be unsuccessful when performed over these adhesions, *B*, but successful when performed over the region of sequestered aqueous, *A*.

lated to the length of time that the chamber remains flat. The time may be as short as 2 to 3 days in some patients and as long as 2 weeks in others. Exacerbating factors include the degree of intraocular inflammation, vitreous loss, and iris prolapse.[58]

Cotlier[26] found that secondary glaucoma did not develop if the anterior chamber was flat for less than 6 days but did develop in 13.5% of his patients when the anterior chamber was flat for longer than 5 days. Kronfeld[76] found a 53% incidence of glaucoma if the chamber was absent for 9 or more days.

In some eyes the elevation of intraocular pressure is lower than one would expect from the apparent extent of the synechiae.[19] In these eyes the peripheral iris is adherent to the peripheral cornea anterior to the meshwork and does not occlude the meshwork itself. Chandler and Simmons[19] believe that bridging synechiae are especially likely when choroidal detachment accompanies a flat anterior chamber.

Nd:YAG Capsulotomy

A number of cases of acute angle-closure glaucoma have been reported after Nd:YAG posterior capsulotomy.[24,82,117,126,134] The angle-closure arises after capsulotomy when vitreous herniates through the capsulotomy and occludes the pupil if an adequate peripheral iridectomy does not exist. An iridectomy should be made at the time of Nd:YAG posterior capsulotomy if not done at the time of cataract extraction.

Neovascular Glaucoma

As in phakic eyes, iris neovascularization leads to elevated intraocular pressure by direct occlusion of the trabecular meshwork and by closure of the angle by peripheral anterior synechiae, which result from contraction of the neovascular membrane. In aphakic eyes, pupillary block caused by iridovitreal synechiae with new vessels is an additional mechanism.

The angle may be open or closed. The central anterior chamber usually remains deep. In those eyes with pupillary block, classic signs such as adherence of the pupil and margins of the iridectomy to the vitreous face, marked iris bombé, and appositional and/or synechial closure of the angle may be observed. Argon laser iridectomy is preferred to Nd:YAG because the risk of hyphema is minimized. Laser iridectomies in eyes with neovascular glaucoma are at greater risk of closing because of chronic low-grade inflammation.

Congenital Cataract and Glaucoma

According to the older literature, glaucoma following surgical treatment of congenital cataract is common.[99] Data is scanty regarding the incidence after present techniques of extraction, but it is felt anecdotally to be less common. Mechanisms for the glaucoma include:

1. Swelling of lens remnants
2. Uveitis
3. Seclusion or occlusion of the pupil
4. Delayed reformation of the anterior chamber
5. Peripheral anterior synechiae
6. Pupillary block
7. Epithelial ingrowth
8. Recurrent hyphema

MANAGEMENT

Gonioscopy should always be performed when elevated intraocular pressure develops, since determining whether the angle is open or closed establishes the glaucoma in one of two broad categories, the approach to which may be quite different. The presence of inflammation, hyphema, lens remnants, or vitreous in the anterior chamber or a history of intraoperative use of hyaluronate or alpha-chymotrypsin will guide the examiner toward the correct management. The interval between cataract extraction and the rise in intraocular pressure is helpful in elucidating the cause of the intraocular pressure rise when the diagnosis is in doubt (see box on p. 1265).

Medical Therapy

The treatment of specific entities is discussed above and in the appropriate chapters. In this final section we wish to provide a few generalizations.

The medical approach to glaucoma therapy is somewhat altered in aphakia. Cholinesterase inhibitors, which are relatively contraindicated in the phakic eye, may be used in the aphakic eye. Epinephrine compounds may be tried in patients in whom they could not be used preoperatively because of narrow angles. However, one must be alert to the development of epinephrine-induced cystoid macular edema. Although this may be less of a concern in eyes with an intact posterior capsule, no conclusive data are yet available.

In the immediate postoperative period in an otherwise normal eye, open-angle glaucoma, regardless of cause, need be treated only if the intraocular pressure is high enough to cause pain or corneal edema, to threaten the integrity of the incision, or to compromise the vasculature of the optic nerve and retina. If a patient has damage from preexisting glaucoma, however, it becomes imperative to lower the intraocular pressure to prevent further damage. The agents of choice are beta-adrenergic blocking agents and carbonic anhydrase inhibitors. Oral glycerin or isosorbide, or parenteral mannitol can be helpful in blunting spikes of intraocular pressure or when rapid pressure lowering is indicated.

Epinephrine may also be considered on a short-term basis when other agents are contraindicated for systemic reasons. The risk of cystoid macular edema makes epinephrine relatively unsuitable for long-term treatment of glaucoma in aphakic patients.[73,83,88,92,140] The maculopathy is dose related and develops weeks to months after the initiation of treatment. The incidence is approximately 20%

to 30% of patients treated and varies with the concentration of epinephrine used.[73] Fortunately, with rare exception, it is reversible after discontinuation of the drug.[83] The incidence of epinephrine maculopathy after ECCE appears to be lower than that after ICCE. This incidence and that with the use of dipivefrin need further elucidation.

When inflammation is judged to contribute to an elevation of intraocular pressure, intensive steroid treatment is indicated. Some patients may develop a secondary steroid-induced elevation of intraocular pressure with prolonged or intensive use.

Miotics do not have a place in the treatment of early-onset open-angle glaucoma, since these tend to exacerbate intraocular inflammation. Nevertheless, the use of echothiophate to control open-angle glaucoma in the early postoperative period has been advocated.[44]

In intermediate- and late-onset glaucoma, when the eye is no longer inflamed, cholinergic agents can be used effectively when indicated. Strong cholinergics, such as echothiophate, no longer contraindicated on the basis of cataractogenesis, become useful and may have a more potent effect than in the phakic eye.[48] Because the incidence of retinal detachment is higher in the aphakic eye, a thorough peripheral retinal examination should be performed before miotic therapy is initiated.

Laser Treatment

The success rate of argon laser trabeculoplasty in aphakic eyes is approximately 50%.[146] The results in pseudophakic patients are better than those in aphakic patients. This may be related to the degree of tension transmitted to the trabecular meshwork through the iris root by the weight of the lens. It is not successful in those cases in which vitreous fills the anterior chamber.[146]

Successful reduction of intraocular pressure by photocoagulation of the ciliary processes has been reported.[78,87] Because the ciliary epithelium may be capable of regeneration, and because extensive photocoagulation is necessary to achieve a measurable reduction in aqueous production, more experience is necessary before this procedure can be properly evaluated.

Surgical Therapy

Only rarely are open-angle glaucomas in the early postoperative period severe enough to warrant surgical intervention. In cases where surgery appears necessary, a simple anterior chamber paracentesis may suffice to lower intraocular pressure

for a long-enough period to allow the process to abate.

Most patients with glaucoma associated with aphakia who come to surgery do so in the late postoperative period and have either primary open-angle glaucoma or chronic angle-closure glaucoma that cannot be controlled medically.

Trabeculectomy

The success rate of trabeculectomy for glaucoma in aphakia has been reported to range from 32%[55] to 92%.[8] In general, filtering surgery is less successful in aphakic than in phakic eyes. The major cause for failure of filtration surgery in aphakic eyes has been scarring of the conjunctiva, which is more likely in an eye that has previously had intraocular surgery. Other factors include obstruction of the filtration site by vitreous, iris, or lens remnants, increased postoperative inflammation, and technical difficulties encountered in performing the surgery. Filtering surgery appears to be more successful after uncomplicated ECCE than ICCE.

An especially high incidence of postoperative suprachoroidal hemorrhage has been noted in aphakic eyes undergoing filtration.[55,114] The higher the myopia, the more likely is this complication.

The technical aspects of the procedure are essentially the same as in phakic eyes. Preoperative preparation with hyperosmotic agents may aid in keeping the vitreous away from the operative site. Our preference is to operate from below to avoid a previously scarred conjunctiva, unless a corneal incision was used for the cataract extraction. Either a limbus-based or a fornix-based flap may be used. When the latter is the case, we prefer to suture it back to the cornea with several 9-0 nylon sutures.

If vitreous appears initially during iridectomy, an anterior vitrectomy should be performed. Viscoelastic agents may be injected through a paracentesis site between the iris and anterior vitreous face at the selected site for trabeculectomy before excision of the meshwork in order to push the vitreous face away from the iris and to lessen the chance of vitreous loss at the time of iridectomy.

Postoperative inflammation should be vigorously controlled. Gentle massage to keep the filtration site open and the bleb expanded should be used when the intraocular pressure rises above 15 mm Hg postoperatively. The use of subconjunctival injections of 5-fluorouracil in the postoperative period to prevent scarring of the bleb has been reported as highly successful and is our procedure of choice.[51,53,54] Preoperative injection of triamcinolone acetamide has also been advocated.

Glaucoma surgery in the presence of an intraocular lens requires meticulous attention to the anterior chamber depth, intraocular lens position, and iridolenticular touch. Viscoelastic materials should be used without hesitation if needed.

Cyclocryotherapy

Cyclocryotherapy has been primarily advocated for eyes with uncontrolled glaucoma that have undergone unsuccessful attempts at surgery and for eyes with neovascular glaucoma. Its effects are unpredictable, and the procedure is associated with a high incidence of complications. These include cataract formation, phthisis, anterior segment necrosis, intraocular hemorrhage, prolonged intraocular inflammation, and macular edema, particularly in patients with neovascular glaucoma.[8] Many variations of the technique, differing in the temperature and placement of the probe, duration and number of applications, and circumferential extent of treatment, have been reported.

Bellows and Grant[7] recommended cyclocryotherapy as the primary procedure for glaucoma in the nonneovascular aphakic eye. They felt crucial considerations to be placement of the anterior edge of the probe tip 2.5 mm from the limbus to ensure freezing over the pars plicata, a single-freeze technique rather than a freeze-thaw-refreeze technique, and initial treatment over 180 degrees rather than 360 degrees to avoid overtreatment. They hypothesized that after zonular rupture the ciliary processes might retract to a location more readily frozen than that in the phakic patient. The efficacy of cyclocryotherapy after ECCE has not been reported.

Other Procedures

Cyclodialysis for glaucoma associated with aphakia[39,135] has declined in popularity, since its results are highly unpredictable and often temporary. Prolonged hypotony, leading to ciliary detachment, macular edema, and papilledema, is a common complication. Frequently the cyclodialysis cleft seals, resulting in an acute elevation of intraocular pressure.

Transscleral Nd:YAG cycloablation, therapeutic ultrasound, and seton implantation are other surgical alternatives.

REFERENCES

1. Allen, JC: Surgical treatment of pupillary block, Ann Ophthalmol 9:661,1977
2. Anderson, DR: Experimental alpha-chymotrypsin glaucoma studied by scanning electron microscopy, Am J Ophthalmol 71:470, 1971
3. Anderson, DR, Forster, RK, and Lewis, ML: Laser iridotomy for aphakic pupillary block, Arch Ophthalmol 93:343, 1975
4. Barkan, O: Glaucoma induced by air blockade, Am J Ophthalmol 34:567, 1951
5. Barron, BA, et al: Comparison the effects of Viscoat and Healon on postoperative intraocular pressure, Am J Ophthalmol 100:377, 1985
6. Beidner, B, Rothkoff, L, and Blumenthal, M: The effect of acetazolamide on early increased intraocular pressure after cataract extraction, Am J Ophthalmol 83:565, 1977
7. Bellows, AR, and Grant, WM: Cyclocryotherapy of chronic open-angle glaucoma in aphakic eyes, Am J Ophthalmol 83:615, 1978
8. Bellows, AR, and Johnstone, MA: Surgical management of chronic glaucoma in aphakia, Ophthalmology 90:807, 1983
9. Berson, FG, et al: Obstruction of aqueous outflow by sodium hyaluronate in enucleated eyes, Am J Ophthalmol 95:668, 1983
10. Bigger, JF, and Becker, B: Cataracts and POAG: The effect of uncomplicated cataract extraction on glaucoma control, Trans Am Acad Ophthalmol, Otolaryngol 75:260, 1971
11. Bloomfield, S: Failure to prevent enzyme glaucoma, Am J Ophthalmol 65:405, 1968
12. Brown, RH, Lynch, MG, Tearse, JE, and Nunn, RD: Neodymium-YAG vitreous surgery for phakic and pseudophakic malignant glaucoma, Arch Ophthalmol 104:1464, 1986
13. Brown, SVL, Thomas, JV, Belcher, CD, and Simmons, RJ: Effect of pilocarpine in the treatment of intraocular pressure elevation following Nd:YAG laser posterior capsulotomy, Ophthalmology 92:354, 1985
14. Brown, SVL, et al: Effect of cataract surgery on intraocular pressure reduction obtained with laser trabeculoplasty, Am J Ophthalmol 100:373, 1985
15. Campbell, DG, and Grant, WM: Trabecular deformation and reduction of outflow facility due to cataract and penetrating keratoplasty sutures, Invest Ophthalmol Vis Sci Suppl 16:126, 1977
16. Chandler, PA: Glaucoma from pupillary block in aphakia, Arch Ophthalmol 67:44, 1962
17. Chandler, PA, and Johnson, CC: A neglected cause of secondary glaucoma in eyes in which the lens is absent or subluxated, Arch Ophthalmol 37:740, 1947
18. Chandler, PA, and Maumenee, AE: A major cause of hypotony, Am J Ophthalmol 52:609, 1961

19. Chandler, PA, and Simmons, RJ: Gonioscopy during surgery for aphakic eyes with pupillary block, Am J Ophthalmol 74:571, 1972

20. Chandler, PA, Simmons, RJ, and Grant, WM: Malignant glaucoma: medical and surgical treatment, Am J Ophthalmol 66:495, 1968

21. Channel, MM, and Beckman, H: Intraocular pressure changes after neodymium:YAG laser posterior capsulotomy, Arch Ophthalmol 102:1024, 1984

22. Cherfan, GM, Rich, WJ, and Wright, G: Raised intraocular pressure and other problems with sodium hyaluronate and cataract surgery, Trans Ophthalmol Soc UK 103:277, 1983

23. Cleasby, GW: Photocoagulation coreoplasty, Arch Ophthalmol 83:145, 1970

24. Cohen, JS, Osher, RH, Weber, P, and Faulkner, JD: Complications of extracapsular cataract surgery, Ophthalmology 91:826, 1984

25. Cotlier, E: Aphakic flat anterior chamber. II. Effect of spontaneous reformation and medical therapy, Arch Ophthalmol 87:124, 1972

26. Cotlier, E: Aphakic flat anterior chamber. III. Effect of inflation of the anterior chamber and drainage of choroidal detachments, Arch Ophthalmol 88:16, 1972

27. Cotlier, E: Aphakic flat anterior chamber. IV. Treatment of pupillary block by iridectomy, Arch Ophthalmol 88:22, 1972

28. Cotlier, E: Aphakic flat chamber: treatment by anterior vitriotomy, Arch Ophthalmol 86:507, 1971

29. Cotlier, E: Anterior vitriotomy for aphakic flat anterior chamber, Br J Ophthalmol 56:347, 1972

30. Demer, JL, Koch, DD, Smith, JA, and Knolle, GE, Jr: Persistent elevation in intraocular pressure after Nd:YAG laser treatment, Ophthalmic Surg 17:465, 1986

31. Emery, JM, and McIntyre, DJ: Extracapsular cataract surgery, St. Louis, 1983, The CV Mosby Co

32. Epstein, DL, Steinert, RF, and Puliafito, CA: Neodymium-YAG laser therapy to the anterior hyaloid in aphakic malignant (ciliovitreal block) glaucoma, Am J Ophthalmol 98:137, 1984

33. Etienne, R: Conduitée à tenir en presence de l'association glaucome et cataracte, Ann Ocul 196:1154, 1963

34. Fanta, H, and Herold, I: Spatfolgen nachenzymatischer Zonulolyse in histologischen Schnitt, Klin Monatsbl Augenheilkd 142:1011, 1963

35. Flohr, MJ, Robin, AL, and Kelley, JS: Early complications following Q-switched neodymium:YAG laser posterior capsulotomy, Ophthalmology 92:360-363, 1985

36. Forman, JS, Ritch, R, Dunn, MW, and Szmyd, L, Jr: Angle-closure glaucoma in pseudophakia, Ophthal Laser Ther 2:85, 1987

37. Franois, J: Aphakic glaucoma, Ann Ophthalmol 6:429, 1974

38. Galin, MA: Surgical technique of cyclodialysis and lens extraction, Ann Ophthalmol 7:1257, 1975

39. Galin, MA, Barasch, KR, and Harris, LS: Enzymatic zonulysis and intraocular pressure, Am J Ophthalmol 61:690, 1966

40. Galin, MA, Hung, PT, and Obstbaum, SA: Cataract extraction in glaucoma, Am J Ophthalmol 87:124, 1979

41. Galin, MA, Lin, LL, and Obstbaum, SA: Cataract extraction and intraocular pressure, Trans Ophthalmol Soc UK 98:124, 1978

42. Glasser, DB, Matsuda, M, and Edelhauser, HF: A comparison of the efficacy and toxicity of and intraocular pressure response to viscous solutions in the anterior chamber, Arch Ophthalmol 104:1819, 1986

43. Gombos, GM, and Oliver, M: Cataract extraction with enzymatic zonulolysis in glaucomatous eyes, Am J Ophthalmol 64:69, 1967

44. Gorin, G: Echothiophate iodide for glaucoma or flat anterior chamber following cataract extraction, Am J Ophthalmol 67:392, 1969

45. Gormaz, A: Ocular tension after cataract surgery, Am J Ophthalmol 53:832, 1969

46. Grant, WM: Open-angle glaucoma with vitreous filling the anterior chamber following cataract extraction, Trans Am Ophthalmol Soc 61:96, 1963

47. Gressel, MG, Parrish, RK, II, and Folberg, R: 5-fluorouracil and glaucoma filtering surgery. I. An animal model, Ophthalmology 91:378, 1984

47a. Gross, JB, et al: Increased intraocular pressure in the immediate postoperative period after extracapsular cataract extraction, Am J Ophthmol 105:466, 1988

48. Guyton, JS: Choice of operation for primary glaucoma combined with cataract extraction, Arch Ophthalmol 33:265, 1945

49. Haimann, MH, and Phelps, CD: Prophylactic timolol for the prevention of high intraocular pressure after cataract extraction, Ophthalmology 88:233, 1981

50. Handa, J, Henry, JC, Krupin, T, and Keates, E: ECCE with posterior chamber lens implantation in patients with glaucoma, Arch Ophthalmol 105:765, 1987

51. Hein, SR, Keates, RH, and Weber, PA: Elimination of sodium hyaluronate–induced decrease in outflow facility with hyaluronidase, Ophthalmic Surg 17:735, 1986

52. Hervouet, F: Nouvelles précisions histologiques sur l'action de l'alpha chymotrypsine sur les tissues oculaires, An Inst Barraquer 3:194, 1962

53. Heuer, DK, et al: Trabeculectomy in aphakic eyes, Ophthalmology 91:1045, 1984

54. Heuer, DK, et al: 5-Fluorouracil and glaucoma filtering surgery. II. A pilot study, Ophthalmology 91:384, 1984

55. Heuer, DK, et al: 5-Fluorouracil and glaucoma filtering surgery. III. Intermediate follow-up of a pilot study, Ophthalmology 93:1537, 1986

56. Hilding, AC: Reduced ocular tension after cataract surgery, Arch Ophthalmol 53:686, 1955

57. Herschler, J, Claflini, AJ, and Fiorentino, G: The effect of aqueous humor on the growth of subconjunctival fibroblast in tissue culture and its implication for glaucoma surgery, Am J Ophthalmol 89:245, 1980

58. Hitchings, RA: Aphakic glaucoma: prophylaxis and management, Trans Ophthalmol Soc UK 98:118, 1978

59. Hollands, RH, Drance, SM, and Schulzer, M: The effect of acetylcholine on early postoperative intraocular pressure, Am J Ophthalmol 103:749, 1987

60. Hollands, RH, Drance, SM, and Schulzer, M: The effect of intracameral carbachol on intraocular pressure after cataract extraction, Am J Ophthalmol 104:225, 1987

61. Iglesios, FG: La zonulolisis enzimatica de Barraquer, An Inst Barraquer 1:3, 1960

62. Jacklin, HN: Excision of pupillary membrane after cataract extraction with the vitreous infusion suction cutter, Am J Ophthalmol 79:1050, 1975

63. Jaffe, NS: Cataract surgery and its complications, ed. 3, St. Louis, 1981, The CV Mosby Co

64. Jaffe, NS, and Light, DS: The danger of air pupillary block glaucoma in cataract surgery with osmotic hypotonia, Arch Ophthalmol 76:633, 1966

65. Jocson, VL: Tonography and gonioscopy before and after cataract extraction with alpha-chymotrypsin, Am J Ophthalmol 60:318, 1965

66. Kaufman, IH: Intraocular pressure after lens extraction, Am J Ophthalmol 59:722, 1965

67. Kirsch, RE: Glaucoma following cataract extraction associated with use of alpha-chymotrypsin, Arch Ophthalmol 72:612, 1964

68. Kirsch RE: Further studies on glaucoma following cataract extraction associated with the use of alpha-chymotrypsin, Trans Am Acad Ophthalmol Otolaryngol 69:1011, 1965

69. Kirsch, RE: Dose relationship of alpha-chymotrypsin in production of glaucoma after cataract extraction, Arch Ophthalmol 75:774, 1966

70. Kirsch, RE, Levine, O, and Singer, JA: The ridge at the internal edge of the cataract incision, Arch Ophthalmol 94:2098, 1976

71. Kirsch, RE, Levine, O, and Singer, JA: Further studies on the ridge at the internal edge of the cataract incision, Trans Am Acad Ophthalmol Otolaryngol 83:224, 1977

72. Kolker, AE: Visual prognosis in advanced glaucoma: a comparison of medical and surgical therapy for retention of vision in 101 eyes with advanced glaucoma, Trans Am Ophthalmol Soc 75:539, 1977

73. Kolker, AE, and Becker, B: Epinephrine maculopathy, Arch Ophthalmol 79:552, 1968

74. Kornzweig, AC, and Schneider, J: Cataract extraction in glaucoma cases, Ann Ophthalmol 6:959, 1974

75. Kraff, MC, Sanders, DR, and Lieberman, HL: Intraocular pressure and the corneal endothelium after Neodymium-YAG laser posterior capsulotomy: relative effects of aphakia and pseudophakia, Arch Ophthalmol 103:511, 1985

76. Kronfeld, PC: Delayed restoration of the anterior chamber, Am J Ophthalmol 38:483, 1954

77. Lantz, JM, and Quigley, JH: Intraocular pressure after cataract extraction: effects of alpha-chymotrypsin, Can J Ophthalmol 8:339, 1973

78. Lee, PF: Argon laser photocoagulation of the ciliary processes in cases of aphakic glaucoma, Arch Ophthalmol 97:235, 1979

79. Lessell, S, and Kuwabara, T: Experimental alpha-chymotrypsin glaucoma, Arch Ophthalmol 81:853, 1969

80. Leydhecker, W: Histologische Untersuchung am Trabekelsystem nach Kurzfritiger Einwiklung von alpha-chymotrypsin, Klin Monatsbl Augenheilkd 142:554, 1963

81. Linn, JG: Cataract extraction in management of glaucoma, Trans Am Acad Ophthalmol Otolaryngol 75:273, 1971

82. MacEwen, CJ, et al: Angle closure following Nd: YAG laser capsulotomy in the aphakic eye (correspondence), Br J Ophthalmol 69:795, 1985

83. Mackool, RJ, Muldoon, T, Fortier, A, and Nelson, D: Epinephrine-induced cystoid macular edema in aphakic eyes, Arch Ophthalmol 95:791, 1977

84. Mamo, JG: Late effects of vitreous loss, Ann Ophthalmol 6:935, 1974

85. Manezo, JL, Marco, M, and Mascarell, EV: Enzymatic ocular hypertension: a statistical study, J Fr Ophthalmol 1:289, 1978

86. McGuigan, LJB, et al: Extracapsular cataract extraction and posterior chamber lens implantation in eyes with preexisting glaucoma, Arch Ophthalmol 104:1301, 1986

87. Merritt, JC: Transpupillary photocoagulation of the ciliary processes, Ann Ophthalmol 8:325, 1976

88. Michels, RG, and Maumenee, AE: Cystoid macular edema associated with topically applied epinephrine in aphakic eyes, Am J Ophthalmol 80:379, 1975

89. Migliori, ME, Berkman, H, and Channell, MM: Intraocular pressure changes after Nd:YAG laser capsulotomy in eyes pretreated with timolol, Arch Ophthalmol 105:473, 1987

90. Miller, JR, and Morin, JD: Intraocular pressure after cataract extraction, Am J Ophthalmol 66:523, 1968

91. Naeser, K, et al: Intraocular pressure in the first days after implantation of posterior chamber lenses with the use of sodium hyaluronate, Acta Ophthalmol 64:330, 1986

92. Obstbaum, SA, Galin, MA, and Poole, TA: Topical epinephrine and cystoid macular edema, Ann Ophthalmol 8:455, 1976

93. Packer, AJ, Fraioli, AJ, and Epstein, DL: The effect of timolol and acetazolamide on transient intraocular pressure elevation following cataract extraction with alpha-chymotrypsin, Ophthalmology 88:239, 1981

94. Palimeris, G, Chimonidou, E, Magouritsas, N, and Velissaropoulos, P: Cataract extraction in chronic simple glaucoma, Ophthalmic Surg 5:62, 1974

95. Passo, MS, Ernest, JT, and Goldstick, TK: Hyaluronate increases intraocular pressure when used in cataract extraction, Br J Ophthalmol 69:572, 1985

96. Patti, JC, and Cinotti, AA: Iris photocoagulation therapy of aphakic pupillary block, Arch Ophthalmol 93:347, 1975

97. Pearce, JL: Experience with 194 posterior chamber lenses in 20 months, Trans Ophthalmol Soc UK 97:258, 1977

98. Petrelli, EA, and Wiznia, RA: Argon laser photocoagulation of inner wound vascularization after cataract extraction, Am J Ophthalmol 84:58, 1977

99. Phelps, CD, and Arafat, NI: Open-angle glaucoma following surgery for congenital cataracts, Arch Ophthalmol 95:1985, 1977

100. Pollack, IP: Use of argon laser energy to produce iridotomies, Trans Am Ophthalmol Soc 77:674, 1979

100a. Pollack, IP, et al: Prevention of the rise in intraocular pressure following neodymium-YAG posterior capsulotomy using topical 1% apraclonidine, Arch Ophthalmol 106:754, 1988

101. Praeger, DL: The reopening of closed filtering blebs using the Neodymium:YAG laser, Ophthalmology 91:373, 1984

102. Radius, RL, et al: Pseudophakia and intraocular pressure, Am J Ophthalmol 97:738, 1984

103. Ray, RR, and Binkhorst, RD: The diagnosis of pupillary block by intravenous injection of fluorescein, Am J Ophthalmol 61:481, 1966

104. Reese, AB: Herniation of the anterior hyaloid membrane following uncomplicated ICCE, Trans Am Ophthalmol Soc 46:73, 1948

105. Reese, AB: Herniation of the anterior hyaloid membrane following uncomplicated ICCE, Am J Ophthalmol 32:933, 1949

106. Regan, EF, and Day, RM: Cataract extraction after filtering procedures, Trans Am Ophthalmol Soc 68:96, 1970

107. Rich, WJ: Further studies on early post-operative ocular hypertension following cataract extraction, Trans Ophthalmol Soc UK 89:639, 1969

108. Rich, WJ: Prevention of post-operative ocular hypertension by prostaglandin inhibitors, Trans Ophthalmol Soc UK 97:268, 1977

109. Rich, WJ, Radtke, ND, and Cohan, BE: Early ocular hypertension after cataract extraction, Br J Ophthalmol 58:725, 1974

110. Richter, CU, et al: Intraocular pressure elevation following Nd:YAG laser posterior capsulotomy, Ophthalmology 92:636, 1985

111. Richter, CU, et al: Prevention of intraocular pressure elevation following neodymium-YAG laser posterior capsulotomy, Arch Ophthamol 103:912, 1985

112. Ritch, R, and Podos, SM: Argon laser treatment of angle-closure glaucoma, Perspect Ophthalmol 4:129, 1980

113. Rothkoff, L, Beidner, B, and Blumenthal, M: The effect of corneal section on early increased intraocular pressure after cataract extraction, Am J Ophthalmol 85:337, 1978

114. Ruderman, JM, Harbin, TS, and Campbell, DG: Postoperative suprachoroidal hemorrhage following filtering procedures, Am Ophthalmol 104:201, 1986

115. Ruiz, RS, et al: Management of increased intraocular pressure after cataract extraction, Am J Ophthalmol 103:487, 1987

116. Samples, JR, and Van Buskirk, EM: Open-angle glaucoma associated with vitreous humor filling the anterior chamber, Am J Ophthalmol 102:759, 1986

117. Samples, JR, et al: Pupillary block with posterior chamber intraocular lenses, Arch Ophthalmol 105:335, 1987

118. Savage, JA, Thomas, JV, Belcher, CD, and Simmons, RJ: ECCE and posterior chamber intraocular lens implantation in glaucomatous eyes, Ophthalmology 92:1506, 1985

119. Scheie, HG, and Ewing, MQ: Aphakic glaucoma, Trans Ophthalmol Soc UK 98:111, 1978

120. Scheie, HG, and Frazier, W: Ocular hypertension induced by air in the anterior chamber, Arch Ophthalmol 44:691, 1950

121. Schulze, RR, and Copeland, JR: Posterior chamber intraocular lens implantation without peripheral iridectomy: a preliminary report, Ophthalmic Surg 13:567, 1982

122. Schwartz, LW, et al: Argon laser iridotomy in the treatment of patients with primary angle-closure or pupillary block glaucoma: a clinicopathologic study, Trans Am Acad Ophthalmol Otolaryngol 85:294, 1978

123. Schwartz, LW, et al: Nd:YAG laser iridectomies in glaucoma associated with closed or occludable angles, Am J Ophthalmol 102:41, 1986

124. Selinger, E: Ocular hypertension induced by air in the anterior chamber after cataract extraction, Am J Ophthalmol 20:827, 1937

125. Sharpe, ED, and Simmons, RJ: Argon laser therapy of occult recurrent hypthema from anterior wound neovascularization, Ophthalmic Surg 17:283, 1986

126. Shrader, CE, et al: Pupillary and iridovitreal block in pseudophakic eyes, Ophthalmology 91:831, 1984

127. Simmons, RJ: The vitreous in glaucoma, Trans Ophthalmol Soc UK 95:422, 1975

128. Simmon, ST, et al: Extracapsular cataract extraction and posterior chamber intraocular lens implantation combined with trabeculectomy in patients with glaucoma, Am J Ophthalmol, 104:465, 1987

129. Smith, CB: Effect of Neodymium-YAG laser posterior capsulotomy on outflow facility, Glaucoma 6:171, 1984

130. Speakman, JS: Recurrent hyphema after surgery, Can J Ophthalmol 10:299, 1975

131. Spector, SM, et al: The effect of extracapsular cataract extraction with posterior chamber intraocular

lens insertion through a corneal incision on filtration in patients with functioning blebs, Invest Ophthalmol Vis Sci Suppl 28:273, 1987

132. Stark, WJ, Fagadau, WR, Stewart, RH, et al: Reduction of pupillary constriction during cataract surgery using suprofen, Arch Ophthalmol 104:364, 1986

133. Stark, WJ, et al: Neodymium:YAG lasers: an FDA report, Ophthalmology 92:209, 1985

134. Sugar, HS: Pupil block in aphakic eyes, Am J Ophthalmol 46:831, 1958

135. Sugar, HS: Pupillary block and pupil-block glaucoma following cataract extraction, Am J Ophthalmol 61:435, 1966

136. Swan, KC: Relationship of basal iridectomy to shallow chamber following cataract extraction, Arch Ophthamol 69:191, 1963

137. Swan, KC: Hyphema due to wound vascularization after cataract extraction, Arch Ophthalmol 89:87, 1973

138. Theodore, FH: Complications after cataract extraction, Boston, 1965, Little, Brown & Co

139. Theodossiadis, G, Kouris-Borgkati, E, and Velissaropoulos, P: Clinical and pathologic-anatomical results following the application of a mobile argon-laser beam in aphakic pupillary block glaucoma, Klin Monatsbl Augenheilkd 175:180, 1979

140. Thomas, JV, Gragoudas, ES, Blair, NP, and Lapus, JV: Correlation of epinephrine use and macular edema in aphakic glaucomatous eyes, Arch Ophthalmol 96:625, 1978

141. Thomas, JV, Simmons, RJ, Belcher, CD: ALT in the presurgical glaucoma patient, Ophthalmology 89:187, 1982

142. Van Buskirk, EM: Pupillary block after intraocular lens implantation, Am J Ophthalmol 95:55, 1983

143. Weinreb, RN, Wasserstrom, JP, Forman, JS, and Ritch, R: Pseudophakic pupillary block and angle-closure glaucoma in diabetics, Am J Ophthalmol 102:325, 1986

144. Wiesel, J, and Swan, KC: Mydriatic therapy of shallow chamber after cataract extraction, Arch Ophthalmol 58:126, 1957

145. Willis, DA, Stewart, RH, and Kimbrough, RL: Pupillary block associated with posterior chamber lens, Ophthalmic Surg 16:108, 1985

146. Wise, JB, and Witter, SL: Argon laser therapy for open-angle glaucoma, Arch Ophthalmol 97:319, 1979

147. Worthen, DM: Scanning electron microscopy after alpha-chymotrypsin perfusion in man, Am J Ophthalmol 73:637, 1972

148. Wyman, GJ: Glaucoma induced by air injections into the anterior chamber, Am J Ophthalmol 37:424, 1954

Chapter 72

Glaucoma and Intraocular Lens Implantation

Deen G. King
William E. Layden

Lens implantation in glaucoma patients is gaining widespread acceptance, although its efficacy still is difficult to ascertain from the literature. Glaucoma was initially considered an absolute contraindication to intraocular lens implantation because of the high rate of complications.[8,24] Improved lens design and implantation techniques have markedly diminished the incidence of intraocular lens-induced glaucoma compared to this earlier literature[4] (Table 72-1). The overwhelming acceptance of pseudophakic correction for cataract patients has led to an increase in the number of intraocular lenses placed in patients with glaucoma.

Table 72-1 *Pseudophakia and glaucoma: secondary glaucoma*

Author	Eyes (lens type)	Incidence (%)
Smith and Anderson[61]	26/606 iris	4.3
Phyodorov et al.[48]	6/2700 iris	0.3
Binkhorst[8]	6/500 iris	1.2
Tennant[64]	0/160 anterior chamber	0
Kern[29]	6/200 iris	3
Taylor and Stein[63]	0/100 iris	0
Drews[13]	21/300 iris	0.7
Praeger[49]	8/300 iris	0.3
Shephard[58]	5/500 iris	1
François[15]	(Review of aphakic glaucoma)	0.7 to 7 (range)

It is important to distinguish between intraocular lens placement in eyes with preexisting glaucoma and the development of secondary glaucoma as a result of intraocular lens implantation. The efficacy of lens implantation in glaucoma patients should be determined from data evaluating current surgical technique and lens design, as there has been a great diversity of intraocular lens designs and techniques for cataract extraction over the past two decades. In addition, the biologic response of the eye to lens implantation may depend on the mechanical and biochemical properties of the particular intraocular lens.

LENS IMPLANTATION IN PATIENTS WITH PREEXISTING GLAUCOMA

Lens implantation in glaucoma patients should maximize the patient's visual potential without making intraocular pressure more difficult to control. The long-term effect of cataract surgery on intraocular pressure is difficult to assess because of the contradictory data arising from variability in surgical technique. Several studies noted a sustained reduction in intraocular pressure after cataract surgery alone[7,19,31,59] (Table 72-2). The use of an intraocular lens does not appear to significantly alter the effect of lens extraction on intraocular pressure control.[10,12,38,40,44]

The advent of surgical microscopes, smaller incisions, and fine suture materials has not affected the long-term pressure effects from cataract sur-

Table 72-2 Pseudophakia and glaucoma: preexisting glaucoma

Author	Eyes	Precontrol	Postcontrol
Smith and Anderson[61]	24	23/24*; 1/24	14/24*; 8/24 (2 lost)
Clayman et al.[10]	48	36/48*; 12/48	18/48*; 30/48
Taylor and Stein[63]	43	(O) 31/32*; 1/32	24/32*; 8/32
		(N) 6/11*; 5/11	4/11*; 7/11
McMahan et al.[34]	46	46/46*	19/46*; 37/46
McGuigan et al.[33]	50	43/50*; 7/50	50/50*
Handa et al.[18]	43	43/43*	31/43*; 12/43

*Medical therapy required.
O, Open-angle glaucoma; N, narrow-angle glaucoma.

gery; but the tighter wound closure tends to produce a higher incidence of postoperative pressure spikes.[51,62] Transient pressure elevation after intraocular lens implantation is frequently encountered and is usually well tolerated by nonglaucomatous patients. This intraocular pressure rise can have devastating results in a patient with preexisting glaucomatous damage and can cause loss of fixation or reduction in the remaining visual field. The elevation is of greater magnitude and duration in patients with preexisting glaucoma.[58] This serious complication can occur in patients who ultimately manifest lower intraocular pressures than before cataract extraction. Thus the overall safety of intraocular lens implantation should be evaluated by reviewing changes in the intraocular pressure, progression of visual field loss, increased cupping of the optic nerve head, and changes in medical therapy of the glaucoma rather than the effect on intraocular pressure alone.[33,53,57,58] Successful lens implantation implies a lack of damage to the optic nerve and visual field.

Postoperative pressure elevations may be more prolonged and of greater duration if a viscoelastic substance is used in surgery; therefore, routine evacuation of these substances at the end of the procedure is recommended.[17] Management of postoperative pressure spikes is best accomplished by close monitoring during the first 24 to 48 hours after surgery and aggressive medical therapy to control the intraocular pressure.[41] An additional margin of safety can be attained with the use of combined cataract surgery and filtration procedures in patients with advanced glaucomatous damage.

Combined cataract extraction with an intraocular lens and filtration surgery should be strongly considered if the cataract patient has moderate to advanced glaucomatous damage, even if well controlled by medications. Combined procedures also produce more uniform long-term intraocular pressure control than cataract surgery alone and may prevent the transient pressure rise after cataract surgery.[22,25,33,47,49] Combined procedures are accompanied by a higher incidence of complications such as flat anterior chamber, hyphema, and corneal decompensation; thus, they should not be used for every patient with ocular hypertension or glaucoma.[26,32] Pretreatment with argon laser trabeculoplasty has shown significant benefit when combined with cataract extraction and intraocular lens implantation but is less protective against the immediate postoperative pressure spikes.[9,58]

Cataract surgery with or without lens implantation in patients who have previously undergone filtration surgery results in a loss of filtration in 25% to 40% of the patients.[1,2,28] Alpar reviewed 40 patients who had previously undergone filtering surgery: 15 patients who subsequently underwent intraocular lens implantation were compared with 25 patients who underwent routine cataract extraction without intraocular lens implantation.[1] The study involved intracapsular lens extraction and four types of intraocular lenses including anterior chamber and iris supported types. Scarring of the bleb occurred in 40% of the patients receiving the lens implant and in a similar number of patients not receiving implants. Cataract extraction appears to induce scarring of the bleb in a significant proportion of patients with previously successful filtration surgery without regard to whether an intraocular lens was implanted.

The reported effect of intraocular lens implantation on intraocular pressure in glaucoma patients is quite variable.[16,33,50,61] Initial studies found that most patients had no response or a detrimental response after implantation of an intraocular lens, versus cataract surgery alone, which led some investigators to recommend against pseudophakia in glaucoma patients.[20] More recent studies indicate that less than 10% of glaucoma patients who undergo cataract extraction with intraocular lens implantation will experience greater difficulty with control of their glaucoma.[34,36,58] The majority of recent papers describe pseudophakia as having little influence or even a positive effect on the postoperative intraocular pressure control, especially with the use of extracapsular surgery and posterior chamber lenses. Several studies indicated that postoperative pressure control was adequate with fewer medications than required preoperatively for approximately 50% of glaucoma patients undergoing cataract surgery with an intraocular lens.[34,36,42,58]

The decision to implant an intraocular lens in glaucoma patients requires careful preoperative patient selection and certain modifications in postoperative therapy. Preoperative evaluation requires particular attention to the degree of pupillary dilation obtained after instillation of mydriatic agents, which will determine the extent of iris surgery necessary to perform the cataract extraction and lens implantation.

Gonioscopy is also useful in determining the position of synechiae, which would affect implantation of anterior chamber lenses. The decision to implant an anterior chamber lens remains controversial, as the haptics may produce trabecular damage at the point of contact and induce frequent peripheral anterior synechiae and vascular proliferation around the haptics.[30,45] The extent of trabecular damage will vary with lens design, but all anterior chamber intraocular lenses have the theoretical disadvantage of compromising outflow in an eye with already inadequate trabecular function. The anterior chamber lens also presents a greater possibility of endothelial contact should the eye require filtration surgery.[27,43] Implantation of a posterior chamber lens has the theoretical advantage of less possibility of corneal endothelial contact if filtration surgery becomes necessary, and the haptics will not be in contact with trabecular meshwork.

Chronic miotic therapy increases the technical difficulty of cataract extraction and intraocular lens implantation, and miotics should be discontinued several days before surgery if the patient's pressure control allows it.[10] Many patients will require iris manipulation, sphincterotomies, and possibly a radial iridotomy to facilitate removal of the lens nucleus and avoid excessive iris trauma or possible disinsertion.[10,13] Multiple sphincterotomies will allow additional dilation in a marginal pupil. The extremely miotic pupil often requires a radial iridotomy to afford adequate dilation for the lens extraction and implantation of an intraocular lens.

Viscoelastic substances can be used to facilitate mechanical dilation of the pupil in marginally dilated patients or in conjunction with the previously mentioned iris surgery. The integrity of the pupil can then be restored if necessary with the use of a 10-0 prolene iris suture (Fig. 72-1). Closure of the iridotomy is often not required and should be assessed on a patient-to-patient basis.[10,13] This maneuver is helpful to control the position of the posterior chamber lens in some instances. Suturing the iris increases the technical difficulty of the procedure, and the additional manipulation of the iris increases the chance of vitreous loss and corneal endothelial damage.

The postoperative control of intraocular pressure may be indirectly affected by the presence of a lens implant, which may require modifications in the glaucoma medications. The use of miotic agents after lens implantation may produce synechiae and inflammatory membranes on the surface of the implant if postoperative inflammation is present. The accelerated synechia formation can then lead to pupillary block. Posterior angulation may help decrease synechia formation if using posterior chamber lenses. Inflammation may necessitate the heavy use of steroids in the postoperative period, which can cause steroid-induced pressure elevation in patients with preexisting open-angle glaucoma. Careful monitoring of the postoperative pressures should be conducted in all patients, particularly while they are receiving topical steroids, which should be restricted to the minimum effective doses.

Cataract extraction and lens implantation in patients with angle-closure glaucoma has been reported to improve intraocular pressure control after surgery, and there appears to be no adverse effects.[63] However, the influence of lens implantation on intraocular pressure in patients with angle-closure glaucoma has not been fully elucidated, as only a small number of cases have been reported. Implantation of intraocular lenses in children with glaucoma is not advised at this time. The placement of intraocular lenses in patients with secondary glaucoma must be made on a case by case basis. Uveitic glaucoma is a relative contraindication for

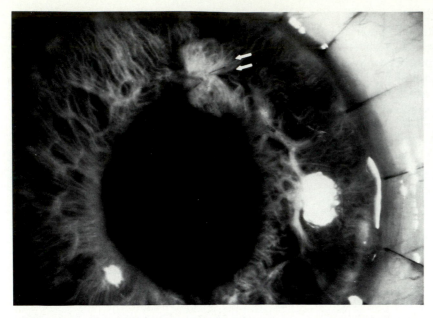

Fig. 72-1 The integrity of the pupil has been restored after cataract extraction by closure of the radial iridectomy with a 10-0 prolene suture *(arrows).*

Table 72-3 Pseudophakia and glaucoma: core study (FDA)

Control	Lens type			
	AC*	IF*	ICF*	PC*
3132	6650	14,360	5722	1182
Pupillary block (%) 0.4	0.6	0.3	0.3	0.0
Secondary glaucoma (%) 3.6	6.3	3.9	2.1	3.5
Hyphema (%) 2.4	5.0	3.3	2.7	0.9
Uveitis (%) 1.7	2.3	1.7	1.3	0.8
Macular edema (%) 3.2	4.9	3.0	2.2	4.3

*AC, Anterior chamber; IF, iris fixation; ICF, iridocapsular fixation; PC, posterior chamber.
From Worthen, DM, et al: Ophthalmology 87:267, 1980. Published courtesy of Ophthalmology.

lens implantation because the implant can significantly complicate the postoperative management. Eyes with glaucoma secondary to trauma must be evaluated for angle recession and zonular damage, which may complicate the placement of certain types of implants.

INTRAOCULAR LENS-INDUCED GLAUCOMA

The intraocular lens is responsible for secondary glaucoma in some individuals; the problem is more common with anterior chamber lenses than iris fixated lenses or posterior chamber lenses[68] (Table 72-3). Pressure elevation can occur from mechanical problems induced by the implant as in

pseudophakic pupillary block or lens induced pigment liberation from the posterior surface of the iris. The eye can react to the implant material with synechia formation at points of contact in the angle. Improper positioning or excessive movement of the implant can lead to chronic iritis and secondary intraocular pressure elevation. The intraocular lens can induce neovascularization, which may lead to recurrent hyphema and cause intraocular pressure elevation. Intraocular lens coatings and lens breakdown products are also potential sources of toxic materials, which could damage the trabecular meshwork. Identification of the offending process is critical in the management of lens-induced intraocular pressure elevation.

CLINICAL PICTURE AND PATHOPHYSIOLOGY OF INTRAOCULAR LENSES AND GLAUCOMA

Visual Acuity

Implantation of an intraocular lens avoids the optical aberration of aphakic eye glasses and the potential difficulties associated with contact lens wear. The lens properties of aphakic spectacles may compound the patient's difficulty with coping with a diminished visual field from glaucoma. Contact lens wear is sometimes impossible in patients with filtering blebs and may lead to trauma to the filtering bleb and secondary infections. Thus, lens implantation frequently offers the optimal visual rehabilitation for glaucoma patients.

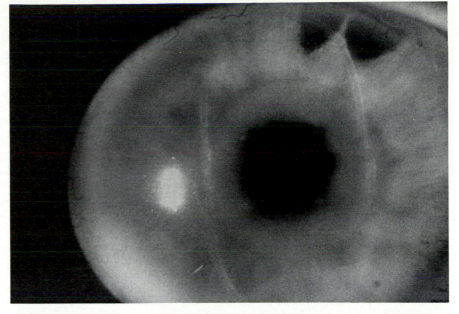

Fig. 72-2   Corneal edema with an intraocular pressure of 40 to 45 mm Hg in eye with anterior chamber IOL.

The overall results of lens implantation in glaucoma patients appears promising; in one study 89% of patients achieved a visual acuity of 20/20 to 20/40.[10] Pupillary membranes, macular degeneration and corneal edema were cited as causes for decreased vision. In another series 20 of 32 eyes with chronic open-angle glaucoma, and intraocular lens implantation had a vision of 20/40 or better.[63] Visual acuities of 20/60 or less were thought to result from macular degeneration or glaucomatous optic atrophy. It appeared that the postoperative vision was consistent with the status of the posterior segment and not a consequence of the surgical procedure or of complications. In the same report, 9 of 11 eyes with open-angle glaucoma and lens implantation demonstrated a postoperative vision of 20/40 or better. In another series eight of 16 glaucoma patients had postoperative vision of 20/40 or better and in three instances visual function was worse after the procedure.[13] It appears in the majority of cases visual acuity is not adversely affected by lens implantation in eyes with preexisting glaucoma. The postoperative vision appears to correlate well with the preoperative status of the cornea, optic nerve head, visual field, and retina.

Cornea, Iris, and Pupil

Postoperative corneal edema has occurred in some patients with elevated pressure after lens implantation. (Fig. 72-2) This is more likely to occur when pressure elevations are in the range of 35

mm Hg or higher after surgery. The edema may result from corneal endothelial damage from the cataract surgery, from elevated pressure, or from a combination of both factors. The use of viscoelastic substances will help to minimize corneal endothelial damage but may contribute to marked pressure elevation in the immediate postoperative period. The viscoelastic substance should be removed at the end of the procedure to reduce the duration of the pressure rise, although Berson et al.[6] found no immediate improvement in outflow after evacuation of Healon from the anterior chamber of cadaver eyes. This may indicate an inability to clear the substance from the trabecular meshwork.

Extracapsular lens extraction requires that the pupil be large enough to perform an adequate anterior capsulotomy, extract the lens nucleus, and insert a posterior chamber lens implant. Iris surgery is necessary if vigorous preoperative dilation fails to produce an adequate opening. Excessive iris manipulation is a source of inflammation and should be avoided. The intraocular lens should be positioned so that iris contact is minimized, as this can lead to pigment release and uveitis.

Anterior Chamber and Angle

Preoperative evaluation of the anterior chamber angle is imperative when considering lens implantation. Identification of synechiae using accurate drawings is necessary to facilitate positioning an anterior chamber lens in an area free of synechiae.[53] If this cannot be accomplished, it is often necessary to avoid insertion of an anterior chamber lens. Positioning the haptics in synechiae can lead to chronic irritation with vascularization around the haptic and may lead to chronic low grade iritis or the UGH (uveitis-glaucoma-hyphema) syndrome.

Misdirection of aqueous flow is a complication of cataract surgery that can occur with or without the presence of an intraocular lens (Table 72-4). The resulting anterior bowing of the iris and shallowing of the anterior chamber can induce extensive synechia formation in the angle and frequently

secondary glaucoma (Fig. 72-3). Misdirection of aqueous flow is most often due to pupillary block but can occur even in the presence of patent iridectomies.[60] The anterior vitreous appears to be the culprit in the former situation, although the pathophysiology of posterior aqueous misdirection is unknown.

Pupillary block is more commonly encountered after anterior chamber lens implantation but can also be seen with posterior chamber lenses.[14,39,66] The incidence after posterior chamber lens implantation is likely to increase because of the trend of avoiding surgical iridectomy. Vigorous dilation is usually successful in temporarily alleviating pupillary block. The iris should be inspected and the patency of the iridectomy ascertained. If no surgical iridectomy was performed at the time of surgery, a laser iridectomy is best undertaken after the pupillary block has been broken and the anterior chamber deepened. Additional laser iridectomies relieve this configuration in most cases. Nd:YAG laser disruption of the vitreous, posterior to the iridectomy, is sometimes successful in patients with recurrent vitreous occlusion of the iridectomy sites. Patients who develop recurrent iris bombé configuration after the appropriate laser therapy may require anterior vitrectomy to maintain the anterior chamber.

A peripheral iridectomy is strongly recommended if an anterior chamber intraocular lens is implanted. The positioning of the anterior chamber

Table 72-4 *Pseudophakia and glaucoma: pupillary block*

Author	Eyes with glaucoma (lens type)	Pupillary block
Smith and Anderson[61]	26/606 iris	1/26 (1.0%)
Kraff et al.[30]	5/613 iris	5/5 (8.0%)
Binkhorst[8]	— iris	(0.2%)
Nordlohne[40]	— iris	(6.94%)
Phyodorov et al.[48]	3000 (L)* iris	(1.8%)
	2000 (NL)* iris	(0.9%)
Pearce and Ghost[46]	4/537 iris	(0.7%)
François[15]	(Review of aphakic glaucoma)	(1.0% to 7.0%)
Dagasan[11]	Extracapsular	(0.7%)
	Intracapsular	(1.5%)

*L, implantation; NL, no implantation.

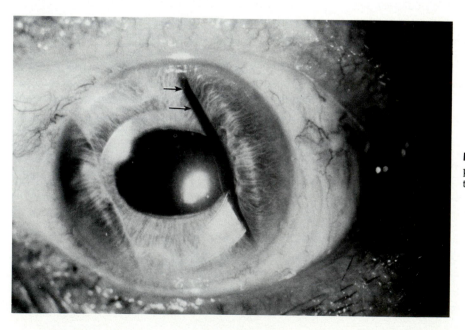

Fig. 72-3 Iris bombé secondary to pupillary block *(arrows)* caused by anterior chamber IOL.

lens is important to avoid occlusion of the iridectomy by the haptics. An iridectomy is not necessary if a posterior chamber intraocular lens is implanted, but pupillary block can still occur even in the presence of an iridectomy, particularly if inflammation is present.[67] Aggressive therapy of postoperative inflammation is necessary to avoid anterior and posterior synechia formation, which may sequester the pupil and lead to secondary angle closure. Persistent inflammation can cause primary trabecular dysfunction and peripheral anterior synechia formation in an otherwise open angle. Angle closure resulting from iritis can be differentiated by the absence of anterior bowing of the iris, deep central anterior chamber, and keratic precipitates on the trabeculum.

The lens implant may be a source of chronic irritation leading to trabecular dysfunction from uveitis or chronic hyphema (Fig. 72-4). The liberation of pigment from mechanical contact with the lens implant may also lead to a secondary pigment dispersion form of glaucoma. Lens implantation can also be a source of epithelial downgrowth, which covers the trabecular meshwork and leads to a persistent, often intractable form of glaucoma. One report noted four to ten eyes enucleated for intractable postoperative glaucoma had epithelization of the anterior chamber angle. Loose or poorly positioned lenses sometimes require removal if the secondary inflammation and corneal trauma is unremitting. Vitreous prolapse into the anterior chamber has been implicated as a source of pressure elevation in some patients and its removal appeared beneficial in one study.[55]

EVALUATION OF PATIENTS WITH ELEVATED PRESSURE AFTER LENS IMPLANTATION

Slit-lamp Examination

Careful examination of the cornea can reveal edema and corneal endothelial abnormality. The presence of inflammatory debris or pigmentation on the endothelium may help identify secondary causes for the pressure elevation. Cells or pigment in the anterior chamber can obstruct aqueous outflow and often arise from contact between the implant and iris.[5,23,35,56] Particular attention should then be directed toward the depth of the anterior chamber, the position of the lens implant, and relative position of the iris.

One should then survey the iris to ascertain patency of a surgical iridectomy if one was performed. Occasionally, the posterior leaf of the iris will be left intact despite what appears to be an adequate iridectomy. This is easily resolved by applying laser to the pigment epithelium to complete the iridectomy. Iris bombé is usually indicative of pupillary block, but in the presence of hypotony, a would leak or inadvertent cyclodialysis cleft must be ruled out (Fig. 72-5). The inflammation must then be controlled and normal aqueous flow restored to prevent peripheral anterior synechia for-

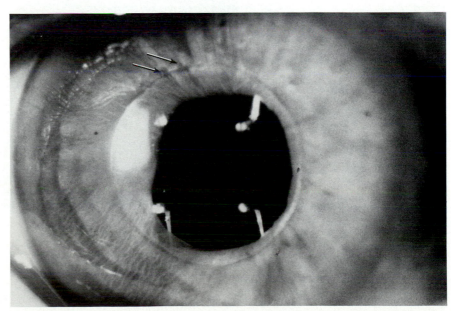

Fig. 72-4 Chronic iritis with metal loop haptic of anterior chamber IOL eroding through iris *(arrows)*.

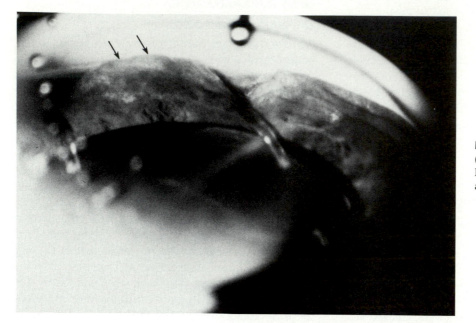

Fig. 72-5 Iris bombé configuration (*arrows*) in eye with anterior chamber IOL with wound leak and shallow anterior chamber.

Fig. 72-6 Synechiae formation (*arrows*) adjacent to the foot of an anterior chamber IOL as a result of pupillary block.

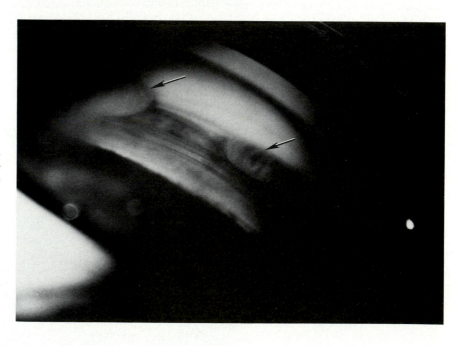

mation (Fig. 72-6). Residual cortical or nuclear material may lead to chronic uveitis and explain persistent inflammation in the postoperative period.

Gonioscopy

Evaluation of the angle is imperative in patients with secondary pressure elevation after lens implantation. Careful attention should be paid to the angle configuration and the appearance of the trabecular meshwork. Neovascularization, debris, pigment and peripheral anterior synechia formation should be carefully noted. A gonioscopic examination of the fellow eye is often useful for comparison in order to identify secondary pigment dispersion related to the lens implantation or a preexisting problem, such as pigment dispersion or exfoliation, which may not have been noted preoperatively. Abnormal positioning of the lens implant can be a source of inflammation, such as in patients with iris tuck, and these individuals may require repositioning of the implant to quiet the inflammation. Vascular tufts can be identified around haptics and in the surgical wound in many patients but seldom cause difficulty.[30] These vascular proliferations sometimes induce recurrent hyphemas, and these vessels should then be ablated with the argon laser (Fig. 72-7).

Attention to the position of the haptics, peripheral anterior synechiae, and any vascular proliferation is necessary before removal of a problem lens implant. Closed haptics should be severed then pulled through any peripheral anterior synechiae, which may have encapsulated them or they should be left in place. Traction should not be applied because many implants attach to the ciliary body and massive hemorrhage will occur if the haptic is disturbed.

Optic Nerve Examination

An accurate description of the optic nerve head using scale drawings or photography is extremely useful in patients with elevated intraocular pressure. Stereoscopic evaluation of the nerve using a contact lens at the slit-lamp allows optimal evaluation of the optic nerve contour. In eyes with extreme miosis, particularly with synechiae to the lens implant, the use of a direct ophthalmoscope and a Koeppe lens may allow visualization of the nerve despite the small pupillary aperture.

DIAGNOSTIC PROCEDURES

A baseline visual field is indicated in patients with persistent pressure elevation after lens implantation, although media opacity can limit the value of this test. Perimetry not only serves as a baseline but may allow diagnosis of previously undetected glaucoma in either eye. A visual evoked response can be very useful in those patients with postoperative media opacity when there is little or no data about the preoperative status of the eye and no visualization of the fundus. This is particularly true in individuals who have an afferent pupillary defect and may have significant optic nerve compromise from glaucoma. Gross color testing is

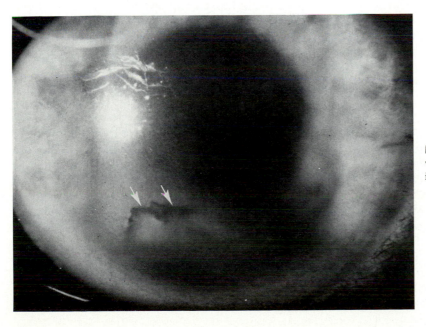

Fig. 72-7 Hyphema (*arrows*) causing elevated pressure and secondary corneal edema in patient with an anterior chamber IOL.

a useful but crude indication of potential function in eyes with media opacities.

Identification of pressure induced damage to the optic nerve is necessary as these patients require aggressive intervention to control the intraocular pressure. Patients with normal findings and moderate pressure elevation need less vigorous intervention, and close observation is often adequate during the immediate postoperative period.

MANAGEMENT OF SECONDARY GLAUCOMA IN PSEUDOPHAKIC PATIENTS

Adequate preoperative examination is extremely useful in determining the cause for secondary pressure elevation after implantation of an intraocular lens. Therapy then begins with medical management of the source of the pressure elevation if possible. The patient should be segregated to an open-angle form of glaucoma or closed-angle glaucoma. Medical therapy seldom succeeds if extensive angle-closure from peripheral anterior synechiae is present. Surgical intervention is dictated by the underlying cause for the pressure elevation, extent of pressure elevation, condition of the optic nerve, and the visual field. Surgical intervention can then be directed at pressure control, repositioning, or removal of the lens.

Medical Therapy

Recognition and treatment of postoperative inflammation is exceedingly important as this may contribute to both closed-angle glaucoma and open-angle glaucoma. The minimum required dose of steroids must be employed as they have a pressure elevating effect in susceptible eyes. The separation of uveitis induced glaucoma versus pressure elevation from steroid use is a difficult determination in patients with long-standing uveitis and steroid use. Control of the uveitis must be attained; then the intraocular pressure is monitored as the steroids are tapered.

Dilating agents are particularly useful in those patients presenting with pupillary block. Release of the pupillary block may be achieved by vigorous dilation of the pupil, but close follow-up must be maintained as the pupillary block often returns after the cycloplegic agent is tapered. Cycloplegia is also useful in lessening the discomfort associated with secondary glaucoma caused by lessening the discomfort associated with secondary glaucoma caused by inflammation.

Beta-blocking agents are generally the first line of therapy if the inciting cause cannot be removed. These agents help control pressure without aggravating postoperative inflammation. Epinephrine derivatives are also useful in reducing postoperative pressure elevation but are generally used in conjunction with other glaucoma medication and seldom as a first line drug. These agents may induce aphakic cystoid maculopathy and can cause pupillary dilation. This last side effect may pose a particular problem in those patients with iris plane lens implants but rarely is sufficient to entrap a posterior chamber lens.

Cholinergic agents are a powerful tool in the control of pseudophakic glaucoma.[54] These agents may increase the postoperative inflammation and synechia formation and should be used with caution in the immediate postoperative period. Cholinergic agents are generally poorly tolerated by patients with chronic postoperative inflammation. The secondary miosis can facilitate posterior synechia formation and increase the possibility of pupillary block. Retinal detachment is also a rare complication in patients using strong miotic agents.

Carbonic anhydrase inhibitors are a valuable tool in the treatment of transient pressure elevations. Their potent pressure reduction properties may be useful in patients requiring chronic pressure control and will also afford reduction of corneal edema in patients requiring laser surgery. Topical glycerine is very beneficial for transient reduction of corneal edema to facilitate diagnostic and therapeutic procedures. Osmotic agents are exceedingly effective in producing a transient pressure reduction in order to clear the cornea in patients requiring laser surgery and will also induce temporary pressure reduction to protect the optic nerve while topical therapy and the carbonic anhydrase inhibitor take effect. The osmotic agent will also afford additional time should secondary surgical intervention be necessary.

Surgical Therapy

Removal of the lens implant is seldom necessary to control pseudophakic glaucoma. Removal of the implant is frequently traumatic and can be associated with vitreous loss, hyphema, iris deformity, peripheral anterior synechia formation, and corneal decompensation. Anterior chamber lenses develop adhesion at the point of haptic contact with the angle, and vitrectomy is often necessary to remove vitreous attachments to the intraocular lens. Careful preoperative inspection of the haptics is necessary to ascertain the technique for the removal of the lens to avoid excessive traction on the eye.

Removal of posterior chamber and iris plane

implants is more difficult than with anterior chamber lens implants. Iris trauma and potential contact with corneal endothelium is likely. It is frequently necessary to severe the haptics rather than to dislodge them. The lens implant must be identified as the source of intractable pressure elevation before removal, and more conservative therapy must have failed.

In those eyes with pupillary block, laser or surgical iridectomy can alleviate the misdirection of aqueous and prevent further damage to the angle. Early detection is necessary to avoid peripheral anterior synechia formation and combined mechanism glaucoma. Disruption of the anterior vitreous using the Nd:YAG laser is sometimes useful in patients with a patent iridectomy and persistent anterior chamber shallowing. Anterior vitrectomy may be necessary if adequate iridectomies do not alleviate the problem, but this is rarely required.

Laser trabeculoplasty is frequently successful in those patients with open angles and medically uncontrolled aphakic glaucoma; thus, many patients can avoid filtration surgery.[52,65] The success rate for patients with uveitis after lens implantation is much lower, but laser trabeculoplasty is sometimes successful in this setting. Those patients not responding to laser therapy should receive appropriate filtration surgery without undue delay.

Trabeculectomy is the most common filtration technique for pseudophakic patients. Shallowing of the anterior chamber can have devastating effects on the pseudophakic eye if the intraocular lens contacts the cornea. Coating the intraocular lens with a viscoelastic substance before opening the fistula will afford some protection to the cornea until the anterior chamber is reestablished at the end of the procedure. Trabeculectomy induces less hypotony and fewer flat anterior chambers than full thickness filtration procedures and produces fewer hyphemas than cyclodialysis. The success rate for filtration in pseudophakic patients is generally less than for phakic patients, and this success rate is further compromised by active uveitis. Trabeculectomy requires adequate unscarred conjunctiva to dissect the bleb and should not be attempted in those patients with extensive conjunctival scarring. Adjunct therapy with antimetabolites, such as 5-FU, appears promising, but the long-term effect on the success of filtration is unknown.[19]

Cyclodialysis with simultaneous extracapsular surgery and intraocular lens implantation has been reported by Montgomery and Gills,[37] who indicate that this combined procedure is relatively safe in experienced hands. Cyclodialysis may be compli-cated by hyphema, sudden closure of the cleft, and rarely with persistent hypotony. The use of Healon through an irrigating cyclodialysis spatula has recently been advocated as a means to lessen complications, particularly bleeding.[3] Transient pressure elevation after cyclodialysis using Healon has occurred; thus, the postoperative pressure must be carefully monitored for several days after surgery.

Cyclocryotherapy is a destructive procedure that decreases aqueous production. Significant anterior chamber and vitreous inflammation accompanies this procedure. It is useful in some individuals with persistent pressure elevation that have not responded to other surgical modalities.[21] Cyclocryotherapy is recommended in eyes with limited visual potential, and it is a useful means of controlling pressure when other modalities have failed.

Control of refractory glaucoma in aphakic and pseudophakic patients remains a difficult problem. No specific procedure is indicated for every patient. The underlying cause for the secondary glaucoma should be isolated and treated if possible. Those patients with uncontrolled pressure elevation should be assessed on an individual basis for the best possible means of surgical pressure reduction when conservative therapy has failed. The surgeon should select the procedure offering the greatest statistical rate of success weighed against the magnitude of potential complications; thus, the ideal procedure will vary with the condition of the conjunctiva, iridocorneal angle, the type of lens implant, and the etiology of the intraocular pressure elevation.

REFERENCES

1. Alpar, JJ: Cataract extraction and lens implantation in eyes with pre-existing filtering blebs, Am Intraocular Implant Soc J 5:33, 1979
2. Alpar, JJ: Personal communication, 1980
3. Alpar, JJ: Sodium hyaluronate (Healon) in cyclodialysis, CLAO J 11:201, 1985
4. Apple, DJ, et al: Complications of intraocular lenses: a historical and histopathological review, Surv Ophthalmol 29:1, 1984
5. Ballin, N, and Weiss, DM: Pigment dispersion and intraocular pressure elevation in pseudophakia, Ann Ophthalmol 14:627, 1982
6. Berson, FG, Patterson, MM, and Epstein, DL: Obstruction of aqueous outflow by sodium hyaluronate in enucleated human eyes, Am J Ophthalmol 95:668, 1983
7. Bigger, JF, and Becker, B: Cataracts and primary open angle glaucoma: the effect of uncomplicated cataract

extraction on glaucoma control, Trans Am Acad Ophthalmol Otolaryngol 75:260, 1971

8. Binkhorst, CD: Ridley's intraocular lens prosthesis: the postoperative reaction: results obtained in 12 cases, Ophthalmologica 133:383, 1957

9. Brown, SVL, et al: Effect of cataract surgery on intraocular pressure reduction obtained with laser trabeculoplasty, Am J Ophthalmol 100:373, 1985

10. Clayman, HM, et al: Lens implantation, miosis and glaucoma, Am J Ophthalmol 87:121, 1979

11. Dagasan, V: Aphakic glaucoma, Ankara Univ Tip Fak Goz Klin Yill 18:135, 1966

12. Dallas, NL: Five year trial of the Binkhorst iris-clip lens in aphakia, Trans Ophthalmol Soc UK 90:725, 1970

13. Drews, RC: Personal communication from transactions of the St. Vincent's Hospital meeting, 1977

14. Forman, JS, Ritch, R, Dunn, MW, and Szmyd, L: Pupillary block following posterior chamber lens implantation, Ophthalmol Laser Ther 2:85, 1987

15. François, J: Aphakic glaucoma, Ann Ophthalmol 6:429, 1974

16. Galin, MA, Lin, LLK, and Obstbaum, SA: Cataract extraction and intraocular pressure, Trans Ophthalmol Soc UK 98:124, 1978

17. Glasser, DB, Matsuda, M, and Edelhauser, HF: A comparison of the efficacy and toxicity of and intraocular pressure response to viscous solutions in the anterior chamber, Arch Ophthalmol 104:1819, 1986

18. Handa, J, et al: Extracapsular cataract extraction with posterior chamber lens implantation in patients with glaucoma, Arch Ophthalmol 105:765, 1987

19. Heuer, DK, et al: 5-Fluorouracil and glaucoma filtering surgery, Ophthalmology 91:384, 1984

20. Herschler, J: Glaucoma and the intraocular lens, Ann Ophthalmol 11:1058, 1979

21. Herschler, J: Personal communication, 1979

22. Hunsaker, J, and Kass, MA: Combined procedures for cataract and glaucoma, Int Ophthalmol Clin 24:33, 1984

23. Insler, MS, and Zatzkis, SM: Pigment dispersion syndrome in pseudophakic corneal transplants, Am J Ophthalmol 102:762, 1986

24. Jaffe, NS: The changing scene of intraocular implant lens surgery, Am J Ophthalmol 88:819, 1979

25. Jerndal, T, and Lundstrom, M: Trabeculectomy combined with cataract extraction, Am J Ophthalmol 81:227, 1976

26. Johns, G, and Layden, WE: Combined trabeculectomy and cataract extraction, Am J Ophthalmol 88:973, 1979

27. Junge, J: Combined intraocular lens implantation and trabeculectomy, Am Intraocular Implant Soc J 3:105, 1977

28. Kass, MA: Cataract extraction in an eye with a filtering bleb, Ophthalmology 89:871, 1982

29. Kern, R: Iridocapsular lenses versus iris-clip lenses: comparison of the results and complications of 100 of each, Ophthalmic Surg 8:82, 1977

30. Kraff, MC, Sanders, DR, and Liebermann, HL: 300 primary anterior chamber lens implantations: gonioscopic findings and specular microscopy, Am Intraocular Implant Soc J 5:207, 1979

31. Laatikainen, L: Late results of surgery on eyes with primary glaucoma and cataract, Acta Ophthalmol 49:281, 1971

32. Luntz, MH, and Berlin, MS: Combined trabeculectomy and cataract extraction; advantages of a modified technique and review of current literature, Trans Ophthal Soc UK 100:533, 1980

33. McGuigan, LJB, et al: Extracapsular cataract extraction and posterior chamber lens implantation in eyes with preexisting glaucoma, Arch Ophthalmol 104:1301, 1986

34. McMahan, LB, Monica, ML, and Zimmerman, TJ: Posterior chamber pseudophakes in glaucoma patients, Ophthalmic Surg 17:146, 1986

35. Masket, S: Pseudophakic posterior iris chafing syndrome, J Cataract Refract Surg 12:252, 1986

36. Monica, ML, Zimmerman, TJ, and McMahan, LB: Implantation of posterior chamber lenses in glaucoma patients, Ann Ophthalmol 17:9, 1985

37. Montgomery, D, and Gills, JP: Extracapsular cataract extraction lens implantation and cyclodialysis, Ophthalmic Surg 11:343, 1980

38. Moses, L: Complications of rigid anterior chamber implants, Ophthalmology 91:819, 1984

39. Naveh-Floman, N, Rosner, M, and Blumenthal, M: Pseudophakic pupillary block glaucoma with posterior-chamber intraocular lens, Glaucoma 7:262, 1985

40. Nordlohne, MD: The intraocular implant lens development and results with special reference to the Binkhorst lens, Doc Ophthalmol 38:1, 1974

41. Obstbaum, SA: Glaucoma and intraocular lens implantation, J Cataract Refract Surg 12:257, 1986

42. Obstbaum, SA, and Galin, MA: Glaucoma, cataract surgery and the intraocular lens, Int Ophthalmol Clin 19:139, 1979

43. Obstbaum, SA, and Galin, MA: The effects of timolol on cataract extraction and intraocular pressure, Am J Ophthalmol 88:1017, 1979

44. Pearce, JL: Long term results of the Binkhorst iris-clip lens in senile cataracts, Br J Ophthalmol 56:319, 1972

45. Pearce, JL: Long term results of the Choyce anterior chamber lens implants Mark V, VII, and VIII, Br J Ophthalmol 59:99, 1975

46. Pearce, JL, and Ghost, T: Surgical and postoperative problems with Binkhorst 2 and 4 loop lenses, Trans Ophthalmol Soc UK 97:84, 1977

47. Percival, SPB: Glaucoma triple procedure of extracapsular cataract extraction, posterior chamber lens implantation, and trabeculectomy, Br J Ophthalmol 69:99, 1985

48. Phyodorov, SN, Yegorov, EV, and Feldman, BG: Analysis of 3000 operations on implantation of intraocular pupillary lens after removal of senile, con-

genital and complicated cataracts (Phyodorov-Zacharov lens), JCE Ophthalmol, June 1979:36

49. Praeger, DL: Combined procedure: sub-scleral trabeculectomy with cataract extraction, Ophthalmic Surg 14:130, 1983
50. Radius, RL, et al: Pseudophakia and intraocular pressure, Am J Ophthalmol 97:738, 1984
51. Rich, WJ: Intraocular pressure and wound closure after cataract extraction, Trans Ophthalmol Soc UK 88:437, 1968
52. Robin, AL, and Pollack, IP: Argon laser trabeculoplasty in secondary forms of open-angle glaucoma, Arch Ophthalmol 101:382, 1983
53. Rousey, JJ: Peripheral anterior synechiae and intraocular lenses, Am Intraocular Implant Soc J 5:307, 1979
54. Ruiz, RS, et al: Management of increased intraocular pressure after cataract extraction, Am J Ophthalmol 103:487, 1987
55. Samples, JR, and Van Buskirk, EM: Open-angle glaucoma associated with vitreous humor filling the anterior chamber, Am J Ophthalmol 102:759, 1986
56. Samples, JR, and Van Buskirk, EM: Pigmentary glaucoma associated with posterior chamber intraocular lenses, Am J Ophthalmol 100:385, 1985
57. Savage, JA, et al: Extracapsular cataract extraction and posterior chamber intraocular lens implantation in glaucomatous eyes, Ophthalmol 92:1506, 1985
58. Shephard, DD: Intraocular lens implantation—analysis of 500 consecutive cases, Ophthalmic Surg 8:57, 1977
59. Sherif, AS, and Dardenne, MU: Posterior chamber lens implantation in patients with glaucoma, Cataract Feb 1984, p. 6
60. Shrader, CE, et al: Pupillary and iridovitreal block in pseudophakic eyes, Ophthalmology 91:831, 1984
61. Smith, JA, and Anderson, DR: Effect of the intraocular lens on intraocular pressure, Arch Ophthalmol 94:1291, 1976
62. Spaeth, GL: Symposium on cataract surgery dedicated to Harold Ridley; the management of cataract in patients with glaucoma, a comparative study, Trans Ophthal Soc UK 100:95, 1980
63. Taylor, DM, and Stein, AL: Long term follow-up of 43 intraocular lenses in eyes with primary glaucoma, Am Intraocular Implant Soc J 5:313, 1979
64. Tennant, JL: Results of primary and secondary implants using Choyce Mark VIII lenses, Ophthalmic Surg 8:54, 1977
65. Thomas, JV, Simmons, RJ, and Belcher, CD, III: Argon laser trabeculoplasty in the presurgical glaucoma patient, Ophthalmology 89:187, 1982
66. Weinreb, RN, et al: Pseudophakic pupillary block with angle-closure glaucoma in diabetic patients, Am J Ophthalmol 102:523, 1986
67. Willis, DA, Stewart, RH, and Kimbrough, RL: Pupillary block associated with posterior chamber lenses, Ophthalmic Surg 16:108, 1985
68. Worthen, DM, et al: Interim FDA report on intraocular lenses, Ophthalmology 87:267, 1980

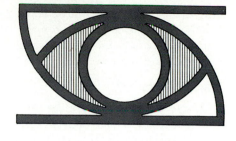

Chapter 73

Epithelial, Fibrous, and Endothelial Proliferation

Patricia Smith
Walter J. Stark
A. Edward Maumenee
William R. Green

Ophthalmologists have long known that epithelium, connective tissue, and endothelium can proliferate in the anterior segment of the eye under the proper conditions. Epithelial ingrowth, fibrous ingrowth and endothelial proliferation are rare but potentially devastating complications of anterior segment surgery or trauma. Despite increased awareness of these entities and surgical innovation, cellular proliferation in the anterior segment remains a diagnostic and therapeutic challenge.

EPITHELIAL PROLIFERATION

Historical Review

After the earlier report of a posttraumatic iris cyst by MacKenzie,[131] there appeared in the nineteenth century German literature numerous case reports of iris cysts or epithelial ingrowth, reviewed by Perera.[166] Rothmund[181] speculated that iris cysts arising after trauma or cataract surgery originated from epithelial implantation into the iris. Collins and Cross[48] confirmed histopathologically the presence of epithelium in the anterior chamber and noted iris incarceration. Guaita[92] first linked ingrowth to postoperative hypotony and the entrance of epithelium through an imperfectly healed wound, confirmed by Meller.[145] Rothmund's "implantation" theory was expanded by the theory of a progressive epithelial lining of the anterior chamber continuous with the ocular surface. In his 1924 textbook, E. Fuchs noted, "the information of an epithelial lining for the anterior chamber cannot be diagnosed clinically, since the epithelium is transparent."[84] However, numerous reports in the first half of this century document the growing awareness of the clinical entity characterized by postoperative hypotony, incarceration of materials in the wound, poor wound coaptation, inflammation, pain, progressive corneal edema and intractable glaucoma.*

Salus[184] gave the first biomicroscopic description of ingrowth. Attempts at experimental reproduction of the disease[44,51,93,163] and interpretation of histopathologic evidence† contributed to the understanding of epithelial ingrowth in 1950, summarized by Calhoun.[30] Calhoun presented 20 cases of epithelial ingrowth of which one in nine eyes treated with x-ray showed "regression" of clinical signs. Nevertheless, he concluded that x-ray therapy offered the only hope for these desperate cases, since surgery had been ". . . unsuccessful and [had] even produced an exacerbation of the epithelial growth."[30] Maumenee emphasized the importance of a biopsy-proven diagnosis in evaluating any method of treatment, and suggested that "if most of the epithelium is removed from the iris and cornea in the case of a downgrowth, the patient might be cured rather than made worse by the surgical procedure,"[140] if treatment were begun early. Surgical extirpation of the epithelial ingrowth, and less frequently of iris cysts, remains the mainstay of current treatment.‡

Most authors have followed Perera's 1937 clas-

---

*References 30, 54, 71, 92, 145, 184.
†References 160, 161, 166, 177, 205, 212, 218, 219.
‡References 22, 23, 81, 130, 135, 136, 139, 207, 211.

sification of epithelial proliferation,[166] as (1) "pearl" tumors of the iris, (2) epithelial cysts, or (3) epithelial ingrowth or downgrowth, because these clinically distinct entities differ greatly in their prognosis and treatment.

Pearl Tumors[140,201]

These rare lesions appear as solid pearly tumors or circumscribed opaque cysts implanted on the iris surface, unconnected with the entrance wound (Fig. 73-1). Resulting from traumatic implantation of skin or hair follicles, pearl tumors are usually small and grow slowly, if at all. Rarely they will enlarge to fill the anterior chamber and extend posteriorly.[201] Mild inflammation may be present. Histologically, these tumors are composed of encapsulated stratified or cuboidal epithelium surrounding keratinized cells or necrotic debris. Occasionally cholesterol, fat, hair follicles, or foreign bodies are found within the core. Total excision is indicated if tumor enlargement or iridocyclitis ensue, generally with good results.

Epithelial Cysts

Perera's review of the historical literature[166] first emphasized the distinguishing presentation and prognosis of epithelial cysts versus sheetlike anterior segment epithelization (ingrowth).

The incidence of epithelial cyst versus ingrowth is difficult to determine from largely histopathologic studies, summarized by Jaffe.[110] An incidence of 0.1% is given by authors who considered cyst and ingrowth as a single entity,[218,219] although cysts are thought to occur more commonly[140] after trauma or cataract surgery. Epithelial cyst formation after penetrating keratoplasty is rare.[11,12,126,189] Epithelial cyst formation has been reported after perforating corneal ulcer,[218] trauma due to prenatal amniocentesis,[53] paracentesis, discission, and iridectomy.[62]

Clinicopathologic features

Clinically, these translucent or gray cysts appear to connect at one point with the surgical or traumatic wound (Fig. 73-2). Rarely, epithelial cysts are discontinuous with the wound and are thought to arise from surface cells implanted by intraocular instruments.[11,21,218] Occasionally they may present in the posterior chamber, having grown through a peripheral iridectomy, and if seen protruding through eroding iris, appear to arise from the iris stroma. The appearance and course of these lesions vary tremendously, some lying dormant for years before enlarging, others growing to considerable size before stabilizing. Pupillary distortion, iridocyclitis, glaucoma, and occlusion of the visual axis may accompany growth of the cyst and indicate treatment. Neither fistula formation with hypotony nor glaucoma is as common as with sheetlike epithelial ingrowth.

It is thought that cystic and sheetlike epithelial invasion of the anterior chamber differ only in mechanical factors, with epithelial cysts entering the anterior chamber as a loop and expanding in a balloon fashion in the anterior chamber.[140] Clinically, evidence for this theory is found in the conversion

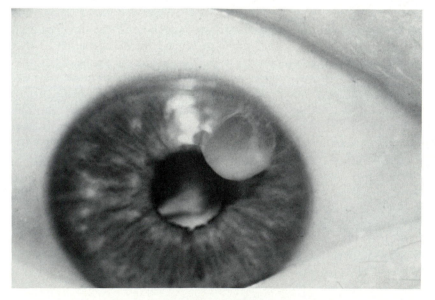

Fig. 73-1 Pearl tumor with desquamative epithelium, 47 years after trauma.

of the cyst to sheetlike ingrowth after surgical intervention.[26,97,117]

Histopathologically, the epithelium comprising cysts and ingrowth is indistinguishable, consisting of one or more layers of squamous or occasionally cuboidal cells, interspersed with goblet cells in some cases (Fig. 73-3). The posterior layer of cells in contact with the iris may be pigmented. The cyst cavity may be filled with serous proteins, mucin,[125] cholesterol, desquamated keratin debris, and/or potentially viable cells.[21] Electron microscopy[21,70] confirms the ocular surface origin of the epithelium, demonstrating cells having a thin basal lamina, desmosomes, tonofilaments, terminal bars, and apical microvilli.

Clinically and experimentally, epithelial cysts are produced when cellular proliferation enters a poorly closed wound, perhaps with iris, lens, or vitreous incarcerated.[44,177,212,219,225] Growth-stimulating factors in a plasmoid aqueous and juxtaposition to the iris for nutrients are thought to determine the size and survival of epithelial cysts.

Clinical clues to the correct diagnosis of epithelial cyst include history of trauma or surgery; evidence of its cystic nature, such as transillumination or tremulousness; lack of vascularity, demonstrable on iris fluorescein angiography[56]; evidence of inflammation accompanying growth; and position on the iris surface versus the stromal or iris pigment epithelial origin of primary iris cysts.[197,198] Shields et al.[198] reviewed the differential diagnosis of iris cysts.

Management

If periodic observation of the epithelial cyst shows sight-threatening complications, antiglaucoma and antiinflammatory medications are used as temporizing measures before definitive treatment. Most authors agree that intervention is warranted only when growth, glaucoma, or iritis affect vision because the cyst can recur as sheetlike epithelial ingrowth.[26,97,117]

Safe, total eradication of epithelial cysts remains an elusive goal. Diathermy[33,220,226]; electrolysis[114,238]; repeated aspiration[87,177,178]; aspiration then diathermy[104]; and irrigation of the cyst with radioactive,[193] corrosive[2,5,116,215,244] or dessicating agents[100] have been successful in isolated cases with limited followup. X-irradiation,[30,58,79,184,217] like the methods previously cited above, has been abandoned as unreliable or unsafe. Cryosurgery has been used to withdraw a collapsed epithelial cyst from the anterior chamber.[78] However, cryothermy's more widespread use has been to destroy residual epithelial cells adherent to the cornea, iris, angle, or vitreous* after cyst aspiration or surgical resection.

Surgical excision of epithelial cysts has undergone numerous modifications, from simple excision of the lesion after aspiration and collapse,[74,140] excision with mechanical or alcohol debridement of the cornea,[139] excision then cryothermy,[26,206] to radical, en bloc resection,[56,210] sometimes including

---

*References 26, 57, 138, 139, 206, 207.

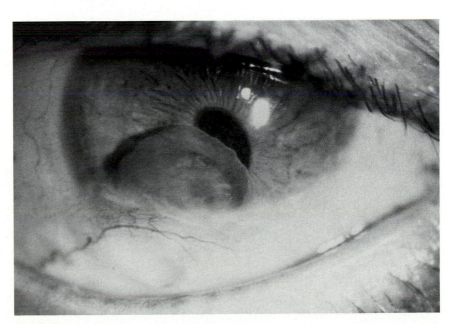

Fig. 73-2 Epithelial cyst in a young man who had undergone corneoscleral transplant for Terrien's marginal degeneration.

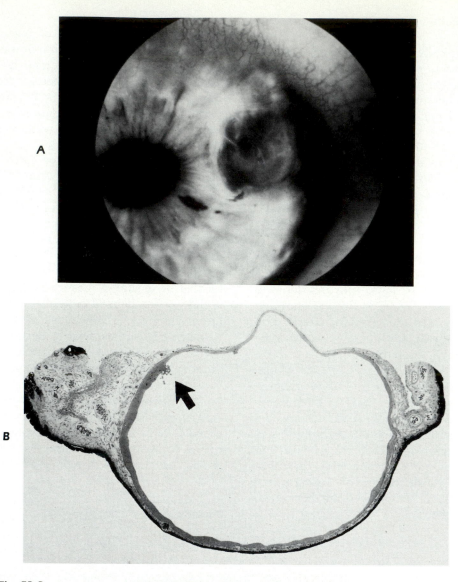

Fig. 73-3 **A,** Appearance of thin-walled iris cyst 22 months after penetrating keratoplasty. **B,** Light micrograph of surgical specimen demonstrates epithelium-lined cyst and its serous contents displacing iris stroma. Arrow indicates desquamating epithelium (paraphenylenediamine, × 16). (From Boruchoff, SA, Kenyon, KR, Foulks, GN, and Green, WR: Br J Ophthalmol 64:440, 1980. Published with permission from the Editor and the British Medical Association.)

vitrectomy.[139,149,207] Excision appears to be the favored approach since the widespread use of the operating microscope and refinement in intraocular surgery and instrumentation. Careful observation of epithelial cysts and awareness of their natural history should prompt earlier, easier intervention and obviate the need for more radical surgical approaches.

Current surgical technique consists of wide excision of the intact cyst, if possible. If the cyst is adherent to cornea, iris, or vitreous face, it is first collapsed by aspiration, using a 25-gauge needle through the limbus at the cyst attachment. We have used a vitreous sweep to peel the cyst away from the cornea. If small, the collapsed cyst is frozen through cornea and limbus after an insulating air bubble is introduced into the anterior chamber. Larger cysts may require the use of vitrectomy instruments, introduced through the limbus or the pars plana, to excise iris and vitreous firmly adherent to the cyst. Freezing over air is then performed, sufficient to briefly form an ice ball involving the adherent epithelial cells. Corneal edema may ensue after cyst excision and freezing; penetrating keratoplasty has been performed to restore good vision in some of these cases.[207]

Photocoagulation has been used to puncture[10,52] and shrink epithelial cysts, although multiple applications are necessary. Meyer-Schwickerath[147] and Cibis[39] used xenon arc laser to treat cysts with results that were "so much better than surgical intervention that a comparison is not possible."[168] The xenon laser was used to "paint" the anterior surface of the cyst[39]; argon laser has been used in later reports.[128] Okun and Mandell[157] reported three cases of epithelial cysts treated with four to six sessions of photocoagulation to the pigmented base, until rapid movement of fine particles within the cyst or iris constriction were noted. The three cysts resolved without sequelae, except for updrawn pupils, at less than 1 year follow-up. Other authors have reported cyst resolution in small series,[10,42,154] with up to 5 years' follow-up.[189] Photocoagulation has the advantage of being relatively less invasive than some surgical procedures. However, when the cyst is not pigmented, when it is firmly adherent to cornea or vitreous, or when it presents in the posterior chamber, photocoagulation may not be useful. In addition, producing a hole in the cyst may externalize it, thereby converting it into sheetlike epithelial ingrowth. Considering the erratic natural history of epithelial cysts, larger series of cases, with long-term follow-up, are necessary before photocoagulation or any treatment modality can be welcomed as a cure.

Epithelial Ingrowth

The rarity of sheetlike epithelial growth into the anterior segment is inversely proportional to the anxiety of the physician who suspects its presence. The treatment of this dread complication, after a century of debate, remains problematic.

Incidence

Figures on the clinical incidence of epithelial ingrowth must be viewed with an awareness of even experienced ophthalmologists' difficulty with its diagnosis. Terry et al.[218] estimated a rate of 0.6% epithelization after traumatic and surgical perforations based on 28 diagnostic laboratory specimens out of 45,500 cases between 1900 and 1939. Theobald and Haas[219] reported an incidence of 1.1% in 8000 cataract extractions, similar to Christianson's incidence of 1.1% for 700 cataract extractions between 1945 and 1951. More recent studies report lower incidences of 0.2%,[158] 0.06%,[13] and

0%.[146] Following a change in surgical technique in 1961, Christensen[37] reported no cases of epithelial ingrowth in over 4000 cataract operations.

The bleak prognosis of eyes failing treatment for ingrowth is reflected in their disproportionate representation in series of globes enucleated after cataract extraction as summarized by Maumenee,[136] Sullivan,[211] and Jaffee.[110] The presence of epithelial ingrowth was detected in an average 17% of eyes enucleated after cataract surgery,[110] ranging from 7.2%[13] to 45.7%.[64] There appears to be no obvious trend in the number of eyes with epithelization coming to enucleation, up to 1969.

Although epithelial ingrowth after penetrating keratoplasty was thought to be quite rare,[35,95,177] several cases have been reported since 1966.[7,120,126,141,209] Sugar has emphasized that ingrowth after keratoplasty may be as frequent as in cataract surgery, with an incidence in his series of 0.25%.[209]

Two cases of bilateral epithelial ingrowth have been reported.[13,30] Epithelial ingrowth has been noted after glaucoma procedures,[219] although, surprisingly, it was not reported in a series of operations for hemolytic glaucoma in which the author produced hypotony by maintaining a conjunctival wick in the anterior chamber.[90] Epithelialization has developed secondary to intraocular lens implantation (AE Maumenee, personal observation), discission of posterior capsule,[246] and McCannel suture.[1]

Some authors have stated that epithelial ingrowth occurs more frequently after intracapsular cataract extraction,[17,145] whereas others note the majority of cases following extracapsular extraction,[37,106] albeit unplanned. Bernardino et al.[73] found the difference in incidence of ingrowth between intracapsular and extracapsular surgery, 0.086% versus 0.13%, nonsignificant. It is now thought that the limbus-based conjunctival flap affords no particular protection against ingrowth, given the current use of microsurgical wound closure.

Clinical findings

The clinical diagnosis of epithelial ingrowth rests on a constellation of signs and symptoms combined with an awareness and suspicion of the disease. The surgery may have been difficult or complicated, perhaps in a young, highly myopic, or diabetic patient.[164] The patient often complains of tearing and dull, aching pain. Photophobia and blurred vision are less frequent complaints.

Examination reveals ciliary injection and, of-

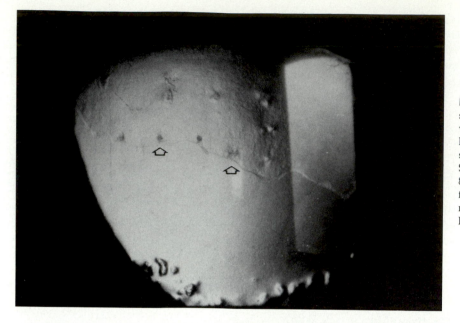

Fig. 73-4 Retroillumination demonstrating posterior corneal epithelial layer with thickened leading edge ("gray line") and focal, pearl-like areas representing heaped-up cells *(arrows)*. (From Stark, WJ, et al: Am J Ophthalmol 85:772, 1978. Published with permission from the American Journal of Ophthalmology. Copyright by the Ophthalmic Publishing Company.)

Fig. 73-5 Scalloped epithelialization of superior one third of cornea.

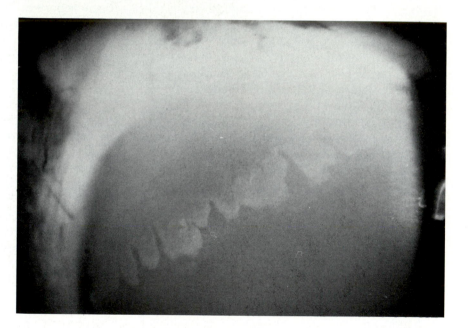

ten, wound gape, bleb, or fistula demonstrable on Seidel testing with 2% fluorescein. Pressure on the globe may be needed to demonstrate a bright green path of aqueous in the fluorescein pool or the presence of conjunctival microcysts. Wadsworth[233] felt that epithelization was rare without a history of delayed reformation of the anterior chamber. A majority of authors note the correlation between postoperative hypotony and epithelial ingrowth, although most authors document hypotony in only one third of cases. Maumenee[136] stated that more

serious cases of epithelial ingrowth were associated with fistula formation.

Band keratopathy is occasionally present.[13,30,221] The cornea may or may not demonstrate edema overlying a posterior corneal membrane demarcated by a gray line, best seen on retroillumination (Fig. 73-4). The gray line, representing the multicellular, thicker leading edge of the epithelial sheet, rarely extends inferiorly past the midcornea. The gray line may be scalloped, with focal pearl-like areas of thickening (Fig. 73-5). Unlike the Khoda-

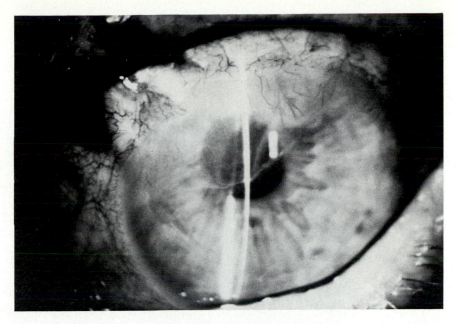

Fig. 73-6 Epithelial ingrowth with prominent corneal vascularization. (From Stark, WJ, et al: Am J Ophthalmol 85:772, 1978. Published with permission from the American Journal of Ophthalmology. Copyright by the Ophthalmic Publishing Company.)

doust rejection line of corneal transplants, keratitic precipitates are not associated with this line.[76] Blomskold[19] reported epithelialization of the entire posterior cornea. Corneal sensation is variably affected. Vascularization of the deep corneal stroma, thought to play a role in nutrition of the ingrowth, is found in about half of cases[30,93,221] (Fig. 73-6); Calhoun[30] associated this vascularization with a more rapid progression of epithelialization. Bernardino et al.[13] demonstrated histopathologic vascularization in all of their cases; in half the cases glaucoma was a presenting sign. Descemet's striae are caused by hypotony and corneal edema. Aqueous flare and cells indicate a variable degree of iridocyclitis. Flare may be disproportionate to ciliary flush or symptoms.[76]

On gonioscopy, wound-incarcerated tissue such as iris, lens cortex or capsule, or vitreous are often seen.[218,219] Epithelium has been observed along suture tracts or lining the internal opening of a bleb or fistula (Fig. 73-7). The epithelium may be seen as a sheet, obscuring details of the trabecular meshwork. Peripheral anterior synechiae (PAS) are often present. Gonioscopy can be used to assess the extent of epithelialization of the angle, through the peripheral iridotomy, on the vitreous face, and sometimes over the ciliary body and retina. Glycerin 50% is used to clear the edematous cornea, if necessary, before gonioscopic examination.

The epithelial sheet grows more rapidly over the iris and ciliary body than down the posterior cornea,[136] perhaps because of nutrients that the uvea provides. Iris details may be obscured, and

infrequently an indentation marks the advancing edge of the tissue, especially in a brown iris. The pupil may be distorted. Membranes over the pupil, on the vitreous face, and enveloping an intraocular lens are seen in advanced cases (Fig. 73-8).

The time of clinical presentation varies tremendously, from 4 days[145] to over 10 years after surgery.[159] Fifteen of Bernardino's 17 cases were diagnosed by 3 years after cataract extraction. All four cases of Sugar et al.[209] were diagnosed by 4 months after keratoplasty. This may reflect the more frequent examinations that are conducted after penetrating keratoplasty.

Histopathology

Histopathologic findings in eyes with epithelial ingrowth typically include one to eight layers of nonkeratinized, stratified squamous epithelium extending over the posterior cornea, lining the surface of the angle or "false angle" created by PAS and continuing over the iris surface. Surface epithelium usually extends deep into the surgical wound, and careful sectioning often reveals its continuity with epithelium lining the anterior chamber (Fig. 73-9). The iris, lens capsule, or vitreous may be incarcerated in the wound. Some reports have noted the presence of goblet cells.[13] Vascularization of the deep corneal stroma, if present, is best seen near the surgical incision. The gray line detected clinically is due to a thicker layer of epithelial cells at the advancing edge of the epithelial sheet (Fig. 73-10). The epithelial layer is thicker and more extensive over the trabecular meshwork (Fig. 73-11)

Text continues on p. 1310.

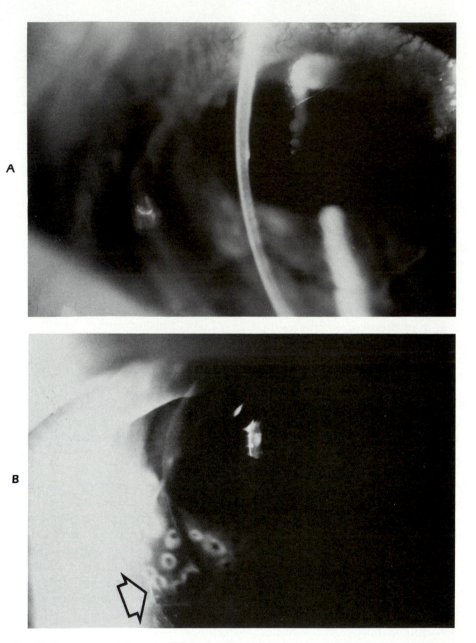

Fig. 73-7 A, Epithelial ingrowth following secondary lens implantation. On gonioscopy, epithelium could be traced to temporal suture tract. **B,** Laser delineates junction between involved and uninvolved iris *(arrow)*.

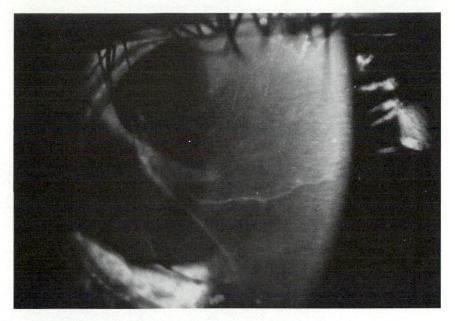

Fig. 73-8 Advanced epithelial ingrowth, with epithelial sheet covering iris, intraocular lens, and vitreous face.

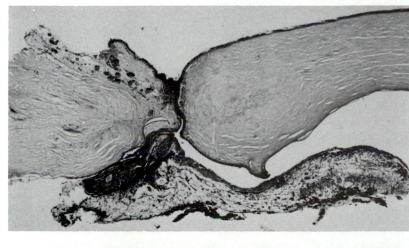

A

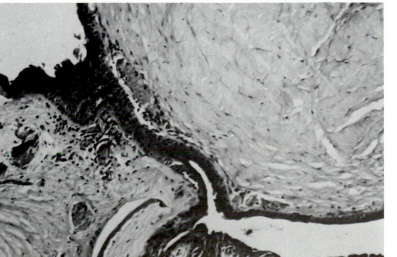

B

Fig. 73-9 Photomicrograph of fistulous tract in cataract wound, demonstrating continuity of nonkeratinized stratified squamous epithelial sheet with conjunctival surface. **A**, Low magnification. **B**, Higher magnification.

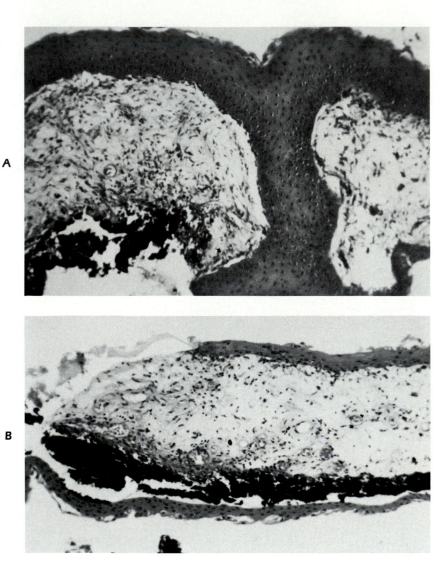

Fig. 73-10 **A,** Epithelium on anterior surface of iris, through iridotomy. **B,** Epithelium continues into posterior surface of iris).

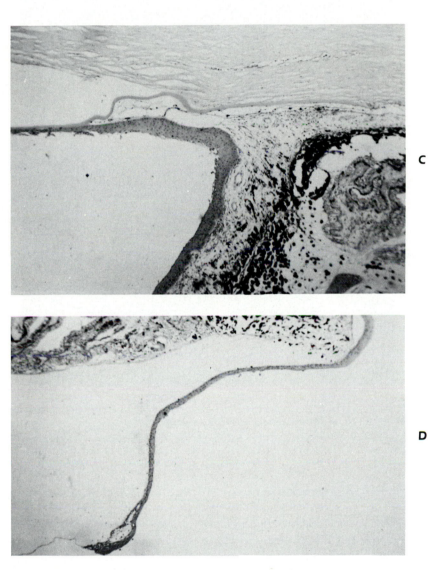

C

D

Fig. 73-10, cont'd   C, Epithelium invests "false angle" formed by peripheral anterior synechiae.
D, Epithelium extends posteriorly, onto vitreous.

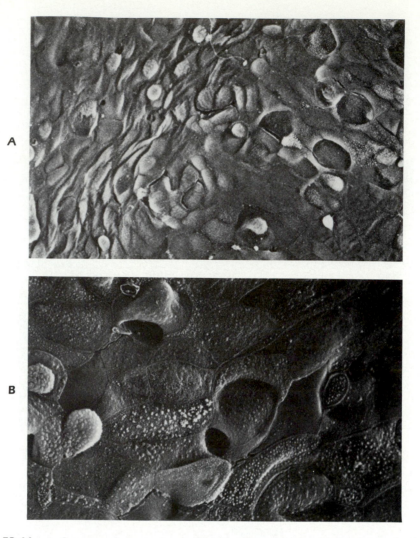

Fig. 73-11 **A,** Scanning electron micrograph of leading edge of epithelium on back of cornea. (×500.) **B,** Microvillous projections are well seen (×1000).

and iris.[37] Often the underlying trabecular meshwork appears sclerotic and focally necrotic. Ectropion uveae is caused by contraction of epithelial tissue coursing around the pupillary margin onto the posterior iris surface. The sheetlike epithelium often appears attenuated when it extends as far as the vitreous, ciliary body, or retinal surface. A chronic inflammatory cell infiltrate is frequently present in the episclera, iris, and ciliary body. Cystoid macular edema is seen in eyes with long-standing inflammation.

Electron microscopy[27,28,108,112,246] demonstrates multilayers of squamous epithelium characterized by numerous surface microvilli; wide intercellular borders; occasional desmosomes; multiple intracellular tonofilaments, most prominent near the leading edge of the sheet; and basal cells containing dense granules (Fig. 73-12). These basal cells are attached by hemidesmosomes to a well-developed basal lamina, which is juxtaposed to a subepithelial connective tissue layer in variable stages of development. Several authors have noted that the corneal endothelium is missing[107] or has undergone epithelial metaplasia[27] in areas of posterior corneal epithelization.

Pathogenesis

Christensen[37] has noted that epithelium is incapable of eroding even a minimal barrier of fibrin in the properly healing wound. In this sense, then, epithelial ingrowth is less an invader and more an invited guest.

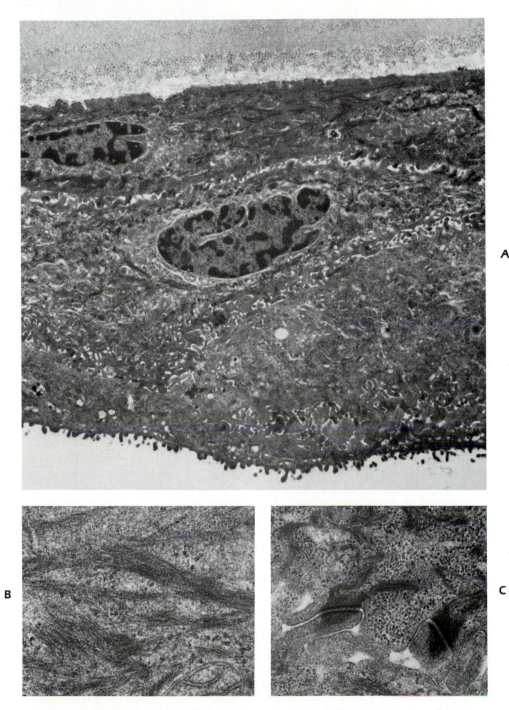

Fig. 73-12   Transmission electron micrograph of ingrowth on the back of the cornea, demonstrating features characteristic of epithelium. **A,** Microplicae between cells and microvilli at anterior chamber surface. (×6500.) **B,** Bundles of 60 to 80 nm tonofilaments. (×60,000.) **C,** Well-developed desmosomes. (×30,000.)

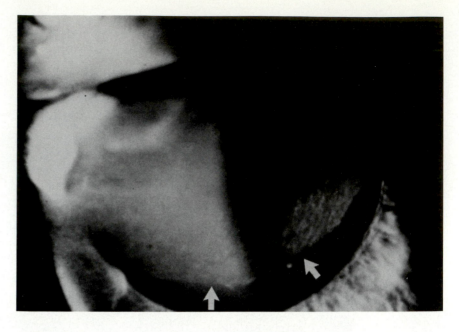

Fig. 73-13 Proliferation of epithelium confined almost entirely to anterior lens surface *(arrows at edge).* (From Bruner, WE, Green, WR, and Stark, WJ: Ophth Surg 17:483, 1986.)

Numerous authors have elucidated the conditions that render the eye receptive to epithelial ingrowth.

1. Complicated surgery, difficult surgery, or faulty surgical techniques, resulting in incarceration of tissue serving as a wick and facilitating postoperative wound gape.
2. Postoperative hypotony is frequently found.
3. Apposition of iris to wound, producing PAS or serving as a nutrient source.
4. The presence of a fistula, or bleb is detected later in one third of eyes.
5. Chronic inflammation plays a role in the establishment of ingrowth, in the poor wound healing leading to fistula formation, in the cyclitis leading to further hypotony, and in later multiple complications of the disease, from cornea to macula.

Experimental efforts to reproduce the clinical spectrum of epithelial ingrowth have met with modest success, at best. In the second half of the nineteenth century, several German authors attempted to produce epithelial cysts by implanting free conjunctiva, cornea, hair and other foreign bodies into the anterior chamber.[61,89,105,181,192] The tissue degenerated or, rarely, formed cysts, and the foreign bodies became encapsulated. Investigators in the 1930s sought to reproduce the clinical substrate of ingrowth by implanting epithelium continuous with its surface origin in hypoto-

nous, inflamed eyes.[51,93,166,212] The more successful experiments[51,212] resulted when the conjunctival or corneal epithelium, contiguous with its surface base, was placed adjacent to the iris, which was thought to play a nutrient role. Proliferation of epithelium only occurred when the eye was maintained in hypotony by nonabsorbed matter in the wound, such as vitreous, lens capsule, or celluloid.[51,166,224] The uninflamed aqueous was thought to be insufficient to maintain the epithelium, much less its proliferation.[44,93]

In the 1940s and 1950s experimental studies rediscovered[134,173] and elaborated the role of epithelial migration into normally[64,80,132] and abnormally healing[15,16,44,66] wounds. Several authors noted that the epithelial sheet seems to "slide" over smooth or fibrin-laden surfaces[44,134,177]; a striking clinical example has been reported where epithelial ingrowth was confined primarily to the lens capsule (Fig. 73-13).[25]

No clear-cut experimental evidence implicated corneoscleral sutures in the establishment of ingrowth, although several authors in the 1950s had attributed a "rising incidence" of ingrowth to the increasing popularity of corneoscleral sutures since the 1930s,[12,17,67,166] which was later refuted.[4] Deep placement of sutures[113,177,219] and the use of silk sutures[67,134,177] have been implicated in the development of ingrowth. The long-standing debate over the role of limbus-based versus fornix-based conjunctival flaps in the pathogenesis of epithelial ingrowth* has been superseded by improvements in wound closure.[13,111,139] The use of a self-sealing biplanar incision, separate closure of the conjunctival and corneoscleral wounds, finer suture material, attention to good wound apposition, and more recently, the use of the operating microscope, refined instrumentation, and decreased vitreous loss have ameliorated the causes of epithelization identified in histopathologic and experimental studies.[4]

There has been an explosion of interest in how cell-extracellular matrix interactions and growth factors affect tissue growth, mobility, and differentiation. More recent reports on epithelial ingrowth, clinical and experimental, discuss the pathogenesis of ingrowth in terms of cell biology made familiar to the physician since the late 1960s.

Theoretically, the breakdown of the blood-aqueous barrier in hypotonous, inflamed eyes provides serum-borne growth factors needed by proliferating epithelium.[171] These factors are not normally present in uninflamed aqueous that will sustain the epithelium[6,202] but not its proliferation. Clinical and experimental studies suggest that healthy cells inhibit the advance of ectopic epithelium[55,199] and, conversely, that damaged or missing endothelium poses an increased risk of epithelialization.† Several authors suggest that a smooth surface and lack of cell-cell inhibition fosters epithelial advance,[25,184] although others note that epithelium has been observed to advance over endothelium[13,245] and believe that additional factors, such as inflammation,[171] must be present.

The availability of a better animal model of the disease[27,28] should encourage research into the cellular and molecular basis of epithelial ingrowth, leading to more effective treatment.

Mechanisms of glaucoma

Intractable glaucoma, long recognized as the final common pathway in enucleated eyes with epithelial ingrowth,[71] has several possible etiologies. Hypotony, inflammation, and shallowing of the anterior chamber lead to broad PAS. Proliferating epithelium covers the trabecular meshwork, as well as lining the false angle created by PAS; and later contraction of this epithelial sheet causes secondary angle closure.[30] Exfoliated epithelial cells and macrophages have been seen to plug the trabecular meshwork.[13,218] Areas of trabecular meshwork un-

derlying the epithelial sheet become sclerosed and necrotic.[112] Chronic inflammation of the uvea leads to trabeculitis and decreased outflow. Rarely, goblet cell secretion leads to mucogenic glaucoma.[125] Chronic steroid use may result in elevated intraocular pressure when a bleb or fistula is not present. Pupillary block glaucoma is produced when the epithelial sheet occludes or secludes the pupil.[34] Hemorrhagic and ghost cell glaucoma may result from repeated hemorrhage from friable neovascularization. Chronic hypotony may progress to intractable glaucoma if the fistula closes, either spontaneously or iatrogenically.

Diagnostic adjuncts

Several clinical tests help confirm the impression of an epithelial ingrowth, in addition to the history, symptoms, and careful examination outlined previously.

Dynamic Seidel test.   Aqueous 2% fluorescein is used, with judicious pressure on the globe, to detect microcyst, bleb, or fistula formation. The dark green appearance of concentrated fluorescein turns bright green when mixed with streaming aqueous (Fig. 73-14).

Specular microscopy.[123,203]   In some cases, a sharply defined border is seen between corneal endothelial cells and the area of epithelial ingrowth, at the level of endothelial focus (Fig. 73-15). Deeper focus brings the interlacing borders of the epithelial cells into view. The endothelium is sometimes missing below the demarcation line.[123]

Argon laser photocoagulation.   Meyer-Schwickerath and Maumenee first described the use of xenon laser for diagnosing the extent of ingrowth.[136,147,148] Stark et al.[207] first described the diagnostic use of the argon laser. It is set at 500 μm, 100 mW, and 0.1 sec initially and aimed at the iris surface in areas of suspected epithelial coverage. A characteristic fluffy white lesion signals the presence of an epithelial layer, versus a well-demarcated slight burn to normal iris (Fig. 73-16). Photocoagulation is used to diagnose ingrowth and to delineate iris involvement preoperatively.

Invasive tests, aimed at histologic confirmation of the diagnosis before surgery, include

1. *Iris biopsy.*[229] Sampling of full-thickness iris to determine the presence of epithelium was described early and remains a diagnostic alternative.
2. *Anterior chamber curettage.*[31,135] Calhoun suggested the use of a 1 mm serrated curette, to obtain tissue for microscopic exam. The

---

*References 4, 37, 40, 167, 177, 213, 216, 219, 222.
†References 32, 55, 83, 108, 121, 123, 218, 245.

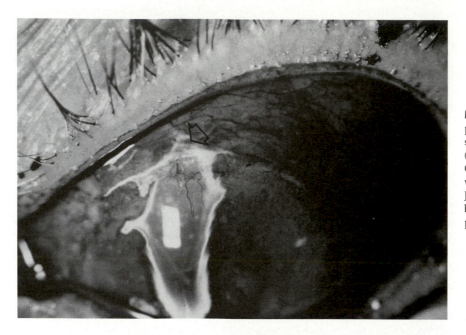

Fig. 73-14 Dynamic Seidel test. Two percent fluorescein is used to demonstrate aqueous leaking through fistula *(arrow)*. (From Stark, WJ, et al: Am J Ophthalmol 85:772, 1978. Published with permission from the American Journal of Ophthalmology. Copyright by the Ophthalmic Publishing Company.)

Fig. 73-15 Specular microscopy across scalloped margin of epithelial ingrowth shows sharp demarcation between normal endothelium, *left*, and ingrowth, *right*. (From Smith, RE, and Parrett, C: Arch Ophthalmol 96:1222, July 1978. Copyright 1978, American Medical Association.)

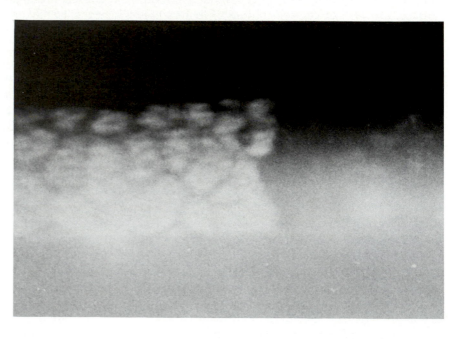

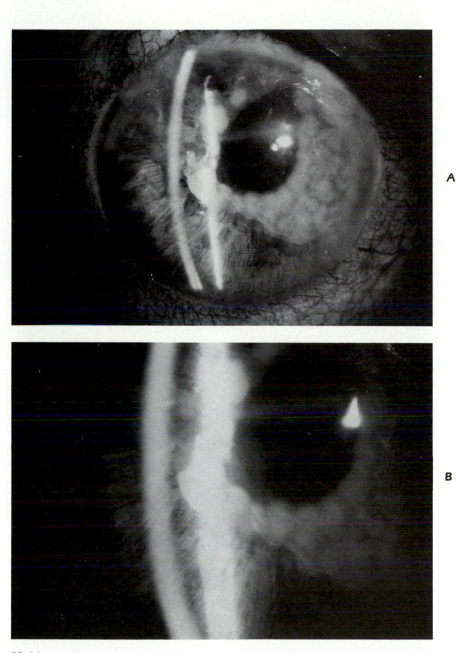

Fig. 73-16 A, Argon laser spots delineate extent of anterior iris involvement by epithelium. Epithelium-covered surface treated with laser turns fluffy white, whereas uninvolved iris surface shows a slight burn. **B,** Closer view of junction between involved *(arrow)* and uninvolved iris. (From Stark, WJ, et al: Am J Ophthalmol 85:772, 1978. Published with permission from the American Journal of Ophthalmology. Copyright by the Ophthalmic Publishing Company.)

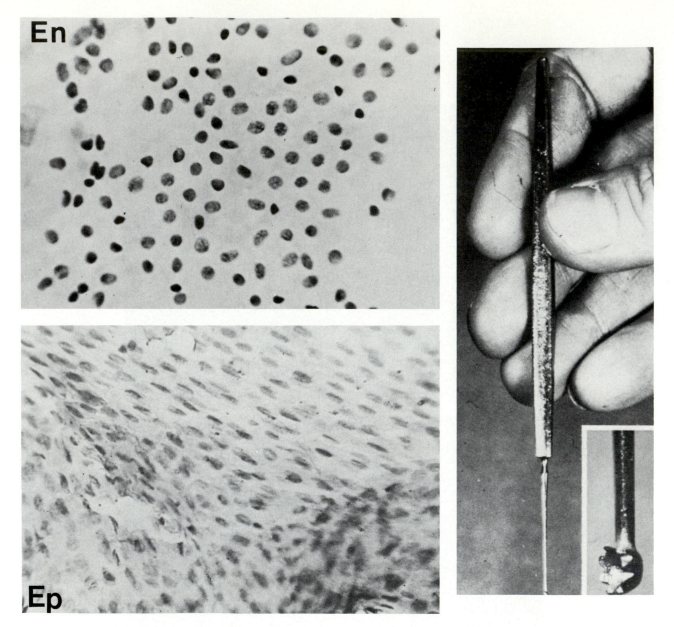

Fig. 73-17 *Right,* Endothelial curette as suggested by Calhoun; *left,* appearance of epithelial cells *(Ep)* compared with endothelial cells *(En).* (From Calhoun, FP, Jr: Am J Ophthalmol 61:1055, 1966. Published with permission from the American Journal of Ophthalmology. Copyright by the Ophthalmic Publishing Company.)

sample is immediately fixed on an albumin-coated slide and stained with hematoxylin and eosin. Epithelial cells are readily differentiated from endothelial cells, being closely packed, spindled, and having denser cytoplasm (Fig. 73-17).

3. *Aqueous aspiration*[228] has been used to diagnose ingrowth, but the numbers of circulating epithelial cells in the aqueous may be insufficient.

4. *Diagnostic vitrectomy.*[72,73,91] The celloidin bag technique is used to confirm the diagnosis of epithelial ingrowth after therapeutic vitrectomy.

Differential diagnosis

Maumenee[136] summarized the differential diagnosis of epithelial ingrowth. It includes (1) glassy membrane (reduplicated Descemet's membrane) occurring in eyes having chronic iridocyclitis; (2)

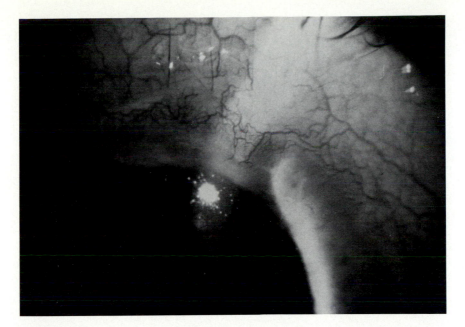

Fig. 73-18 Shelved corneal incision mimicking epithelial ingrowth. By slit-lamp examination, incision can be followed anteriorly into corneal stroma.

fibrous ingrowth (see next section), distinguished by its very slow growth and vascularity; (3) vitreo-corneal adhesions, which may cause corneal edema and have a grayish appearance; (4) an anterior, shelved corneal cataract incision, seen as a diagonal, posteroanterior intrastromal line on careful slit-lamp examination (Fig. 73-18); (5) detachment of Descemet's membrane; and (6) peripheral corneal edema, most likely due to operative endothelial trauma. The first condition, descemetization of the cornea, angle, and iris, can clinically most resemble ingrowth; however, the photocoagulation test is negative.

Management

Surgical extirpation of epithelial ingrowth has become the mainstay of treatment since the pioneering reports of Maumenee[135,136,139,140] and others.[22,23,130,179,207] Before 1950, however, a singular surgical success reported by Fazakus in 1932,[75] scraping combined with diathermy to the wound margins, could not be reproduced; and, based on their experiences, Pincus,[167] Duke-Elder,[62] and others[30] concluded that "operative intervention is of no avail; if anything, it hastens the deterioration of the eye."[167]

Radiation therapy,* using a wide variety of

sources, doses, and regimens, was the treatment of choice for these desperate patients from the 1930s to the mid-1960s, despite uncertain diagnoses and short follow-up. First used in 1924,[96] the confusion regarding dose; the uncertain effects; and the danger to lens, retina, optic nerve, and vasculature led to abandonment of irradiation for ingrowth by the late 1960s. The most recent review of radiation therapy[58] documents the failure of irradiation to affect "diffuse epithelial invasion,"[58] compared to modest success with epithelial cysts.

Surgical intervention for epithelial ingrowth, reintroduced by Maumenee[135,136,140] and others,[130,211] resulted in about 25% of eyes retaining good visual acuity (equal to or better than 20/40), generally in younger patients. Extensive freezing of the cornea to destroy epithelium on its posterior surface[136] resulted in diffuse corneal edema. Localized freezing[139] or wound and iris debridement only without corneal freezing[122,144] were later suggested. Freezing alone without other surgical intervention has failed.[144] Photocoagulation has been employed[136,148] but with variable success and is now used as a diagnostic adjunct preoperatively and postoperatively, to detect the extent of epithelization. Early surgical series demonstrated the poorer prognosis of eyes retaining fistulas after surgical repair.[136] Therefore, fistula repair at the time of initial intervention, using the hinged-flap technique and removing any vitreous wick if necessary,[136,139,179,207] is recommended.

---

*References 30, 54, 58, 184, 217, 224.

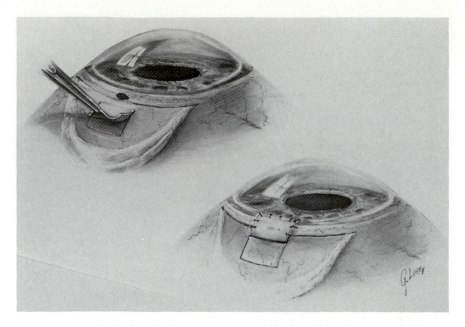

Fig. 73-19 Partial-thickness scleral flap is used to cover external opening of fistula if it cannot be closed with sutures. (From Rice, TA, and Michaels, RG: Am J Ophthalmol 85:656, 1978. Published with permission from the American Journal of Ophthalmology. Copyright by the Ophthalmic Publishing Company.)

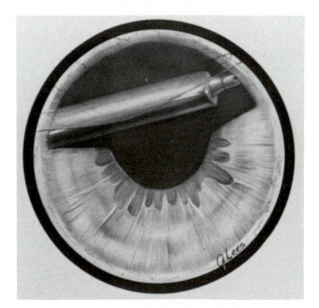

Fig. 73-20 Iris and vitreous involved in epithelial ingrowth are excised, using vitrectomy instrument. (From Stark, WJ, et al: Am J Ophthalmol 85:772, 1978. Published with permission from the American Journal of Ophthalmology. Copyright by the Ophthalmic Publishing Company.)

Maumenee's surgical technique[139] can be outlined as follows:

1. Photocoagulation is used to delineate the extent of iris involvement.
2. Osmotic agents are used preoperatively as needed to produce a soft eye.
3. A Flieringa ring is sutured to the sclera.
4. At surgery, the border of the corneal involvement is marked on the corneal surface using a sharp instrument to scratch the epithelium.
5. A careful intraoperative search for a fistula is made, using 2% aqueous fluorescein.
6. The fistula is excised or a hinged scleral flap prepared, if necessary (Fig. 73-19).
7. If no fistula is present, the anterior chamber is entered posterior to the original cataract wound.
8. Excision of involved iris, ciliary body and anterior vitreous is carried out (Fig. 73-20).
9. The posterior corneal surface is scraped, peeled, curetted, or swabbed free of epithelium, or alternatively, the marked-off area of cornea is frozen on the endothelial side. The ice ball formed is allowed to melt before reapplying the probe, to avoid stripping Descemet's membrane.

With stringent criteria for success (vision better than 20/50 and control of glaucoma), Maumenee et al.[139] had successful results in 11 of 40 of consecutive cases. Complications included persistent, clinically significant corneal edema (20 eyes); glaucoma (17 eyes); hypotony (5 eyes); phthisis (3 eyes); and enucleation (7 eyes).

Modifications of the preceding technique include tectonic "minigrafts" to close fistulae,[211,231] more extensive excision of the angle structures,[22,81,155,211,246] cryotherapy to involved angle structures and ciliary body,[23] cryotherapy to the anterior corneal surface,[57] posterior lamellar keratectomy to remove posterior corneal epithelium,[22,210] use of air tamponade to insulate other structures during corneal cryotherapy,[207] and the use of ultrasonic[88] and vitrectomy instrumentation to remove involved iris and anterior vitreous.[149,179,207]

The currently accepted technique is Stark's and Michels' modification of Maumenee's technique. Preoperatively, the iris is treated by argon laser photocoagulation to define the extent of epithelial involvement. Photocoagulation spots of 500 μm are placed along the advancing edge of the epithelial sheet in such a way that one half of each spot turns white, indicating the presence of epithelium, and the other half turns brown, indicating noninvolved iris tissue. Photocoagulation is performed within 24 hours of the planned surgical procedure because this treatment can cause moderate anterior chamber inflammation.

Traction sutures are placed under each rectus muscle in a transconjunctival fashion, and a conjunctival incision is performed. A limbal-based conjunctival flap is dissected to expose the superior corneoscleral limbus. The fistula is closed, if necessary, using the hinged-flap technique previously described.[136]

When a pars plana approach is used, a sclerotomy is performed 4 mm posterior and parallel to the corneoscleral limbus in the superotemporal quadrant. The vitrectomy instrument, equipped with an overlying fiberoptic sleeve, is inserted into the pupillary space. The area of involved vitreous and iris is excised, a bite at a time, by using an oscillating cutting mode to minimize traction on the iris root. If bleeding occurs, it is controlled by temporarily increasing the intraocular pressure or by applying bipolar diathermy.[151]

After excising the involved vitreous and iris tissue, any vitreous gel remaining in the anterior one half of the vitreous cavity is removed. This provides a fluid space that can subsequently be filled with air to enhance the freezing technique. The vitrectomy instrument is then withdrawn and

the sclerotomy site closed with multiple sutures.

The anterior one half of the eye is filled with sterile air by fluid-gas exchange (Fig. 73-21, A). Air is introduced through the infusion system of the instrument while intraocular fluid is passively displaced through the aspiration system vented to the atmosphere. If a large fistula is present, a partial-thickness scleral flap is reflected over the fistula and sutured to the peripheral cornea. The fundus is examined with indirect ophthalmoscopy with scleral depression. Any retinal tears are treated with cryotherapy and their position marked on the sclera. A silicone-rubber exoplant provides a scleral buckling effect beneath any retinal break.

Cryotherapy is finally applied in a transcorneal and transscleral fashion to devitalize the epithelium remaining on the posterior surface of the cornea, in the anterior chamber angle, and on the ciliary body (Fig. 73-21, B). With the air bubble in place, one can advance the full-thickness freeze from the corneoscleral limbus onto the cornea with considerable precision and extend it just beyond the edge of the epithelial sheet, thus minimizing damage to the adjacent corneal endothelial cells. Part of the air bubble is then removed and replaced by physiologic salt solution if no retinal breaks are present.

Postoperatively, the eye is treated frequently with topical corticosteroids. Posturing of the patient is used, if retinal breaks are present, to position the remaining intraocular bubble against the retinal breaks. Epithelium on the posterior cornea in the treated area typically sloughs during the first few postoperative days (Fig. 73-22).

Using vitrectomy techniques, Stark et al.[207] reported visual improvement in eight of ten consecutive cases, and better than 20/50 vision in four eyes. Penetrating keratoplasties have done surprisingly well in stabilized eyes after treatment for ingrowth.[23]

In some cases where the disease is so extensive that surgical intervention is not considered, closure of the fistula, if present, is contraindicated because the intraocular tension can become unmanageable. One report describes mixed results during attempts at control of glaucoma using the Krupin-Denver valve.[8]

Although the use of antimetabolites against epithelial ingrowth has been suggested,[232] they have never been given a clinical trial. The renewed interest in antimetabolites as therapeutic adjuncts to trabeculectomy, vitrectomy, and lensectomy may lead to investigation of their efficacy in the often frustrating treatment of epithelial ingrowth.

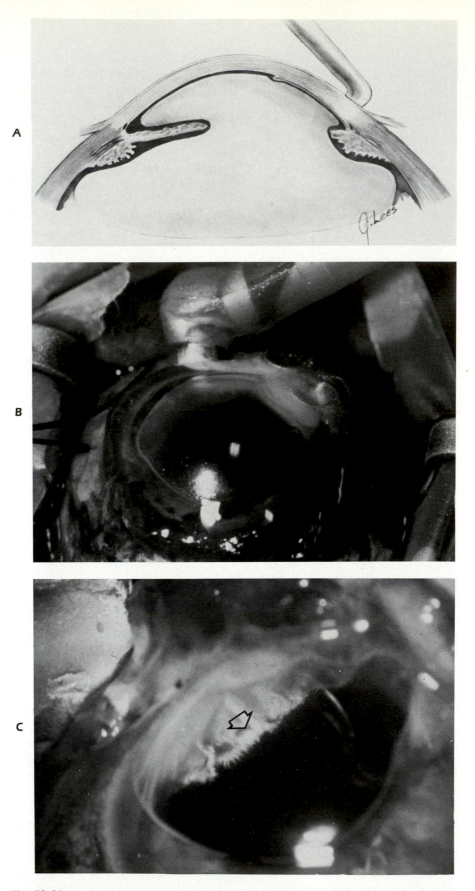

Fig. 73-21 **A,** Air insulates other tissues from effects of transcorneal and transcleral cryotherapy. **B,** Full-thickness corneal freezing can be applied accurately to treat ingrowth and minimize damage to adjacent uninvolved tissue. **C,** Transscleral cryotherapy is used to treat involved ciliary body. Ice is visible on ciliary processes *(arrow).* (From Stark, WJ, et al: Am J Ophthalmol 85:772, 1978. Published with permission from the American Journal of Ophthalmology. Copyright by the Ophthalmic Publishing Company.)

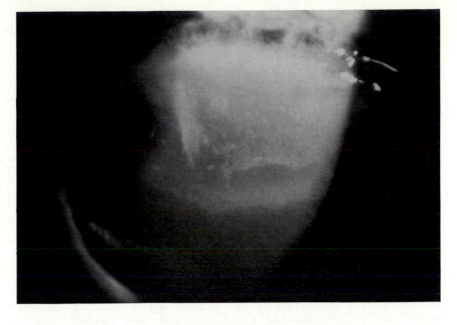

Fig. 73-22 Epithelium on posterior cornea sloughs 1 day after cryotherapy. (From Stark, WJ, et al: Am J Ophthalmol 85:772, 1978. Published with permission from the American Journal of Ophthalmology. Copyright by the Ophthalmic Publishing Company.)

FIBROUS INGROWTH

Fibrous ingrowth, sometimes confused with epithelial ingrowth, is also called stromal ingrowth, stromal overgrowth, fibrous overgrowth, or fibrous metaplasia and is equated with retrocorneal membrane by some authors. Much less has been written about fibrous ingrowth compared to epithelial ingrowth, perhaps because its progression is less spectacular, frequently self-limited, and often better tolerated by the postoperative eye.

Historical Background

Henderson[101,102] observed cataract wound healing in eyes with incarcerated iris or lens capsule, where proliferating subconjunctival connective tissue continuous with the ocular surface extended over anterior chamber structures. He considered fibroblastic ingrowth through faulty limbal incisions to be the counterpart of epithelial ingrowth. Collins[46] rejected the theory of fibroblastic response without concomitant infection. Swan[213] attributed fibroplasia to scleral reaction when lens, fibrin, or vitreous was incarcerated in the wound; whereas Levkoieva[129] and Duke-Elder[62] thought that corneal stroma provided the connective tissue invading gaping, inflamed wounds.

Incidence

There are no solid data on the incidence of clinically recognized fibrous ingrowth. Fibrous ingrowth is seen in 50% to 80% of failed keratoplasty specimens[236] and has been termed "retrocorneal

membrane." Some histopathologic studies of globes enucleated after complications of anterior segment surgery note fibrous ingrowth as frequently as epithelial ingrowth. Dunnington[65] reported an incidence of 33% fibrous ingrowth in 177 eyes, compared to an incidence of 36% epithelial ingrowth. Bettmann[14] reported that 25 of 74 enucleated eyes demonstrated fibrous ingrowth (34%). Allen, including "only those cases in which the stromal ingrowth was extensive enough to close the angle or massive enough to disorganize the eye,"[3] reported an incidence of 36% of 50 eyes enucleated after cataract surgery, 11% of 237 eyes enucleated after trauma, and 15% of 13 eyes enucleated after glaucoma surgery. Other histopathologic studies note that epithelial ingrowth is far more common than fibrous ingrowth in series of enucleated eyes.[18,165,191] Blodi[18] noted a lower incidence of fibrous ingrowth after extracapsular cataract extraction (ECCE) compared to intracapsular cataract extraction (ICCE), attributing it to the proximity of vitreous to the wound after ICCE. In a recent histopathologic study investigating 31 eyes in which vitreous was incarcerated in the cataract wound, fibrous ingrowth was reported in 84%.[142]

Clinical Presentation and Pathologic Correlation

The same predisposing factors for epithelial ingrowth, enumerated in the preceding section, have been associated with the development of fibrous ingrowth: (1) difficult surgery, (2) vitreous loss, (3) incarceration of materials in the wound, (4) poor wound closure, (5) postoperative hypotony, and (6) marked and/or chronic postoperative inflammation. Swan[214] cited suture-induced inflammation, posteriorly placed incisions,[213] and endothelial damage as lesser known factors that contribute to fibrous ingrowth. Trauma[3,62,63,186] and postoperative hyphema[20,214] have also been mentioned as causal factors.

Fibrous ingrowth is most commonly recognized clinically as a retrocorneal membrane developing after penetrating keratoplasty.[120,195,196,237] The presence of a fibrous retrocorneal membrane in failed keratoplasty specimens, first reported by Fuchs,[84] has been noted in 50% to 80% of histopathologic specimens.[24,36,95,183,227] Clinical recognition is not so frequent. The graft-host junction may reveal a plaquelike thickening as early as 2 weeks postoperatively. It may progress to a thickened, opacified and perhaps vascularized crescent or chord, more extensive behind the donor button. Proceeding from a break in Descemet's membrane, this fibrous proliferation can extend into the anterior chamber, appearing as a fenestrated membrane, or it can cover the entire posterior donor button.

Fibrous ingrowth has been noted after cataract extraction, trauma, goniotomy, and filtering surgery.[3,50]

The clinical picture of fibrous ingrowth varies, depending on the severity of the initial insult (Fig. 73-23).[82,214] The patient is often not uncomfortable. A translucent membranous type of fibrous in-

growth, occurring on the posterior cornea in areas of stripped Descemet's or vitreous touch, can have a fairly distinct border and resemble epithelial ingrowth. More commonly, however, the fibrous membrane, located adjacent to the wound, extends onto the posterior corneal surface, appearing as a feltlike or woven gray-white opacity with a frayed leading margin. Fibrous ingrowth secondary to intraocular bleeding may appear straw colored,[20,213,214] because of retained blood breakdown products. Corneal edema usually overlies the involved portion of cornea. Extension of the ingrowth over angle, iris, and vitreous is often easily recognized as a thick enveloping membrane. If attenuated, the membrane resembles the fine gray sheet seen after hyphema or prolonged iridocyclitis. The pupil may be updrawn into a superior fibrous scar.

Inflammation often accompanies fibrous ingrowth and is proportional to the severity and extent of the initial injury. The clinical spectrum of fibrous ingrowth ranges from minimal and self-limited, without significant inflammation, to massive fibrous intraocular proliferation and later retraction, resulting in retinal detachment, hypotony,[14,38] and phthisis bulbi.[14]

Glaucoma, rather than hypotony, can result from fibrous ingrowth, resulting from obliteration of the angle structures, peripheral anterior synechia from persistent flat chamber or inflammation, or recurrent bleeding from friable fibrovascular tissue, occasionally leading to hemolytic glaucoma.[82,214]

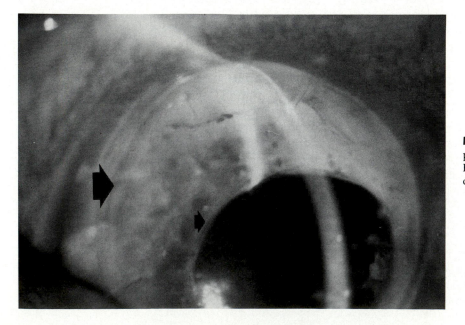

Fig. 73-23 Fibrous ingrowth after penetrating keratoplasty. *Large arrow,* Keratoplasty wound; *small arrows,* edge of retrocorneal tissue.

Differential Diagnosis

The fibrous ingrowth associated with trauma or surgery, most commonly penetrating keratoplasty, should be distinguished from the "retrocorneal membrane" associated with some dystrophies, degenerations, or chemical or inflammatory stimuli. For example, retrocorneal membrane has been described in eyes without a break in Descemet's membrane with various dystrophies and degenerations,[236] in the vitreous touch syndrome[204] after chemical burns,[118,133,152] after corneal freezing,[150] after pars plana vitrectomy,[115] after herpetic keratitis,[223] and after silicone oil tamponade in experimental animals.[208] Waring[236] reviewed the clinical and histologic appearance of Descemet's membrane reaction to a variety of pathologic stimuli. The differential diagnosis of fibrous ingrowth parallels that of epithelial ingrowth: (1) detachment of Descemet's membrane, (2) glass membrane ("descemetization"), (3) vitreocorneal adhesion, and (4) shelved corneal incision.

Diagnosis[213] is based on clinical observation and a knowledge of predisposing factors for fibrous ingrowth. Unlike the helpful diagnostic tests for epithelial ingrowth, there are no specific adjunctive tests to diagnose fibrous ingrowth. In one case, excisional biopsy[20] for visual rehabilitation confirmed a clinical diagnosis of fibrous ingrowth.

Histopathology

Histopathologic examination of fibrous ingrowth from a limbal cataract incision may reveal a poorly coapted wound with surrounding inflammation within sclera and/or corneal stroma (Fig. 73-24). Posterior wound gaping can be inferred from a relatively large space between cut ends of Descemet's membrane, filled in by fibrocellular proliferative tissue. The proliferative tissue may be vascular, especially near the wound margin. Often the origin of the fibrous proliferation—whether stromal, episcleral, or endothelial—is not clear. Bulky or poorly tied sutures can surround areas of focal necrosis and inflammation. Wound-incarcerated iris, lens capsule, vitreous, or lens fragments have been reported, providing a scaffolding for the proliferating fibrous tissue. Endothelium is frequently missing adjacent to the wound, and stripped Descemet's membrane provides additional evidence of intraoperative trauma to the posterior cornea in eyes with posterior corneal fibrous ingrowth. There may be deep vascularization and chronic inflammation of the corneal stroma. Descemet's membrane can be thickened, irregular, and covered by subjacent fibroblastic endothelium. Peripheral anterior synechiae or fibrous tissue may close the trabecular meshwork, which will often incorporate pigment or inflammatory cells and will later demonstrate a sclerotic or atrophic appearance. Corectopia, ectropion uveae, and pupillary membranes can result from more florid fibrous proliferation. Retinal detachment has been reported secondary to massive fibrous ingrowth.

Fibrous ingrowth reported after corneal incisions (i.e., clear corneal cataract sections, or penetrating keratoplasty) differs in its histopathologic appearance from that developing after limbal incisions. The fibroblastic cells appear to originate from metaplastic endothelium or from stromal ker-

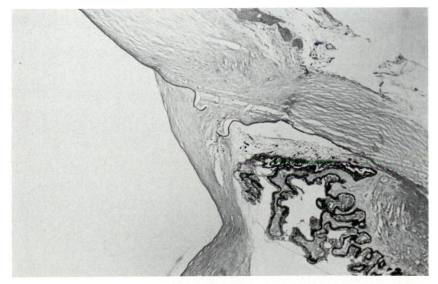

Fig. 73-24 Histopathology of fibrous ingrowth through limbal cataract incision.

atocytes. The retrocorneal membrane, or, as suggested by Waring,[235] the posterior collagenous layer of the cornea, consists of Descemet's membrane, ruptured at the surgical wound, opposed to a multilaminar, PAS-positive layer of variable thickness and cellularity. Endothelium may appear metaplastic, pigment-laden, attenuated, or missing entirely.

Based on his ultrastructural examination of 30 corneas, Waring described three morphologic types of posterior collagenous layers (PCLs): banded, fibrillar, and fibrocellular. The classic "retrocorneal fibrous membrane," connecting to the stroma through a break in Descemet's membrane, was seen in two failed keratoplasty specimens and in one lacerated cornea. Ultrastructurally, the membrane was the fibrocellular type. The fibrocellular PCL was seen on the posterior surface of an intact Descemet's membrane only in one case of herpes simplex keratouveitis.[235]

Pathogenesis

Factors predisposing the eye to fibrous ingrowth are identical to those associated with epithelial ingrowth. In addition, recurrent bleeding into the postoperative eye from a vascularized, inflamed wound is thought to provide a fibrin scaffold for fibrous proliferation into the anterior chamber.[214] Swan[214] implicated suture-induced reactions, scleral incisions, and damage to the endothelium as lesser known factors that contribute to fibrous ingrowth.

Experimental fibrous ingrowth was produced in rabbits by Sherrard and Rycroft,[196] who described the maturation of the tissue from a sheet of fibroblasts to a relatively acellular stroma-like tissue. They noted that (1) healthy stroma, capable of providing collagen-producing keratocytes, (2) a large break in Descemet's membrane, and (3) damage to the endothelium around the posterior wound were important in promoting fibrous ingrowth. Attempts at reproducing fibrous ingrowth from trauma posterior to the limbus have met with limited success.[41]

Retrocorneal membrane (RCM) has been reproduced successfully. Leigh[127] produced RCM when endothelium was removed from one half of a corneal graft. Retrocorneal membrane was produced when blood was injected into the anterior chamber, the donor endothelium was injured, or repeated flattening of the anterior chamber was induced in a group of corneal transplanted rabbits.[29]

The cellular origin of the RCM depends on such factors as the inciting injury and subsequent inflammation, bleeding, and wound apposition. The myriad sources of cells identified include (1) subepithelial connective tissue;[66,82,102,214] (2) corneal stromal fibroblasts,[195,237] which may be of host origin[24] when Descemet's membrane is violated, and endothelium injured; (3) metaplastic corneal endothelium,* which may be of donor origin,[200] especially in the absence of breaks in Descemet's membrane; (4) migratory cells from the anterior chamber angle;[133] and (5) metaplastic monocytes of uveal origin.[170] Bloomfield et al.[20] reported a unique case of RCM after cataract and postoperative hyphema, in which the ultrastructure of the keratoplasty specimen demonstrated a double membrane, probably of two separate origins: (1) an anterior, vascular layer, the capillaries of which resembled those of subconjunctival connective tissue by transmission electron microscopy; and (2) a posterior amorphous layer containing basement membrane, collagen, and fibroblast-like endothelial cells with prominent cytoplasmic filaments, thought to be derived from metaplastic endothelium.[20]

Management

No satisfactory treatment for massive fibrous ingrowth has been proposed except surgical intervention.[20] Medical management is directed toward control of inflammation, glaucoma, or corneal edema as the need arises. Steroid treatment has not been useful in preventing the extension of fibrous ingrowth. Fortunately, many of these eyes remain quiescent and periodic observation often reveals maturation of the fibrous scar without progressive inflammatory damage to the globe. In progressive fibrous ingrowth, radiation therapy has been suggested,[82] but no clinical series are available to support this theory.

Surgical intervention may be attempted to relieve specific consequences of fibrous ingrowth, that is, trabeculectomy or cyclocryothermy for glaucoma, discission for a pupillary membrane, dissection or repeat penetrating keratoplasty for retrocorneal membrane, or vitrectomy of posterior pole fibrous ingrowth.

ENDOTHELIAL PROLIFERATION (DESCEMETIZATION)

Under the proper conditions, the normally staid corneal endothelium slides, divides, and transforms into fibroblastic or myoblastic tissue,

---

*References 115, 120, 133, 137, 150, 153, 170, 204, 208, 223, 236.

which can obliterate normal trabecular structure. This discussion of endothelial proliferation and descemetization of the anterior segment will be directed toward those clinical entities associated with secondary glaucoma.

Historical Background

The origin of the "glass membrane" on the iris surface of an eye with extensive anterior synechiae, first noted by Donders,[60] was elucidated by Wagenmann,[234] who identified the membrane as the product of proliferating corneal endothelial cells. The association of anterior synechiae and glass membranes of the iris surface in glaucomatous eyes was said to be "common"[160,161] earlier this century, but very little mention of this entity is found in the clinical literature.[103,230]

In one histopathologic study, 22 of 100 consecutive enucleated globes were found to have corneal endothelial overgrowth of the angle.[49] In another study, nearly half of 31 eyes enucleated for posttraumatic angle recession glaucoma demonstrated endothelization of the angle; one half of these had anterior synechiae, and one half did not.[124]

Clinical Spectrum

Descemet's tubes or glassy cones[230] are transparent tubes connecting the corneal endothelium with its scaffolding of vitreous or lens zonules. Associated with needling operations for congenital cataracts, perforating corneal injuries, or rarely, with cataract surgery, they are associated with nei-

ther anterior synechiae nor inevitable glaucoma.*

In contrast, sheetlike endothelial proliferation and migration across the trabecular meshwork has been described in numerous clinical entities often associated with glaucoma: blunt trauma, with or without angle recession;† perforating injury;[174,241,242] with anterior chamber IOLs;[143,182] with chronic iridocyclitis;[103,124] congenital glaucoma;[47] open-angle glaucoma;[175] anterior chamber cleavage syndromes;[9,49,86,118,176] with retinopathy of prematurity;[236] posterior polymorphous dystrophy;[180] iridocorneal endothelial syndromes, such as the iris nevus syndrome,[45,69,187,243] Chandler's syndrome,[162,172] and essential iris atrophy;[68,94,99,156,188] and with iris neovascularization in chronic retinal detachment,[98,242] in central retinal vein occlusion,[190] and in diabetic rubeosis iridis.[86,98,190] Discussion of the clinical and histopathologic features of many of these entities is found elsewhere in the text.

Pathophysiology

Corneal endothelium is derived from embryonic neural crest cells. It can undergo fibroblastic and myofibroblastic transformation. Corneal endothelial cells, unlike vascular endothelial cells, lack Weibel-Palade bodies (an ultrastructural marker for vascular endothelium) and are negative for factor VIII antigen.[194] The presence of both neuron-specific enolase and S-100 protein indicates the neuronal origin of the corneal endothelium.[194]

---

*References 59, 111, 119, 236, 240, 241.
†References 5, 98, 107, 109, 124, 239, 242.

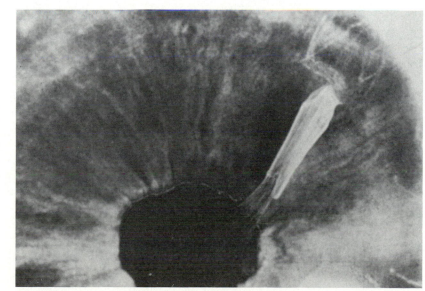

Fig. 73-25 Descemet's membrane tube in a man who had had multiple discissions for congenital cataract 60 years previously. A strand of vitreous is adherent to end of tube near pupil. (From Donaldson, DD, and Smith, TR: Trans Am Ophthalmol Soc 64:89, 1966. Used with the permission of the American Ophthalmological Society.)

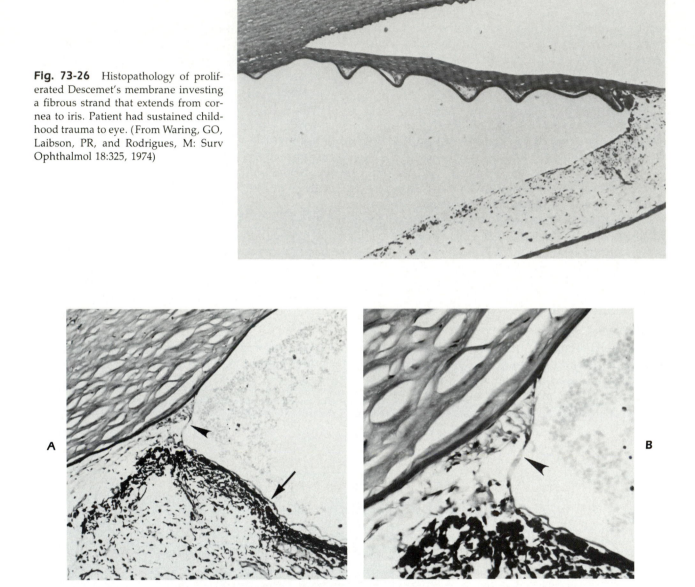

Fig. 73-26 Histopathology of proliferated Descemet's membrane investing a fibrous strand that extends from cornea to iris. Patient had sustained childhood trauma to eye. (From Waring, GO, Laibson, PR, and Rodrigues, M: Surv Ophthalmol 18:325, 1974)

Fig. 73-27 Iris neovascularization with endothelialization. **A,** Fibrovascular membrane (arrow) covering anterior iris surface and false angle formed by peripheral anterior synechiae. A single layer of cells (arrowhead) that is continuous with corneal endothelium extends across false angle and onto anterior iris surface. (Periodic acid-Schiff, ×100.) **B,** Higher magnification shows endothelial cells bridging false angle. (Periodic acid-Schiff, ×240). (From Harris, M, et al: Ophthalmology 91:1154, 1984)

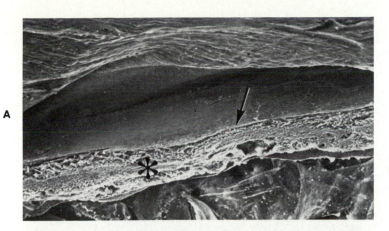

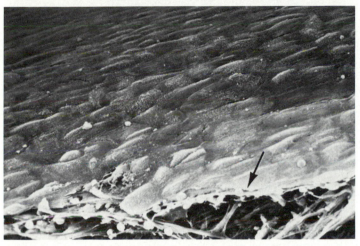

Fig. 73-28 Scanning electron microscopic appearance of anterior surface of iris. **A,** View showing cut surface of iris *(asterisk)* and cellular membrane on anterior iris surface *(arrow)*. (×57.) **B,** Higher power shows mosaic of endothelium on anterior iris surface. Arrow marks cut edge of membrane. (×570.) **C,** Transmission electron microscopy of false anterior chamber angle formed by peripheral anterior synechiae. Corneal endothelium *(arrow)* extends over false angle onto anterior iris surface *(arrowheads)* covered by thick fibrovascular membrane *(FM)*. *Asterisk,* Descemet's membrane. (×2500). (From Harris, M, et al: Ophthalmology 91:1154, 1984)

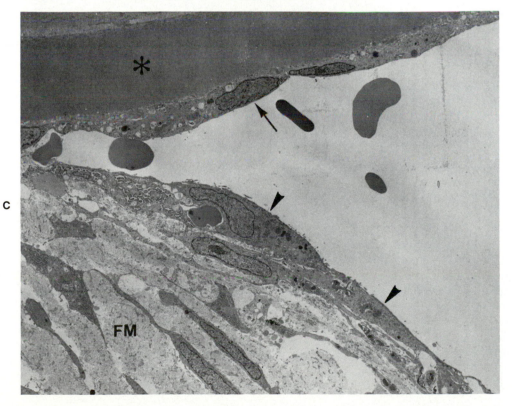

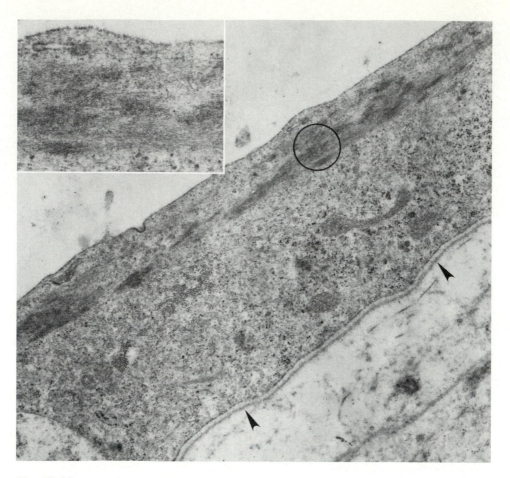

Fig. 73-29   Corneal endothelium on anterior iris surface with apical subplasmalemmal micro-filaments (measuring about 5 nm) with fusiform densities (*circle* and *inset*) and prominent basement membrane (*arrowheads*) (×30,000; inset ×50,000). (From Harris, M, Ophthalmology 91:1154, 1984)

Normally rarely mitotic in vivo,[16,35,43,232] with stimulation (surgical wound, inflammation, apposition of iris after injury to the cells) the endothelium undergoes mitotic cell divisions.[16] Waring reviewed the processes of endothelial proliferation, metaplasia, and elaboration of Descemet-like basement membrane.[236] The endothelium can regain a relatively normal appearance after the reparative process.

Light microscopic studies of endothelial proliferation typically show a fusiform proliferation of fibroblastic cells over the area of original injury, with extension of a fibroblastic cell layer, continuous with corneal endothelium, over the adjacent angle, and onto the iris. This layer can envelop broken ends of Descemet's membrane, scrolls of Descemet's membrane, foreign bodies, iris, ciliary body, zonules, vitreous and even extend onto the retina (Figs. 73-25 and 73-26).[236,241] Endothelial proliferation readily extends over a "false angle"

formed by peripheral anterior synechiae; however, in eyes with traumatic angle recession, PAS are not necessary for angle endothelization and subsequent glaucoma.[124] The layer of cells lining the angle and anterior iris can be thick and fibrovascular (Fig. 73-27).[98] There is a variable amount of basement membrane material subjacent to the metaplastic endothelial layer; generally, the younger the patient at the time of injury, the more exuberant the elaboration of a Descemet-like structure.[111]

An important insight into the processes involved in endothelialization of the angle, formation of anterior synechiae, and production of glaucoma was provided by Harris et al.[98] Ultrastructural studies of four eyes with either iris neovascularization or contusion injury demonstrated myofibrillar structures within metaplastic endothelial cells (Fig. 73-28). This myoblastic differentiation of endothelial cells not only helps explain their mobilization across an injured angle, but also the contractile quality of the proliferating tissue as it matures. Thus, the PAS seen in various clinical entities associated with endothelial proliferation may be the result of inflammatory scarring or of ectopic endothelial contraction. Fibrocytes of other origin besides the endothelium may contribute to the angle-closure process.

Management

Medical and surgical management of the myriad clinical entities associated with endothelial proliferation are detailed elsewhere in the text. Recent advances, such as local antimetabolite therapy in conjunction with glaucoma filtering procedures, the use of Nd:YAG laser trabeculoplasty, and goniosynechialysis may become standard in our armamentarium for treating these often difficult forms of glaucoma.

REFERENCES

1. Abbott, RL, and Spencer, WH: Epithelialization of the anterior chamber after transcorneal (McCannel) suture, Arch Ophthalmol 96:482, 1978
2. Alger, EM: Large implantation cyst of the iris treated by aspiration and injection of iodine, Arch Ophthalmol 7:984-986, 1932
3. Allen, JC: Epithelial and stromal ingrowths, Am J Ophthalmol 65:179-182, 1968
4. Allen, JC, and Duehr, PA: Sutures and epithelial downgrowth, Am J Ophthalmol 96:293-294, 1968
5. Alper, MG: Contusion angle deformity and glaucoma; gonioscopic observations and clinical course, Arch Ophthalmol 69:445-467, 1963
6. Arkin, W: Reverse experimental corneal transplantation, Post Okul 1:120-124, 1954
7. Avni, I, Blumenthal, M, and Belkin, M: Epithelial invasion of the anterior chamber following repeated keratoplasty, Metab Pediatr Syst Ophthalmol 6:337-341, 1982
8. Bacin, F, and Kantelip, B: Tentative de traitement des complications de l'invasion epitheliale par la valve de Krupin-Denver, Bull Soc Ophtalmol Fr 83:519-521, 1983
9. Ballantyne, AJ: Multiple congenital anomalies of the eyes, Proc R Soc Med 42:756-762, 1949
10. Bec, P, Philippot, AV, and Secheyron, P: La photocoagulation au laser des kystes de l'iris, Bull Soc Ophtalmol Fr 77:863-864, 1977
11. Bennett, T, and D'Amico, RA: Epithelial inclusion cyst of iris after keratoplasty, Am J Ophthalmol 77:87-89, 1971
12. Berliner, ML: Epithelial downgrowth into the anterior chamber, Am J Ophthalmol 34:899-900, 1951
13. Bernardino, VB, Kim, JC, and Smith, TR: Epithelialization of the anterior chamber after cataract extraction, Arch Ophthalmol 82:742-750, 1969
14. Bettman, JW Jr: Pathology of complications of intraocular surgery, Am J Ophthalmol 68:1037-1050, 1969
15. Bick, MN: Heparinization of the eye, Am J Ophthalmol 32:663-670, 1949
16. Binder, RF, and Binder, HF: Regenerative processes in the endothelium of the cornea, Arch Ophthalmol 57:11-13, 1957
17. Blodi, FC: Failures of cataract extractions and their pathologic explanation, J Iowa Med Soc 44:514-516, 1954
18. Blodi, FC: Causes and frequency of enucleation after cataract extraction, Int Ophthalmol Clin 5:257-269, 1965
19. Blomskold, G: Epitheleinwanderung in die vordere Augenkammer nach Katarakt Extraktion, Acta Ophthalmol 32:669-678, 1954
20. Bloomfield, SE, Jakobiec, FA, and Iwamoto, F: Fibrous ingrowth with retrocorneal membrane, Ophthalmology 88:459-465, 1981
21. Boruchoff, SA, Kenyon, KR, Foulks, GN, and Green, WR: Epithelial cyst of the iris following penetrating keratoplasty, Br J Ophthalmol 64:440-445, 1980
22. Brown, SI: Treatment of advanced epithelial downgrowth, Ophthalmology 77:618-622, 1973
23. Brown, SI: Results of excision of advanced epithelial downgrowth, Ophthalmology 86:321-328, 1979
24. Brown, SI, and Kitano, S: Pathogenesis of the retrocorneal membrane, Arch Ophthalmol 75:518-525, 1966
25. Bruner, WE, Green, WR, and Stark, WJ: A case of epithelial ingrowth primarily involving the lens capsule, Ophthalmic Surg 17:483-485, 1986
26. Bruner, WE, Michels, RG, Stark, WJ, and Maumenee, AE: Management of epithelial cysts of the anterior chamber, Ophthalmic Surg 12:279-285, 1981
27. Burris, TE, Rowsey, JJ, and Nordquist, RE: Model of epithelial downgrowth: II. Scanning and transmission electron microscopy of corneal epithelialization, Cornea 3:141-151, 1984
28. Burris, TE, Nordquist, RE, and Rowsey, JJ: Model of epithelial downgrowth: III. Scanning and transmission electron microscopy of iris epithelialization, Cornea 4:249-255, 1985
29. Bushmich, DG, and Stepanik, J: Clinical and morphologic investigation of retrocorneal membranes after keratoplasty, Oftalmol Zh 4:223, 1963
30. Calhoun, FP Jr: The clinical recognition and treatment of epithelialization of the anterior chamber following cataract extraction, Trans Am Ophthalmol Soc 47:498-553, 1949
31. Calhoun, FP Jr: An aid to the clinical diagnosis of epithelial downgrowth into the anterior chamber following cataract extraction, Am J Ophthalmol 61:1055-1059, 1966
32. Cameron, JD, Flaxman, BA, and Yanoff, M: In vitro studies of corneal wound healing: epithelial-

endothelial interactions, Invest Ophthalmol 13:575, 1974

33. Chailous, MJ: Traitement par l'électrolyse des kystes transparents de la chambre antérieure, Bull Soc Franc Ophthalmol 31:450-451, 1914

34. Chandler, PA, and Grant, WM: Lectures on glaucoma, Philadelphia, 1965, Lea & Febiger

35. Chi, HH, Teng, CC, and Katzin, HM: Healing progress in the mechanical denudation of the corneal endothelium, Am J Ophthalmol 49:693, 1960

36. Chi, HH, Teng, CC, and Katzin, HM: Histopathology of the corneal endothelium, Am J Ophthalmol 53:215-235, 1962

37. Christensen, L: Epithelialization of the anterior chamber. In Transactions of the New Orleans Academy of Ophthalmology: Symposium on cataracts, St Louis, 1965, The CV Mosby Co

38. Christensen, L: Pathogenesis of surgical complications—the role of fibroplasia. In Transactions of the New Orleans Academy of Ophthalmology, Symposium on cataracts, St Louis, 1965, The CV Mosby Co

39. Cibis, PA: Symposium: photocoagulation, Trans Am Acad Ophthalmol Otolaryngol 66:71, 1962

40. Cinotti, AA, and Jacobson, JH: Complications following cataract extraction, Am J Ophthalmol 36:929, 1953

41. Cleary, PE, Jarus, G, and Ryan, SJ: Experimental posterior penetrating eye injury in the rhesus monkey: vitreous-lens admixture, Br J Ophthalmol 64:801, 1980

42. Cleasby, GW: Photocoagulation of iris-ciliary body epithelial cysts, Trans Am Acad Ophthalmol Otolaryngol 75:638, 1971

43. Cogan, DG: Applied anatomy and physiology of the cornea, Ophthalmology 55:329, 1951

44. Cogan, DG: Experimental implants of conjunctiva into the anterior chamber, II, Am J Ophthalmol 39:165, 1955

45. Cogan, DG, and Reese, AB: A syndrome of iris nodules, ectopic Descemet's membrane, and unilateral glaucoma, Doc Ophthalmol 26:424-433, 1958

46. Collins, ET: Discussion on postoperative complications of cataract extraction, Trans Ophthalmol Soc UK 34:18, 1914

47. Collins, ET: The anatomy and pathology of the eye, Lancet 1:435, 1900

48. Collins, ET, and Cross, FR: Two cases of epithelial implantation cyst in the anterior chamber after extraction of cataract, Trans Ophthalmol Soc UK 12:175, 1892

49. Colosi, NJ, and Yanoff, M: Reactive corneal endothelialization, Am J Ophthalmol 83:219, 1977

50. Contreras, CF: Retrocorneal membranes. In Polack, FM, editor: Corneal and external diseases of the eye, Springfield, 1970, Charles C Thomas

51. Corrado, M: Glaucoma secondario a penetrazione e proliferazione di epitelio in c.a. in occhio operato di cataratta, Ann di Ottal e Clin Ocul 59:706, 1931

52. Coston, T: In discussion of Okun, E, and Mandell, A: Photocoagulation treatment of epithelial implantation cysts following cataract surgery, Trans Am Ophthalmol Soc 72:181, 1974

53. Cross, HE, and Maumenee, AE: Ocular trauma during aminocentesis, Arch Ophthalmol 90:303, 1973

54. Custodis, E: Ueber die Epithelauskleidung der Vorderkammer, Klin Monatsbl Augenheilkd 89:612, 1932

55. Davanger, M, and Olsen, EG: Experimental epithelial ingrowth. Epithelial/endothelial interaction through a corneal perforation, studied in organ culture, Acta Ophthalmol 63:443, 1985

56. Demeler, U, and Hinzpeter, EN: Fluoreszenzangiographische und histopathologische Befunde bei nicht pigmentierten und Iris, Klin Monatsbl Augenheilkd 172:720, 1978

57. Dixon, WS, and Speakman, JS: Epithelial downgrowth following cataract surgery. Cryotherapy for an intraocular foreign body, Arch Ophthalmol 84:303, 1970

58. Dollfus, MA, and Vail, D: Roentgen therapy of epithelial invasion of the anterior chamber, Trans Am Ophthalmol Soc 64:50, 1966

59. Donaldson, DD, and Smith, TR: Descemet's membrane tubes. Trans Am Ophthalmol Soc 64:89, 1966

60. Donders, FC: Beiträge zur pathologischen Anatomie des Auges. III. Neubildung von Glashäuten im Auge,v Graefes Arch Ophthalmol 3(pt 1):150, 1857

61. Dooremaal, JC: Die Entwickelung der in fremden Grund ver setzten lebenden Gewebe, Arch Ophthalmol 19:359, 1873

62. Duke-Elder, S: Textbook of ophthalmology, part VI: injuries. London, 1954, Henry Kimpton

63. Duke-Elder, S: System of ophthalmology, vol 14, part 1: injuries-mechanical, London, 1972, Henry Kimpton

64. Dunnington, JH: Ocular wound healing with particular reference to the cataract incision, Arch Ophthalmol 56:639, 1956

65. Dunnington, JH: Complications of wound healing after cataract surgery. In Haik, GM: Symposium on diseases and surgery of the lens, St Louis, 1957, The CV Mosby Co

66. Dunnington, JH, and Regan, EF: The effect of sutures and of thrombin upon ocular wound healing, Trans Am Acad Ophthalmol 55:761, 1951

67. Dunnington, JH, and Regan, EF: Absorbable sutures in cataract surgery, Arch Ophthalmol 50:545, 1953

68. Eagle, RC Jr, Font, RL, Yanoff, M, and Fine, BS: Proliferative endotheliopathy with iris abnormalities. The iridocorneal endothelial syndrome, Arch Ophthalmol 97:2104, 1979

69. Eagle, RC Jr, Font, RL, Yanoff, M, and Fine, BS: The iris naevus (Cogan-Reese) syndrome: light and electron microscopic onservations, Br J Ophthalmol 64:446, 1980

70. Eiferman, RA, and Rodrigues, MM: Squamous epithelial implantation cyst of the iris, Ophthalmology 88:1281, 1981

71. Elschnig, A: Epithelauskleidung der Vorder—und Hinterkammer als Ursache von Glaukom nach Staroperation, Klin Monatsbl Augenheilkd 41:247, 1903

72. Engel, HM, et al: Cytopreparatory techniques for eye fluid specimens obtained by vitrectomy, Acta Cytol (Baltimore) 26:551, 1982

73. Engel, HM, et al: Diagnostic vitrectomy, Retina 1:121, 1981

74. Farmer, SG, and Kalina, RE: Epithelial implantation cyst of the iris, Ophthalmology 88:1286, 1981

75. Fazakus, S: Epitheliosis of the anterior chamber of the eye following cataract operation, Orv Hetil 76:776, 1932

76. Feder, RS, and Krachmer, JH: The diagnosis of epithelial downgrowth after keratoplasty, Am J Ophthalmol 99:697, 1985

77. Ferry, AP: The possible role of epithelial-bearing surgical instruments in pathogenesis of epithelialization of the anterior chamber, Ann Ophthalmol 3:1089, 1971

78. Ferry, AP, and Naghdi, MR: Cryosurgical removal of epithelial cyst of iris and anterior chamber, Arch Ophthalmol 77:86, 1967

79. Fields, HM: Traumatic cyst of the iris, Am J Ophthalmol 26:193, 1943

80. Friedenwald, JS, and Bushke, W: Mitotic and wound healing activities of the corneal wound, Arch Ophthalmol 32:410, 1946

81. Friedman, AH: Radical anterior segment surgery for epithelial invasion of the anterior chamber: report of three cases, Trans Am Acad Ophthalmol Otolaryngol 83:216, 1977

82. Friedman, AH, and Henkind, P: Corneal stroma overgrowth after cataract extraction, Br J Ophthalmol 54:528, 1970

83. Fry, WE: In discussion of Perera, CA: Epithelium in the anterior chamber of the eye after operation and injury, Trans Am Acad Ophthalmol Otolaryngol 42:142, 1937

84. Fuchs, E: On keratoplasty, Z Augenheilkd 5:1, 1901

85. Fuchs, E: Textbook of ophthalmology, ed 8, Philadelphia, 1924, JB Lippincott Co

86. Gartner, S, Taffet, S, and Friedman, AH: The association of rubeosis iridis with endothelialisation of the anterior chamber; report of a clinical case with histopathological review of 16 additional cases, Br J Ophthalmol 61:267, 1977

87. Gifford, H: In discussion of Okun, E, and Mandell, A: Photocoagulation as a treatment of epithelial implantation cysts following cataract surgery, Trans Am Ophthalmol Soc 72:170, 1974

88. Girard, LJ, Nieves, R, and Hawkins, RS: Ultrasonic fragmentation for vitrectomy and associated surgical procedures, Trans Am Acad Ophthalmol Otolaryngol 81:432, 1976

89. Goldzieher, W: Ueber Implantationen in die vordere Augenkammer, Arch Exper Path Pharmakol 2:387-404, 1874

90. Gradle, HS: Conjunctival drain of the anterior chamber, Trans Soc Ophthalmol AMA 329, 1927

91. Green, WR: Diagnostic cytopathology of ocular fluid specimens, Ophthalmology 91:726, 1984

92. Guaita, M: Proliferation de l'endothélium cornéen sur l'iris et le champ pupillaire après l'extraction de la cataracte, Arch d'opht 13:507, 1893

93. Gundersen, T: Results of autotransplantation of cornea into the anterior chamber: their significance regarding corneal nutrition. Trans Am Ophthalmol Soc 36:207, 1938

94. Günther, G: Uber die Verdoppelung der Descemet'schen Membran. Beitrag über Anomalie der hinteren Glashaut der Cornea, Ophthalmologica 131:410, 1956

95. Hales, RH, and Spencer, WH: Unsuccessful penetrating keratoplasties. Correlation of clinical and histologic findings, Arch Ophthalmol 70:805, 1963

96. Handmann, M: Disparition complète d'un Kyste traumatique de l'iris après roentgenthérapie, Klin Monatsld Augenheilkd 72:111, 1924

97. Harbin, TS Jr, and Maumenee, AE: Epithelial downgrowth after surgery for epithelial cyst, Am J Ophthalmol 78:1, 1974

98. Harris, M, et al: Corneal endothelial overgrowth of angle and iris, Ophthalmology 91:1154, 1984

99. Heath, P: Essential atrophy of the iris: a histopathologic study, Trans Am Ophthalmol Soc 51:167, 1953

100. Henderson, JW: In discussion of Okun, E, and Mandell, A: Photocoagulation as a treatment of epithelial implantation cysts following cataract surgery, Trans Am Ophthal Soc 72:179, 1974

101. Henderson, T: A histological study of the normal healing of wounds after cataract extraction, Ophthalmology Review 26:127, 1907

102. Henderson, T: Postoperative complications of cataract extraction, Trans Ophthalmol Soc UK 34:88, 1914

103. Herbert, H: Glass membrane foration in chronic iridocyclitis, Trans Ophthalmol Soc UK 47:155, 1927

104. Hogan, MJ, and Goodner, EK: Surgical treatment of epithelial cysts of the anterior chamber, Arch Ophthalmol 64:286, 1960

105. Hosch, F: Experimentelle Studien ueber Iriscysten, Virchows Arch [A] 99:448, 1885

106. Irvine, AR: Round table discussion. In Transactions of the New Orleans Academy of Ophthalmology: Symposium on cataracts, St Louis, 1965, The CV Mosby Co

107. Iwamoto, T, and DeVoe, AG: Electron microscopic studies on Fuchs' combined dystrophy. I. Posterior portion of the cornea, Invest Ophthalmol 10:9, 1971

108. Iwamoto, T, Srinivasan, BD, and DeVoe, AG: Electron microscopy of epithelial downgrowth, Ann Ophthalmol 9:1095, 1977

109. Iwamoto, T, Witmer, R, and Landolt, E: Light and electron microscopy in absolute glaucoma with pigment dispersion phenomena and contusion angle deformity, Am J Ophthalmol 72:420, 1971

110. Jaffe, NS: Epithelial invasion of the anterior chamber. In Jaffe, NS: Cataract surgery and its complications, St Louis, 1981, The CV Mosby Co

111. Jaffe, NS: Corneal endothelial proliferation. In Jaffe, NS: Cataract surgery, St Louis, 1984, The CV Mosby Co

112. Jenson, P, Minckler, DS, and Chandler, JW: Epithelial ingrowth, Arch Ophthalmol 95:837, 1977

113. Kara, GB: Histologic appearance of an eye four days after cataract extraction, Arch Ophthalmol 49:285, 1953

114. Kennedy, PJ: Treatment of cysts of the iris with electrolysis, Arch Ophthalmol 55:522, 1956

115. Kenyon, DR, Stark, WJ, and Stone, DL: Corneal endothelial degeneration and fibrous proliferation after pars plana vitrectomy, Am J Ophthalmol 81:486, 1976

116. Kerby, DB: Discussion of Vail D: Treatment of cysts of the iris with diathermy coagulation, Trans Am Ophthalmol Soc 51:380, 1953

117. Kinoshita, A: A case of traumatic iris cyst, Folia Ophthalmol Jpn 18:776, 1967

118. Koucek, F: The corneal endothelium, Acta Univ Carol [Med] (Praha) 13:321, 1967

119. Kroll, AJ: Proliferation of Descemet's membrane, Arch Ophthalmol 82:339, 1969

120. Kurz, GH, and D'Amico, RA: Histopathology of corneal graft failures, Am J Ophthalmol 66:184, 1968

121. Kuwabara, T, Quevedo, AR, and Cogan, DG: An experimental study of dichloroethane poisoning, Arch Ophthalmol 79:321, 1968

122. Laflamme, MY: L'invasion epitheliale de la chambre antérieure: à propos de 8 cas opérés selon la technique de Maumenee, Can J Ophthalmol 11:17, 1976

123. Laing, RA, Sandstorm, MM, Leibowitz, HM, and Berrospi, AR: Epithelialization of the anterior chamber: clinical investigation with the specular microscope, Arch Ophthalmol 97:1870, 1979

124. Lauring, L: Anterior chamber glass membranes, Am J Ophthalmol 68:308, 1969

125. Layden, WE, Torczynski, E, and Font, RL: Mucogenic glaucoma and goblet cell cyst of the anterior chamber, Arch Ophthalmol 96:2259, 1978

126. Leibowitz, HM, Elliott, JH, and Boruchoff, SA: Epithelialization of the anterior chamber following penetrating keratoplasty, Arch Ophthalmol 78:613, 1967

127. Leigh, AG: Complications of corneal grafting, Int Ophthalmol Clin 2:776, 1962

128. L'Esperance, FA: Ocular photocoagulation: an atlas, St Louis, 1975, The CV Mosby Co

129. Levkoieva, E: The regeneration of wounds of external membrane of the eye in the light of new pathologico-anatomical results, Br J Ophthalmol 31:336, 1947

130. Long, JC, and Tyner, GS: Three cases of epithelial invasion of the anterior chamber treated surgically, Arch Ophthalmol 58:396, 1957

131. MacKenzie, W: A practical treatise on the diseases of the eye, London, 1830, Longman, Rees, Orme, Brown & Green

132. Mann, I: A study of epithelial regeneration on some experimental variables on the epithelial movements in the healing of corneal wounds, Br J Ophthalmol 28:26, 1944

133. Matsuda, H, and Smelser, GK: Endothelial cells in akali-burned corneas. Ultrastructural alterations, Arch Ophthalmol 89:402, 1973

134. Matsumoto, S: Contribution to the study of epithelial movement: the corneal epithelium of the frog in tissue culture, J Exp Zool 26:545, 1918

135. Maumenee, AE: Epithelial invasion of the anterior chamber, Trans Am Acad Ophthalmol Otolaryngol 61:51, 1957

136. Maumenee, AE: Treatment of epithelial downgrowth and intraocular fistula following cataract extraction, Trans Am Ophthalmol Soc 62:153, 1964

137. Maumenee, AE: Histopathology of corneal grafts. In King, JH, Metigue, JW, (editors): The Cornea World Congress, Washington DC, 1965, Butterworth

138. Maumenee, AE: In Emery, DM, and Paton, D, editors: Current concepts in cataract surgery. Selected proceedings of the Third Biennial Cataract Surgical Congress, St Louis, 1974, The CV Mosby Co

139. Maumenee, AE, Paton, D, Morse, PH, and Butner, R: Review of 40 histologically proven cases of epithelial downgrowth following cataract extraction and suggested surgical management, Am J Ophthalmol 69:598, 1970

140. Maumenee, AE, and Shannon, CR: Epithelial invasion of the anterior chamber, Am J Ophthalmol 41:929, 1956

141. Mazow, ML, and Stephens, RW: An unusual complication after keratoplasty, Surv Ophthalmol 11:205, 1966

142. McDonnell, PJ, de la Cruz, ZC, and Green, WR: Vitreous incarceration complicating cataract surgery, Ophthalmology 93:247, 1986

143. McDonnell, PJ, Green, WR, Maumenee, AE, and Iliff, WJ: Pathology of intraocular lenses in 33 eyes examined postmortem, Ophthalmology 90:386, 1983

144. McLean, J: Discussion of Maumenee AE: Treatment of epithelial downgrowth and intraocular fistula following cataract extraction, Trans Am Ophthalmol Soc 62:164, 1964

145. Meller, J: Ueber Epitheleinsenkung und Cystenbildung im Auge, Arch F Ophth 52:436, 1901

146. Merenmies, L, and Tarkhanen, A: Causes of enucleation following cataract surgery, Acta Ophthalmol 55:347, 1977

147. Meyer-Schwickerath, G: Light coagulation, St Louis, 1960, The CV Mosby Co

148. Meyer-Schwickerath, G: Discussion of Maumenee AE: Treatment of epithelial downgrowth and intraocular fistula following cataract extraction, Trans Am Ophthalmol Soc 62:165, 1964

149. Michels, RG: Vitreous surgery, St Louis, 1981, The CV Mosby Co

150. Michels, RG, Kenyon, KR, and Maumenee, AE: Retrocorneal fibrous membrane, Invest Ophthalmol 11:822, 1972

151. Michels, RG, and Rice, TR: Internal-external bimanual bipolar diathermy for treatment of bleeding from the anterior chamber angle, Am J Ophthalmol 83:873, 1977

152. Mochizuki, K, Murakomi, M, and Kitano, S: Experimental studies on burns of the cornea. Report I. Histological findings on burns of the cornea with NaOH and HCL, Acta Soc Ophthalmol Jpn 71:1112, 1967

153. Morton, PL, Ormsby, HL, and Basu, PK: Healing of endothelium and Descemet's membrane of rabbit cornea, Am J Ophthalmol 6:62, 1958

154. Moschos, M, Baltatzis, S, and Theodosiadis, G: Traitement des kystes epitheliaux de l'iris par le laser, J Fr Ophtalmol 2:539, 1979

155. Naumann, G, and Volcker, HE: Block Exzision intraokularer Prozesse. II. Epithelein Wachsung in das vordere Augensegment, Klin Monatsbl Augenheilkd 166:448, 1975

156. Oh, JO: Changes with age in the corneal endothelium of normal rabbits, Acta Ophthalmol 41:568, 1963

157. Okun, E, and Mandell, A: Photocoagulation treatment of epithelial implantation cysts following cataract surgery, Trans Am Ophthalmol Soc 72:170, 1974

158. Otradovec, J, and Zicha, Z: Epithelial invasion into the anterior chamber after cataract extraction, Cesk Oftalmol 16:131, 1960

159. Papolczy, F: Partielle Epithelauskleidung der vorder Kammer nach graefescher Starextraktion, Klin Monatsbl Augenheilkd 84:266, 1930

160. Parsons, J: The Pathology of the Eye, vol I, New York, 1904, GP Putnam's Sons

161. Parsons, JH: The pathology of the eye, London, 1904, Hodder & Stroughton

162. Patel, A, et al: Clinicopathologic features of Chandler's syndrome, Surv Ophthalmol 27:327, 1983

163. Patz, A, Wulff, L, and Rogers, S: Experimental production of epithelial invasion of the anterior chamber, Am J Ophthalmol 47:815, 1959

164. Paufique, L, and Hervouet, F: L'invasion epitheliale de la chambre antérieure après l'opération de cataracte, American Oculist 197:105, 1964

165. Payne, BF, Simonton, JT, and Cury, D: Some causes of enucleation after cataract extraction, Trans Am Ophthalmol Soc 53:231, 1955

166. Perera, CA: Epithelium in the anterior chamber of the eye after operation and injury, Ophthalmology 42:142, 1937

167. Pincus, MH: Epithelial invasion of the anterior chamber following cataract extraction: effect of radiation therapy, Arch Ophthalmol 43:509, 1950

168. Pischel, DK: Symposium: photocoagulation, Trans Am Acad Ophthalmol Otolaryngol 66:70, 1962

169. Polack, FM: Clinical and pathologic aspects of the corneal graft reaction, Ophthalmology 77:418, 1973

170. Polack, FM, and Kanai, A: Electron microscopic studies of graft endothelium in corneal graft rejection, Am J Ophthalmol 73:711, 1972

171. Puck, A, Tso, MO, and Yue, B: Cellular deposits on intraocular lenses, Acta Ophthalmol [Suppl] (Copenh) 170:54, 1985

172. Quigley, HA, and Forster, RF: Histopathology of cornea and iris in Chandler's syndrome, Arch Ophthalmol 96:1878, 1978

173. Ranvier, ML: Une théorie nouvelle sur la cicatrisation et le role de epithelium antérieur de la cornée dans le guérison des plaies de cette membrane, Compt Rend Acad Sci 123:1228, 1896

174. Redslob, E, and Brini, A: Proliferations de l'endothelium cornéen et de la membrane de Descemet, Ann Ocul 186:969, 1953

175. Reese, AB: Deep-chamber glaucoma due to the formation of a cuticular product in the filtration angle, Am J Ophthalmol 27:1193, 1944

176. Reese, AB, and Ellsworth, RM: The anterior chamber cleavage syndrome, Arch Ophthalmol 75:307, 1966

177. Regan, EF: Epithelial invasion of the anterior chamber, Arch Ophthalmol 60:907, 1958

178. Reid, C: cited by Duke-Elder S: Textbook of ophthalmology, vol 3, St Louis, 1941, The CV Mosby Co

179. Rice, TA, and Michels, RG: Current surgical management of vitreous wick syndrome, Am J Ophthalmol 85:656, 1978

180. Rodrigues, MM, et al: Glaucoma due to endothelialization of the anterior chamber angle; a comparison of posterior polymorphous dystrophy of the cornea and Chandler's syndrome, Arch Ophthalmol 98:688, 1980

181. Rothmund, A: Ueber Cysten der Regenbogen haut, Klin Monatsbl Augenheilkd 10:189, 1872

182. Rowsey, JJ, and Gayler, JR: Intraocular lens disasters: peripheral anterior synechia, Ophthalmology 87:646, 1980

183. Rycroft, PV: Corneal graft membranes, Trans Ophthalmol Soc UK 85:317, 1965

184. Salus, R: Geheilte Epithelaus-Kleidung der Vorderkammer, Klin Monatsbl Augenheilkd 78:368, 1927

185. Samples, JR, and Van Buskirk, EM: Epithelial ingrowth on an intraocular lens, Ophthalmic Surg 15:869, 1984

186. Sannwald, PM, and Knobel, HH: Zur Entstehung der retrokornealen Membran nach Trauma, Klin Monatsbl Augenheilkd 183:28, 1983

187. Scheie, HG, and Yanoff, M: Iris nevus (Cogan-Reese) syndrome; a cause of unilateral glaucoma, Arch Ophthalmol 93:963, 1975

188. Scheie, HG, Yanoff, M, and Kellogg, WT: Essential iris atrophy; report of a case, Arch Ophthalmol 94:1315, 1976

189. Scholz, RT, and Kelley, JS: Argon laser photocoagulation treatment of iris cysts following penetrating keratoplasty, Arch Ophthalmol 100:926, 1982

190. Schulze, RR: Rubeosis iridis, Am J Ophthalmol 63:487, 1967

191. Schulze, RR, and Duke, JR: Causes of enucleation following cataract extraction, Arch Ophthalmol 73:74, 1965

192. Schweninger, E: Ueber Transplantation und Implantation von Haaren, Ztschr Biol 11:341, 1875

193. Shaffer, RN: Alpha irradiation. Effect of astatine on the anterior segment and on an epithelial cyst, Trans Am Ophthalmol Soc 50:607, 1952

194. Shamsuddin, AKM, Nirankari, V, Purnell, DM, and Chang, SH: Is the corneal posterior cell layer truly endothelial? Ophthalmology 93:1298, 1986

195. Sherrard, ES, and Rycroft, PV: Retrocorneal membranes. I. Their origin and structure, Br J Ophthalmol 51:379, 1967

196. Sherrard, ES, and Rycroft, PV: Retrocorneal membranes. II. Factors influencing their growth, Br J Ophthalmol 51:387, 1967

197. Shields, JA: Primary cysts of the iris, Trans Am Ophthalmol Soc 79:771, 1981

198. Shields, JA, Sanborn, GE, and Augsburger, JJ: The differential diagnosis of malignant melanoma of the iris. A clinical study of 200 patients, Ophthalmology 90:716, 1983

199. Sidrys, LA, and Demong, T: Epithelial downgrowth after penetrating keratoplasty, Can J Ophthalmol 17:29, 1982

200. Silbert, AM, and Boum, JL: Origin of the retrocorneal membrane in the rabbit, Arch Ophthalmol 97:1141, 1979

201. Sitchevska, O, and Payne, BF: Pearl cysts of the iris, Am J Ophthalmol 34:833, 1951

202. Smith, DR, Somerville, GM, and Shew, M: An experimental model of epithelialization of the anterior chamber, Can J Ophthalmol 2:158, 1967

203. Smith, RE, and Parrett, C: Specular microscopy of epithelial downgrowth, Arch Ophthalmol 96:1222, 1978

204. Snip, RC, Kenyon, ER, and Green, WR: Retrocorneal fibrous membrane in the vitreous touch syndrome, Am J Ophthalmol 79:233, 1975

205. Speciale-Cirincione, F: Glaucoma provoked by epithelial chamber investment of the anterior chamber following cataract operation, Atti d Cong Soc ital oftal 180, 1924

206. Stark, WJ: Management of epithelial ingrowth and cysts, Dev Ophthalmol 5:64, 1981

207. Stark, WJ, Michels, RG, Maumenee, AE, and Cupples, H: Surgical management of epithelial ingrowth, Am J Ophthalmol 85:772, 1978

208. Sternberg, PJ, Hatchell, DL, Foulks, GN, and Landers, MB III: The effect of silicone oil on the cornea, Arch Ophthalmol 103:90, 1985

209. Sugar, A, Meyer, RF, and Hood, CI: Epithelial downgrowth following penetrating keratoplasty in the aphake, Arch Ophthalmol 95:464, 1977

210. Sugar, HS: Further experience with posterior lamellar resection of the cornea for epithelial implantation cyst, Am J Ophthalmol 64:291, 1967

211. Sullivan, GL: Treatment of epithelization of the anterior chamber following cataract extraction, Trans Ophthalmol Soc UK 87:835, 1968

212. Suzuki, J: Experimentelle Studien ueber die Entstekung der traumatischen seroesen Iriscysten, Acta Soc Ophth [Suppl] 34:107, 1930

213. Swan, KC: Some contemporary concepts of scleral disease, Arch Ophthalmol 45:630, 1951

214. Swan, KC: Fibroblastic ingrowth following cataract extraction, Arch Ophthalmol 89:445, 1973

215. Swan, KC: Epithelial cell cysts of the anterior chamber treated by acid injections, Doc Ophthalmol 18:363, 1979

216. Swan, KC, and Christensen, L: The half-lap incision and closure in cataract surgery, Am J Ophthalmol 61:1330, 1966

217. Tanew, N: cited in Calhoun FP: The clinical recognition and treatment of epithelialization of the anterior chamber following cataract extraction, Trans Am Ophthalmol Soc 47:498, 1949

218. Terry, TL, Chisholm, JF, and Schonberg, AL: Studies on surface epithelium invasion of the anterior segment of the eye, Am J Ophthalmol 22:1083, 1939

219. Theobald, GD, and Haas, JS: Epithelial invasion of the anterior chamber following cataract extraction, Ophthalmology 52:470, 1948

220. Thilliez: Traitement des kystes de l'iris par l'électrolyse, Bull Soc Franc Ophthalmol 25:490, 1908

221. Thomas, CI: The cornea, Springfield, IL, 1955, Charles C Thomas

222. Townes, CD, Moran, CT, and Pfingst, HA: Complications of cataract surgery, Trans Am Ophthalmol Soc 49:91, 1951

223. Townsend, WM, and Kaufman, HE: Pathogenesis of glaucoma and endothelial changes in herpetic keratouveitis, Am J Ophthalmol 71:904, 1971

224. Vail, D: Epithelial downgrowth into the anterior chamber following cataract extraction: arrest by radium treatment, Arch Ophthalmol 15:270, 1936

225. Vail, D: Discussion of of Perera CA: Epithelium in the anterior chamber of the eye after operation and injury, Ophthalmology 42:163, 1937

226. Vail, D: Treatment of cysts of the iris with diathermy coagulation, Trans Am Ophthalmol Soc 51:371, 1953

227. Velter, SL: Pathologic anatomy of corneal transplantation in man, Zbl Ges Ophthal 46:532, 1941

228. Verrey, F: Cytologie de l'humeur aqueuse et invasion epitheliale de la chambre antérieure, Ophthalmologica 154:310, 1967

229. Voerhoff, A: In discussion of Vail, D: Epithelial downgrowth into the anterior chamber following cataract extraction arrested by radiation treatment, Trans Am Ophthalmol Soc 33:306, 1935

230. Vogt, A: Lehrbuch und Atlas der Spaltlampenmikroskopie des legenden Auges mit Anleitung zur Technik und Methodik der Untersuchung. Hornhaut und Vorderkammer, vol 1, Berlin, 1930, Julius Springer Verlag

231. Volcker, HE, and Naumann, GO: Exzentrische tektorrische mini-Keratoplastik bei kernealen, korneoskleralen und skleralen Prozessen, Klin Monatsbl Augenheilkd 185:158, 1984

232. von Sallman, L, Caravaggio, LL, and Grimes, P: Studies on the corneal endothelium of the rabbit. I. Cell division and growth, Am J Ophthalmol 51:955, 1961

233. Wadsworth, JAC: Complication following cataract extraction, Am J Ophthalmol 37:672, 1954

234. Wagenmann, A: Weitre Mittheilungen über Glashäutige Neubildungen an der Descemet'schen Membran und auf der Iris und über Veränderungen des Hornhautendothels, v Graefes Arch Klin Exp Ophthalmol 38:90, 1892

235. Waring, GO: Posterior collagenous layer of the cornea, Arch Ophthalmol 100:122, 1982

236. Waring, GO, Laibson, PR, and Rodrigues, M: Clinical and pathologic alteration of Descemet's membrane: with emphasis on endothelial metaplasia, Surv Ophthalmol 18:325, 1974

237. Werb, A: The postgraft membrane, Int Ophthalmol Clin 2:771, 1962

238. Wilson, W: Iris cyst treated by electrolysis, Br J Ophthalmol 48:45, 1964

239. Wolff, SM, and Zimmerman, LE: Chronic secondary glaucoma associated with retrodisplacement of iris root and deepening of the anterior chamber angle secondary to contusion, Am J Ophthalmol 54:547, 1962

240. Wolter, JR: Descemet's membrane tubes on the zonular fibers of the lens, J Pediatr Ophthalmol 6:153, 1969

241. Wolter, JR: The histopathology of Descemet's membrane tubes, J Pediatr Ophthalmol 9:39, 1972

242. Wolter, JR, and Fechner, PU: Glass membranes on the anterior iris surface, Am J Ophthalmol 53:235, 1962

243. Wolter, JR, and Makley, TA Jr: Cogan-Reese syndrome; formation of a glass membrane on an iris nevus clinically simulating tumor growth, J Pediatr Ophthalmol 9:102, 1972

244. Wright, RE: Cyst of the iris, Br J Ophthalmol 9:454, 1925

245. Yamaguchi, T, Polack, FM, and Valenti, J: Electron microscopic study of epithelial downgrowth after penetrating keratoplasty, Br J Ophthalmol 65:374, 1981

246. Zavala, EY, and Binder, PS: The pathologic findings of epithelial ingrowth, Arch Ophthalmol 98:2007, 1980

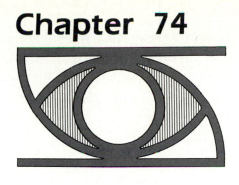

Chapter 74

Glaucoma Associated with Penetrating Keratoplasty

Randall J. Olson
Julie S. Lee
Thom J. Zimmerman

For many years very little was known about the intraocular pressure after penetrating keratoplasty, mainly because there was no accurate technique for determining the intraocular pressure in corneal graft patients. With the development of electronic applanation tonometers, studies in the late 1960s suggested that the intraocular pressure can sometimes be very high after keratoplasty[8] (Table 74-1). Initially, no obvious cause was apparent, but it was noted that the postoperative pressure elevation tended to occur most often in aphakic patients.

Postkeratoplasty glaucoma is defined as an acutely elevated intraocular pressure after penetrating keratoplasty, with or without optic nerve and visual field changes. In some patients this acute rise in intraocular pressure persists to become a chronic problem.

Table 74-1 Comparison of groups in study of intraocular pressure the first week after penetrating keratoplasty

Patient group	No. of patients	Average age (years)	Average maximum intraocular pressure (mm Hg)
Phakic	16	33	24
Aphakic	18	70	40
Lens extraction and keratoplasty	10	70	50

From Irvine, AR, and Kaufman, HE: Am J Ophthalmol 68:835, 1969

CLINICAL PRESENTATION

Postkeratoplasty glaucoma usually presents with a clear graft, which is thinner than a graft in an eye with a normal intraocular pressure. However, this presentation is dependent on an otherwise normal donor epithelium (Table 74-2).[13] The intraocular pressure is markedly elevated to levels between 40 and 50 mm Hg.

In the early postoperative period, postkeratoplasty glaucoma, especially in the aphakic eye, usually responds very poorly to medical therapy.[15] Although the elevated pressure usually resolves spontaneously by the end of the first postoperative week, it can become a chronic problem.

The extremely high postoperative pressure may be caused by angle-closure, which is often difficult to diagnose in postkeratoplasty patients. The peripheral cornea (recipient bed) is often distorted and edematous, resulting in a limited and distorted gonioscopic examination.

MECHANISMS OF SECONDARY GLAUCOMA

Frequently encountered causes of elevated intraocular pressure following penetrating keratoplasty include
1. Preexisting glaucoma
2. Distortion of the trabecular meshwork
3. Angle-closure
4. Postoperative inflammation
5. Retention of a viscoelastic substance
6. Malignant (ciliary block) glaucoma

Table 74-2 Results for all patients studied

	Group 1*		Group 2*		Combined groups 1 and 2	
	High pressure range	Low pressure range	High pressure range	Low pressure range	High pressure range	Low pressure range
No. of measurements	20	20	39	39	59	59
No. of patients	14	14	29	29	43	43
Mean intraocular pressure	48.4	21.2	31.1	17.7	36.9	18.9
with standard deviation (mm Hg)	±15.4	±12.2	±9.1	±8.6	±14.1	±10.0
Mean corneal thickness	0.587	0.631	0.611	0.636	0.601	0.635
with standard deviation (mm)	± 0.078	±0.084	±0.089	±0.096	±0.085	±0.091
P value for corneal thickness	.025		.031		.012	

From Olson, RJ, and Kaufman, HE: Am J Ophthalmol 86:97, 1978
*Group 1: patients with IOP ≥ 20 mm Hg during first postoperative week; group 2: patients with IOP 10 to 19 mm Hg during first postoperative week.

Table 74-3 Effect of suture placement on outflow facility*: combined penetrating keratoplasty and cataract extraction on eye bank eyes

Experiment no.	Baseline	Outflow facility, μl/min/mm Hg	
		Through-and-through suture	Conventional depth suture
1	0.35	0.42	0.25
2	0.28	0.41	0.12
3	0.61	0.58	0.42
4	0.25	0.16	0.10
5	0.24	0.48	0.15
6	0.21	0.28	0.15
7	0.14	0.18	0.11
Mean	0.30	0.36	0.19†
SEM	±0.06	±0.06	±0.04

From Zimmerman, TJ, Krupin, T, Grodzki, W, and Waltman, SR: Arch Ophthalmol 96:505, 1978
*Measured by constant pressure perfusion at 20 mm Hg.
†Significant change from baseline value, paired-t $p < 0.005$.

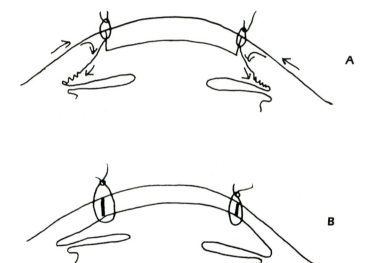

Fig. 74-1 Penetrating keratoplasty in aphakic eyes. **A,** Conventional sutures with posterior gape. **B,** Through-and-through sutures preserving the integrity of the anterior support. (From Zimmerman, TJ, et al: Ann Ophthalmol 11:809, 1979)

7. Enzyme glaucoma
8. Steroid-induced glaucoma

These different mechanisms must be recognized and treated appropriately. Many of these problems are not unique to keratoplasty and are discussed in detail in other chapters. The discussion in this chapter will concentrate on the mechanisms of intraocular pressure elevation that appear to be directly related to the corneal graft procedure.

Distortion of the Trabecular Meshwork

Research by Zimmerman et al.[23] on perfused human autopsy eyes, suggested that alterations occur in the aqueous outflow apparatus of aphakic eyes that lead to a decrease in outflow facility (Table 74-3). Collapse of the trabecular meshwork was proposed as the mechanism of outflow obstruction. The decrease in outflow obstruction in perfused eyes was greater after the lens was removed. This suggested that aphakia resulted in a greater loss of posterior support (especially after intracapsular cataract surgery) for the trabecular meshwork and/or Schlemm's canal, which could account for the higher occurrence of glaucoma after aphakic corneal transplantation.

Zimmerman et al.[23] suggested that through-and-through sutures might alleviate the loss of pos-

Table 74-4 Intraocular pressure in aphakic eyes after penetrating keratoplasty

Patient	Preoperative IOP (mm Hg)	Postoperative IOP (mm Hg) Day 1	Day 2	Day 3	Day 4	Day 5	1 month
CONVENTIONAL SUTURING							
1	16	50 D*	55	50	46	40	14
2	19	42	60 N†	29	40	—	24
3	16	39	44 D*	32	22	—	20
4	21	34	33	—	45 N†	35	22
5	20	22	18	—	21	18	20
6	17	28	36 N†	26	28	32	30
7	17	45 D*	38	32	40	40	38
8	17	46	47 N†	40	37	—	28
9	16	40	42 D*	30	42	30	28
10	24	26	14	18	20	—	—
11	18	28	35	22	14	—	17
12	19	26	33	37 N†	26	—	26
13	17	50 N†	50	42	32	33	26
14	18	40	25	20	35	36	23
15	20	35	50 N†	38	40	36	16
Mean	18.33	36.73	38.67	32.00	32.53	33.33	23.75
SEM	±0.58	±2.36	±3.38	±2.58	±2.61	±2.22	±1.69
THROUGH-AND-THROUGH SUTURING							
1	18	29	27	28	28	—	24
2	17	24	18	18	40	39	24
3	16	27	30	24	22	—	20
4	18	15	19	16	18	18	‡
5	18	8	20	18	22	20	18
6	14	24	22	28	26	24	25
7	17	27	24	16	16	—	15
8	16	18	34	300	27	—	26
9	17	17	20	20	32	24	19
10	17	28	—	28	26	30	30
Mean	16.8	21.70	23.78	22.60	25.70	25.83	22.33
SEM	±0.39	±2.18	±1.83	±1.77	±2.19	±3.12	±1.55

From Zimmerman, TJ, Waltman, SR, Sachs, U, and Kaufman, HE: Ophthalmic Surg 10:49, 1979
*Acetazolamide (Diamox) regimen begun and continued throughout the study.
†Methazolamide (Neptazane) regimen begun and continued throughout the study.
‡Regrafted at 10 days postoperatively because of graft failure which was thought to be unrelated to the suturing technique.

terior support to the trabecular outflow channels (Fig. 74-1). A clinical study did indeed show a marked reduction in the occurrence of glaucoma after aphakic keratoplasty when through-and-through sutures were used (Table 74-4).[26] This study was discontinued, however, when it was found that a number of the patients had persistent aqueous leakage around the through-and-through suture tracks, which could have been the mechanism for the reduced intraocular pressure. Zimmerman et al.[24] showed in perfused aphakic human autopsy eyes that a donor button 0.5 mm larger than the recipient bed had the same effect as through-and-through sutures in preventing the loss of posterior trabecular support. The decrease in outflow facility in eyes with the larger donor buttons was less than in eyes with same-sized grafts (Table 74-5).

Table 74-5 The effect of a larger corneal button on outflow facility in aphakic penetrating keratoplasty

Experiment number	Outflow facility (µl/min/mm Hg)* Baseline	Postoperative
1	0.26	0.22
2	0.27	0.30
3	0.51	0.50
4	0.24	0.25
5	0.15	0.16
6	0.26	0.28
Mean ± SD	0.28 ± .12	0.29 ± .12

From Zimmerman, TJ, et al: Ann Ophthalmol 11:809, 1979
*Outflow facility measured by constant pressure perfusion at 20 mm Hg on human eye bank eyes.

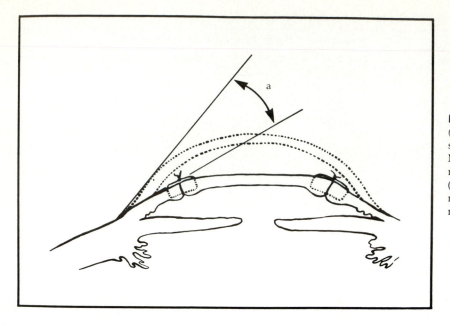

Fig. 74-2   Change in corneolimbal angle *(a)* after penetrating keratoplasty using same-sized donor button as recipient bed. Note crowding of iridocorneal angle, which may cause decrease in outflow facility. (From Zimmerman, TJ, Olson, RJ, Waltman, SR, and Kaufman, HE: Arch Ophthalmol 96:2231, 1978)

Fig. 74-3   Relationship of wound compression and angle (12.0 mm corneal diameter). (From Olson, RJ, and Kaufman, HE: Invest Ophthalmol Vis Sci 16:1085, 1977)

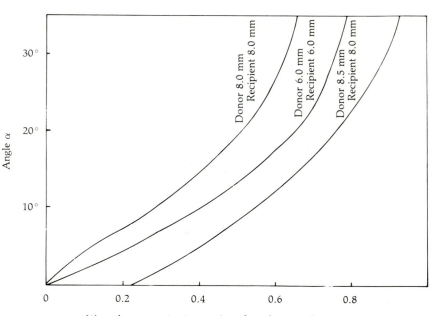

Wound compression in mm (equal on donor and recipient side)

Olson and Kaufman[12] used mathematical modeling to suggest that in aphakic keratoplasty with tight sutures, distortion of the angle resulted in decreased outflow facility (Figs. 74-2 and 74-3). The exact mechanism for the angle distortion was not apparent, although it seemed to be minimized by using the larger donor corneal button.

Based on the previous observations, a prospective, randomized clinical trial was carried out[25] (Tables 74-6 to 74-9). This study revealed a marked decrease in the postoperative intraocular pressure elevation in aphakic eyes when a donor button 0.5 mm larger in diameter than the recipient bed was used, as compared with eyes with the same-sized donor grafts. Several subsequent studies[3,9,17] were unable to confirm these findings, showing no significant difference in postoperative intraocular pressure between eyes having an oversized or a same-sized donor button. None of the patients in these studies, however, showed significant elevations in intraocular pressure. Another prospective, randomized trial suggested that aphakic oversized

Table 74-6 Postoperative intraocular pressure (group averages) after penetrating keratoplasty with 7.5 mm recipient bed

Condition of eye	Group	No. in group (average age, yr)	Preoperative IOP, mm Hg*	No. with glaucoma	1	2	3	4	5	6	Average IOP for all days, mm Hg	Average maximum IOP for each patient, mm Hg
Aphakic	A†	12 (74.9)	18.0	3	18.5	20.3	19.3	17.3	15.3	17.5	18.3	23.7
	B‡	12 (62.8)	20.9	4	25.7	31.8	26.4	27.7	27.9	27.9	26.6	37.7
Combined procedure§	A	5 (65.4)	16.4	0	19.0	22.9	22.0	20.0	22.0	22.0	21.2	24.0
	B	7 (59.0)	18.4	2	37.0	40.6	39.1	28.0	33.5	31.4	34.4	43.7
Phakic	A	6 (29.0)	15.8	0	21.0	15.8	16.5	22.0	22.0	20.0	19.0	22.8
	B	8 (41.2)	16.1	0	23.4	21.6	21.5	22.3	19.2	18.0	21.1	25.7

From Zimmerman, TJ, Olson, RJ, Waltman, SR, and Kaufman, HE: Arch Ophthalmol 96:2231, 1978
*IOP is intraocular pressure.
†Donor button was 0.5 mm larger than recipient bed.
‡Donor button was same size as recipient bed.
§Eyes that had combined keratoplasty and lens extraction.

Table 74-7 Maximum postoperative intraocular pressure after penetrating keratoplasty with 7.5 mm recipient bed

Condition of eye	Group	No. in group	Maximum IOP* >25 mm Hg	>30 mm Hg	>40 mm Hg	>50 mm Hg
Aphakic	A†	12	5	2	0	0
	B‡	12	8	5	5	5
Combined procedure§	A	5	2	0	0	0
	B	7	6	4	3	3
Phakic	A	6	2	0	0	0
	B	8	3	1	1	1

From Zimmerman, TJ, Olson, RJ, Waltman, SR, and Kaufman, HE: Arch Ophthalmol 96:2231, 1978
*IOP is intraocular pressure.
†Donor button was 0.5 mm larger than recipient bed.
‡Donor button was same size as recipient bed.
§Eyes that had combined keratoplasty and lens extraction.

Table 74-8 Postoperative intraocular pressure (group averages) after penetrating keratoplasty with 8.0 mm recipient bed

Condition of eye	Group	No. in group (average age, yr)	Preoperative IOP, mm Hg*	1	2	3	4	5	Average IOP for all days, mm Hg	Average maximum IOP for each patient, mm Hg	Vitrectomy
Aphakic	A†	6 (71.7)	17.8	37.5	39.0	34.7	29.0	30.0	34.0	42.5	5
	B‡	8 (79.8)	16.8	39.3	42.6	40.0	36.9	37.1	39.2	45.5	7
Combined procedure§	A	9 (73.9)	16.4	36.2	35.9	33.8	33.1	32.5	34.3	39.0	0
	B	8 (69.4)	15.4	54.4	49.6	49.6	47.9	48.3	50.0	54.4	0

From Zimmerman, TJ, Olson, RJ, Waltman, SR, and Kaufman, HE: Arch Ophthalmol 96:2231, 1978
*IOP is intraocular pressure.
†Donor button was 0.5 mm larger than recipient bed.
‡Donor button was same size as recipient bed.
§Eyes that had combined keratoplasty and lens extraction.

Table 74-9 Maximum postoperative intraocular pressure after penetrating keratoplasty with 8.0 mm recipient bed

Condition of eye	Group	No. in group	Maximum IOP*		
			>30 mm Hg	>40 mm Hg	>50 mm Hg
Aphakic	A†	6	6	3	1
	B‡	8	8	7	3
Combined procedure§	A	9	9	6	0
	B	8	8	8	8

From Zimmerman, TJ, Olson, RJ, Waltman, SR, and Kaufman, HE: Arch Ophthalmol 96:2231, 1978
*IOP is intraocular pressure.
†Donor button 0.5 mm larger than recipient bed.
‡Donor button same size as recipient bed.
§Eyes that had combined keratoplasty and lens extraction.

Table 74-10 Incidence of glaucoma after aphakic keratoplasty (without preoperative glaucoma)

Graft/ recipient size (mm)	No.	IOP > 40 mm Hg first five days	Glaucoma 13 months postoperative
7.5/7.5	13	6 (46%)	4 (31%)
		$P = 0.01$	$P = 0.08$
7.5/8.0	18	1 (6%)	1 (6%)

From Bourne, WM, Davison, JA, and O'Fallon, WM: Ophthalmology 89:242, 1982

grafts were associated with lower postoperative intraocular pressure, although no statistical significance was demonstrated.[6] A prospective, randomized study by Bourne et al.[1] showed a significant lowering in the postoperative intraocular pressure course when a larger donor button was used with aphakic grafts (Table 74-10). These findings were also supported in a retrospective study by Foulks[4] who showed that oversized donor buttons reduced the incidence of postkeratoplasty glaucoma in both aphakic or pseudophakic patients.

Angle-closure Mechanism

Three studies have suggested that progressive synechial angle-closure is the cause for persistent glaucoma after keratoplasty.[2,10,20] Gnad[5] reported loss of support of angle structures, as well as a forward shift of the intact hyaloid face after posterior vitreous detachment, causing progressive flattening of the anterior chamber. He proposed prophylactic anterior vitrectomy in aphakic patients undergoing corneal grafting to prevent postkeratoplasty glaucoma.

Cohen et al.[2] suggested performing an iridoplasty by placing sutures near the iris sphincter to maintain a mechanically rigid iris diaphragm.

This iridoplasty may prevent postoperative anterior synechiae and progressive angle-closure. Other measures to prevent angle-closure include iridectomy and anterior vitrectomy, especially if there is an unusual forward shift of the vitreous during surgery.

Although a definitive study to determine the exact pathophysiology has not been performed, this speculated collapse of the angle structures would explain the variation from normal pressure to the exceedingly high pressure that occurs postoperatively. Moreover, trabecular collapse seems to occur only when the posterior pull of the lens zonules is lost in conjunction with a marked anterior distortion of the angle associated with an undersized donor button and very tight sutures. Despite the lack of supporting clinical data, many surgeons feel that patients with extracapsular cataract extractions are less likely to develop postkeratoplasty glaucoma compared to patients with intracapsular cataract extractions. Foulks[4] found the incidence of postkeratoplasty glaucoma in aphakic patients to be 39%, compared to 16% among pseudophakic patients.

It appears that chronic damage can occur from early postkeratoplasty glaucoma, resulting in a persistently elevated pressure. Many patients who have severely elevated intraocular pressures after penetrating keratoplasty often develop chronic glaucoma.[1,14] These studies indicate that many of these patients require medical or surgical treatment for glaucoma control (Tables 74-11 and 74-12).

MANAGEMENT

Computer models of penetrating keratoplasty suggest that the distortion in the anterior chamber angle, with the subsequent reduction in aqueous outflow, may be minimized by considering the following factors.[12,14]

Table 74-11 Intraocular pressure (mm Hg) before and after keratoplasty in aphakia or combined keratoplasty and cataract extraction

	Without preoperative glaucoma		With preoperative glaucoma	
	Aphakic	**Combined**	**Aphakic**	**Combined**
No. of eyes	21	23	26	11
Mean age	67.9	69.3*	65.2	59.4*
Preoperative IOP	17.4†	16.5‡	22.7†	30.2‡
Postoperative IOP				
Day 1	26.6	24.6	28.8	27.3
Day 2	29.6	24.5	26.6	29.9
Day 3	27.1	25.1	23.7	27.5
Day 4	23.5	23.3	21.8	22.0
Day 5	23.7	24.7	25.2	25.3
Mean IOP, Days 1-5	26.2	24.4	25.2	26.4
Maximum IOP, Days 1-5	32.1	30.6	34.8	34.0
IOP, 2-4 wks	24.8	23.7	28.3	29.8
IOP, 2-3 mos	22.9	21.1	25.4	27.3
IOP, 5-7 mos	22.4	23.9	22.5	22.4
Mean IOP, 2 wks-7 mos	23.3	22.8	25.4	26.4
Maximum IOP, 2 wks-7 mos	30.5§	29.0	38.3§	33.7

From Olson, RJ, and Kaufman, HE: Am J Ophthalmol 86:510, 1978
*P = .031.
†P = .002.
‡P = .00004.
§P = .017.

Table 74-12 Outcome after keratoplasty in aphakia or combined with cataract extraction in patients with maximum pressure more than 35 mm Hg during first postoperative week

	Without preoperative glaucoma		With preoperative glaucoma	
	Aphakic (N = 10)	**Combined (N = 8)**	**Aphakic (N = 15)**	**Combined (N = 4)**
Glaucoma medication needed				
At discharge from hospital (%)	10 (100)	8 (100)	14 (93)	4 (100)
Six months postoperatively (%)	7 (70)	6 (75)	11 (73)	4 (100)
Cyclocryotherapy (%)	2 (20)	1 (12)	3 (20)	1 (25)
Maximum IOP > 35 mm Hg during late postoperative period* (%)	6 (60)	2 (25)	7 (47)	3 (75)
Vitrectomies (%)	8 (80)	6 (75)	14 (93)	2 (50)

From Olson, RJ, and Kaufman, HE: Am J Ophthalmol 86:510, 1978
*Two weeks to seven months postoperatively.

Relative size of graft. Undersized donor tissue is an aggravating factor and this is, in fact, what usually occurs when the same trephine is used for the donor button and recipient bed dissection. When the recipient bed dissection is approached from the anterior surface, the cornea can balloon inside the trephine, resulting in a cut slightly larger than the diameter of the trephine. Most donor tissue, on the other hand, is punched from the posterior side; thus, the tissue will flatten slightly before penetration, resulting in a button often smaller than the diameter of the trephine. This size differ-ence, when using the same trephine, may vary from surgeon to surgeon, although the difference between the diameters of host and donor buttons, as determined in one in vitro study,[11] is approximately 0.25 mm when a 7.5 mm trephine is used (Table 74-13).

Trephine diameter. A smaller graft, for example 7.0 mm, results in less angle distortion than a larger 8.5 mm graft (Fig. 74-4). Smaller corneal diameters also tend to result in more angle distortion and possible trabecular collapse.

Suture tension. Tight sutures are a significant

Table 74-13 Human corneal tissue size with trephination from endothelial side and from epithelial side on intact globes

Category	No. of eyes	Mean diameter, mm		
		Epithelial side	Endothelial side	Epithelial plus endothelial sides
McCarey-Kaufman (M-K) corneas				
Dull trephine	2	7.57 ± 0.051[1]* (12)†	7.59 ± 0.055[2] (12)	7.58 ± 0.053[3] (24)
Fresh trephine	2	7.42 ± 0.063[1] (12)	7.47 ± 0.055[2] (12)	7.45 ± 0.064[3] (24)
Total	4	7.49 ± 0.094[4] (24)	7.53 ± 0.079[5] (24)	7.51 ± 0.088[6] (48)
Intact globes	11	7.80 ± 0.18[4] (66)	7.73 ± 0.20[5] (42)	7.77 ± 0.19[4] (108)

From Olson, RJ: Arch Ophthalmol 97:1323, 1979, Copyright 1979, American Medical Association
*All superscripts represent comparisons whose measurements are significantly different at .05 level or less.
†Number in parentheses represents number of measurements used to determine mean.

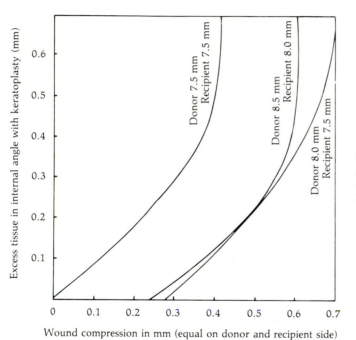

Fig. 74-4 Relationship of wound compression and internal angle relaxation (11.0 mm corneal diameter). (From Olson, RJ, and Kaufman, HE: Invest Ophthalmol Vis Sci 16:1085, 1977)

aggravating factor; the tighter the suture the more pronounced the distortion of the chamber angle (Fig. 74-5).
Peripheral corneal thickness. Peripheral corneal edema, or any factor resulting in a thicker peripheral cornea, also causes increased distortion of the trabecular areas (Fig. 74-6).

The use of an oversized donor button and adjustment of suture tightness are the most significant clinical factors in avoiding elevated pressure postkeratoplasty.[1,6,24,25,26] Both of these factors correlate with the data from the mathematical modeling studies.[12,14]

In summary, several factors may be useful in preventing postkeratoplasty glaucoma in aphakic patients.
1. Oversized donor cornea
2. Suture technique
3. Peripheral iridectomy
4. Anterior vitrectomy
5. Iridoplasty

The key to managing postkeratoplasty glaucoma is the understanding that the pressure increase is usually self-limited, lasting approximately 5 to 7 days. Miotics are usually ineffective in lowering the early increase in intraocular pressure after

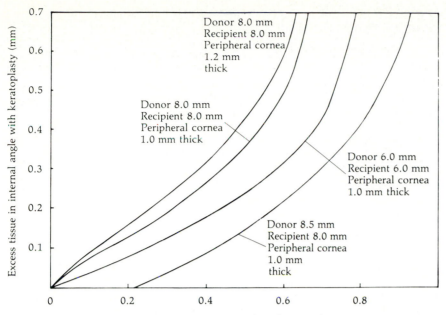

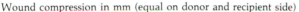

Fig. 74-5 Relationship of wound compression and internal angle relaxation (12.0 mm corneal diameter). (From Olson, RJ, and Kaufman, HE: Invest Ophthalmol Vis Sci 16:1085, 1977)

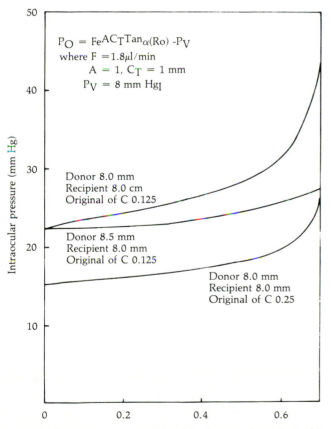

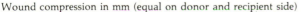

Fig. 74-6 Hypothetical relationship of wound compression and intraocular pressure. (From Olson, RJ, and Kaufman, HE: Invest Ophthalmol Vis Sci 16:1085, 1977)

keratoplasty and may aggravate postoperative inflammation and predispose to synechia formation. Therefore, the preferred medical approach is to decrease aqueous humor formation. Topical beta-blockers should be used initially, supplemented with systemic carbonic anhydrase inhibitors if necessary. However, one study[15] showed that neither of these agents, when used separately or in combination, significantly lowered the pressure (Table 74-14). If beta-blockers and carbonic anhydrase inhibitors do not significantly lower the pressure, then the intermittent administration of hyperosmotic agents must be used until the problem resolves.

Transient intraocular pressure elevations may be tolerated in many eyes if the optic nerve is healthy. Also, many patients are often surprisingly pain free with high intraocular pressures. However, pressures of 50 to 60 mm Hg on a continuous basis may be associated with ischemic optic neuropathy and central retinal vein and central retinal artery occlusion. One study of patients with aphakic keratoplasty glaucoma suggested an increased incidence of ischemic optic neuropathy during the phase of elevated pressure.[14] Therefore, lowering the intraocular pressure to a more normal level is usually prudent.

Many investigators have studied the effects of increased intraocular pressure on the corneal endothelium. Svedbergh[19] showed that moderately

Table 74-14 Effect of timolol and daranide on IOP of patients with elevated pressures after aphakic penetrating keratoplasty and PKP combined with cataract extraction

Group	Age	Postoperative IOP (mm Hg)			Max IOP (Day 2+)	Total No. IOP measurements	Patients removed*
		Day 1	Day 2	Day 2+			
Timolol (N = 5)	71.2 ± 10.6	39.6 ± 10.7	38.4 ± 13.8	27.9 ± 12.7	38.8 ± 13.1	12	2 (40%)
Daranide (N = 4)	72.0 ± 8.3	44.5 ± 11.2	40.0 ± 14.2	28.6 ± 12.7	40.0 ± 14.2	11	2 (50%)
Timolol + Daranide (N = 8)	57.8 ± 21.2	43.9 ± 10.2†	36.6 ± 16.6	23.9 ± 12.3‡	36.6 ± 16.6	29	3 (37.5%)
Placebo (N = 6)	66.7 ± 12.5	34.5 ± 11.9†	32.8 ± 13.5	31.1 ± 12.3‡	35.8 ± 14.3	15	3 (50%)

From Olson, RJ, Kaufman, HE, and Zimmerman, TJ: Ann Ophthalmol 11:1833, 1979
*Patients removed from study because of uncontrolled IOP.
†P = .138
‡P = .070
No differences were statistically significant.

elevated intraocular pressure causes corneal endothelial thinning and morphologic signs of damage. Vannas et al.[21] found a decrease in endothelial cell count in the glaucomatous eyes of 15 of 27 patients with unilateral glaucoma. Other studies[16,18] have clinically documented the association of glaucoma with a poor prognosis for the corneal graft.

A chronically elevated intraocular pressure requires consideration of other therapeutic modalities. Miotics may be beneficial at this stage if there is sufficient trabecular meshwork not involved with peripheral anterior synechiae. Suppression of aqueous humor formation with carbonic anhydrase inhibitors and beta-blockers may also be effective in lowering the pressure. Surgical means of controlling the elevated pressure must be considered if medical therapy is unsuccessful. Foulks[4] found that surgical therapy was necessary in 24% of the cases of postkeratoplasty glaucoma. Cyclocryotherapy[22] is the usual mode of treatment in aphakic postkeratoplasty glaucoma. Foulks[4] has reported the use of argon laser trabeculoplasty in three patients, with no effect on the elevated pressure postkeratoplasty. He also reports that using argon laser iridoplasty, treating the base of the iris at the edge of progressive angle closure, is usually ineffective. Insler et al.[7] reported seven cases of combined keratoplasty and trabeculectomy with controlled postoperative intraocular pressure in five of the seven eyes.

Filtration surgery may be less successful because of peripheral anterior synechiae and an inability to perform a limbal sclerostomy to communicate with the anterior chamber. The use of seton tube devices (see Chapter 39) may be beneficial in these eyes. Increased failure may also be related to enhanced postoperative inflammation in

the eye with previous keratoplasty. The use of pharmacologic agents to control wound healing after filtration surgery (see Chapter 33) may increase the rate of filtration success.

REFERENCES

1. Bourne, WM, Davison, JA, and O'Fallin, WM: The effects of oversize donor buttons on postoperative intraocular pressure and corneal curvature in aphakic penetrating keratoplasty, Ophthalmology 89:242, 1982
2. Cohen, EJ, Kenyon, KR, and Dohlman, CH: Iridoplasty for preventing postkeratoplasty angle closure and glaucoma, Ophthalmic Surg 13:994, 1982
3. Foulks, GN, Perry, HD, and Dohlman, CH: Oversize corneal donor grafts in penetrating keratoplasty, Ophthalmology 86:490, 1979
4. Foulks, GN: Glaucoma associated with penetrating keratoplasty, Ophthalmology 94:871, 1987
5. Gnad, HD: Athalamia as a late complication after keratoplasty on aphakic eyes, Br J Ophthalmol 64:528, 1980
6. Heidemann, DG, Sugar, A, Meyer, RF, and Musch, DC: Oversized donor grafts in penetrating keratoplasty. A randomized trial, Arch Ophthalmol 103:1807, 1985
7. Insler, MS, Cooper, HD, Katz, PE, and Caldwell, DR: Penetrating keratoplasty with trabeculectomy, Am J Ophthalmol 100:593, 1985
8. Irvine, AR, and Kaufman, HE: Intraocular pressure following penetrating keratoplasty, Am J Ophthalmol 68:835, 1969
9. Karesh, JW, and Nirankari, VS: Factors associated with glaucoma after penetrating keratoplasty, Am J Ophthalmol 96:160, 1983
10. Lass, JH, and Pavan-Langston, D: Timolol therapy in secondary angle-closure glaucoma post penetrating keratoplasty, Ophthalmology 86:51, 1979
11. Olson, RJ: Variation in corneal graft size related to trephine technique, Arch Ophthalmol 97:1323, 1979

12. Olson, RJ, and Kaufman, HE: A mathematical description of causative factors and prevention of elevated intraocular pressure after keratoplasty, Invest Ophthalmol Vis Sci 16:1085, 1977
13. Olson, RJ, and Kaufman HE: Intraocular pressure and corneal thickness after penetrating keratoplasty, Am J Ophthalmol 86:97, 1978
14. Olson, RJ, and Kaufman, HE: Prognostic factors of intraocular pressure after aphakic keratoplasty, Am J Ophthalmol 86:510, 1978
15. Olson, RJ, Kaufman, HE, and Zimmerman, TJ: Effects of timolol and Daranide on elevated intraocular pressure after aphakic keratoplasty, Ann Ophthalmol 11:1833, 1979
16. Paton, D: The prognosis of penetrating keratoplasty: based upon corneal morphology, Ophthalmic Surg 7:36, 1976
17. Perl, T, Charlton, KH, and Binder, PS: Disparate diameter grafting: astigmatism, intraocular pressure, and visual acuity, Ophthalmology 88:774, 1981
18. Robinson, C: Indications, complications and prognosis for repeat penetrating keratoplasty, Ophthalmic Surg 10:27, 1979
19. Svedbergh, B: Effects of artificial intraocular pressure elevation on the corneal endothelium in the vervet monkey, Acta Ophthalmol 53:839, 1975
20. Thoft, RA, Gordon, JM, and Dohlman, CH: Glaucoma following keratoplasty, Trans Am Acad Ophthalmol Otolaryngol 78:352, 1974
21. Vannas, A, Setala, K, and Ruusuvaara, P: Endothelial cells in capsular glaucoma, Acta Ophthalmol 55:951, 1977
22. West, CE, Wood, TO, and Kaufman, HE: Cyclocryotherapy for glaucoma pre or post penetrating keratoplasty, Am J Ophthalmol 76:485, 1973
23. Zimmerman, TJ, Krupin, T, Grodzki, W, and Waltman, SR: The effect of suture depth on outflow facility in penetrating keratoplasty, Arch Ophthalmol 96:505, 1978
24. Zimmerman, TJ, et al: Size of donor corneal button and outflow facility in aphakic eyes, Arch Ophthalmol 96:505, 1978
25. Zimmerman, TJ, Olson, RJ, Waltman, SR, and Kaufman, HE: Transplant size and elevated intraocular pressure postkeratoplasty, Arch Ophthalmol 96: 2231, 1978
26. Zimmerman, TJ, Waltman, SR, Sachs, U, Kaufman, HE: Intraocular pressure after aphakic penetrating keratoplasty: through-and-through suturing, Ophthalmic Surg 10:49, 1979

Index

Straining, 302
Streptomycin sulfate, 1174
Stress
  acute angle-closure glaucoma and, 841
  open-angle glaucoma and, 815
Stretch burn
  iridectomy and, 585, 586
  iridoplasty and, 599
Stretching, corneal, 773
  megalocornea, 766-767
Stroma
  ciliary, 85
  conjunctival epithelium and, 22
  cornea development and, 8-9, 22
  fluorescence in, 340
  iris
    aqueous humor and, 41-42
    congenital glaucoma and, 765
  laser iridectomy and, 590
  mid limbal, 20, 22
  Peters' anomaly and, 897, 898
  scleral, 22
  uveal, 1119
Strontium 90, 674
Strophanthidin, 213
Stump of iris, 874
Sturge-Weber syndrome, 25, 30, 31, 32-33, 913-920
  episcleral venous pressure and, 1133-1134
  filtration surgery and, 672-673
  surgery and, 727
  tumors and, 1123
Subacute angle-closure glaucoma, 860
Subconjunctival fistula, 647
Subconjunctival injection, 1207
Subendothelial membrane, 43
Subendothelium, 167, 171
Subluxation, lens, 1028
  blunt trauma and, 1228
Substance P, 260
Substance P immunoreactive nerve fiber, 264-265
Sub-Tenon injection, 1207
Succinylcholine, 1177-1178
  anticholinesterase agents and, 520
  filtration surgery and, 659
  intraocular pressure and, 302
Suction effect, 347
Sulcus, ciliary, 77
Sulfa drug, 1173-1174
Sulfite oxidase deficiency, 1041
Sulfonamide
  carbonic anhydrase inhibitors and, 541
  structures of, 545
Sulfur hexafluoride, 1054-1055
Sulindac, 673
Summation
  kinetic perimetry and, 374
  perimeter and, 373
Superior cervical ganglion, 258
Superior ophthalmic vein, 1127
Superior vena cava syndrome, 1134-1135
Suprachoroidal fluid, 285-286

Suprachoroidal hemorrhage, 1255
  aphakic eye undergoing filtration and, 1279
  expulsive, 682, 683
Suprachoroidal space
  anatomy and, 241
  sclerotomy and, 1258
Supraciliary fluid, 285
Supraciliary space, 241
Suprathreshold screening, 381-382
  stepped, 411
Surface layer of nerve fiber, 135
Surgery
  angle-closure glaucoma and nanophthalmos and, 1050
  aniridia and, 881-882
  aphakia and, 1279
  Axenfeld-Rieger syndrome and, 895
  ciliary body and, 738
  congenital glaucoma and, 707-727, 781-782; see also Congenital glaucoma
  cyclodialysis and, 284-285
  episcleral venous pressure and, 1135, 1137
  epithelial cyst and, 1301-1303
  epithelial ingrowth and, 1317
  exfoliation syndrome and, 1011
  fibrous ingrowth and, 1324
  filtering; see Filtration surgery
  ghost cell glaucoma and, 1244-1245
  glaucoma associated with, 1249-1347
    aphakia and, 1265-1283; see also Aphakia
    intraocular lens implantation and, 1285-1297
    malignant glaucoma and, 1251-1262
    penetrating keratoplasty and, 1337-1347
    proliferation and, 1299-1335
  glaucoma treatment and, 631-749
    cataract and, 697-706
    congenital glaucoma and, 707-727
    conventional iridectomy and, 645-651
    cyclodestructive, 729-740
    filtration and, 653-696
    setons in, 741-748
    wound healing and, 633-643
  hypotony and, 287
  iridectomy; see Iridectomy
  laser, 565-629; see Laser
  neovascular glaucoma and, 1095
  neurofibromatosis and, 913
  open-angle glaucoma and, 818-819
  phacoanaphylaxis and, 1024
  phacolytic glaucoma and, 1020-1021
  pigmentary glaucoma and, 994
  pseudophakic glaucoma and, 1294-1295
  retinal detachment and, 1054-1055
    neovascular glaucoma and, 1090
  uveitis and, 1209

Suture
  bridle, 660, 661
  corneoscleral, 1267
  releasable, 675
  tension of, 1343-1344
  through-and-through, 1339
Suture-cutting, laser 626-627
Suxamethonium, 302
Swan-Jacob lens, 713
Sympathectomy, chemical, 529
Sympathetic nerve
  ciliary body and, 84-85
  intraocular pressure and, 269-270
Sympathomimetic agent, 1175-1176
  uveitis and, 1207
Synapse, 89
Synechia, 1206
  angle-closure glaucoma and, 1053
  neovascular glaucoma and, 1067, 1073
    treatment of, 1095
  peripheral anterior; see Peripheral anterior synechia
  Peters' anomaly and, 899
  posterior, 594
Synthetic drainage device, 784
Syphilis, 1213-1214
  interstitial keratitis and, 1203
Syringomyelia, 1211

T
Tapetoretinal degeneration, 939
Tear
  ciliary body and, 1230
  congenital glaucoma and, 773
  Descemet's membrane and, 784
Telangiectasia-cataracta syndrome, 938
Telangiectasis, 1155
TEM; see Transverse electromagnetic mode
Temperature
  cyclocryotherapy probe and, 732-733
  irradiated tissue and, 573
Temporal angle, 349-350
Temporal coherence, 571
Temporal contrast sensitivity, 189
Temporal vision, 187-189
Tendon, ciliary muscle, 47
Tenon's capsule
  cyst and, 685-687
  filtration surgery and, 659
  posterior lip sclerectomy and, 676
  sclerotomy and, 1258
Tenonectomy, 673
Tenon's flap, 721-725
Tension
  intraocular; see Intraocular pressure
  suture, 1343-1344
Terbutaline, 342
Testing
  color vision, 183-185
  functional, 179-197
  visual field, 369-380; see also Perimetry; Visual field
Tetracaine, 520
Tetracycline, 1173-1174